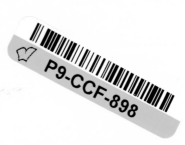
P9-CCF-898

The
Well-Managed
Community
Hospital

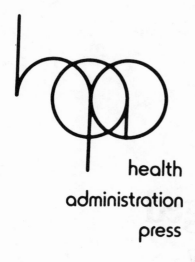

health
administration
press

John R. Griffith

The Well-Managed Community Hospital

Health Administration Press
Ann Arbor • Michigan
1987

Library of Congress Cataloging-in-Publication Data

Griffith, John R.
    The well-managed community hospital.

    Includes bibliographies and index.
    1. Hospitals—Administration.   2. Community health services—
Administration.   I. Title. [DNLM: 1. Hospital Administration—United States.   2.
Hospitals, Community—United States. WX 150 G853w]
RA971.G76   1987   362.1'1'068   87-17710
ISBN 0-910701-25-3

Health Administration Press
A Division of the Foundation of the
American College of Healthcare Executives
1021 East Huron Street
Ann Arbor, Michigan 48104-9990
(313) 764-1380

Dedicated to my father, Richard R. Griffith, FACHE, and his colleagues. They were the first generation of hospital executives, and they placed the keystones for the well-managed community hospital.

Contents

List of Figures

List of Tables

Foreword

This book arises from a deep conviction in the worth—indeed even the inevitability—of locally managed health care and a respect for the voluntary hospitals that have emerged as central to that care. I believe that these institutions are improvable, and better than most alternatives. Their most impressive strength is the underlying commitment of their communities. In most places the citizens will rally quickly against any outside threat to their hospital; "our hospital" is always a good hospital, worth defending to the extreme.

This commitment may be as foolish as the critics allege it to be, but it is a central measure of the success of these institutions. Commitment is infinitely better than the detachment and cynicism which surround too many of the nation's other social organizations, both public and private. It is the thread that binds the individual to the society. Local commitment to a hospital has intrinsic worth beyond health care itself. The urge to help is an expression of universal concern, transcending the race, religion, age, and income distinctions which fractionate our society. The community hospital, well-managed or not, is usually the most visible single expression of this Samaritan motive. As such, it should be strengthened and expanded.

The book offers what I hope are practical suggestions to that end. Somewhat to my surprise, these suggestions are often technical, rigorous, and complex. I suppose this is because the world is complex, from medical technology to health insurance to legal constraints. The book is best taken in small doses, "p.r.n.", as the doctor orders, except for those hardy souls who choose to become health care executives. I hope they will find these suggestions useful enough to master in their entirety, and valuable enough to create more well-managed hospitals.

Too many people helped me to begin to list. Virtually every thought in the book I learned from someone else. I would like to thank three whose encouragement was particularly important: John K. Kerr, Gail L. Warden, and Thomas A. D'Aunno. I also thank my secretary, Angela Hochstetler Fretz, who spent many evenings to help produce a finished manuscript.

JOHN R. GRIFFITH
University of Michigan

Ann Arbor
May 1987

Introduction

The Expanding Community Hospital

Americans consider the community hospital a part of the good life. There are several in every city and one in all but the smallest towns. Each typically employs over 20 different professions and an equal variety of nonprofessional trades and contracts with several dozen doctors. It identifies and responds to patients' needs, and the needs of their families, from conception through life to death. There is scarcely a family whose members or friends will not be either patient or visitor in the course of a year. The price of running community hospitals is so high that each working American will work an average of two and one-half hours a week to support them.[1] Perhaps only supermarkets reach as many people, only courts and churches touch them at such personal moments of their lives, and only national defense takes as much of their money. Probably none of these is as complicated.

The Trend Toward Larger Organizations

The role of the community hospital has been expanding through most of this century into several different dimensions. Socially, the hospital has evolved from a place to die to a well-justified source of hope. Legally, the obligations of the hospital now include far greater responsibility for quality of care. Many federal and state regulations covering general commerce have been extended to hospitals, and specific regulations have been added. Technologically, hospitals have been the obvious location for capital-intensive developments in medicine. Both lifesaving and life-improving services have resulted. Economically, hospitals now account for almost half of all expenditures on health care. Major shifts are occurring to accommodate prospective and comprehensive pricing, so far without reducing the total economic commitment. Responding to these shifts, the emphasis on inpatient care has begun to diminish, the scope and location of outpatient services to increase, and the commitment to quality and patient satisfaction to be expanded and formalized.

The latest development is the trend to health care systems that transcend or incorporate the traditional hospital. Single hospitals have merged in multihospital groups, acquired related services such as home care and nursing homes, and begun to share the risk of the cost of illness through health maintenance organizations (HMOs) and other devices integrating the hospital with insurance carriers. The new systems are changing the fundamentals of the service hospitals provide, including the point of sale, the price, the point of selection of physician, and the incentives of the individual doctor.

It is not likely that this trend will be reversed. It has resulted in central financing mechanisms serving large markets and forcing greater uniformity. It adds to the momentum of the past, suggesting that the future may hold even larger units integrating medical care, related services, and health insurance in comprehensive organizations. One plausible scenario holds that these organizations will replace hospitals, but that replacement is likely to be more a matter of symbol than of substance. *Subsume* is a more likely outcome than *replace,* because most of the functions that hospitals perform will still have to be performed by the new organization, and the way in which they are performed will not differ from the way they are now performed by the well-managed hospital.

The Health Care Transaction

One aspect of health care is not likely to change. The central transaction remains the one-to-one interchange between the patient and the professional providing care. In most cases, the professional is a doctor, but nurses and several other healing professions also engage in that transaction. The success of any organization selling health care services depends now, and will increasingly depend, on fulfilling health care transactions in ways that satisfy the patient in terms of quality, amenities, and economy. The community hospital has a long-standing commitment to managing the health care transaction. It is the leading employer of many of the health care professions, including physicians, and it provides essential support to doctors in private practice. Most important, both the courts and the national organization recognizing good management, the Joint Commission on Accreditation of Hospitals (JCAH), have pressed the hospital to control the quality of the health care transaction. The marketplace has demanded control of its cost.

As a result, the hospital has developed organizational structures that are equally useful for controlling cost and quality. It is true, of course, that the hospital record on quality is imperfect and on cost is as yet unproven. The same can easily be said of other proposals to address these complex and intransigent issues, however, and there is to date no compelling alternative. The most promising of the alternatives is probably an HMO structure like that of Group Health Cooperative of Puget Sound. This structure extends the control function more deeply into the outpatient arena, but it has many management parallels to hospitals and has only recently been modified to make it as broadly attractive in the marketplace.

Thus, although the hospital organization is likely to be enlarged, revised, or even subsumed, it is not likely to be replaced, because it is ubiquitous, popular, flexible, partially successful, and readily improvable. Two demands of the marketplace are central to its survival: the ability to incorporate most of the sources of primary care, including office and home care, nursing homes, preventive services, pharmacies, laboratories, and emergency services; and the ability to improve its mechanisms for cost and quality control.

Conceptualizing the Well-Managed Hospital

This book is designed to help managers, trustees, doctors, and other interested professionals understand the complexities of the hospital, make better informed and more satisfactory decisions, and improve the management of their hospital. Given the central transaction, and the popularity of hospitals at managing and supporting that transaction, it should be useful to many other health care institutions, especially larger clinics and HMOs, which share the task of managing health care. The subject seems timely, not so much because hospitals are badly managed —they are frequently criticized, but neither more severely nor with more justification than many other industries and organizations—but because both the need and the opportunity to improve are there. This book attempts to supply the concept of the opportunity required for improvement.

The well-run hospital is the result not of good fortune or accident, but rather the repeated application of well-established management principles. In this book I develop these principles into models for the solution of recurring questions of hospital management. The models are drawn from observation of successful hospitals and checked against the results of general research into organizations.

It is not so much that these models are right as that they are useful as templates to focus discussion, stimulate consensus, avoid unnecessary disagreement, and speed decision making. The book therefore anticipates a pluralistic approach to hospitals and health care. The responsiveness to the market that pluralism engenders is an essential component of the American health care system. The system that has resulted from this premise emphasizes free choice of physician, local governance, high technical quality, convenience, and generous amenities. Many people disagree with both the premise and the result, noting that the system is expensive and far from flawless, but the system and the premise have strong, widespread political and economic support, which, despite criticism, has not significantly diminished. With all its inequities and inefficiencies, the system that supports the hospital is not something the American people seem willing to sacrifice; nonetheless, both supporters and critics would welcome improvement.

Open System and Exchange Theory: Identifying Goals

The **open system** model likens organizations in their social environment to organisms in their biological one. The organization's basic motive is survival, which is achieved by reaching the most rewarding possible equilibrium with its environment. The organization requires certain resources, such as land and people's time. It acquires these resources by providing useful services, or benefits, in return. The transactions that result are called **exchanges**. Typical exchanges include sales to customers, employment of workers, and purchase of supplies. Although most permanent organizations have a complex array of exchanges, hospitals are exceptional. Their more unusual exchanges include the acceptance of charitable donations, the unique "privilege" contract with many of their physicians, complicated and unique mechanisms for financing the purchase of service, and, most important, a relatively vague contract between them and their patients.

In spite of these complexities, the hospital under the open systems concept must be responsive to the environment that supports it. It has as one of its primary tasks the identification and achievement of mutually beneficial exchanges. Success for a hospital is measured by the willingness of the outside world to support and expand the exchange relationships. Success occurs because the organization is able to identify, evaluate, and respond to the complex and changing exchange opportunities.

Closed System Theory: Achieving Goals

Closed system models also apply to all organizations. They describe ways in which the organizations generate responses to external, or open system, opportunities. Predictable responses are necessary to sustain large volumes of exchanges among many different people.

Hospitals rely on a great diversity of effort by many people. The key to predictability lies in coordinating these efforts and motivating these individuals to work toward common goals. Closed systems respond to the relatively uncertain, shifting conditions in the environment by creating more stable, focused working conditions that permit improvement by learning, specialization, and standardization. Hospitals rely heavily upon learning, specialization, and standardization to achieve success. They establish uniformity while maintaining the flexibility necessary to respond to the external environment by periodically setting **expectations**, that is, highly specific statements about the working conditions of their smaller units and individual members.

Both open and closed systems are **cybernetic** in that they continually adjust in search of an improved, more successful solution. Success is characterized by a surplus, or reward. Just as successful exchange is one that rewards both parties, a successful organization is one that uses rewards of successful exchanges to attract additional opportunities for exchange. The concepts of open and closed systems are discussed at length in chapters 2 and 3, respectively.

Characteristics of Well-Managed Hospitals

For each of the problems hospitals face, there are better solutions, solutions more likely to lead to successful exchange relationships. Over many years and many trials, there have emerged approaches and processes that increase the probability of success. This book seeks these solutions, identifying them as those of the well-managed hospital. In the sense used here, the well-managed hospital is an ideal rather than a reality. It is a description of the state which is most likely to make the hospital successful. Real hospitals lie on a continuum. The better ones conform to the ideal more closely, more often, and for more important activities. They can often be identified by their popularity, prestige, and financial solvency, for these are the outward signs of successful management.

There are many relatively well-managed hospitals. In fact, many sections of this book were written by considering the question, "What hospitals do this activity best, and how do they do it?"

Certain philosophical principles motivate well-managed hospitals, among them:

1. The well-managed hospital always operates in a morally constructive way; that is, the first ethical test of any proposed action is that it do no harm.

2. Consistent with the first premise, clinical services of well-managed hospitals always meet basic levels of quality. The frontier of quality improvement is almost always well past the minimum standards reflected in licensure, certification, and accreditation guidelines.

3. A desire to improve the quality of life in the community and a respect for the rights of all individuals motivate the actions of a well-managed hospital. These rights embrace patients, employees, doctors, and families.

4. People who are involved in the well-managed hospital are motivated by a process of participation, education, and reward. Since the resources for reward are available only by satisfying the community, the seeking of rewards reinforces the well-managed hospital's commitment to the general good.

5. Sanctions and negative corrective action must be used promptly, judiciously, and equitably, when required. Although these punitive actions protect and defend the organizational structure and the rights of individuals in it, their utility is limited and their application is rare.

Successful hospitals differ from others in their processes and their results, but the distinctive difference seems to be willingness to work at getting better. Commitment to improvement is as important as any accident of location, endowment, or quality of people. Successful hospitals aspire to be better and are never fully content with their achievements. If they are asked whether they are well-managed, they usually reply, "There's a lot more to do."

As a result of continued pursuit of improvement using concepts from open and closed system theories, well-managed hospitals share some common solutions. These appear at the broadest levels of consensus, such as criteria, agendas, and measures. They also appear in a similar yearly cycle of events.

Well-managed hospitals tend not to dispute the following assumptions:

— The most important *measure of success* is long-term market share, because it reflects the real response of the people served. This measure is the proper focus of all management decisions, and is comparable to the profit criterion of for-profit enterprises. (Of course, neither of these measures is perfect, nor complete, nor easy to apply.)

— The *mission* guides the decision making of the well-managed hospital. To do this, the mission must concisely and realistically identify an intended community, market share, and scope, or segment, of service.

— *Resource allocation and quality control,* and the political stress that inevitably accompanies them, are managed by pushing decisions forward in time, emphasizing planning, budgeting, and future improvements and de-emphasizing current performance as a topic of group discussion. The well-managed hospital talks about how it will do better, not about how it did not do well. The detailed steps taken to achieve this comprise the budget cycle:

- Annual environmental assessment is used to identify progress toward the mission and marketplace comfort with the mission.

- The five-year plan and the five-year fiscal plan are updated on the basis of the assessment.

- The major parameters of next year's budget are set at the governance level from the revised plans.

- The budget, expanded to include cost, marketing, quality, and productivity goals, is negotiated upward, beginning at the lowest supervisory levels and involving the medical staff as much as practical. The major parameters guide the budget discussions. It becomes a set of *expectations* for improvements next year.

- The capital and new programs budget is developed from employee and doctor proposals, negotiated through the organization, and presented to the board as a ranked list of recommended projects.

— *Human resources, supervisory, and medical staff policies* are scrutinized to make sure they encourage personal growth, loyalty to the organization, and respect for others. In particular, those in positions of authority are encouraged to view themselves as accountable to their superiors but responsible to their subordinates.

— *Information systems* are recognized as the key to improvement. Data on achievement of (or, rarely, departure from) expectations is disseminated widely and promptly. Information systems provide detail and analysis to identify opportunities and design improvements.

Figure 1

Annual Cycle of a Well-Managed Hospital

Month	Task
1	New officers and committee members Staff preparation for environmental assessment
2	Board and staff retreats for environmental assessment
3	Development of budget guidelines Beginning of competitive review of new programs and capital requests
4	Development of operating budget
5	Development of operating budget
6	Board approval of budgets
7	Review of future projects and charges to ad hoc committees and task forces
8–12	Work of ad hoc committees and task forces

— *Rewards* of all kinds are generously distributed for achievement of expectations. Sanctions are used promptly but only when essential. Any individual whose behavior threatens the organization is strongly encouraged to leave.

One way to deal with the unpredictability created by encouraging health care professionals to respond flexibly to their patients is to make predictable as much of the rest of the work setting as possible. Thus a hallmark of the well-managed hospital is the predictability of its systems. In many hospitals this has evolved into a clearly recognizable cycle, with annual and multiyear components.

The cycle can be said to begin at the start of the budget process, as shown in figure 1. Because the decisions are difficult and properly require the advice of many different people associated with the hospital, it takes most hospitals about six months to complete the budget. Several other events, such as the appointment of new board members and members of standing committees, must be fit appropriately into the annual calendar.

The remaining months become the interval for developing new improvements to be implemented in the next budget. Ideas too complex to be negotiated in the budget process are pursued as projects to evaluate new programs, new investments, closures and terminations of programs, and new methods. The cycle provides time for everyone affected by the proposal to participate in identification and resolution of conflicts, and prudent forecasting of results. The most complex ideas spill into the next budget cycle or remain on the agenda for several years, but there is a natural motivation to finish a project before the budget cycle decisions are made.

The cycle permits the integration of individual diversity into hospitalwide consensus, and it allows each participant in the organization to know not only how decisions are made, but when.

How the Book Can Be Useful

This book focuses on how a hospital can be responsive to its community by identifying and making a series of exchanges that are necessary and efficient and, as a result, popular. How to find the right thing to do, how to make sure it happens as intended, and how to make it happen at the lowest possible cost are recurring themes.

Although the discussion will be directed toward community hospitals, it is applicable to other institutions directly involved in the health care transaction, as noted above. It will require varying degrees of modification for differing situations. Certainly much of what is true about community hospitals is true about other short-term general hospitals, such as university teaching hospitals and federal short-term hospitals. Large and complex outpatient clinics are now indistinguishable from their hospital counterparts in all respects except the lack of overnight care. HMOs and insurance carriers which operate hospitals and clinics will find most of the book directly applicable. Those that purchase services from hospitals will find it a useful guide to their hospital suppliers. Long-term care institutions and special mental and substance abuse programs may find the concepts in this book useful, but the specifics will require much modification.

The book is written in sufficient depth to serve the needs of full-time hospital management personnel. Persons with a part-time interest, such as doctors and trustees, may find selected sections useful. At the expense of some redundancy, an effort has been made to make each chapter useful in its own right.

Part I expands upon the key concepts. Chapter 1 discusses the definitions and classifications commonly used for hospitals. Chapter 2 develops the application of exchange theory to hospitals. Chapter 3 describes closed system modeling and provides a classification of the kinds of quantitative measures that are available to implement the model in hospital settings. Chapter 4 expands the ethical assumptions of well-managed hospitals, elaborates the activities of the five systems more fully, and describes the issues in organization design.

The following three parts of the book address the major components of the well-managed hospital. The review of the components of the hospital is organized according to the five major system groups by which the hospital carries out its exchanges.[2]

— **Governance,** which monitors the outside environment, selects appropriate alternatives, and negotiates the implementation of these alternatives with others inside and outside the hospital.

— **Finance,** which collects and manages the funds the organization needs, but which also monitors the proper use of resources and maintains much of the internal information system.

— **Clinical,** which is the hands-on patient care activity and the monitoring and controlling activities that ensure both the quality and effectiveness of that care.

— **Human resources,** which recruits and supports the hospital's employees.

— **Plant,** which operates and maintains the physical facilities and equipment of the institution.

Governance and finance are discussed in Part II. The clinical operations, which are at the heart of any hospital, are described in Part III. The supporting organizations for human and plant resources are reviewed briefly in Part IV.

Obviously there are book-length works devoted to each system, and, for the clinical activities, whole libraries. The effort here has been to identify those components of each system which affect the ability of the hospital to form an integrated whole. With minor modifications, the clusters identify the purpose and functions of each system from the perspective of its contribution to the whole. These are followed by a discussion of the organizational and human resource requirements, specific measures which evaluate the system's contribution, and finally, a discussion of some important issues that well-managed systems are currently facing.

Notes

1. National Health Expenditures, published annually in *Health Care Financing Review* by the Health Care Financing Administration, U. S. Department of Health and Human Services. See also *Hospital Statistics,* published annually by the American Hospital Association, Chicago, and U. S. Bureau of Census, *Current Population Reports,* Series P-60, No. 151, *Money Income of Households, Families and Persons in the United States, 1984* (Washington, D.C.: Government Printing Office, 1986).

2. American Hospital Association, *Program of Institutional Effectiveness Review* (Chicago: AHA, 1979).

The Infrastructure of the Well-Managed Hospital

Introduction to Part I

The hospital, like any other organization, must have certain characteristics—a recognizable definition or identity, a method of gaining outside support, a method of assigning tasks and responsibilities, and an established network for communication. Well-managed hospitals have developed these characteristics in subtle, sophisticated, and extensive ways. Part I describes the characteristics that underpin the success of the enterprise as a whole and that are often invisible to or overlooked by the casual observer. Because of the subtlety of these characteristics, it is helpful to have a theory to explain what lies behind the evidence of good management. This book uses two theories, open systems and closed systems, each of which provides the framework for a chapter.

— *Identifying the Community Hospital: Definitions, Taxonomies, and Scope.* Chapter 1 notes that structural definitions of hospitals, while necessary for statistical and regulatory purposes, fail to capture the true extent or meaning of most well-managed institutions. A functional definition that matches more closely the mission statements of leading institutions is developed. Methods of classifying hospitals are discussed, including the definition of the community hospital. The issue of ownership is discussed briefly, identifying the few but often consequential places where it is likely to affect operations.

— *Understanding the Hospital Organization: Open Systems Concepts.* Chapter 2 develops the idea of the hospital as an organism sustained by and therefore responsive to its environment.

Open systems theory explores the interface between the hospital and the rest of the world. It identifies *exchanges,* the specific transactions the hospital must make to acquire patients, funds, and staff. Five things that motivate people to support hospitals are identified. A brief history traces how these motivations have shaped the development of community hospitals, with emphasis on the years since World War II.

— *Controlling Hospital Organizations: Closed System Concepts.* Chapter 3 develops the theory of the bureaucratic organization in a hospital context. The parts of the organization, the roles of the participants, and the incentives for compliance with expectations are reviewed. Emphasis is placed on quantifying performance, reflecting current public demand and the expanded capability of computers. Performance measures useful for all parts of the hospital are identified and classified according to closed system theory.

— *Foundations of the Hospital Organization.* Chapter 4 examines organization as a process, beginning with ethical assumptions. It reviews the role of the smallest unit of the organization and its leader in terms of their response to the closed system measures. Alternative *accountability hierarchies* are described as are the roles of *middle management.* The inevitability of difficulties in designing the hierarchy is noted, and collateral mechanisms for overcoming them are suggested.

1

Identifying the Community Hospital: Definitions, Taxonomies, and Scope

Most of us think we know what a hospital is until we try to define it. It's a place. It's an organization. It's an institution. It has a certain atmosphere about it, but that atmosphere is very difficult to describe. Yet one could hardly manage a hospital if it could not be defined, for a definition includes a statement of function or purpose.

Most of mankind's creations can be defined both by what they are and what they do, that is, by their structure and by their functions. Structural definitions are particularly useful for legal and statistical purposes; functional definitions are important in understanding what lies behind the structures.

Structural Definitions

The structural definition of a hospital begins with the hospital's historically most prominent characteristic, inpatient beds, and proceeds from there. Thus most legal and statistical definitions begin, "An institution (or a facility) providing inpatient care. . . ."

Because hospitals are licensed, they must be legally defined. Most states use language such as the following:

> Hospital means a facility offering inpatient overnight care and services for observation, diagnosis and active treatment of an individual with medical, surgical, obstetrical, chronic, or rehabilitative condition requiring the daily direction or supervision of a physician.[1]

The National Center for Health Statistics and the American Hospital Association (AHA) use the following phrases to distinguish hospitals from other health care facilities in registering and counting the number of hospitals:

1. At least six beds for the care of patients who are non related, who are sick, and whose average stay is in excess of 24 hours per admission
2. In those states and provinces having licensing laws, licensed
3. Doctors of medicine, osteopathy, and dentistry admitting patients
4. An organized medical staff
5. Evidence of regular care by a doctor
6. Records of clinical work available for reference
7. Registered nurse supervision and patient care around the clock
8. Operating and delivery rooms or relatively complete diagnostic and treatment facilities
9. Diagnostic X-ray services
10. Clinical laboratory services[2]

The AHA defines community hospitals as all those offering "short-term general and other special" services, and owned by groups other than the federal government. The "other special" hospitals are a small group of principally pediatric and obstetric hospitals.[3] Federal, state mental, and specialty hospitals that limit their service to mental health, substance abuse, and rehabilitation are excluded. Otherwise, the statistical definition is accepted as reasonable even though it does not exactly match the concept. Difficulties occur in classifying certain individual institutions, for example state-owned university hospitals (included) and federal Indian hospitals (excluded). Private cancer research hospitals are included; federal ones are not.

Structural definitions are useful for differentiating hospitals from other institutions and organizations, but they have a static, taxonomic quality that limits their use in the context of open systems management. For example, the only way one can expand the statistical definition above is to add to the list of services. Since even a moderate-sized hospital will have several dozen specific services, the definition soon becomes unwieldy. As a result, functional definitions assume much greater importance in hospital operations.

Functional Definitions

A functional definition identifies by purpose rather than by parts. The purpose of the modern community hospital is an issue worthy of careful thought. One might suspect that so complicated an organization would have several purposes, and indeed, the community hospital does. By far the most important is to support the health of individuals in the community. Certainly it is inconceivable to think of a community hospital which does not have this purpose. But if the structural definition was too specific and inflexible, this is too broad and too vague. Doctors' offices, sewers, and even highways can be said to "support the health of individuals in the community."

The confusion with sewers and highways can be eliminated if the definition is shifted to "provide personal health care." Public health and safety are collective functions excluded from the term "personal health care." Most hospitals have limited their focus to "personal health care" and away from collective health functions.

How can one escape the confusion with the doctor's office, or, for that matter, with the nursing home and other places providing personal health care? The first step is to recognize that the community general hospital is a collective institution even though it gives a personal service. It uses funds from, operates for the benefit of, and is usually owned by a community. Thus some community or collective benefit would be an appropriate criterion for exactly what personal health care will be provided. The functional definition can be expanded:

> A community hospital is an institution to provide personal health care for the community's benefit.

The above is actually a common definition of community hospitals. Many people use the term "need" in place of "benefit," but the word "need" creates semantic difficulties and may not reflect real hospital actions as well as "benefit." A fuller statement of the criteria determining which personal health services the hospital will provide is probably in order. Many services may provide benefit, so some rank ordering of relative benefit will be necessary. This ranking is usually based, at least intuitively, on a benefit-cost ratio. Decisions that pursue the least costly route to a given benefit use resources most effectively. The functional definition used in this book is:

> **A community hospital is an institution whose purpose is to provide personal health care in a manner which uses the available resources most effectively for the community's benefit.**

Under this definition, the distinction between a hospital and a doctor's office or a nursing home exists only if the hospital management chooses to make it. Community hospitals often include both these activities: they operate offices for doctors under a wide variety of arrangements, including salaried employment, and they own and run nursing homes. They also do things which blur the boundary between personal and collective health activities, such as antismoking education and nutrition classes. They make decisions which stretch the boundaries of the definition in any direction that improves their responsiveness to the community's benefit. In adopting this definition, one explicitly acknowledges three conclusions:

1. The owners and managers of a community hospital define the scope of services that will be offered.

2. Community benefit and cost-effectiveness are the criteria for that selection.

3. Optimization of the open systems exchanges is an inherent part of the definition of the community hospital.

Distinguishing Community Hospitals from Other Hospitals

It also follows from the definition that any community hospital must have an identifiable community or group of individuals who benefit from the services. The nature of the definition and the open systems process suggests that, in order to thrive, the typical community hospital will offer a relatively complete range of services to that group of individuals.

It is necessary to define the hospital's community geographically, because community hospitals must be accessible to their patients. Most community hospitals serve a catchment area, or trading area—that is, the population living in and around the town where the hospital is located. The limit of the catchment area is usually established by people's actual habits of use. The catchment area ends where the hospital no longer commands a majority or a plurality of hospitalizations. The geographic definition must be expanded for hospitals that serve special populations. An Indian hospital or a veteran's hospital serves a community defined by population status in addition to geography. Similarly, some hospitals serve only persons with certain health insurance, such as only members of a health maintenance organization, but practicality would add a geographic dimension to those hospitals' communities as well.

Many community hospitals find that, because their community is limited in size by geography, they must provide a wide scope of services. Under open systems theory, an organization must find constituencies that will exchange with it to provide the necessary resources. The geographic community thus becomes the focus of exchange transactions. The hospital extends and shapes its functional definition to find as many services as possible that are beneficial and cost-effective for its specific community. Normally, the services will include all those for which hospitalization is frequently sought and will provide for the needs of all age groups. A typical community hospital offers surgical, medical, pediatric, obstetrical, and emergency service.

There are several conditions under which a hospital may limit its services, but these occur rarely. Almost all of them represent special cases of the beneficial and cost-effective criteria. A community hospital may also close or discontinue services under certain circumstances. For example, it might discontinue a common service such as obstetrics or emergency care if other community hospitals were available to provide that service. In large cities, a community hospital might elect to specialize. Women's hospitals and children's hospitals were once common, but the trend has been away from specialization for some years. (Emerging environmental constraints may bring a return to specialization, however.) In theory, whether or not a specific hospital wishes to consider itself a community hospital is up to its management to decide. Although a not-for-profit hospital providing the only source of inpatient care in a small town would have great difficulty *not* calling itself a community hospital, the question would generate important debate in a large teaching hospital owned by a state university.

Who Owns the Community Hospital?

Major Types of Ownership

Hospitals in the United States are owned by a wide variety of groups and are even occasionally owned by individuals. There are three major types of ownership.

— **Government** hospitals are owned by federal, state, or local governments. Federal and state institutions tend to have special purposes, such as the care of special groups (military, mentally ill) or education (hospitals attached to state universities). Local government includes not only cities and counties, but also, in several states, hospital authorities that have been created from smaller political units. Local government hospitals in large cities are principally for the care of the poor, but many in smaller cities and towns are indistinguishable from not-for-profit institutions. Both are counted as community hospitals. Government hospitals are not as numerous as not-for-profit hospitals. State mental hospitals and federal hospitals are not classed as community hospitals.

— **Not-for-profit** hospitals are owned by corporations established by private (non-governmental) groups for the common good rather than for individual gain. As a result, they are granted broad federal, state, and local tax exemptions. Although they are frequently operated by organizations which have religious ties, secular, or nonreligious, not-for-profit hospitals constitute the largest single group of community hospitals, both in number and in total volume of care, exceeding religious not-for-profit, government, and for-profit hospitals by a wide margin.

— **For-profit** hospitals are owned by private corporations, which are allowed to declare dividends or otherwise distribute profits to individuals. They pay taxes like other private corporations. These hospitals are also called *investor-owned.* They are usually community hospitals, although there has been rapid growth in private psychiatric hospitals. Historically, the owners were doctors and other individuals, but large-scale publicly held corporations now own most for-profit hospitals. Although the amount of care given by for-profit hospitals is smaller than that given by government or not-for-profit hospitals, it has grown rapidly since 1970.

Table 1.1 shows community hospital statistics compiled by the American Hospital Association. Because the AHA plays a major role in collecting statistics about hospitals, its classification system is used for most purposes.[4] Several measures of volume are shown in the table, in addition to the number of institutions in each ownership class. Beds, admissions, and expenses can be used to classify hospitals by size. Discharges, which are virtually identical to admissions in the course of a year, and revenue, differing from expenses only by profit or loss, are also used. The difference between discharge and admission and between revenue and expense rarely affects the classification. A small hospital will count equally with a big one, but it will be much less important in number of beds or admissions. Usually it will be even less significant in expense, because a small hospital provides less expensive and less elaborate care than a large one.

Implications of Different Types of Ownership

Both for-profit and not-for-profit ownerships are sometimes referred to as private, to distinguish them from public, or government hospitals. However, as a consequence of their commitment not to distribute prof-

Table 1.1   Statistics on U.S. Community Hospitals, 1985

Ownership	Number	Beds (thousands)	Admissions (thousands)	Expenses ($ billions)
Nongovernment				
Not-for-profit	3,349	707	24,179	96.2
For-profit	805	104	3,242	11.5
State and local governments*	1,578	189	6,028	22.9
Total	5,732	1,000	33,449	130.6
Percentage Distribution (rounded)				
Nongovernment				
Not-for-profit	58%	71%	72%	74%
For-profit	14%	10%	10%	9%
State and local governments*	28%	19%	18%	18%
Total	100%	100%	100%	100%

Source: American Hospital Association, *Hospital Statistics* (Chicago: AHA, 1986), table 1, p. 5.

*Although the detail is not conveniently available, over 90 percent are owned by local governments.

its or assets to any individual, not-for-profit hospitals are legally dedicated to the collective good. Thus for the vast majority of community hospitals in the United States, the owners, in the sense of beneficiaries, are the communities they serve. The owners of record hold the assets, including any accumulated profits, in trust for the citizens of the community.

In part because of the trust relationship, but perhaps in larger part because of the need to be responsive to the same exchange opportunities, ownership of community hospitals is rarely critical in their overall management. Many hospitals owned by local governments are indistinguishable from not-for-profit hospitals in similar settings. In the courts, government hospitals are generally held to slightly higher standards of public accountability and conformity to the Constitution. Because they must honor any citizen's economic rights and religious freedom, they are obliged to provide abortions (if they provide related services),[5] to have open medical staffs, and to respect constitutional guarantees of freedom from participation in religious activities. Private hospitals are obliged simply to use due process and not to discriminate on grounds of age, sex, race, or creed. Other ownership distinctions make similarly minor differences. The only difference in the rights and obligations of religious versus nonreligious not-for-profit owners is that religious owners may favor persons sharing their own beliefs. (In practice, this privilege is rarely exercised.) Except for the obvious right to distribute dividends and the obligation to pay taxes, so are those of for-profit owners.

Given the narrow range of these distinctions, it is not surprising that studies of the effectiveness of various types of ownership rarely reveal major differences. If the open systems model is correct, all community hospitals are led to seek similar exchange opportunities. How well a hospital carries out the process of benefit assessment and program development depends much more on who manages it and how well than it does on who owns the property. A community hospital can be successful under any ownership if it is effectively managed. The most significant difference is that the results of that success accrue to a community in the case of not-for-profit hospitals and to the stockholders in the case of for-profit hospitals.

Distinguishing Between Ownership and Governance

While community hospitals are owned by various groups, they are almost all governed by a governing board. The function of the governing board is subtle and complex, but, in the broadest possible terms, the board decides what exchange transactions are appropriate, both in type and in quantity, and it resolves conflicts among various constituencies of the community. For example, the governing board will decide what services will be offered, how many people will be employed, and what restrictions will be put upon physicians granted privileges to practice in the hospital. If there are conflicting interests, as for example between the doctors and the employers who pay insurance premiums, the governing board will decide between them.

The owner's principal job is to select the governing board or to set up the mechanism by which the board will be selected. Governments usually do this either by direct election or by nomination from elected officials. Secular not-for-profit boards are most commonly self-appointing. The original incorporators formed the first board many years ago, and they appointed their successors. Religious hospitals frequently have board members nominated from the sponsoring religious organization. They often balance these members with others selected to represent the community. The owners of for-profit hospitals are stockholders. They or their employed representatives usually serve as the governing board. Some religious and for-profit hospitals use community advisory groups to supplement boards comprised solely of owners' representatives.

The governing board or its equivalent is the organizational unit ultimately responsible for success or failure. It is the board's responsibility to perceive and assess community benefits and exchange opportunities, to select all those the hospital can effectively fill, and to hire a capable management group. Hospitals in which these jobs are done well tend to thrive. They are the successful, well-managed hospitals.

Various studies have shown quite clearly that major differences exist in the operation of community hospitals. Some hospitals serve their communities for only half the cost of other ostensibly similar hospitals.[6] Similar patients undergoing surgery have nearly half again the risk of death in some hospitals that they do in others.[7] Presumably, with such wide variation on such fundamental issues, there are corresponding differences in success. Unfortunately, no particular group seems to have found the key. There is little direct connection between ownership and available measures of success. As is often the case, simple answers are not helpful: finding the well-managed hospital is more than identifying a specific kind of ownership.

Notes

1. Michigan Public Act 368, 1978, as amended.

2. National Center for Health Statistics, Vital and Health Statistics, series 1, no. 3, *Development and Maintenance of a National Inventory of Hospitals and Institutions* (Washington, D.C.: Government Printing Office, 1965), p. 9.

3. American Hospital Association, *Hospital Statistics,* 1983 (Chicago: AHA, 1984), p. ix.

4. American Hospital Association, *Hospital Statistics.*

5. Arthur F. Southwick, *The Law of Hospital and Health Care Administration* (Ann Arbor, MI: Health Administration Press, 1978), pp. 272–76.

6. J. R. Griffith, et al., "Measuring Community Hospital Services in Michigan," *Health Services Research* 16 (1981):135–60; J. Wennberg and A. Gittelsohn, "Small Area Variations in Health Care Delivery," *Science* 182 (1973): 1102–8.

7. Stanford Center for Health Services Research, "Comparisons of Hospitals with Regard to Outcomes of Surgery," *Health Services Research* 11 (1976): 112–27.

Suggested Readings

American Hospital Association. *Guide to the Healthcare Field.* Chicago: AHA, published annually.

Program of Institutional Effectiveness Review. Chicago: AHA, 1981.

Hospital Statistics. Chicago: AHA, published annually.

Wilson, F. A., and Neuhauser, D. *Health Services in the United States,* 2d ed. Cambridge, MA: Ballinger, 1982.

2

Understanding the Hospital Organization: Open Systems Concepts

Introduction

The Open and Closed System Concepts

This chapter and the one that follows develop in some detail a philosophy, or way of looking at the hospital. The philosophy is based upon two concepts that have been found useful in a wide variety of fields, one of which is the study of organizations. One concept is that of **homeostasis,** in biology a "state of physiological equilibrium produced by a balance of functions and of chemical composition within an organism"[1] and more generally a "tendency towards relatively stable equilibrium between interdependent elements."[2] The second concept has to do with how that equilibrium is achieved, or **cybernetics,** "the science of systems of control and communications."[3]

Homeostasis provides both a way of identifying an organization's objective or purpose and a model of the organization's behavior in relation to its environment. Most living organisms strive for homeostasis. Under the open systems concept, it is assumed that organizations, including hospitals, also strive for homeostasis, that is, that their overriding goal is a mutually satisfactory relationship with the society in which they are located. The organization identifies the needs or desires of its environment and establishes exchanges, or relationships, with it. Environments are constantly changing so the search for equilibrium is an ongoing one. **Open systems** activities are outwardlooking, those through which the organization selects its exchanges. These activities define more precisely what the organization must do to thrive in the environment and what expectations the organization must establish and fulfill in order to succeed. Success is the fulfillment of a set of exchanges which satisfies all parties; the broader the response, the greater the success and the broader and more stable the homeostasis.

How the expectations are fulfilled is described by the closed system model discussed in chapter 3. The closed system senses the difference between the expectations and the actual performance of the organization. It looks inward on what the organization is doing and compares that to the expectation. It then strives to bring the two into agreement by manipulating various parts of the organization. Its success must be fed back to the open system as one consideration in the adjustment of exchanges.

Both open and closed system theories are properly described as cybernetic in the sense that both use systems of control and communications to achieve homeostasis. In this book they are viewed as sequentially linked, the outward-looking, broader reaching, more ambiguous open system identifying the potential directions, and the more immediate, narrow, and precise closed system providing practical ways in which the expectations can be met. In this way, the open system serves as a buffer or intermediary between the day-to-day actions of the organization and the changing needs of the outside world.

This chapter explores the implications of open systems and exchange theory. It:

1. Identifies the many exchange partners of the modern hospital, labeling and grouping them for convenient reference throughout the book

2. Discusses how systems theory reflects failure and success in hospitals

3. Discusses a strategy for managing exchanges that distinguishes well-managed hospitals

4. Reviews the multiple goals that community exchange partners have and relates them to five underlying motivations

5. Traces how these motivations have influenced hospital activities through the past 100 years

The Importance of Systems Concepts

As applied to organizations seeking long-term survival such as hospitals, the concepts of open and closed systems mean the following:

— All objectives, goals, or purposes, except the mission of the hospital, are set by a search and evaluation process that focuses on mutually acceptable exchanges between society's resources and what the hospital can do. The best exchanges are those that society wants most, as measured by its willingness to commit resources, and that the hospital can deliver better than any other source.

— Control of the organization is achieved by detailed expectations derived from the exchanges. Expectations are used constantly to steer the organization toward fulfillment of the agreed-upon exchanges.

— Success is the reward for fulfilling the exchanges. Fulfilling the exchanges society sees as most useful assures the organization of the largest continuing stream of resources and thus the best opportunity for survival.

— Failure can occur in four ways:

1. the hospital can misread society's wants and select the wrong exchanges;

2. the translation of exchanges to expectations can contain errors;

3. the units of the hospital can fail to meet their expectations; and

4. the demands of society can move away from any the hospital can fulfill.

This view of the hospital is significantly broader than most, and it is consistent with the definition of the hospital established in chapter 1. Some people would argue that it is too broad. One such argument suggests that the theory gives the hospital very few limits; the hospital may try to do anything society wants. If society wanted the hospital to operate a bank, for example, it could try. This statement is literally correct. The theory encourages hospitals to contemplate such an idea, but to do it only when it would be successful. What hospitals will actually do, rather than just think about doing, under these models is limited by the need for success. There are tricks to every trade, and hospitals know the tricks of health care. They do not know the tricks of banking and would probably fail at it. In practice, there are limits on what society will actually request and even more on what the hospital can deliver. One function of the organization is to find those limits.

A second argument suggests that under this theory the wishes of owners are ignored. This is actually a misreading of the theory, which says only that the hospital should seek mutually satisfactory exchanges.

Do Catholic hospitals have to provide abortions under this model? Legally in the United States, government-owned hospitals must provide abortions, but others have a choice. Does a hospital incorporated for sick children have to care for adults? Only if it chooses to. The owners have the privilege of limiting the mission on moral or even esthetic grounds. Of course if they are not successful at their chosen mission, they face a more serious choice—they can revise their morals or esthetics or they can disband the organization. A well-chosen mission is based on extensive open systems review of real and perceived community needs. In general, the better the hospital carries out its open systems activities, the broader the range of exchange choices it will have; the better it carries out its closed system activities, the broader the range it will be able to handle successfully.

Identifying the Well-Managed Hospital

There are also persons who deny that real hospitals work according to these models, principally because these persons see confusion, variability, and conflict in hospitals. Such conditions actually support the validity of the models: confusion inevitably occurs when the process of open systems analysis and exchange identification is incomplete. If not resolved, expectations are left vague, or are not coordinated among units. The hospital's response becomes variable, and too many responses will be unsatisfactory. Conflict arises because different participants put different priorities on exchange opportunities. Like confusion, it is natural, but it must be resolved.

As modeled in open systems theory, poorly run hospitals are more prone to misread opportunities, leave society's wants unmet, argue inconclusively over their selections, and create confusing or conflicting expectations among operating personnel. In closed system theory, they leave some expectations unstated, fail to quantify expectations when they can, and tolerate wide variations in performance. The well-managed hospital does the opposite: it excels at these tasks. Throughout the text, examples of specific areas in which the well-managed hospital gains its advantages will be noted.

Exchanges and Exchange Partners

An exchange is a mutual or reciprocal transfer that occurs when both parties believe themselves to benefit from it. Exchanges occur constantly in society, and in a certain sense they ultimately can occur only between individuals. As a practical matter, a great many exchanges occur through formal groups of people such as governments and organizations that represent and have the commitment of their members.

Exchange partners can be either individuals or groups. Partners can be classified according to the nature of their exchange, although many individuals and some groups will be in several categories of exchanges simultaneously.

Members. Group exchanges are fruitful for individuals because they can meet some wants that would otherwise go unmet. The set of exchanges that commits the individuals to their groups is central; the success of the groups depends upon these exchanges. The most fundamental exchange of an organization, therefore, is between it and its **members**, those people who either give or withhold their participation in it. For hospitals, members are employees, doctors, trustees, and other volunteers. In most community hospitals, there are other, nonemployed providers of care, chiefly dentists, psychologists, and podiatrists.

Member Groups. Members are often organized into groups, and their exchanges are arranged to some extent collectively. There are unions and professional associations for members, and any subunit of the hospital—the doctors specializing in neurology, for example—can become a group representing its members to the hospital.

Government agencies of various kinds monitor the rights of member groups. Occupational safety, licensure, and equal employment opportunity agencies are among those entitled to access to the hospital and its records. The hospital is obligated to collect Social Security and federal income taxes. Records and taxes are examples of exchanges with member groups. The strategy of most well-run hospitals is to minimize disagreement with members and their representative groups by complying with existing agreements.

Patients and Families. Members of an organization only join it in the hope of some reward. Where the participation is vocational, as it is for doctors and employees, that reward must include economically competitive compensation. The hospital, however, cannot provide compensation unless it sells the services of the doctors and the employees to patients. (The fact that many doctors sell their hospital services directly to patients changes the details, but not the concept.) Patients, then, are the second most important exchange partners.

Most patients are aided in their hospitalization by friends and family. In some cases, hospitals must establish close and direct relations with friends and family (for example, with the fathers of newborn, the next-of-kin of dying, and the family of chronically impaired patients). In all cases, the hospital is responsible for amenities, safety, parking, and on-site mobility for these people. These are exchanges as well.

Payment Partners. In modern industrial societies, patients rely on a variety of insurance mechanisms to pay for care. Insurance carriers are essential exchange partners. Carriers differ by locale, but the Blue Cross–Blue Shield plan is usually important.

Newer forms of insurance have created many alternative delivery systems. Most are commonly referred to by their initials: **HMOs**, health maintenance organizations, are usually broad-benefit health insurance plans that work through salaried rather than fee-for-service doctors (HMO is sometimes used in a broader sense to cover all alternative delivery systems); **IPAs**, independent practice associations, are groups of doctors providing care for an annual premium like an HMO, but paying their affiliated doctors on a fee-for-service basis; **PPOs**, preferred provider organizations, are insurance plans that pay on a fee-for-service basis, but only to selected hospitals, doctors, and other providers with whom they have established a contract; **PROs**, peer review organizations, which are led by doctors, do not insure or provide care, but audit the use of insurance benefits for Medicare and other insurers; and **TPAs**, third-party administrators, process claims and sometimes also audit use for insurance companies or employers who are carrying their own insurance.

Two large governmental insurance programs are direct exchange partners with most hospitals. Medicare deals with hospitals through the **Medicare intermediary**, usually the local Blue Cross–Blue Shield plan. Medicaid, a state-federal program financing care for the poor, is run through the state **Medicaid agency**.

Much insurance is provided through employment. Since hospitalization insurance is an increasingly expensive employment benefit, employing corporations have become important exchange partners. A major reason for arranging insurance through employment in the past was unions.

Regulatory Partners. Most insurers mandate two outside audits of hospital performance, one by the **Joint Commission on Accreditation of Hospitals** or its osteopathic counterpart, the **Osteopathic Hospital Association**, and the other by a public accounting firm of the hospital's choice. Hospitals have exchange relationships with these agencies.

The health care hospitals provide is judged by society to require collective supervision via government regulation. As a result, governmental regulatory agencies are exchange partners. Licensing agencies and rate-regulating commissions are common. Most states have certificate of need laws, requiring permission for hospital construction or expansion. These are administered through a complex network of state and local **health systems agencies** (HSAs).

Community Partners. The hospital as an organization makes certain exchanges with other organizations, governments, and informal groups. These are numerous, varied, and far-reaching. Taken as a whole they constitute the **community**, the individuals, groups, and organizations (including members) who have or may have exchanges with the hospital.

Hospitals use significant quantities of goods and services. The suppliers of these, from artificial implants to banking, are exchange partners. Morticians are a special class of suppliers; they are employed by patients' families, but work closely with the hospital. Many supplies face unique problems. Electrical power, communications, and human blood are three examples.

Hospitals provide babies for adoption; receive the victims of accidents, violent crimes, rape, and family abuse; and attract the homeless, the mentally incompetent, and the chronically alcoholic. These activities draw them into exchange relations with police, mental health clinics, mental hospitals, and social service agencies.

Hospitals require land and zoning permits; they use water, sewer, traffic, electronic communications, fire protection, and police services. Hospitals often present special problems in these areas which must be negotiated with local government.

Hospitals take United Fund charity; they facilitate baptisms, ritual circumcisions, group religious observances, and rites for the dying. They provide educational facilities and services to the community. These activities make them partners of charitable, religious, educational, and cultural organizations, and the citizenry at large.

Influence

Beyond the partnerships involving frequent and continuing exchanges are less frequent ones between the hospital and its community or society. The many groups involved can be classified by their **influence**, that is, by their ability to affect the hospital's success. Influence is gained by controlling a resource. The more complete the control and the more critical the resource, the greater the influence. Member partners with critical skills, such as doctors, have considerable influence, as do partners with whom there are frequent exchanges, such as payment partners; however, a group or even an individual who relates to the institution only infrequently can sometimes acquire startling influence. Public health licensure officials, for example, can close a hospital for an emergency situation. Partners having above average influence are sometimes called **influentials**.

Influence is relative among the partners and variable across time and place, although national, regional, and community trends and events dictate considerable similarity at any particular time. The history of the modern hospital can generally be described as one of steadily increasing numbers of influentials. The "doctors' workshop" of the first decades of the twentieth century accurately captures the influence existing then—influence limited almost exclusively to members, particularly physicians. The problems attending the development of technology, the growth of health insurance, government subsidies through Hill-Burton and other legislative vehicles, and government finance through Medicare and Medicaid, led to demonstrable increases in the lists of influentials.

In the early 1980s, the relative influence of the partners of the typical community hospital was again substantially revised. The federal government changed the method of payment for Medicare, dropping the phrase "reasonable cost" and stating explicit limits for government payment. Since Medicare revenue constituted 35 to 40 percent of most hospitals' income, the government's influence was unquestionable. At the same time, and driven by some of the same underlying causes, employing corporations began to exert their influence to reduce cost. They became more aggressive in using their governing board membership positions, created community groups to supplement trustees' and regulatory agencies' control of costs, and generated market support for the newer forms of payment. The net results of these actions was to significantly raise the influence of payment partners. At the same time, certain kinds of government regulatory agencies, particularly the health systems agencies, lost influence. In short, a consensus among influentials created a buyer's market for the purchase of hospital services.

This change in the influence structure has spread across most of the United States, and it appears to be permanent. The result was to require substantial improvements in and extensions of the closed system models in order to control costs more closely. Since the costs of hospital care involve not only the efficiency of operation of individual activities but also the clinical decisions about what services to use, these reorganizations focused heavily upon the medical staff. The well-run hospitals were in a position to respond to the new needs more rapidly and more effectively than others. In general, they achieved that position by maintaining sound, constructive, and forward-looking relationships with all of their exchange partners. They entered the period of extreme change with three assets: first, they had the resources which accrued to successful institutions prior to the change; second, they had a background of goodwill and effective communications with their exchange partners; and third, they had better sensing and forecasting mechanisms, which allowed them to see the extent and permanence of the change faster.

Optimizing Exchange Relationships

It is clear that the exchange relationships supporting community hospitals are extensive and complicated. One way to consider how to optimize them would be to explore the tasks involved in identifying, selecting, and negotiating the relationships themselves. These tasks can be classified as environmental surveillance, planning, and marketing, respectively. They are the function of several components of the governance system of hospitals, and much of Part II is devoted to an exploration of them.

On the other hand, one might search not for tasks, but for principles that well-run hospitals follow in optimizing their exchanges. Several principles can be identified, particularly if one notes that the exchanges can be roughly divided into two categories. One category is all those people who take services and provide support, that is, the patient and community partners; the other is those who provide services and require support, that is, the members.

The first step to success is recognizing the duality of exchanges. It is best to assume that any exchange must benefit both members and community or it will sooner or later be changed. In a free society, the exploited group will gain the political, economic, or social strength to redress its disadvantage. If one also recognizes that no exchange is ever perfect, the world can be understood as a continuing struggle for equilibrium. The well-managed hospital not only recognizes but incorporates that struggle. It devises formal systems to resolve the inevitable conflict in the most constructive manner. To put it another way, both well-run and poorly run hospitals have agendas of unsatisfactory exchanges, but the well-run hospital manages its list more effectively. It removes items faster, adds items more promptly and selectively, and as a result sustains a larger set of satisfactory exchanges. More specifically, well-managed hospitals constantly pursue the six steps identified below.

Responding to the Needs of Members

The hospital is a creation of its members. If they fail to make exchanges with it, it will pass from existence, or be forced to find new members. On the other hand, members depend upon the rewards of those exchanges and are willing to sacrifice their time and energies for them. Thus there exists an equilibrium between the two. In general, the relationship benefits from clear presentation of the needs of community partners and by an orderly, candid exploration of potential conflicts. This allows members to explore their own wants and contributions and to develop their own adaptations gradually. Failures of this process are marked by strikes, low morale, high turnover, recruitment difficulty, and low productivity. One measure of success is the quality of recruited members. A hospital which responds to its own members attracts strong recruits. This is one of several ways in which success feeds upon itself in the well-managed hospital.

Responding to the Needs of Community Partners

As a rule, the larger the number of community partners, the more successful a hospital will be; that is, for most hospitals, the larger the market share, the better. Not only is there a wider support base for resources, there is more diversification and therefore more protection against adversity. There are obvious limits. Some patients may be better served by other hospitals: price, distance, quality, amenities, ability to pay, and religious preference are common factors in a patient's choice of hospital. Although price was unimportant from 1967 to 1982, it has emerged as a major concern since then. Distance is very important. Few people wish to travel very far for hospital care, and doctors must minimize travel time. Quality and amenities may conflict with price. A hospital that reduces these conflicts—by being more efficient, for example—can serve a larger share of the market.

Hospitals should seek to satisfy a high percentage of the needs of their closest partners. Geographically, this usually means meeting the needs of a high share of nearby markets. Hospitals that allow dissatisfaction to mount in their immediate area or among their important partners risk serious consequences. Creation of new organizations and firing of executives are related to the emergence of an effectively large, dissatisfied group of either community partners or members. Both exchange groups are important. Community partners have better access to resources, but both groups have exchange relationships outside the hospital, permitting dissatisfied members to gain community support.

Although a large number of partners is usually desirable, if there are too many commitments to community partners, some exchanges go unfulfilled, promoting dissatisfaction with service. If there are too many members, costs rise, promoting dissatisfaction. The well-run hospital maintains close surveillance in both areas and tries to plan in a way that ensures balance.

Understanding the Multiple Nature of Networks

In addition to the complexities suggested by a listing of the hospital's exchange partners, most of these partners have relationships with exchange partners of their own; thus, the hospital is located in a web of networks. Respect for these networks is one of the keys to success. Exchange partners can reward more generously services which do not require them to revise other relationships that are important to them.

The most important of the networks is that between doctor and patient. Patients visit doctors much more often than they are admitted to hospitals. Several specialties of doctors—mainly the primary care doctors in family practice, general internal medicine, pediatrics, and psychiatry—derive more income from work in their office than from work in the hospital. Their exchange relationships with the hospital will be different from those of specialists who rely on referral from primary care and who use hospital resources more heavily.

The relationship among employers, unions, and insurance carriers of various kinds is another network. For many hospitals, direct relations with insurance carriers yield their largest single source of revenue. Yet the carrier is only the point of contact; if wants of employers and unions are not met, carriers can be changed. The proliferation of alternative delivery systems and the decline of Blue Cross–Blue Shield in the marketplace was associated with profound shifts in the exchanges between employers and unions. These, in turn, were driven by changes in the general economy, chiefly in the diminished ability of the United States to compete in world trade.

A third important network is the one relating to government. Governments have multiple exchanges with hospitals, as well as exchanges among themselves (for example, state and federal governments) and between units of government (such as Medicaid and the regulatory agencies). There are obvious relations among governments and employers, unions, and the citizenry. When people are dissatisfied with their exchange relationship with hospitals, they can choose either governmental or nongovernmental routes to relief. The growth in governmental regulation that has occurred in the past decade is related partly to citizen dissatisfaction with hospital cost increases and partly to government difficulty with Medicaid and Medicare costs.

There are many other networks between exchange partners of hospitals. Identifying and understanding them in the local setting is an essential skill of well-run hospitals.

Sensing Change Promptly and Evaluating It Correctly

Extensive environmental surveillance results in a steady stream of information, and modern life is such that most of this information will reflect a desire, or even a need, for change. Yet some evaluation of this information must occur, because it is very likely that nothing will come of most of it. There are, for example, several thousand bills introduced in each session of Congress and several hundred in each session of the state legislatures. Dozens relate to the exchange relationships important to hospitals. If a hospital tried to prepare for all these proposals, or even to comment on them, it might do nothing else. Only a handful of the proposals will ever get to committee hearing, and most will not survive to enactment. A similar, though less visible, overload occurs in economic arenas. Thus effective surveillance is timely and wide-ranging, but it is also selective. Opportunities and threats are carefully judged, both on importance and on likelihood of occurrence, and attention is focused on the probable and the important.

Ironically, what is probable and important is likely to have been around for a while. Many leaders define prudence as waiting for an idea to be tested and to mature. Brand-new ideas, therefore, tend to lack sufficient support to make them probable. An important function of surveillance is not so much the identification of every single new idea as the tracking of trends in maturing ideas. The well-run hospital strives to recognize when an idea's time has come and be prepared for it.

Identifying the Underlying Forces

A second important characteristic relating to environmental surveillance is its search for major trends and underlying factors. Individual ideas and proposals are followed as they mature, and the totality of ideas is evaluated for content and direction—that is, the extent to which new thinking has emerged, new consensus has formed, new influentials have emerged, or interest in certain values has increased or diminished. The best surveillance takes into account non-health-related events and even international events. Walter McNerney, a noted health care leader, once remarked that a test of insight was the ability to answer the question: "What is the connection between the Arab-Israeli war of 1973 and U.S. national health insurance?" There is an answer, and those who saw it first understood first that there would be no national health insurance for the United States in the 1970s, or in all probability the 1980s.[4]

Responding Effectively to Opportunities

It is never enough just to know what is happening; organizations must change their actions effectively in response. Through the governance system, the proper response must be selected and developed into changes in the expectations of each small work unit affected. The expectations must be detailed and thorough, specifying new processes, volumes, resources, financing, and quality considerations for each unit.

Effective response for individuals is a two-step process of decision and reaction. For organizations, it is a multistep process. Like individuals, organizations must decide what should be done. Unlike individuals, they must then gain acceptance of the solution from their members and coordinate many different actions. In organizations as large and complicated as hospitals, this process takes time. Well-run hospitals perceive important trends far enough in advance to explore thoroughly both the possible solutions and the opinions of their members about these solutions. This permits debate and development of internal consensus, which clarifies and simplifies the final step. Often it permits testing, modification, and gradual adjustment.

The Wellsprings of Exchange: What Is a Community Seeking?

Hospitals have been a part of community life since antiquity. There have always been individuals who were willing to work in them for economic and other personal reward. But if exchange theory is correct, community partners must also have perceived the exchanges to answer certain needs. Community partners supported hospitals because they met those needs more effectively than available alternatives. Something as commonplace as hospitals must be responsive to needs that are nearly universal. At the same time, needs and effective responses are not all alike, and certainly they have changed through history. By studying changes in needs and tracing their impact upon hospitals, one may hope to identify what community partners were seeking.

In fact, the history of hospitals clearly reveals multiple and powerful motivations in the communities that built them. Although other taxonomies could be created, it is useful to think of these motivations in five groups:

1. *Samaritanism and government support of the poor*, a desire to aid the sick and needy because the aid itself has value or intrinsic merit. In advanced industrial nations, Samaritanism has two forms: the larger part is government programs supported by tax dollars; the smaller is personal, voluntary charity.

2. *Personal health*, a desire to improve the health of oneself and one's loved ones, to be able to deal more effectively with disease, disability, and death.

3. *Public health*, a desire for health as a collective or social benefit, to reduce contagion, assure a healthy workforce and military force, and reduce the tax burdens associated with disease, disability, and death.

4. *Economical health care*, a desire to control the costs of the health care endeavor so that personal and public funds are available for other goals.

5. *Economic gain for the community,* a desire to make the community as a whole and its individual citizens economically successful.

These five motivations are complex in themselves, and they tend to interact with one another in real situations. Also, of course, they interact with motivations having to do with other human wants. To understand how these interactions might occur, and as a result shape a specific hospital in a given community or the 6,000 hospitals across the United States, each motivation requires some amplification.

Samaritanism and Government Support of the Poor

Whether Samaritanism deserves first place in a list of motivations for hospitals is debatable, but a claim for prominence can be based on the long history and diversity of examples.

The urge to help one's fellow man is widespread, although it appears to wax and wane at various times and places. It is, however, one of the characteristics that distinguishes man from animals, and it is strongly endorsed by most of the major religions of the world. Charity to the sick and injured is particularly appealing to many citizens of the community. The sick have an obvious need, and concerns with the worth of the recipients can be set aside more easily than they can, for example, in the case of criminals or unwed mothers. The word *hospital* has the same root as the words *host, hospitality,* and *hotel,* reflecting the ancient role of places called hospitals as refuges. In the twentieth century, places called hospitals range from simple refuges, in emerging nations, to citadels of high technology where refuge is not often considered. Samaritanism occurs in both, however.

Government programs to help the poor, distinguished from programs to help all citizens or other special groups, can also be viewed as Samaritan; in fact, they are often justified politically in that way. They also may have more mundane motives. Supporting the poor creates jobs, wins votes in some districts, and helps prevent riots. Many governments have diminished the role of charity and eliminated support for the poor by establishing universal health insurance. The United States has been uniquely reluctant to pursue such a course. Instead, it has Medicaid, a state-federal program with widely varying impact on hospitals, averaging about 5 percent of revenues. For many hospitals, Medicaid is trivial. For others, it can amount to more than a third of all revenues. Many states and large cities have other programs of charitable care as well, but these are almost always smaller.

"It is more blessed to give than to receive" is an important principle in most major religions and ethical systems. A world without charity would be palpably less civilized. It is also likely that not all charitable motives are altruistic: donations to hospitals are a way to relieve feelings of guilt about wealth, advertise the better characteristics of the donor, and, since 1913, reduce income taxes.

It is easy to be cynical about the power of Samaritanism, but it may be unwise. Donated funds amount to less than 2 percent of all income, but those funds can be used flexibly, in ways that directly express the wish or even the whim of the donor or the recipient. Thus hospitals cultivate donations in order to have unrestricted sources of capital, and donors seek hospitals to meet needs that could be more those of the giver than of the recipient. For example, children's hospitals are more appealing to donors than an objective observer might expect. Donor satisfaction is as important to the exchange as the use to which the gift is put: if donors are not satisfied, gifts will not continue.

Not all charity is in dollars or property. Service is often contributed. Volunteers provide important amenities and assistance in most community hospitals. Although real value exists for the hospital, it is not the full measure of the exchange. The opportunity to serve is also important. The service of trustees is almost entirely volunteered; tax law requires that they receive no direct profit from their efforts. Many hours of medical staff activity are unpaid as well, although one can argue that doctors are compensated by the privilege of using the hospital in caring for patients. Often overlooked is the charitable impulse of employees at all levels in hospitals. Aiding the sick is in itself a reward of their job, a compensation that sometimes offsets low wages. Whenever a hospital employee or doctor spends time at activities that would be better compensated elsewhere, a charitable donation has occurred.

Personal Health

Although most Americans would say that hospitals exist to provide personal health care, this purpose is more recent than Samaritanism. Until a century ago, hospitals had almost no contribution to make toward restoring health, and the actual lifesaving abilities of a hospital are probably still less than most people think. Personal health care comes from several sources: the individual, family and friends, and doctors are all important. The hospital supplements these sources; it supplies personal health services that they either cannot or prefer not to provide. What the community expects of the hospital, therefore, is the difference between what the community wants in total and what it is willing to provide elsewhere. It is this difference that makes community hospital resources so variable. What communities can provide elsewhere tends to be simpler and more individualized, pushing the hospital contribution inevitably toward complex and expensive technology. Several elements go into the final equation: community size, wealth, diversity, and attitude toward health care on the one hand, and changes in technical capability on the other.

High-Tech Health Care. The hospital's contribution to personal health care became more complicated, expensive, and high-tech as its services became more readily available and valuable. The operating room was the first such service to emerge. By 1870, new technology was providing safe and pain-free surgery, greatly improving the patient's chance of surviving what today are routine procedures. Cesarean section ceased to be immediately fatal to the mother. Hernia repairs, trauma repairs, and removal of diseased organs in the abdominal cavity became dramatically safer. The cost, difficulty, and need for trained personnel put this technology out of reach of most individual doctors. The new opportunities for truly valuable care via the hospital led to the first great growth period for American hospitals.[5]

Many more recent hospital services reflect this pattern: new and expensive technology arises and is provided centrally for the community by the hospital. Often the hospital's role shifts over time as the new technology becomes less costly and easier to use. A typical pattern is for the new service to leave the research stage as an activity that occurs solely on an inpatient basis in the hospital, is changed to an outpatient hospital activity, and finally migrates to the doctor's office, at least for the less complicated cases. Many of the surgical procedures responsible for the rise in the hospital's contribution to personal health care a century ago are now done without overnight hospitalization. Some are done in doctors' offices, and some have been replaced by nonsurgical treatment.

A community's investment in hospitals is dramatically affected by its view of the desirability of new technology. A community that is slow to adopt the fruits of research may invest little or nothing in early stage, hospital-centered technology. A community with a bias toward rapid adoption of technology will invest much more in hospitals and will pay much more for hospital care. Within surprisingly broad ranges, these choices are not reflected in measurable differences in health. One reason is that the health care services of hospitals have a wide variety of benefits and are difficult to measure. Another is that the technology is usually available at some more distant place.

Technology is attractive in the local community because it provides comfort, convenience, reassurance, or some other important, but less than vital, benefit. It is also related in important ways to three other motives: Samaritanism, economy of health care, and community gain and prestige. Thus when communities bias their hospital plans toward or away from high-tech investment, they are dealing with matters below the threshold of differences in personal health. It may be less convenient to drive Grandmother to the state university hospital for care, but it does not measurably affect her health, and it clearly does not affect her longevity. The bias in most communities through 1982 was in favor of high technology. It is likely that a strong demand continues to exist, only temporarily dampened by concerns about economy.

The High-Touch Alternative. The hospital is usually pictured in terms of its dramatic conquests over disease, death, and disability, and the reality and importance of such services is indeed a major role. Stopped hearts are restarted, airways are reopened, arteries are sewn, babies are rescued by Cesarean section, rampant infection is overcome. People are snatched from the shadow of death dozens of times each day.

What is important to understand is that this is only a minor part of hospital activity. The patient with cardiovascular disease is much more often in the hospital for continuing support of an impaired heart than immediate treatment of a heart attack. Chronic lung disease is more important than the occasional dramatic stoppage of breathing. Alcoholism, a principal cause of accidents, remains after the artery is sewn. Most mothers deliver babies virtually unaided, and many infections are defeated by the body itself with only modest technology.

The popular raison d'être of the hospital may be dramatic lifesaving, but the day-to-day reality is relief of distress that is not life-threatening. Increasingly, the hospital's services are part of a program of care of chronic illness, a fact that will assume more importance as the population ages. Not only are few patients at death's door when they arrive, few are cured when they leave. Most are better off in some important ways, and a very small percentage leave dead. Many will return in months or years with a new manifestation of a continuing, underlying disease. A growing role of the hospital is to support the optimal management of the chronically sick. This generally requires more human services and less dramatic technology; such services are high-touch in contrast to high-tech. High-touch services will compete increasingly with high-tech ones in community motivations.

Toward a More Comprehensive View of Hospital Contributions. There are other ways to look on hospital contributions than the high-tech–high-touch duality. The following are examples of hospital activities which show the diversity and complexity of the personal health service motives.

— Care of the dying is a very important example. About 25 percent of hospital expenditures go for care of people who will not survive a year.[6] Often the terminal nature of their illness is known. Although the amount and kind of care given by hospitals to the dying is now a matter of debate, a pattern of maximal response is traditional. This tradition has encouraged the use of technology even past the point where a chance of life remained. The hospital has been assigned an important role because people believe that it will prolong life if possible, handle the responsibility ethically and humanely, and reduce the burden on the family. People feel better if Grandmother dies in the hospital.

— Obstetrics and newborn care provide another numerically important example. Well over 99 percent of births in this country occur in hospitals. In the Netherlands, less than half of the births occur in hospitals, yet the safety of comparable populations of mothers and babies is the same. In Great Britain, home birthing was the rule, as it is in the Netherlands, but it has become less popular. At the same time, modest trends toward home birthing have developed in the United States. Attitudes determine the differences in the three countries, not technology or safety.

— Communities, and as a result hospitals, differ in their views of the importance of services for chronic disease. Nursing homes are frequently associated directly with community hospitals in Wisconsin, though they rarely are in other states. Alcoholism and substance abuse programs are more popular in some areas than in others. Many communities have begun to emphasize disease prevention and health promotion, but the vigor of their pursuit has differed.

— Both the relative attractiveness of outpatient care and the length of recuperative stay associated with each hospitalization appear to be sensitive to social issues, such as changes in family structure, as well as to disease and technology. Small houses unequipped for home nursing, the decline of the extended family as a result of a more mobile middle class, and the growth of families where both adults work promote the attractiveness of hospitals for inpatient care of the sick. These factors have supported more use of hospitals as the century progressed. Concern over cost appears to have reversed the trend.

— Although most patients contract with their physicians directly, in some circumstances the doctor is an employee of the hospital or a closely related corporation. In such cases, the hospital is the direct provider, rather than simply a support for the doctor. Hospitals traditionally provided direct medical care in clinics for the poor and in emergency rooms. Emergency rooms frequently treat patients who do not have personal physicians, even though they are not emergency cases. It is more and more common for hospitals to employ physicians or to form close affiliations with them. The changes of the 1980s appear to be supporting closer relations between doctors and hospitals.

— Hospitals must provide a level of comfort and convenience which matches the life-style of the community. In the postwar decades, as Americans grew rapidly wealthier, hospitals were pressured to provide single rooms, more toilets and showers, carpeting, and air conditioning. Although some of these are viewed as necessities (toilets in patient rooms and air conditioning are specified in the national Life Safety Code), they are more accurately amenities to which Americans have become accustomed. Other advanced nations have made other choices, with no loss of health.

Values that communities place on benefits like these clearly differ by time and place. The differences are generated by complex, not easily modified phenomena. Age, education, and religion are known to be important in establishing attitudes. Economic factors are also influential, and two different ones can be identified: the general level of wealth supports a larger, more high-tech, more costly hospital system, yet poverty also appears to stimulate hospital growth. Communities with more poor persons tend to use more hospital beds and to spend more on hospital operation.

Public Health

The distinction between public and personal health is conceptually clear but sometimes hard to trace in real situations. Personal health care is that which is given directly to the individual. Public health emphasizes activity for groups, such as maintaining a pure water supply. A public benefit also occurs when care is given to individuals. The clearest examples are care of contagious disease. Immunization helps the group because epidemics are impossible when a large fraction of the population is immunized, even if that fraction is less than 100 percent. Immunizations are usually provided by private doctors, but hospitals assist. Quarantine for the sick prevented the spread of disease, at least theoretically; in fact, quarantine of persons with a contagious disease was one of the important exchange contributions of hospitals until this century. Hospitals were relied upon for care of persons with a long list of contagious diseases, beginning with tuberculosis and leprosy and including scarlet fever, polio, and infant diarrheal diseases. None of these diseases is of major importance in U.S. hospitals today, having been nearly eliminated by vaccine or reduced greatly in severity by antibiotics. Treatment for alcoholism, smoking cessation programs, and other substance abuse programs have dramatic effects beyond the individual. They are among the modern epidemics with which hospitals deal.

If one adopts the position that any sickness is to the community's disadvantage as well as to the individual's, then the hospital's contribution to public health parallels its contribution to personal health. Prompt, effective treatment meets the needs of both. Maintenance of a healthy work force, and traditionally a healthy army, are important public goals. Minimizing expenditures necessary to deal with sickness is also important. Dollars spent on the care of the sick and disabled are not available for other social goods and services. For this reason, prevention of disease is particularly valued for its public contribution.

Hospitals have a strong contribution to make in prevention. They normally reach people when they are especially receptive to learning better health habits, improved nutrition, and the best care of their continuing disease or disability. Thus many hospitals provide pre- and postnatal education for parents: safe pregnancy, avoidance of drugs injurious to the infant, nutrition and breast feeding, psychological aspects of child rearing, the importance of immunization, and family planning are topics frequently covered. In each case, parental failure can create a child who may be a great financial burden on the state.

In addition to preventive services for patients, hospitals are reaching out with preventive services for the general public. Hospitals and doctors are accepted as authorities on health care. Hospital support helps persuade people of the value of programs. In addition, contact with well people is a form of advertising for the hospital. Four health promotion programs have a reasonable chance of reducing disease and disability. They are, in order of effectiveness: hypertension control, smoking cessation, alcoholism treatment, and nutrition and weight control. Well-run hospitals now support programs in several of these areas.

Economical Health Care

The operation of a hospital can be viewed as having an opportunity cost. That is, funds put toward its support are not available for new production investment, purchase of raw materials, education, or some other use leading more directly to increased gross national or community product. This leads some members of the community to say the proper hospital expenditure is the absolute minimum necessary to maintain public and private health. What they are seeking is *economy* rather than strictly *efficiency*.

Although it is true that the most economical system must be the most efficient one, it is possible to be efficient but not economical, as the following situation makes clear. Consider a hospital which is currently operating at 80 percent of achievable efficiency. If it can reduce its expenditures on the present number of patients, it can reach greater efficiency and achieve greater economy. If it treats new patients and its expenditures remain the same, economy has not been gained even though efficiency has been improved. What has happened is that the role of the hospital as a supplement to family and doctor care has been redefined. The new definition may be more convenient or have important other benefits, but it is not more economical.

The motivation toward economy runs counter to many other motivations. Presumably levels of hospital care that impaired individual or public health would be uneconomical because they were self-defeating, but many of the factors affecting the choice of the hospital as supplement, do not obviously improve health. An extreme position in favor of economy (for example, Ivan Illich's[7]) would advocate dying at home, birthing at home, deferring surgery that makes only slight improvements in comfort, and in general pursuing a Spartan philosophy. Correctly implemented, such views would not be dangerous or unhealthy. They would be unpopular, and a massive shift toward Spartanism is unlikely. An increasing number of critics of the health care system wants some Spartanism, however. Since the hospital is the most expensive sort of care, it is the focus of these efforts toward economy.

Economic Gain for the Community

Diametrically opposed to motivations toward economy are desires for non-health-related economic gains that occur to communities spending funds on hospitals. These gains occur both directly and indirectly. Directly, hospitals create jobs, particularly for unskilled workers, who are difficult to employ in modern society. Hospitals also generate income for some local suppliers. If the money that pays for these expenditures comes from outside the community, the community as a whole benefits. Hospital care can be sold as interstate or even foreign exchange. Rochester, Minnesota; Cleveland, Ohio; and Boston, Massachusetts are extreme examples of a much more widespread desire to attract dollars to the community through hospital operation. There are four basic ways a hospital can attract outside dollars: by the sale of services to patients from other communities, by attracting federal grants and donations from individuals, by providing service to local people whose insurance is paid by others and by attracting new industry to a community. An example of the last would be if a community treats more Medicare patients in its hospitals than other communities do. Although the Social Security tax supporting the cost is uniform, more of the dollars flow into the high-volume community, where they create jobs and other desirable things. Another example exists where a plant or division of a large corporation shares a common health insurance cost with other units in other communities. Then an increase in hospital expenditures, with direct and indirect benefits for the community, is not offset by an increase in the health insurance premium the community pays.

Indirectly, hospitals help local economies by making it much easier to recruit doctors and by being one of the things an attractive community should have. Many U.S. communities have aggressive programs to recruit new industry. New industry brings new people and new wealth to town, but the new people want satisfactory hospitals and doctors. An attractive, well-equipped hospital is an asset in an industrial recruitment program. Concerned industrialists are now seeking economy more than attractiveness, but both goals will remain important.

Summary

The motivations supporting any real hospital are complex, deeply rooted in community and individual needs, and economically conflicting. Different mixes of the five major motives, and differing emphases on the various perspectives of personal health service, shape the way hospital resources are translated into programs. To the extent that there is a typical community hospital, it modestly encourages Samaritanism, provides technically oriented, supportive personal health care, discourages alcoholism and cigarette smoking, is a point of pride and employment for its community, and costs more than it needs to. But there are so many exceptions to each of these five statements that the profile is a potentially misleading stereotype.

The complexity and sensitivity of finding the proper balance among these motives are a very strong argument for local management, and so far Americans have concluded that variety is desirable and a local governing board is important in reaching an adequate solution. One of the critical functions of the governing board is to evaluate and implement the motivations of its particular community. Clearly, this is not an easy task, and one of the key executive functions is to help it.

People rarely, if ever, state their motivations clearly in the context of the five categories constructed above. Rather, they express their wants through demands for services, endorsement of legislative positions, donations, and opinions on specific propositions. To identify and evaluate motivations in real communities requires detailed understanding of the origins and implications of specific proposals. One way to begin developing an understanding is to analyze past actions in terms of these five motivational groups. This will be done in the following sections, first showing how the modern hospital emerged and then reviewing in more detail the changes of the last 30 years.

How Community Motivations Have Shaped
Community Hospitals

Over the years, both the relative strength of the five motivations and the capability of the hospital to satisfy them has varied. People built hospitals for centuries before any real impact on personal health could be identified. Their actions testify to the importance of Samaritanism and of the desire to respond in the face of disease and disability. Hospitals, like witch doctors and faith healers, tap powerful motivations that are independent of their primary objective. The ability of hospitals to control contagious disease was speculative, but their provision of refuge was real and important.[8] Economic aspects, both cost avoidance and local gain, were probably very much on the minds of the builders. There is a clear reference to excessive use and cost of hospitals in the reign of Henry VIII, 400 years ago.[9]

When a motivation becomes stronger, it is translated into programs or actions that condition the environment surrounding the hospital, making it easier for the hospital to move in certain directions and more difficult to move in others. These actions can occur in any of several different settings. New laws are common. New administrative regulation by the executive branch of government is relatively recent as an important vehicle. The marketplace, what people want to buy and do not want to buy, may be the most powerful expression of motivation. Donors can occasionally impose their motivations upon everyone else, but more often they tend to express a collective will. The courts have had a significant impact on hospitals in the last three decades. Finally, hospital people themselves—doctors, nurses, and managers—make their own positions clear.

Hospitals tend to respond to these changes, growing in some ways and shrinking in others. Those hospitals which do not respond to the changes do not flourish; patients, doctors, donors, and public programs leave them for other, more receptive organizations. The history of U.S. hospitals shows this process in action, whether it is examined over decades and centuries, or over months and years. The public debate over the numbers, kinds, costs, quality, location, and finance of hospitals is continuous. It is the process by which changes in motivation begin, become a consensus, are translated into action, and change the shape of hospitals.

Benjamin Franklin, conducting the fund drive for the first community hospital in North America, The Pennsylvania Hospital, founded in 1760, eloquently built his case on five arguments. They parallel exactly the five motivational groups:

1. We need a refuge for the unfortunate, and Christianity will re- ward you for your generosity to this cause. (Although Franklin did not say so, Judaism, Islam, and Buddhism also praise chari- table behavior.)
2. You might need it yourself this very night.
3. Among other things, we can keep contagious people off the streets.
4. We can certainly handle this better as a community than as individuals.
5. Grants from the Crown and the Commonwealth will lower the out-of-pocket costs. (He might have added that the grants were "new money" that would eventually end up in Philadelphians' purses.)[10]

Little has changed in 225 years except the language; four of these arguments appear in most twentieth century fund-raising literature. Only control of contagious disease is no longer appealing.

About 100 years after Franklin's effort, hospitals' ability to im- prove personal health began to increase. Consequently, that motivation and the sum of all the motivations became more powerful. Health in- surance began to develop as a way to finance the newly desirable hospi- tal service. A growing benefit unevenly distributed leads a progressive society to set up programs for reaching the poor. The combination of private and government funds pouring into the health care sector led, not surprisingly, both to higher costs and to an influx of funds into local economies. As costs mounted, interest in gaining access to local funds grew, but so did interest in economizing. That sequence summarizes the second century of community hospitals. It is useful to examine the last 30 years in detail, to establish a basis for understanding the future.

On balance, the exchange relationships established by the Ameri- can people for their hospitals after World War II were highly expansion- ist. The concept of Samaritanism was expressed in private charity and the Medicaid program of governmental support for the poor. Local communities were enthusiastic in their support for newer, bigger, and better hospitals. The public health motivation and the desire for econo- mizing became noticeably less popular. Costs rose at rates well over growth in gross national product: hospital care as a share of GNP more than tripled, and the share for all health care costs more than doubled. Only in the 1980s did substantial public support for economy make it- self felt.

The postwar actions in health care were very dependent upon the environment. There was great faith in American technology generally. The nation's extraordinary success in World War II, not only on the battlefield, but in factory and farm, had swept away most of the self-doubts of the Depression. Yet fears about that era remained, so Congress sought opportunities to stimulate the economy. It was willing to assume debt in order to avoid unemployment. The baby boom opened new markets, attracting private investment and creating new jobs. Population growth, and later the increased number of women in the work force, provided new workers. Had any of these elements been missing, the recent history of hospitals would have been quite different.

Samaritanism and Government Support of the Poor

After 20 years of national debate, both state and federal programs for the poor were significantly expanded by Public Law 89-97, the 1965 amendment to the Social Security Act that established Medicare and Medicaid. Title 18, Medicare, is a government insurance program based on Social Security taxes rather than charity or Samaritanism. Title 19 created Medicaid as a new and greatly expanded program of governmental support for the poor. Although the realities of implementation were less grandiose than the words of the act, hospitals began to receive much larger amounts of money than they had previously. A series of Great Society programs for the poor was also enacted in the late 1960s. These programs contained a number of health initiatives, but their impact was brief. Within 12 years, most had been substantially eliminated.

Perhaps the most important statement about Samaritanism was a negative one. Unlike most other countries of the Western world, the United States rejected universal entitlement to health care under national health insurance. In repeated congressional struggles, the view which prevailed was that hospital care is a local and private obligation. Only limited support is available to the poor after they have established their poverty by a means test.

At the same time, charity to hospitals continued to be privately popular and publicly encouraged. The annual fund drive is a thriving institution for many community hospitals, as is a program to encourage trusts and bequests. As stated earlier, charity is a small but important percentage of hospital income. It provides for some free care, but it is used in many cases as a margin to support innovation.

Personal Health

The Growth of Health Insurance. The set of exchange relationships which best reflects the willingness of Americans to support personal health care is the demand for private health insurance. Hospitalization insurance grew dramatically from 1945 to 1965 and more slowly thereafter. In the 1980s, about 85 percent of hospital care for the nonpoor is financed through insurance and prepayment. More than half these funds are privately purchased, usually as a benefit of employment. Medicare, the compulsory federal health insurance program for the aged, is the largest single source of funds, but even the aged purchase private insurance. In fact, most Medicare recipients also carry supplementary private insurance.[11]

The demand remained strong through the early 1980s. By then, virtually every American who could afford hospitalization insurance had bought it. There was also a steady increase in benefits, particularly under union contracts. By 1984, many industries and individuals were interested in forms of health insurance that would emphasize economy. Important labor groups resisted the notion of reduced expenditure, however, and overall demand for the kind of comprehensive insurance that had been popular in the preceding decades persisted.

As is the case with charity to hospitals, demand for health insurance benefits is supported by highly favorable tax provisions. For most Americans, a dollar spent on health insurance escapes taxation, while a dollar spent directly on health care does not. This means that it is cheaper to pay costs of handling insurance than to pay cash and taxes. Some believe that the incentives provided by the tax law are dysfunctional, encouraging excessive insurance, frivolous benefits, and unnecessary use of health services. Political support for this feature of the tax law is strong, however. Efforts to amend it were begun around 1980 but were dropped from active consideration in the major 1985 tax revision proposals.

Support for New Technology. Americans continued their enthusiastic support for new health care technology throughout the postwar era. A demand approaching fascination with the best and the newest in health care has been a permanent feature of exchange relationships at the local hospital level. Development of new technology is actively supported through the National Institutes of Health (NIH), funded entirely from federal taxes. Americans support the training of doctors, nurses, and other skilled clinical personnel through federal and state subsidies for education. From 1945 to 1970, Americans actively encouraged the construction of hospitals through the Hill-Burton program of federal subsidies for construction. Even after the end of Hill-Burton, indirect subsidies remained in the form of tax-exempt bond programs. These programs allow governmental and not-for-profit—sometimes even for-profit—community hospitals to borrow money at substantially lower rates of interest than are available to non-health-related commercial enterprises.

So strong is American support for high technology that any hospital which ignores it can exist only in a marginal exchange relationship to society as a whole. Although the British may queue up for advanced X ray and surgery and the Dutch may have their babies at home, Americans want a CAT scanner (an expensive but very promising imaging technology for viewing internal organs), cardiovascular surgery, and intensive neonatal care right in their own home towns. When those attention-getters are replaced by some new advance from NIH, they will want it, too. Profound arguments have been made that this fascination with high technology is outrageously expensive and even useless in some cases, but any hospital that ignores it does so at its peril.

Equity of Access to Hospitals. Support for uniform access and reasonable control of quality has been less visible than programs to enhance technology, but the expression of will has been clear. Strong sanctions exist in federal law to discourage hospitals from discrimination on the basis of race, sex, ethnic origin, or handicap. A federal regulation even requires hospitals that received Hill-Burton support to care for the poor using funds from charity or paying patients. Federal subsidies encouraging doctors and other health personnel to work in underserved areas have been useful to hospitals in those areas.

Quality of Service. When hospital service has little effect on illness, quality tends to be viewed as less important; but when success is the rule, concerns about ensuring quality develop. These concerns have been expressed in two ways. Day-to-day measurement and control of quality are provided by peer review, a system that has doctors and nurses evaluate one another's work. The Joint Commission on Accreditation of Hospitals became the principal vehicle for the development of peer review, and the complexity and rigor of the system have increased steadily. Second, the malpractice lawsuit became the vehicle for gaining compensation when poor quality had been delivered, causing the threat of malpractice suits to become an important pressure to maintain quality.

The notion of peer review, that a group of doctors can assist themselves in improving quality, received strong impetus from the American College of Surgeons shortly after World War I.[12] The ACS, a voluntary association of surgeons seeking to improve their profession, began to certify hospitals whose activities included keeping adequate records and routinely reviewing at least the more serious results of care. Not incidentally, certification also required that surgical practice be limited to qualified surgeons. Membership in the ACS was not the sole measure of qualification, but it certainly was an acceptable one. Much is made of the self-serving character of the ACS concepts. On the other hand, it was the only group providing guidance on the qualifications of surgeons. Nonsurgical specialists (internists) were few in number and had no formal program for this task. The ACS program was also successful. Hospitals became steadily safer places, and under ACS leadership much surgery by unqualified surgeons was eliminated.

By 1951 it had become clear that the American College of Surgeons was not big enough to manage the certification program. At its invitation, a joint commission made up of the American Medical Association, the American Hospital Association, and the American College of Physicians was formed to accredit (rather than *certify*) hospitals. A process of extending and improving the criteria for accreditation was begun, and the program assumed considerable importance when Blue Cross included accreditation as a condition for payment of insurance benefits. By the late 1950s, Blue Cross had become the dominant private insurance carrier, and its endorsement of accreditation meant that few hospitals could do without it. The vast majority of community hospitals were accredited by the time Medicare was enacted, and the act recognized the voluntary system of accreditation as one of two ways in which a hospital could be certified to receive Medicare funds. It is almost impossible for a community hospital to survive without Medicare certification, and well over 95 percent choose to become accredited by JCAH.

The standards for accreditation grow steadily more complex, reflecting JCAH's consensus of exchange relationships relating to quality of care. Arguments that the commission was biased toward providers led to the appointment of consumer representatives in the early 1970s, although the practical impact of that action is unclear. The commission represents the view of the leadership of the health care world, and it has the authority to enforce that view on every community hospital. It is clear that unresponsive behavior on the part of this leadership would lead to replacement of the Commission, for example, by a federal licensing program.

While licensing programs have the appeal of democratic control, their record is unattractive. Many states did not attempt to license hospitals until they were forced to by Medicare law. An earlier federal effort to force state licensure as a condition of receiving funds under Hill-Burton failed. Under Medicare, the states wrote different standards and enforced them even more differently. Licensure also focuses heavily on fire safety and sanitation. While these are important in hospitals, as they are in other dormitory settings, the major risks in hospitals lie in the practice of medicine and nursing. Only the joint commission and its members have seriously addressed those risks.

A strong public interest has been expressed in protection of individuals who might have received injury through the health care system.

Relief is provided through the courts, where suit can be brought against both the hospital and the doctor for malpractice. The trend of malpractice decisions has been steadily toward increased responsibility for the community hospital. Charitable immunity and governmental immunity protected hospitals from malpractice liability through World War II. Beginning about 1950, the courts began holding hospitals financially responsible for the consequences of their negligent acts. The number of suits won by former patients increased, but the number instituted rose even more spectacularly. By 1980, community hospitals were clearly responsible not only for any negligence of their employees, but also for any negligence of their physicians, and monetary judgments were increasingly levied against the hospital as well as the doctor. These changes in the legal exchange relationships had profound implications for the organization of hospitals. They forced the development of means for controlling physician behavior and encouraged consensus on standards of practice for diagnosis and treatment. Most hospitals chose to respond by using peer review, reinforcing the JCAH quality assurance structures.

Economical Operation

One would expect a system that chooses tax-subsidized finance; directly subsidizes technological development, education, and expansion; insists on minimum levels of quality and access; and demands high-tech services to be expensive. It is not surprising that the U. S. health care system is among the most expensive in the world. The final decision on how much to pay is quite beyond the scope of hospital management or even health care management. The amount of money to be devoted to health care is a function of income and the desire for health care relative to the desire for other services such as food, defense, and education. This means that many characteristics of the system—its rules for charity, fascination with technology, and attitude toward malpractice liability, for example—are statements from the environment rather than issues to be debated in community hospital management.

At the same time, one repeatedly hears a demand for economy. Advocates of economy have a serious political problem: the economy they seek involves the loss of somebody's job in some local community. By 1970, it was becoming clear that the price for the American way was not going to be cheap, and concerns for economy began to be expressed under the guise of efficiency. (From a politician's point of view it is wise to blur the distinction between economy and efficiency so as not to appear in favor of cutting back, or removing local gains. Managers, however, cannot afford to be confused.)

Planning Regulation. One important early expression of concern over costs was that for planning capital expansion and facility construction. Public Law 89-749, the Community Health Planning Act, was passed only a year after Medicare and Medicaid. It established a set of locally oriented review boards for hospital capital expansion. Public Law 93-641 and Public Law 93-602, enacted eight years later, reinforced local review board decisions by requiring state certificates of need for construction and federal approval for Medicare and Medicaid payments. Thus in most states, hospitals could not construct additional facilities or open new services without approval.

Utilization Review. Public Law 93-602 took an additional step: it established **professional standards review organizations**, local physician-controlled groups responsible for monitoring both the quality and the appropriateness of hospital care. The activity was called utilization review. The notion that economy in hospital care might relate to the doctor's actions in admitting, discharging, and designing specific treatments had attracted state insurance commissioners more than a decade before, and prototypes of PSROs existed in Western states. The fundamental contribution of PSROs was to extend the concept of peer review beyond quality to efficiency of medical and hospital care.

Unfortunately, neither planning nor PSROs worked particularly well. Repeated studies had trouble demonstrating that gains exceeded program costs.[13] Thus the drive for economy was blunted. The motivation became stronger as costs continued to mount.

Rate Regulation. After 1975, the states developed a strong interest in hospital economy, not only because of the views of their citizens, but more directly because of difficulties in funding their share of the Medicaid program. Over half the states had rate regulation programs by 1980, and they differed markedly. By far the most rigorous as well as the oldest was New York's. After several modifications, the New York program was structured so that it was one of the few that measurably achieved its stated purpose. It actually reduced real dollar expenditures. Many others were apparently designed more to slow the increase in costs than to stop expansion. Using persuasion, public disclosure, reviews of budgets, limits on price increases, and other devices, the public made clear its diminishing appetite for the very rapid expansion that had prevailed from 1967 to 1977.

It is noteworthy that the places which had most enthusiastically supported expansion had the highest costs and most enthusiastically supported regulation. New York City had built a large public hospital system in the 1930s, and New York State wrote one of the broadest interpretations of Medicaid benefits. Massachusetts, another state which adopted rigorous rate regulation, had developed a broad spectrum of tax-supported benefits for its citizens, including Medicaid. It ended the 1970s with one of the highest tax burdens of the 50 states, as well as one of the heaviest burdens of hospital costs. Rate regulation in other states was a less pressing issue. As a result, legislation gathered less widespread support, and the programs were weaker in design and less effective in cost control. It is tempting to conclude that these programs failed because they did not reduce costs, but such value judgments are dangerous. Another perspective might be that they more effectively represented the collective will of the people, who in the main did not want cost reduction.

The Competitive Movement. The most striking change in the expression of motivation for economy came after 1980, with the rapid growth of interest in organizations directly controlling the cost of care and guaranteeing a certain insurance premium. These are marketplace expressions of motivation, as opposed to regulatory approaches. Prepaid group practices, the first model for such activity, had existed for generations but had not been popular except in the western states. They were relabeled health maintenance organizations in the late 1960s. A limited total cost per person per year, or capitation, is central to the concept. Efforts by several states and the federal government to stimulate HMO growth in the late 1960s, had modest success.

The recession of 1981–1983, combined with the implications of international manufacturing competition, stimulated significant market demand for controlled mechanisms of care delivery. The original HMO capitation concept, plus the newer ones of IPAs and PPOs, became the talk of the marketplace. In addition, difficulties in funding the Social Security Trust Fund for Medicare led the federal government to limit payment to hospitals (by means of the *prospective payment system* in Public Law 98-21, Social Security Amendments of 1983). The federal program was a payment program, not rate regulation. It differed from the capitation approach by focusing on each hospitalization, setting a price based upon categories of illness called *diagnosis-related groups* (DRGs).

The organizational implications of these changes for hospitals were profound. Under both the HMO and the DRG approach, the organization as a whole takes financial responsibility for the quantity of care provided to a patient. Just as a few years previously hospitals had taken responsibility for quality of care, they now had to assume responsibility for appropriateness. Clinical organizations had to be extended to monitor actual care delivery and intervene when unnecessary care was provided. Governance and finance organizations had to be extended to support these expansions.

The Future

One result of the last century's growth has been an increase in the amount of exchange activity. Ben Franklin's hospital, once built, took little of his time, but today's hospital is discussed constantly in the marketplace, the legislature, the courts, and the press. There is little chance that this situation will change. Institutionalized expression of viewpoints—by consumer groups, unions, voluntary committees and coalitions, auditors and inspectors, regulatory agencies, legislative appropriations, and the courts—will continue. The agenda will get longer, not shorter.

Forecasting the nature of public concerns is difficult. It appears, however, that motivations for personal health, local economic gain, and high technology will predominate by a much smaller margin than in the past. Low-cost hospital insurance will continue to be an important, competing motivation. Subsidies for research, education, and hospital construction will continue, although less lavishly than in the past. The courts will impose responsibility for quality upon health care providers and will make special demands upon hospitals. Various kinds of regulation will continue imperfectly to express consensuses on quality, access, and cost. The market for HMO approaches of all kinds will grow. Peer review mechanisms to meet these demands will continue, but they will be applied through formal organizations, not through loose associations of individual professionals. The difficulty of meeting these conflicting goals, or indeed even of understanding their relative strength, will make hospital management a challenging field. The demand for personal service, particularly as driven by the aging of the population and by new, subsidized technology, will make it a growing field.

Two areas may be less prominent, although they will continue as motivations. They are the two which formed the foundation of motivations before the current century, Samaritanism and public health. Immunization and antibiotics have considerably reduced the threat of contagion in this country. Their contribution will continue and perhaps expand under genetic technology. Other aspects of public health tend not to involve the hospital. One exception, which can be expected to receive increased attention over the coming decades, is health promotion and health education. Statements by hospital personnel are taken as authoritative, and patients upset by a medical problem are disposed to avoid repetition of it.

It seems unlikely that a major effort will be made on behalf of the poor or that Americans will increase their charity for health care beyond current levels. National health insurance, an idea which has had some support throughout this century, seems to regain center stage at about 15-year intervals, making it due back in 1990. In 1986, it is difficult to see widespread support. The great consensus for collective action on social issues which swept the North Atlantic nations after World War II has significantly weakened under the pressures of inflation, unemployment, and taxation. The importance of meeting other needs of the disadvantaged has been gaining ground. The study of history suggests, however, that collective charity for health care will return to popularity.

Notes

1. *American Heritage Dictionary*, New College Edition (Boston: Houghton-Mifflin, 1979), p. 630.
2. *Concise Oxford Dictionary of Current English*, 6th ed. (Oxford: Oxford University Press, 1976), p. 514.
3. *Concise Oxford Dictionary*, p. 254.
4. Answer: The war led to an oil embargo and later a pricing cartel which disrupted the world economy, causing a full decade of turmoil. Oversimplified, when energy prices went up, the United States could no longer afford national health insurance.
5. Paul Starr, *The Social Transformation of American Medicine* (New York: Basic Books, 1982), pp.145–79.
6. Anne A. Scitovsky, "The High Cost of Dying: What Do the Data Show?" *Milbank Memorial Fund Quarterly* 62 (Fall 1984):591–608.
7. Ivan D. Illich, *Medical Nemesis* (New York: Pantheon, 1976).
8. G. Rosen, *The Hospital: Historical Sociology of the Community Institution in the Hospital and Modern Society*, ed. E. Freidson (New York: Free Press of Glencoe, 1963), pp. 1–36.
9. Rosen, *The Hospital*, p. 15.
10. B. Franklin, *Some Account of the Pennsylvania Hospital*, ed. I.B.Coker (Baltimore: The Johns Hopkins Press, 1954).
11. U. S. Department of Health and Human Services, Health Care Financing Administration, *Health Care Financing Review*, reports annually on sources and uses of health care funds.
12. P. A. Lembcke, "The Evolution of the Medical Audit," *Journal of the American Medical Association* 199 (1967): 543–50.
13. K. Lohr and R. H. Brook, *Quality Assurance in Medicine, Experience in the Public Sector* (Santa Monica, CA: Rand, 1984).

Suggested Readings

Aldrich, H. E. *Organizations and Environments*. Englewood Cliffs, NJ: Prentice-Hall, 1979.
Katz, D., and Kahn, R. L. *The Social Psychology of Organizations*. New York: Wiley, 1966.

Laumann, E., and Pappi, F. *Networks of Collective Action: A Perspective on Community Influence Systems.* New York: Academic Press, 1976.

Pfeffer, J., and Salancik, G. R. *The External Control of Organizations: A Resource Dependence Perspective.* New York: Harper & Row, 1978.

Thompson, J. D. *Organizations in Action.* New York: McGraw-Hill, 1967.

3

Controlling Hospital Organizations: Closed System Concepts

Concepts of Responsiveness and Control

Theory of Cybernetic Control

If, as the preceding chapter has described, organizations are created by a series of exchanges between individuals and groups who view the transactions as mutually beneficial, how does it happen that the transactions occur as desired? This does not seem difficult in a simple society where two or three citizens are involved in some gainful exchange, but it seems quite challenging when hundreds of people with dozens of sets of technical skills coordinate their activities toward several different rewards. Such is the case in the modern hospital. Patients are seeking care; employees are seeking wages; professionals are seeking personal rewards from their work; volunteers and donors are seeking the satisfactions of altruism; and the community is seeking security against the risks of disease. Given that there is much disparity within these major groups, confusion seems inevitable.

In fact, the function of the organization is to keep that confusion from occurring. The contribution of modern bureaucratic organizations is that they allow society to attain such complex objectives as open-heart surgery or a flight to the moon. The first step is to translate the desired objective into a set of specific expectations. Each expectation must be clear, complete, sufficiently detailed that an individual doing a small part of the total can carry it out, and integrated to produce the desired result. The expectations for lunar landings are not just "build a rocket for $20 billion." They include thousands of pages of detail at an extraordinary level of precision. The same is true for open-heart surgery.

The job and the rewards of each individual on the team are defined by relevant parts of the expectations. Similar individual expectations are grouped together under a leader, and similar groups are aggregated in hierarchies of accountability until the total set is reassembled. These expectations and hierarchies of accountability make it possible for reasonable people to agree upon what the job is and whether or not it has been done. The agreements, the mutual acceptance of the expectations, allow the bureaucratic organization to exist. When our ability to specify in advance falls short of what we need, we turn to professionals, whose training allows them to make important decisions on their own but in a manner consistent with the overall objective. Thus each lunar flight has a pilot, who is usually a senior military officer, and each open-heart operation has a chief surgeon with analogous credentials and authority.

It is possible to describe the activity of each individual or any related group of individuals in a hospital in terms of expectations for the resources required (often called costs), for how the work is done (activity), and for the results (outcomes). A simple drawing is often used to show this concept:

$$\text{Resources} \longrightarrow \boxed{\text{Activity}} \longrightarrow \text{Outcomes}$$

Costs will include personnel, supplies, and capital (buildings and equipment). Activity expectations are work methods and procedures. Outcomes expectations usually include several measures of quality and efficiency. In many cases, the outcomes generated revenues. There may also be by-products and even the avoidance of unexpected or undesired results, such as pollution or accidents.

In order to make the expectations occur, one needs a monitor, whose job it is to compare actual performance to expectations and to take actions necessary to achieve the desired result. In effect, the monitor contracts with the organization to see that the expectations are met. The monitor's activities center ideally on two tasks:

1. Helping the work group achieve the expectations

2. Considering how the expectations can be improved or exceeded

These concepts are shown in figure 3.1 which represents the primary work group of a hierarchical organization.

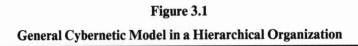

Figure 3.1

General Cybernetic Model in a Hierarchical Organization

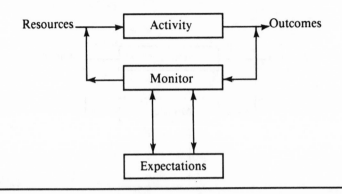

The concept of expectations, activities using resources, and a monitor modifying the activity to improve the fit with expectations, is called the cybernetic model of behavior. It fits a great deal more than simply organizations. The word *cybernetic* comes from the Greek *cybernos,* or helmsman, who guided sailing vessels. In addition to sailing ships and lunar rockets, biological organisms, psychological conditioning, and automatic heating systems are cybernetic. The monitor obviously need not be human; but for organizations the expectations are always set by human beings, and for hospitals the important monitors are always human.

In hospital applications it is frequently useful to modify the diagram to reflect the role of the patient in the activity. Few important hospital activities can be carried out without a specific patient either physically present or close by. There must be demand for hospital activities; the work cannot be done for inventory and used at a later date. Let us label this aspect of the requirements for a hospital activity *demand,* and show it as part of the cybernetic model; the more complete cybernetic model for hospitals is shown in figure 3.2.

Applying the Cybernetic Model

Even for a small, simple activity, full description of the six parameters shown in figure 3.2 (resources, demand, activity, outcomes, monitor, and expectations) is often impractical. Many of the descriptions of the activity, that is, what is done and how it is done, are highly technical and are embedded in certain equipment designs. At the same time,

Figure 3.2

Cybernetic Model for Hospitals

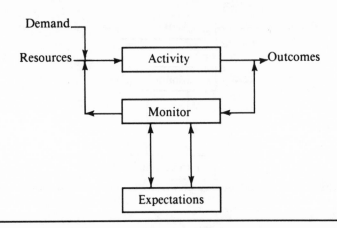

many descriptions are established by the traditions of the organization and what is sometimes called *organization culture*. What normally happens is that an experienced monitor and an experienced team develop subtle and sensitive insights which guide them to the routine production of outcome in a manner satisfactory to the larger unit. If the world were stable rather than dynamic, this would be enough. The understanding might exist entirely in people's memories; the written record is not necessary for what everyone knows.

Although one sometimes encounters effective units with only rudimentary formal statements, the well-managed hospital formalizes as much as possible of the important aspects of the expectations. It is now routinely the case in the well-managed hospital that expectations of demand, outcome, and resources are specified in the annual budget. Critical elements in the work methods, capital facilities, and materials to be used are specified in procedural manuals and similar documents.

It is the statements of expectations for resources, demand, and outcomes that constitute the principal link between the activity shown in figure 3.2 and the open system. Figure 3.2 is closed in the sense that it is partially isolated from the outside exchange environment. Open systems activities identify and evaluate pressures and opportunities for exchange from the outside world. They tailor the general response of the hospital to these pressures and opportunities. The nature of that response, in turn, affects the expectations of the closed system. Buffering permits the closed system to proceed on a stable basis for considerable periods of time. Adjustment to changes which have occurred in the out-side world must come through the annual renegotiations of expectations centered around the budget process. In the well-managed hospital, the budget process results in formal statements of expectations for the re-sources, demand, and outcomes parameters. It also serves as a focus for broader considerations, including the unmeasured and unmeasurable aspects of the activity. The expectations themselves result from a care-ful negotiation which recognizes both the needs and skills of members and the needs and opportunities presented by the outside environment. In well-managed situations, the negotiating of these expectations is more important than their achievement; so carefully are they set, their achievement becomes almost automatic.

Nesting Cybernetic Systems

Once an achievable expectation is set, the entire process reflected in fig-ure 3.2 can be considered all or part of a larger activity that can itself be modelled and monitored. In this way the small components of lunar landings or open-heart surgery are pulled together into increasingly meaningful blocks called the National Aeronautics and Space Adminis-tration or the well-managed community hospital. Thus, one application of the model would be to the operation of a single nursing unit. There are usually several such units in a hospital, and they are specialized in various ways. The specialization is reflected in different statements for the six parameters. The component units can be nested within the broader activity which aggregates them all, usually called the nursing department.

The parameter expectations for an aggregate such as a nursing de-partment are compiled from those of its components. Resource require-ments, demand, and outcomes, for example, include those of all component nursing units. The activities include not only component activities, but probably new ones, unique to the aggregate, as well. The monitor would be a different person (the director of nurses as opposed to the several head nurses). Expectations can be aggregated by achieve-ment counts, such as, "Achieve a state in which all the component units reach 90 percent of their expectations"; where common measurement units permit, one might add, "Employ 40 registered nurses." It is im-portant that aggregate expectations be coordinated with those of the components. If they differ too much, higher levels of the organization work toward different goals than lower levels, and the organization may fail. (At the same time, the goals of various levels are rarely identical. Among other factors, higher levels must deal more with changing ex-change needs.)

Importance of the Cybernetic Model

Examples fitting the cybernetic model are so ubiquitous in nature and in human affairs that its use is probably inescapable in hospitals. Any time a supervisory person states an expectation, returns later to see if it has been done, and praises or criticizes the result, a feedback situation resembling the model has been established. The question is not whether to use the model, but how well it can be used.

In the chapters that follow, I rely heavily on both the open and the closed system models, trying to describe the hospital as a bureaucratic organization in an exchange environment and tracing the implications of changes in the environment upon the closed systems which carry out the work. Of course, these models have limitations. They are imperfect and incomplete representations of reality. At the same time, these concepts allow one to reduce the apparent chaos of a busy emergency room to a series of realistic understandings about what it does, why it does that, why it costs what it does, who works in it, what outcomes are expected, and what possibilities there are for either not having one at all or designing one that is completely different.

The following sections of this chapter describe the process by which expectations are set and the kinds of measures that make the cybernetic model work by providing feedback. They are the compass readings for *cybernos,* the helmsman or manager of the closed system organization. It is by following these processes more carefully and more rigorously that the well-managed hospital achieves much of its excellence.

Using the Cybernetic Model

Correct operation of formal cybernetic systems is only one of two critical management tasks. Open systems issues are equally important. A well-run closed system, however, reduces open systems concerns, particularly those relating the organization to its members—that is, creation of a work environment which supports and encourages people at all levels to find personal and psychological rewards in, as well as economic gain from, their work. Recruitment and such important matters of management style as delegation, communication, and participation are also affected.

The contribution of workers and managers is also enhanced by well-designed systems. More accurately specified goals provide them an opportunity to demonstrate their capabilities, an opportunity that is missing when expectations are poorly defined. Few people can work well with a vague charge, particularly when they must coordinate their work with that of others who have similarly vague instructions. Many people can complete and enjoy specific charges, and can use more imagination, in a defined situation. Properly supplemented with other policies and procedures, well-designed, formal cybernetic systems can support professional rewards and job satisfaction better than poorly designed ones.

Using cybernetic systems well, creating a smoothly running, responsive, efficient organization, is a matter of managing the expectations, the reporting and monitoring systems, and the incentives or rewards. Managers at all levels of the organization have a responsibility to sustain the closed system by making it work effectively.

Role of Monitors in Nested Cybernetic Systems

The smallest aggregate of organizational activity modeled is usually the first level at which a human monitor appears. That unit has several labels, **responsibility center** probably being the clearest. Primary work group is also used, and the first-level monitor is called the **primary monitor** or first-line supervisor. Monitors of aggregates such as nursing departments are sometimes called **supercontrollers,** managers, or, at the highest level, executives.

Much of the job of monitors and supercontrollers involves the study and improvement of the expectations for specific applications. Are they clear? Consistent with community objectives? Consistent with other activities? Are the resources adequate, or excessive? Could costs be lowered by a different combination of resources? Can the demand be changed? Are the work methods correct? Were the desired outcomes achieved? Is the quality satisfactory? Did the monitor perform as well as possible? These are the abstract versions of the questions hospital managers ask themselves continuously about the many activities they guide. So complex is the modern world that the asking and answering of these questions become activities in themselves, performed by analysts, consultants, task forces, study teams, and committees.

Role of the Primary Monitor. The primary monitor or first-line supervisor of a unit or activity has a detailed factual grasp of that activity which is both more comprehensive and more current than any automated control system or higher level supervisor can ever maintain. When the monitor knows and subjectively accepts the expectations, he or she will detect variations as they occur or before they occur and will correct those in her or his power. The primary monitor knows beforehand what the formal report will say, and if it contains an unfavorable variation he or she will have ideas about how to correct it. Any surprises call for extensive reexamination of the activity, the resources, the demand, the monitoring system itself, and the expectations. It is at the point of surprises, or at the point of repeated, uncorrected signals of error, that the supercontroller correctly enters the monitoring process.[1]

When expectations are well set, the day-to-day activity of hospitals can proceed smoothly. Much more of the time of management goes to expectation setting than to monitoring, and departures from expectations are rare. Thus, because of what is sometimes called the "principle of no surprises," the attention of the primary monitor is directed toward correcting variation from expectation before it can be reported in formal monitoring systems.

Role of Middle and Upper Management. Supercontrollers, or middle managers, deal more with integration, coordination, and goal setting and less with error detection and correction than primary controllers. Their role in detection should be limited to those cases where the primary controller has failed to correct the error, and their role in correction should stress those interunit activities beyond the authority of the primary controller. Many errors occur in the interunit category and will come to the lower levels of middle management.

The responsibilities of middle managers can be summarized as follows:

1. *Systems design*—All questions of assigning accountability lie above the level where the accountability will rest and thus fall to middle managers. Organizational structures are defined by assuming accountability (see chapter 4). In addition, many policies governing the activities of the units—hours of operation, scheduling rules, work procedures, and so on—are the responsibility of middle and upper management because they require extensive coordination.

2. *Systems maintenance*—This includes everything necessary to make and keep the system operational. Many of these needs are met by other major systems, such as plant for facilities and equipment, human resources for personnel, finance for key reports, and governance for open systems assessment and exchange needs.

3. *Managing interunit difficulties*—These include relating clinical units to activity in planning and human resources, coordinating units in these two groups with each other, and resolving problems of control when the variation originates in several different units.

4. *Information systems design and maintenance*—Most information system improvements involve several units and are therefore the domain of middle management.

5. *Expectation setting*—Middle management is responsible for encouraging the primary controllers to consider new methods and higher expectations and for encouraging coordination among units to improve collective expectations. Middle management must effectively communicate both lower-level views upward and top management views downward.

6. *Fitting expectations to outside exchange needs*—Middle management at all levels shares with the planning staff the responsibility for identifying and correcting situations in which community wants differ from expectations.

7. *Managing the incentive system*—Middle management evaluates progress towards goals and disburses both tangible and intangible rewards.

It is important to emphasize that the closed system theory of the role of middle management is contrary to the folklore of the boss. That image of the boss is one of an authority figure who issues orders and enforces compliance. Closed system theory proposes that expectations are set by mutual understanding and are driven not by middle management views, but by open systems exchange needs. Furthermore, the manager does not enforce compliance, but rather supplies training, equipment, supplies, and other resources so that the worker has no difficulty in meeting expectations. Far from enforcing, the manager must respond to any unmet worker need or question. Although cynics and sophomores frequently argue to the contrary, well-managed organizations, including hospitals, reject the folklore and adhere to the theory: its value has been repeatedly proven both by formal research and by realities of the marketplace.

The Importance of Role Distinction. A recurring problem in hospitals relates to the proper role of primary controllers and various levels of supercontrollers. It is common in poorly run hospitals to find several levels of management involved in error detection and correction for single units or groups of units well below their total span of authority. Two serious problems result. One is that the time of middle managers is consumed in unnecessary activity, usually to the detriment of their other responsibilities. Perhaps even more important, the effectiveness of primary controllers is destroyed. If a supercontroller does what a primary controller is supposed to do, there is nothing left for the primary controller to do. Some hospitals have created whole cadres of redundant managers by this process.

Setting Expectations

Intuitively, many people think that setting clear and complete expectations for each member of the organization reduces job content and freedom. They fear that overspecification may interfere with quality of work life; however, if expectations and policies describing work activities are truly well designed, the opposite can occur. Many of the constraints and frustrations of hospital work have to do with the integration of different tasks and work groups. Doctors frustrate nurses, nurses frustrate admitting officers, laboratory technicians and medical records personnel frustrate doctors. The key to minimizing these frustrations is specifying and completing the individual tasks effectively, because the conflicts often arise from incomplete, ambiguous, and competing expectations. The result of improved specification is twofold: opportunities for confusion between units are removed, and opportunities to improve internal performance are increased.

The parts of cybernetic systems are a chain that is formed by expectation setting. Obviously, expectations may be set unrealistically high. Other potential errors which are frequently just as serious include ambiguity, conflict, impracticality, irrelevance, and redundancy. Expectation setting is a complex, ongoing process that is unique to each hospital. It is an important test of organizational design and managerial effectiveness.

A checklist for managing under cybernetic systems can be remembered by its four Cs: cooperation, conflict resolution, comprehensiveness, and clarity. The key to the process is an organization of open, two-way communication. The best goals are set by a wide-ranging process of discussion and debate, carried on essentially continuously at all levels of the institution. Discussion is foreclosed by conflict, and unresolved conflict eventually disables expectation setting. Thus procedures for conflict resolution are an important part of the overall expectation-setting process.

Cooperation: Participation in Setting Expectations. A well-designed goal-setting process becomes comprehensive by developing goals simultaneously throughout the organization. Goal setting occurs neither from the bottom up nor from the top down, but in both directions. In a well-designed system, unit managers are encouraged to think of improvements in their current goals. At the same time, planning and marketing staffs, financial staffs, and board-level committees are encouraged to consider what the outside environment demands. The board coordinates the effort by maintaining a mission statement and a long-range plan, concise but comprehensive documents indicating as clearly as possible who the exchange partners are and what services can be provided them (see chapters 5 and 7). The chief executive officer (CEO) also co-ordinates expectation setting by translating certain key environmental demands into quantitative expectations. An overall profit expectation, a total cost expectation, and expectations for a few major demand aggregates are often set by a board committee at the start of each budget cycle (chapter 8).

When expectations are developed simultaneously, the role of the various levels of middle management is a coordinating one. Individual unit expectations must be coordinated with broader needs, and units must be integrated with each other. Effective middle managers carry out this task by encouraging participation and communication of differing viewpoints rather than by disposing authoritatively of conflicting views. Through discussion, each participant is encouraged to see the perspectives of others.

The process is not in any sense democratic, because the objectives of the organization prevail. The ultimate determination of an organization's expectations is the view of its most powerful exchange partner, almost always its customers. Members, that is, employees and doctors, are also important exchange partners. Their views must somehow be incorporated in the final expectations. The process of communicating, understanding, and integrating these views is a complicated and time-consuming one.

One perspective of a hospital organization is that it has an entire set of committees, conferences, task forces, and retreats solely for the purpose of gaining widespread participation in expectation setting. That broad group of organizational activities is called the **collateral organization** in this text and discussed in chapter 4. The collateral organization always works well in a well-managed hospital. It permits the views of lower-level members to be heard by governing board and top executives and at the same time it permits members of the organization to see the exchange demands being imposed by customers and government. Thus attending physicians see the interests of other specialties and nursing, plant managers see radiology's needs for imaging services, human resources learns of changing needs for employment benefits, while all discover growth opportunities for the organization as a whole. Over time, knowledge and respect for various views lead the participants to grow together, rather than apart.

Resolving Conflict Among Members. Conflicting views among participants are natural, and it is inevitable that in the process of setting expectations some participants will be disappointed. Each participant, after all, is rewarded for rigorously pursuing his or her specialty—whether nursing, cardiology, or cost control. It is useful to think of these conflicts as having two parts. One part, the process part, involves the discussion itself. The other part, conflicts over resources, involves the final decision. Well-run hospitals recognize, accept, and deal constructively with process conflicts by:

— Creating an open process of debate and decision, so that everyone who is interested understands each position

— Managing the debate in ways which emphasize content rather than rank and which do not tolerate personal attacks

— Establishing clearly the central governing board's authority to make the final decision

— Making the decision in a manner that demonstrates, if not wisdom, at least good faith and consistency

Conflicts over the resources themselves must also be resolved by process. Well-run hospitals follow these guidelines:

— The process for resource allocation is rigorously followed in order that every member has the opportunity to understand how, where, and by whom the decision will be made.

— The governance structure deliberately assists members in requesting resources (see chapters 7 and 8).

— The criteria for a resource allocation decision are specified in the mission, the long-range plan, and the long-range financial plan and are well publicized.

— There is sufficient participation in the resource allocation process that any member can assure himself or herself of consistency and equity.

— In cases of severe disagreement there is a well-understood and respected appeals process.

Conflict is avoided and resolved by open processes, candid discussion, clear criteria, and well-understood decision and appeal mechanisms. Conflict can be seriously disabling, and the hospital which uses secrecy, ambiguity, and expediency is not well-managed.

Comprehensiveness: Tying Expectations to Goals and Exchanges. In the open systems processes, community wants and available resources must be identified, translated into organizational goals, qualified, and expanded to specify what outcomes are expected. The activities for carrying out this process are described in the preceding chapter and in chapter 7. A variety of errors occurs when the outcome expectations are not carefully coordinated with each other and with exchange needs. Omission of important exchange needs may be a fatal error. Redundancy or duplication of activities creates inefficiency. The error known as *suboptimization* can be avoided by paying attention to the hierarchy of expectations within the organization. Suboptimization occurs when a unit increases its achievement in a direction not consistent with the whole. The X-ray department, for example, may reduce its costs by reporting results of examinations once daily instead of twice daily. If the slower reporting is out of phase with the activities of attending physicians and if the doctor waits for the X-ray report before initiating the next phase of care, increased length of stay can result. Errors similar to suboptimization occur when one unit is organized for more or less comprehensive service than another that feeds it. A cardiology unit may expect a great volume of referrals, but the internal medicine and family practice unit may be too small to provide these referrals.

Clarity: Sources of Expectations. Vague and ambiguous expectations divert workers' attention from their work to an effort to understand their limits. These probings to clarify expectations frequently create general adversarial conditions between workers and management (or doctors and management), causing relations to become highly dysfunctional. To paraphrase Robert Frost, good expectations make good workers (and good managers). Often the clarity of an expectation can be improved by making it quantitative. Thus one of the efforts of the well-run hospital is to steadily quantify its expectations. The management record of hospitals since World War II has emphasized quantification of cost, demand, output, efficiency, and quality. As a specific expectation becomes more precise and more quantitative, managers try to gain a measurable, if small, improvement by changing the expectation with each budget cycle. So important is the quantification of measures in closed systems, it is a major theme in the balance of this chapter.

No matter what expectation-setting process is used, there are only four broad sources of inspiration:

1. *Subjective*—Subjectively, one can build an expectation on one's desires or philosophic commitments. ("Next year we will care for 2,000 poor people in our primary care clinics," or "Next year we will decrease our surgical mortality to half its current level.") An exchange partner may establish a subjective expectation and enforce it by the exchange requirements. ("Unemployment is so high we must care for 2,000 poor people next year," or "An additional family practitioner will require a $50,000 net income guarantee," or "The major employers in town insist that cost increases be held to 5 percent next year.")

   There need be no scientific support for subjective goals. Many important ones have been achieved on faith and willpower alone. Subjective external expectations are usually the result of considerations well beyond the health care field. Examples in the 1970s included sharp increases in fuel prices, higher standards for environmental health, and a "crisis" in malpractice liability insurance. In the 1980s, Congress's action limiting Medicare expenditures to a fixed percentage of the federal budget is a striking example with far-reaching ramifications.

2. *Historical*—The hospital's history is usually available and can serve as the source of expectations. Forecasts from history need not repeat last year's values; it is usually better if they carry forward past trends. ("Surgical mortality has been falling 10 percent per year for several years, so we expect it will fall 10 percent next year.") This is the *ceteris paribus,* or other things being equal, forecast. ("Our primary care staff can support a maximum of 1,500 poor people next year.") Even the best designed and best motivated changes often require time to achieve, and thus the short-range expectations are a blend of history and the other sources of expectations.

3. *Comparative*—The achievements or expectations of others are often a guide. ("Average costs of laboratory tests in this area are $7.86.") In a competitive environment, it is occasionally necessary to consider the expectations of other hospitals. ("Crosstown Hospital has published a charge of $40 per emergency room visit, $10 lower than our charge.") It is not always necessary to match the expectations of others, even in a competitive situation. In fact, for a variety of reasons, this may be the least rewarding source of expectations.

4. *Scientific*—One may establish standards by careful, objective study, such as cost analysis, time and motion study, or the results of scheduling systems used as simulators. Willingness to investigate and use objective sources of expectations seems to characterize well-run hospitals. The science of others may suggest new expectations. ("Massachusetts General Hospital reported in the *New England Journal of Medicine* that it reduced intensive care unit usage by 22 percent using patient classification systems.[2] We should do that here.")

Scientific and objective expectations should be adopted with care. In addition to allowing time to achieve a better position, management needs to consider its finite resources. Realistically, the profile of real achievement is almost always below what is the scientifically possible. Priority must be given to those deficiencies that most seriously impair exchange relationships—and they are not always the largest or most obvious.

Since the ultimate test of an expectation is not where it came from but how well it serves the organization in its exchange setting, there can be no ranking of these four sources of expectations. Expectations not subjectively accepted by participants are rarely achieved, but ideals uninformed by science or unaccepted by the customer are foolishness. A historical trend can be healthy or destructive. What others do is interesting, but it may not fit local history or exchange needs. Even exchange needs can be misinterpreted. Major employers who hold too rigidly to limited cost increases could find themselves with a shortage of doctors or labor strife.

The obvious answer is that well-run hospitals use all four of these sources of expectations, and crosscheck them thoroughly. Probably the best expectation is one that is a philosophic commitment, consistent with science and history and broadly shared in the local community. It need not be consistent with any other community or hospital; in fact, if it is truly innovative, it will be unique. On the other hand, a well-run hospital will note what other hospitals are doing to make sure no new advance escapes its attention.

Monitoring Performance

Functions. An unmonitored system will drift unpredictably, even if expectations are clearly set. The functions of monitoring are as follows:

1. To provide unambiguous measures of achievement so that every member of the organization knows not only his or her own performance, but also that of relevant other members
2. To identify correctable errors or deviations from plan so that additional resources may be brought to bear
3. To provide an objective basis for rewarding members of the organization
4. To provide data useful in setting new expectations
5. To permit members to deal with the more complex and less well understood goals and problems of the organization

These functions can often be fulfilled by formal written reports, but it is wise to remember that the primary monitor's understanding is both quicker and broader than any possible formal reporting. Much of the organization's responsiveness depends upon unwritten and even unmentioned understandings. A sound view of closed system theory is that formal reports supplement rather than replace these understandings. Unambiguous expectations and formal reports permit members of the organization to focus their attention on the frontier of unresolved issues, the fifth and final function.

Components. In cybernetic theory, the monitoring reports are called *signals,* and the subsystems creating them, *signal detectors.* Because any real system contains a certain amount of *noise,* that is, variation that cannot be corrected with current technology, variations are assigned to two categories—*significant,* or likely to be correctable, and *not significant.* Significant variations can be called *error signals.* This terminology is not common in hospitals, but it pays to remember that noise does exist and that not all variations are worth correcting. A monitoring system has five parts:

1. *Signal detection*—collecting, entering, and processing the necessary information
2. *Signal evaluation*—comparing the signal to its expectation and its noise content to decide whether the variation is significant or not
3. *Analysis*—identifying possible causes and corrections
4. *Correction*—acting to reduce future variation
5. *Reporting*—integrating the preceding four steps to suggest revised expectations

Data Systems. Monitoring is principally a human activity, but automation has greatly increased the possibilities for control. The first two parts of the monitoring system are increasingly susceptible to automation. Speed, reliability, validity, and economy of operation are generally enhanced by using routine transactions in automated systems as the basis for monitoring and further using the computer to identify error signals. The role and use of information systems is developed in detail in chapter 7. The principal data systems that provide monitoring information are the following:

1. *Patient order entry or order communications systems*—These capture original entries into the accounts receivable system and identify the necessary descriptive characteristics of the patient (age, sex, disease, major procedures, residence, referral source, discharge destination, payment source, and treating physicians), the demand (specific service requested), and the service (location, time of completion). They are now automated for many inpatient applications.
2. *Patient medical records*—These are archival documents which are created in part by order entries and results, but which also contain other information. They are rarely automated, but increasingly detailed, electronically readable abstracts are being drawn from them for quality and utilization control.

3. *Departmental service and reporting systems*—These monitor all the internal activities of departments, including many aspects of detailed efficiency and quality control. They include patient scheduling and personnel scheduling. They also produce reports on patient services for clinical departments. Many are now partially automated, with laboratory and pharmacy systems leading in computerization.

4. *Accounts receivable systems*—These are fully automated and supply not only revenue information, but also counts of services used by each patient.

5. *Payroll systems*—These are fully automated for purposes of compensating workers and accounting labor costs. The better systems have been extended to report personnel usage to primary control units in both real and dollar terms and to provide a factual basis for analysis and control of other employment benefits.

6. *Materials management systems*—These monitor supplies, purchase costs, inventory levels, and usage. Automation progressed rapidly in the early 1980s, but few hospitals had current systems.

7. *Physical plant management systems*—These support maintenance, cost accounting, space assignment and planning, energy management, and equipment maintenance and replacement. Much automation has been through departmental or specialized systems. The static nature of the activity permits continued reliance on manual systems.

8. *General accounting systems*—These are usually fully automated to perform a variety of accounting and financial calculations, including cost accounting and financial analysis.

The output of each of these systems now meets its first objective, providing data for monitoring specific activities. Increasingly, output is also being summarized and fed to analytic and integrative systems developing clinical expectations at several levels, budgets, long-range plans, and long-range financial plans.

Incentives for Achieving Expectations

Cybernetic systems involving human behavior must include rewards or positive incentives for desired behavior and sanctions for undesired behavior. Rewards yield better results than sanctions. It is theoretically possible to build some kinds of organizations on sanctions alone, but it is foolish to use them heavily in hospitals. There are three reasons for this. First, the sensitivity and variability of patient care is such that only those who seek to do it well will succeed. Second, rewards can be broader, longer lasting, and more flexible. Third, systems built on sanctions are inherently regressive rather than progressive. The attention of management is diverted from improvement to enforcement.

Well-managed hospitals assume that expectations will be met in the vast majority of cases. Even a few cases of failure require so much energy to investigate and correct that they endanger the entire system. Sanctions are a part of the well-designed system that is clearly understood but rarely used. Sanctions must be quickly and judiciously applied whenever necessary, but their basic purpose is to protect the organization from destructive behavior.

Incentives can be divided into two groups, those that are psychological, or *intangible,* and those that are monetary, or *tangible.* Although most individuals work for money, that is, they require a certain tangible compensation, well-run hospitals gain their distinction by more effective management of intangible incentives. They typically rely on a combination of tangible and intangible incentives which capitalizes on all of the following kinds of rewards and uses each as frequently as possible.

1. *Inherent satisfactions in treating the sick*—Both the caring role and the curing role are rewarded in human societies. Religious recognition is particularly strong. A surprising number of hospital workers at all levels feel God will reward them for their efforts or believe their work is part of a good life and therefore wish to do their jobs well.

2. *Acceptance by the work group*—Work is an important social event for most people, and the comradeship of the work group is an important reward. To use this reward for the benefit of the organization as a whole requires extensive socialization of the work groups, but it is not impossible. Hospitals have advantages over many kinds of commerce in that their professional groups already share a common socialization and in that they can attract people who share a Samaritan motive.

3. *Professional rewards*—The procedures for many of the activities occurring in hospitals are incorporated in professional education. Rewards may be recognition and honorary promotions in professional organizations. Merit pay increases or salary scale changes can reinforce these. The principal sanction is denial of access, as in loss of admitting privileges for physicians, or discharge for other professions.

4. *Job evaluations, promotions, and salary adjustments*—Promotion and merit increases may depend upon favorable evaluations. Ideally, these evaluations should be linked to the unit expectations; individuals who help units achieve their expectations should get a tangible reward. Tangible sanctions are rare, but the power of poor evaluations as an intangible sanction should not be underestimated.

5. *Prizes and special recognition*—Important intangible rewards can be achieved by special awards, such as Employee of the Month. Many employees expect praise and will work to avoid criticism. Cash bonuses, prizes, and other tangible rewards can be added, but they are probably less important. There are no corresponding sanctions.

Tangible incentives in the form of salary adjustment, bonuses, and prizes are assuming increasing importance in hospitals but only as supplements to effective programs of closed systems management and intangible incentives. Formal wage programs such as piece rates and productivity incentive pay systems are rare, for several reasons. Incentive pay has had an equivocal effect upon production. The systems themselves are expensive; hidden costs in labor relations and grievances are frequently overlooked. They require extensive quality control and monitoring systems to be effective in complex activities. Hospitals' complex problems of coordination make attribution of improvement difficult, reducing the reliability of assigning rewards. Unit production incentives may draw a group's attention away from the need for cooperation with other units.

A number of very well-run hospitals exist without direct incentive pay systems. While many are interested in finding incentive pay systems, and there have been numerous experiments, it is accurate to say that no convincing model suitable for widespread application currently exists.

Limitations of the Incentives. The list of incentives available to hospitals has some notable deficiencies. There appears to be a wide variety of relatively weak but highly flexible rewards and a few sanctions, which seem to be mostly strong and irreversible. The natural result of having sanctions like dismissal and loss of privileges is that they will be used only sparingly. It is clearly a challenge to use the variety of incentives in an effective package, yet similar problems afflict other kinds of organizations, and on the whole, the hospital's list is as long and as powerful as that of many other complex organizations.

Hospitals that have difficulty motivating their personnel often have problems outside the incentives themselves. Lack of clear expectations and consensus on goals are probably the most common causes of disincentive. A feeling that the real rewards will be handed out on a basis other than achievement of the publicly stated goals may be the most destructive counterincentive. Boards and executive officers whose actions are unpredictable or inconsistent are in danger of generating this result. Cynical statements such as, "It's not what you do, but who you know," or "The doctors (or the surgeons, or the unions, or any other special-interest group) really run this place; they get what they want, and the rest of us get leftovers," reflect the alienation that causes cybernetic systems to fail. There is further discussion of incentives and programs for building an effective work force in chapter 14. The correction of many problems lies not only in incentives, but in the management structure itself.

Developing Measures for Closed System Performance

The closed system model will work better when as many expectations as possible are specified in quantitative terms. Although it is often necessary to substitute words and subjective judgments for quantitative measures, simply because a concept is too complex for measurement, the use of subjective measures increases the possibility of delay and dispute. Thus one dimension of effective hospital management is the constant search for ways to quantify objectives and performance.

Whether a quantitative measurement exists or not, any real activity must monitor all of the closed system elements. It is often easier to monitor a quantitative measure than one that requires study and subjective evaluation. Measurement and quantification help the monitor keep track of what is going on.

Substantial gains have been made in our ability to measure closed system parameters in the past several decades. The gains are the result of three major external forces: scientific advances in medicine and our understanding of the "right" thing to do for each clinical symptom or condition; improvements in general management applications of cybernetic models; and the development of computers that allow easy capture, storage, and recovery of voluminous quantitative information. There is every reason to think these three trends will continue.

Figure 3.3 classifies the measures used to quantify closed system expectations. Issues in the selection and design of measures are discussed below, and later in this chapter each parameter in the figure is discussed in terms of definitions, characteristics that affect ability to maintain control, and examples.

Figure 3.3

Classification of Measures of Hospital Performance

Demand Measures
    Counts
    Time distribution
    Market share

Outcomes Measures
    Outputs
        Counts
        Duration
        Intensity weights
    Efficiency
    Quality
        Statistical characteristics
            Attributes
            Variables
        Conceptual characteristics
            Outcomes
            Process
            Structural

Resource Measures
    Resource consumption
        Physical values
        Cost values
            Labor
            Supplies
            Plant and equipment
    Resource conservation
        Revenue
        Revenue proxies
        Profits

Measurement and Scaling Alternatives

The activities of health care rarely lend themselves easily to measurement. They are often continuous rather than discrete. Individual differences are important. No two patients or treatments are ever alike; two activities with the same name are quite different when performed on different patients. Quantifying the closed system parameters is a matter of continually searching for measures that usually evolve from crude, almost subjective beginnings. There are four measurement categories, or scales. All are useful, and measurement may evolve through several before reaching the most useful, ratio scales.

    1. *Nominal scales*—These identify categories that represent reliable differences, such as sex, race, or specific diagnoses. Classifi-

cations for disease, procedure, and prescription drugs are all nominal scales underpinning health care computerization. (The International Classification of Diseases is now used almost universally to describe the illnesses leading to hospitalization. Often several categories are necessary to describe a real patient, and the order of these categories is also important.) Account classifications, both for functions and responsibility centers, are nominal scales.

2. *Ordinal scales*—These identify categories that move reliably in a uniform direction, so higher numbers represent consistently different situations from lower ones. (Nominal scales are assigned arbitrarily so that high numbers have no intrinsic meaning.) The five numerical classes of Papanicolaou smears, for example, indicate progressively more serious disease as the numbers get higher. Burns, respiratory distress, infant distress, and several other clinical characteristics are quantified by ordinal scales. In a recent application related to quality and appropriateness of care, intensive care units have been using an ordinal scale to determine necessity for admission.[3] Individual patients' daily nursing requirements are usually assessed with ordinal scales.[4] Satisfaction questionnaires use ordinal scales.

3. *Interval scales*—These are ordinal scales that have uniform values between entries (so that differences may be compared). The usual example of a scalar measure, temperature, is easily recognized, because two popular scales, celsius and fahrenheit, have two different, equally arbitrary zero points.

4. *Ratio scales*—A ratio scale fulfills all the requirements of interval measures but has in addition a nonarbitrary zero value. This permits the use of percentages. Height, weight, and percentile standing on comparative distributions are all ratio scales. In accounting, dollars are a ratio scale. Most outputs of closed system processes, such as discharges, patient-days, and treatments, can be processed as ratio scales, but nominal or ordinal scales must be used to group them into comparable sets.

The problem of too many measures is a serious one. Purely redundant or conflicting measures can be eliminated, and competing alternatives can be evaluated, as suggested by the criteria that follow. The problem of summarizing or aggregating multiple parameters in a single-dimensional concept of performance, in order to avoid an unmanageably large amount of data at high management levels, must also be addressed. For closed systems, multiple measures are a serious problem. Given two measures of different elements of closed system performance, any evaluation requires implicitly or explicitly weighting the two equally, or one of the two more heavily. In some cases, the weights are clearly understood. It is easy to aggregate costs and revenues, even for activities of very different character. Dollars serve as weights, for example, for radiologists' hours and raw food. Other dimensions of expectation and achievement aggregate badly because there is no agreed-upon weighting. One avoidable infant death and one failure to pursue preventive care in an elderly man do not clearly add to anything. Neither can one comfortably average "66 percent efficiency in the operating room" and "95 percent achievement of expected raw food costs."

Conceptually, there are three ways around the dilemma of multiple measures:

1. Rank the various measures by importance, and concentrate on a manageable number of the most important. Those omitted are not lost, they are just removed from the routine reports; they would still be available for special study and for setting future expectations. The ranking should follow the importance of the activity to the mission of the hospital.

2. Find acceptable weights to permit aggregation. There must be several of these because there are several different aggregation problems. Often an arbitrary weight is used, because the cost of more precise work exceeds the value of the measure.

3. Sample the measures, either at random or by identifying those that are representative of their group.

All three of these approaches are required, in combinations. Well-run hospitals are more aggressive and more ingenious than others in their pursuit of opportunities for condensing multiple measures. Most hospitals start with rank ordering, using weighting and sampling as adjunct tools. Although the actual rank order depends on the mission, suppose a criterion for assigning rank could be established for each of the major groups of measures. In some cases, this criterion would suggest the number and kind of measures as well. Then weighting and sampling or elimination of the measures could be decided on the basis of their importance as well.

Criteria for Selecting Measures

One judges the acceptability of a measure by its value and its cost. Value is the measures contribution to performance. Value stems from systems of application, including the measure itself, expectations, and reporting. Selecting a measure, therefore, means selecting a measurement system. In most situations, the monitor is able to achieve some level of performance without a particular measure and a better level of performance with it. On the other hand, providing the measure involves certain costs. Conceptually, both values and costs must be measured against the mission of the organization. If the measure contributes more to achievement than it costs to maintain, it is desirable. Often there are several possible measurement schemes differing in reliability, validity, timing, and, as a result, both in costs and in value. Thus the design of a measurement system involves the selection of the best alternative.

Value. Measures are valuable because they assist the monitor in achieving control. If, for example, a given system for reporting budgeting and payroll costs allows the monitor to maintain operations while reducing labor costs by $5,000 per year, that is its value. Generally speaking, the more reliable, valid, and timely the measure is, the greater its value will be—up to the point where the monitor can change actual performance. As a result of this limit, the value of measurement systems is always constrained by a variety of other factors and characteristics of the organization.

Cost. The cost of a measurement system is a combination of two elements, the resources consumed in obtaining, processing, reporting, and setting expectations for it and the opportunity costs of incorrect reports. It is convenient to label the first group *accounting costs* and the second *hidden costs.* Thoughtful measurement design must always address both.

Accounting costs tend to increase with improvements in reliability, validity, and timeliness, but automation has generally permitted great reductions in accounting costs of measurement. Often accounting costs can be reduced at the same time the accuracy of the measure is increased, by a combination of automation and integration. If a large number of measures is generated from the same basic collection and processing system and the output is used frequently, the result is a relatively large number of accurate and inexpensive measures. Measurement system design, therefore, frequently involves seeking ways to integrate several different measures.

The cost of a measure can also be reduced by sacrificing accuracy and timeliness, although these sacrifices risk increasing the hidden costs. Hidden costs occur because of two possible incorrect interpretations of the error signal. *False negatives* occur when a correctable condition is not reported to the monitor, and therefore the monitor achieves less than he or she might. *False positives* occur when the measurement system reports a correctable situation when in fact none exists; the monitor must investigate the finding, and that investigation is costly.

Reliability. A measure is conceptually reliable if repeated application to an identical situation yields the same value. The repetition may be either in time, space, or detection system; test and retest and substitution of observers are frequently used to measure reliability. Lack of reliability impairs precision of measurement. Although reliability in excess of the monitor's ability to respond is valueless, it is also true that the monitor can only respond within the limits of the measurement's reliability. Allowance must be made for measurement error. If the goal is 200 units of output, but the reliability of the measure is only ±10 percent, all values from 180 to 220 must be interpreted as achieving the goal.

Reliability is enhanced by clear definitions of what is to be counted or measured, good measuring tools, audits, and training of observers. A measurement that is used routinely is likely to improve in reliability because it is used frequently.

Validity. A measure is said to be valid if the reported value is true as defined by the exchange objectives. If an invalid measure is used in a cybernetic system, the energies of the unit can be directed toward achieving high scores on that measure rather than achieving the unit's true goals. The result may be a seriously disabling distortion of intended activity.

An anecdote may be the best way to illustrate the question of validity. A factory produced nails, and someone wished to improve its performance by setting output goals for the employees. So a goal was set at a certain number of nails per hour. After a short time, the goal was exceeded, but the factory was producing mostly tacks. So the goal was changed to a certain number of *pounds* of nails per hour. Again the goal was exceeded, but this time the factory was producing spikes. The moral is that validity of measurement depends upon what the goals are. If one wants a variety of nails, one's measures and expectations in cybernetic systems must reflect that.

Timeliness. There are two important criteria of timeliness: frequency and delay. Particularly at lower levels of the organization, the monitor must react quite quickly. The measurement system that reports too late for the monitor to respond is at best useless and at worst costly, because it generates hidden costs by prompting improper responses.

Measures also differ in how frequently they usefully can be reported. Reports that are too infrequent allow correctable conditions to exist, yet reports can come too often. There is a finite time attached to a response cycle. Reporting more frequently than once per response cycle is not useful. In some of the complex issues of quality and efficiency the response cycles are quite long. For example, changing physical facilities may be possible only at intervals of many years. Interim reports on the cost of physical facilities will be of little value. Several dimensions of quality require extensive and careful responses and as a result tolerate infrequent measurement.

Special Studies. A special study is basically an infrequent, or nonrecurring measurement system. It is a relatively low-cost, useful means of evaluating and selecting measures. Using research techniques, measurements can be as reliable and valid as desired, within the limits of current technology. The results can be considered in terms of the monitor's ability to respond, the potential value of the response, and both the accounting and hidden costs of a continuing or more frequent measurement system. Special studies are useful for a variety of purposes, including verifying assumptions about improvement in performance, evaluating changes in systems, evaluating changes in measurement systems, and collecting very expensive performance measures. The most common examples of special studies in hospitals are measures of quality, because both their accounting and their hidden costs are frequently quite high. Surveys of doctor, patient, and community attitudes are another example. Special investigations of medical and nursing care of specific kinds of cases are yet another.

Importance of Output Measures

Although many closed system parameters can be measured, the extent to which hospital organizational units have a countable product or output is particularly critical in the design of cybernetic systems. Having countable outputs greatly simplifies the management task. Not only demand and volume, but efficiency, revenue, profit, and at least one measure of quality are easily quantified as a result. Efficiency, the ratio of output to inputs, is measurable only when output can be measured. Revenue can be posted only when a unit of service has been defined. The measurement of profit depends upon revenue. A pass-fail judgment on work by inspection of a sample of output constitutes a basic measure of quality.

Obstetrical deliveries and appendectomies are discrete, unambiguous events, archetypes of countable outputs. Complications are relatively rare and can be handled by establishing a separate, much smaller count. In contrast, many hospital activities are quite difficult to count. Clinical services such as psychiatry and social work and support services such as housekeeping are more continuous than discrete. Managerial support services with infrequent or intermittent end points, for example planning and marketing, essentially cannot be measured by output. There is no meaningful analogy in these departments to number of births.

Operating rooms, delivery rooms, clinics, kitchens, laboratories, pharmacies, laundries, and X-ray and physical therapy units all have measures of output and, as a result, measures of most of the closed system parameters. Continuous service activities such as medical care, nursing, housekeeping, and plant maintenance, require major adjustments. Counselling services (for example, personnel, social service, and psychology) present serious measurement problems that reduce the contribution of quantitative approaches. Such staff services as planning and public relations are very difficult to measure. The cybernetic process still works, but words and concepts must be substituted for measures and expectations. The clearer expectations can be made, however, the better the cybernetic process will work.

Measures of Demand

Kinds of Demand Measures

Demand can be categorized as unrecognized, unexpressed, unmet, and filled. The combination of unmet and filled is the total requested service. As a practical matter, requests for service are often the best available measure of demand. Conceptually, one might include unexpressed demand, a service not requested, possibly because of barriers to access. Similarly, one might include unrecognized demand, a needed service not perceived as such. Such problems are relatively severe in medical care, but they are difficult to identify and measure except through special study of the population.

Even when service is requested, there is frequently a mechanical problem of measurement—the request is not actually tallied until it has been scheduled, if not filled. In such situations, accepted requests (or scheduled requests) and output (or requests filled) are proxies for requests. Most accepted requests in hospitals are also requests filled, thus the two proxies are usually the same. The difference between accepted requests and total demand is more serious. Reduced requests for service from hospital units can result from unsatisfactory service, delays, or quality, and from unattractive amenities. Units can increase the number of requests for their service by responding promptly and positively. A key marketing and planning question—the difference between potential demand and the number of requests—cannot be measured directly by request counts; it must be assessed by special studies.

There are several other ways of classifying demand. Most units provide several kinds of service, often requiring several counts of requests. In addition, demand is sometimes categorized as *appropriate* or *inappropriate*. Inappropriate demand is by definition inefficient and can represent serious quality problems. Demand can also be classified by its position in the patient care process. A great many kinds of demand within the hospital are dependent upon or derived from the admission of the patient or the initiation of treatment in the physician's office. By extension, concepts of demand can be developed for activities that do not serve patients directly, but rather serve other units of the hospital. Plant, human resources, and finance systems frequently fall in this category. For example, the demand for housekeeping is generated by other members of the hospital organization.

Market share is becoming increasingly important in measuring demand. It requires that demand for other hospitals or providers be measured in order to calculate the fraction of total demand accruing to the study hospital. Output is almost always used as a proxy for requests in constructing measures of market share. Even so, the data collection requirements are formidable, and special studies are often required.

Characteristics of Demand Measures

Arrival patterns of requests for service are frequently critical. Demand can be *stationary,* that is, arriving at a stable, continuous rate, or *cyclical,* arriving at a regularly recurring rate. It also may be *stochastic,* arriving at unpredictable intervals with little notice, or *deterministic,* arriving at predictable intervals. Special studies are usually necessary to determine arrival patterns.

Urgency of requests is also important. Requests that can be deferred can be accommodated at much lower cost than those that must be handled immediately. It is common to classify urgency in three categories: **emergency, urgent**, and **elective**. The categories are defined by the length of delay acceptable without impairing quality of service. They differ depending upon the demand being studied.

Requests that are cyclical, stochastic, and emergency require resources to meet the highest possible arrival rate and complex schedules to tailor resources to the cycle. Efficiency will be low, because most of the time the highest possible rate will not occur. Hospital emergency rooms have that kind of demand. Most hospital activity is elective, however. This means that, even if the underlying demand is stochastic and cyclical, the service can be provided smoothly and efficiently by scheduling patients or relying upon acceptably brief delays.[5]

Examples of Demand Measures

The following are examples of measures of demand:

1. Emergency room arrivals—stochastic, cyclical, and all categories of urgency (emergency, urgent, and elective)
2. Obstetrical deliveries—stochastic, stationary, and emergency
3. Admission requests—stochastic, cyclical, and about 60 percent elective in most hospitals
4. Specialty clinic visit requests—stochastic, usually stationary, and elective
5. Periodic physicals for employees—deterministic, stationary, and elective
6. Equipment maintenance (an internally generated demand)—preventive maintenance, cyclical and elective; breakdowns, stochastic and all three categories of urgency

Measures of Outcomes

The outcomes, or results, of a hospital activity can be measured along several different dimensions: *outputs,* the products or services themselves; *efficiency,* output per unit of input; and *quality* are the most common. Others, such as by-products and contaminants, occur rarely and are not discussed here.

Output Measures

Specification and measurement of output are essential to improving the performance of a closed system activity. Most actions directed at economy, efficiency, and quality depend upon an understanding of what constitutes output and, in many cases, a specific and reliable measure of it.

Because of the nested character of hospital activities and systems, few outputs are truly final. Most hospital activities result in an output that is simply an input to something else. One of the most important distinctions is between final products and intermediate products:

— **Final products** are the delivery of completed packages of services or achievement of generally recognized end points in the process of care. Final products are generally discharges, disease episodes, or, occasionally, ambulatory visits. The word *final* is used in the context of the patient's total contact with the institution. It does not necessarily mean the cure or death of the patient.

— **Intermediate products** are the outputs of component processes of care, such as admissions, patient-days, inpatient meals, and laboratory tests. Although intermediate products may be sold for revenue and may in some circumstances be appropriately viewed as final products in themselves, they are most commonly treated as inputs to final products. Thus the cost per discharge is frequently described as the sum of all of the intermediate products involved in hospitalization.

These concepts can also be applied to support services within the hospital. Thus it can be said that each small work group or activity modelled as in figure 3.2 has an output, but that for most activities the output is an intermediate product. While there should be assessments of quality and efficiency of each intermediate product as an independent output, there must also be assessments of quality and efficiency of the final products. In particular, efforts to improve intermediate products can never be assumed to transfer to improvements in final products.

Kinds of Output Measures. The following are commonly used measures of output:

— *Counts* are of either final or intermediate products and are normally undertaken for different categories of episodes (such as obstetrical discharges or inpatient meals), particularly when they differ in duration or intensity.

— *Duration* is obtained by weighting counts on the basis of the extent of time involved in the service.

— *Intensity* is obtained by weighting either counts or duration on the basis of level of resource required for the service. An example of weighting counts is laboratory tests weighted by the American College of Pathologists' scale of personnel requirements; an example of weighting duration measures is patient-days weighted by level of nursing care required.

— *Case-mix categories*, such as diagnosis-related groups, are often used for weighting. Resource requirements (for example, total costs, labor costs, patient-days, and number of tests) are used as weights for each category of treatment.

Characteristics of Output Measures. Output measures are usually characterized like demand measures. This is useful when they serve as a proxy for demand. It is also useful in establishing efficiency expectations, where it is important to recognize the stochastic and cyclical nature of some outputs. Nominal and ordinal scaling are frequently used to establish either homogeneous or comparable groups of outputs.

Examples of Output Measures. The following are examples of measures of output:

1. Pounds of clean laundry—count
2. Discharges by DRG—count by a nominal intensity category
3. Patient-days by DRG—duration by an intensity category
4. DRG-weighted discharges—weighted count, where each nominal category is weighted by some measure that reflects differences between categories. The weight is usually the average value of the category divided by the average value of *all* categories; for example,

$$(\text{Average Cost per Discharge for DRG 222})$$
$$\div (\text{Average Cost per Discharge for All DRGs}).$$

   The products of category weights times category counts are added to get the weighted total.
5. Recovery room hours by surgical procedure—duration weighted by nominal category. Recovery room use is likely to vary by surgical procedure, and the measure is more reliable when categorized.

Efficiency Measures

Kinds of Efficiency Measures. Efficiency measures are usually ratios of inputs to outputs (or occasionally the reciprocal, outputs to inputs, when that form is more convenient; there is no real difference between the two). Both final and intermediate products can be said to have efficiency, thus "tests per patient-day" is a measure of efficiency, just as "hours of labor per test" is. (That is, tests are an input to patient-days, an output. Therefore the ratio of the two is an efficiency measure.)

A second form of efficiency measure, which incorporates a standard and is expressed as a percent, is

$$(\text{Actual Output per Input Unit}) \div (\text{Standard Output per Input Unit}).$$

Characteristics of Efficiency Measures. The concept of efficiency is disarmingly simple compared to its reality. In general, efficiency is irrelevant unless the output goals are valid. The nail factory in the anecdote above became very efficient twice, but in neither case did it produce the right product. This problem affects hospitals as well. Given the interrelated character of hospital activities, the first problem is to produce what the patient really needs, that is, the appropriate mix of intermediate products for the desired final product. Intermediate product efficiency is secondary, and it must often be sacrificed to overall or final product efficiency. The process of improving efficiency can be viewed as having two stages. In the first stage, the appropriate set of intermediate products for a given final product is identified. This frequently results in changes in demand for intermediate product activities. Many changes will be reductions. A reduction in demand for an intermediate product usually reduces the efficiency as well. The second stage, then, is to reduce inputs to the intermediate products and return efficiency to a high level.

In hospitals, there are two other important characteristics that make measurement and expectation setting for intermediate product efficiency a demanding task. The first is the stochastic nature of demand, noted above. Where demand is both unpredictable and emergency, workers must be ready to meet it, even if there is no alternative but to sit idle until it occurs. This happens frequently in the emergency room, the delivery room, and the coronary care unit.

The second problem is more widespread but less clearly recognized. Many hospital workers are professionals who legitimately define their jobs as well as do them. Physicians' care and services with a counselling component (nursing, social work) have this characteristic, but so do many physical care activities, such as the rehabilitation therapies, intensive care nursing, and surgery. In a different but no less important way, diagnostic services such as laboratory and X-ray can generate their own demand by poor quality of output, requiring retests.

It is possible for all three of these intermediate product problems to exist simultaneously. An X-ray department, for example, could theoretically produce the wrong product (doing dye studies of soft tissue when ultrasound or tomography is preferred), need a substantial allowance for emergencies (on the night shift, when there is little else to do), and generate its own work (by producing poor-quality images or reporting false diagnoses). Fortunately, such complexity is relatively rare. Before any efficiency expectation is set, however, these three issues should be carefully reviewed. Otherwise, achievements of expectations by the unit will be dysfunctional to achievement of expectations by the organization as a whole.

Examples of Efficiency Measures. The following are examples of measures of efficiency:

1. Patient-days and discharge (length of stay)—A measure of clinical intermediate product efficiency usually specified for a certain kind of case, such as by DRG, to increase reliability. Patient-days of care is also a durational measure of output, especially for nursing.

2. Laboratory tests per labor-hour—A common measure of intermediate labor efficiency, often stated as its reciprocal (labor-
   hours per test). Similar measures are used wherever the output
   of the department can be quantified, for example, nurse-hours
   per patient-day. The measure becomes meaningless where output cannot be quantified, for example, hours of counselling per
   counselling hour.

3. Standardized efficiency of laboratory labor—The second form
   of intermediate efficiency measure, using standard times for
   laboratory outputs. This measure is complex because it must
   include an intensity weight on the output. In the simple hypothetical case where the laboratory did only one kind of test, the
   formula would be

$$\text{(Labor-Hours)} \div \text{(Standard Hours per Test) (Number of Tests Performed)}.$$

   In practice, both terms of the denominator would have to be
   measured for each kind of test and summed for all kinds.

4. Laboratory tests per discharge—A component of final product
   efficiency. Note that laboratory hours per discharge is similar.
   Laboratory tests, an output of the laboratory, are an input to
   the final product.

5. Patient-days per bed-day (occupancy)—One of several common
   measures of intermediate efficiency of use of physical resources,
   called facility load factors. Where the time period (day, in this
   example) is the same for both the numerator (use) and the denominator (availability), a simple ratio suffices.

6. Computer load factor—A related measure of physical resource
   capacity, used when it is necessary to translate availability into
   potential units of service, using a standard output per resource-
   hour:

$$\text{(Actual Computer Transactions)} \div \text{(Standard Transaction per Hour)}$$
$$\text{(Hours of Computer Availability)}.$$

7. Radiation therapy machine load factor—An example of a complex intermediate efficiency measure, in which treatments
   would have to be weighted by kind because they have different
   machine time requirements. The formula would be

$$\sum_{i-1}^{n} [(\text{Actual Treatments})_i (\text{Standard Hours per Treatment})_i] \div (\text{Hours Machine Available}).$$

Quality Measures

Concepts of quality are complex and ambiguous.[6] In health care, the term includes a number of considerations from the patient's perspective —access, comprehensiveness, acceptability, prevention, continuity, and satisfaction—in addition to measures of how well specific tasks were performed from a professional perspective. Formal questionnaires and surveys are increasingly common devices for assessing quality, as are inspections.

Special studies, samples, and proxies are used frequently. A readily available, but less reliable, inexpensive measure may be used to approximate a much more complex concept. In both inspections and surveys, only a random sample of outputs may be evaluated in order to reduce costs. In many cases, items that are representative of concepts of quality will be used. In effect, this represents sampling of the measures themselves.

While quality assessment is particularly demanding in clinical areas, it applies elsewhere in hospitals as well. Meals served and trash removed can be accomplished at high or low levels of quality, just as open-heart operations can. Patient satisfaction with parking cannot be ignored.

Cybernetic systems operated without measurements of quality tend to deteriorate to minimal or unacceptable levels. The greater the incentives to perform well on other measures, the more rapidly this deterioration can be expected to occur. For protection, all cybernetic systems should include at least rudimentary expectations and measures of quality.

Kinds of Quality Measures. The construction of quality measures in hospitals follows two dimensions, one statistical and the other conceptual. The statistical dimension has to do with whether the assessment of an individual piece of work results in a count or a score:

— *Attributes measures* are counts of the number of output units possessing a certain characteristic, divided by the total output count. Typical attributes are "good," "survived," "accepted," "on time," "appropriate," and their opposites. Ordinal categories are also possible, such as "good," "fair," "poor," "unacceptable." Although the assessment itself can be quite subjective, each unit of output must be unambiguously assigned to a single category.

— *Variables measures* are interval or ratio scores applicable to each unit of output. Typical scores are dimensions (weight of newborns) and multi-item evaluations (professional examination scores of personnel). Variables measures tend to be more reliable and valid than attributes measures, and they introduce the possibility of assessing the variability of a product within a given period. They are also more expensive. A variables measure can be reduced to an attribute by putting it on a pass-fail basis, but there is no way to create a variables measure from an attribute except by revising the assessment process.

The conceptual dimension is concerned with the assessment of structure, process, or outcome. Although this dimension is often thought of as relating only to clinical concerns, it has a far broader application, and in fact was first described outside the health care field.[7]

— *Outcomes measures.* Conceptually, the output of a hospital unit should be measured in terms of its contribution to the larger goal. ("Outcomes" is an evaluative term, involving some judgment of the utility or contribution of the output, or product itself.) If the patient got better or the department using the service was pleased with it or donations to the hospital went up, quality was high. These are outcomes measures of quality. They apply to both intermediate and final outputs, and they can be either attributes or variables measures. There are a great many of them in hospitals, and they are inherently valid. Because of their validity, they are the preferred measure of quality.

— *Process measures.* Process measures of quality represent interim points short of the outcome. They can be variables measures, but they are more often attributes. They are more numerous in hospitals than outcomes measures, and in fact constitute the bulk of quality assessment measures, particularly for the clinical activities. Process measures are defined by establishing a standard of practice: coffee should be over 150° Fahrenheit when served; each new patient should have height, weight, and blood pressure recorded; a plan for nursing care should be developed for every patient within 24 hours of admission; all trash cans should be emptied by 3 p.m.

— *Structural measures.* **Structural measures** are counts of relatively fixed attributes of the organization and the physical facility. They tend to be static or very slow in changing, and their relationship to good outcomes is often highly attenuated. It is often true that places which fail to comply with structural measures of quality have poor outcomes, but many that do comply also have poor outcomes. Thus good structural measures tend to be necessary but not sufficient conditions for good results, a starting point rather than a complete quality assessment program.

Two serious problems limit the use of outcomes measures of quality. First, the outcome may not be immediately perceptible. The patient may be discharged alive, but die later. Second, and more common, the success of the outcome may be caused by factors outside the control of the activity. The patient may die, but he would have died anyway, (or he might have lived anyway). In fact, the complexity of health care is such that it is rare that an outcome can be unambiguously linked to an activity. Extensive research is often necessary to specify what the relationship is.

Attributes counts can be constructed from rates of compliance with these standards. Variables scores can be constructed whenever several similar attributes can be collected together or whenever a continuous interval or ratio measurement is available. A variables measure could be constructed for coffee served, recording the actual temperature of each cup, although an attributes measure is cheaper and more appropriate for this relatively trivial matter. More sensibly, several similar attributes could be combined to evaluate a whole patient food tray on various attributes, yielding a percentage score for each tray. Nursing quality scores are frequently built in this manner. Several attributes constituting a "good" patient care plan are counted, and the number of successes is expressed as a ratio of all opportunities. The ratio can be treated as a variables measure.

The critical question regarding process measures of quality is their validity. They are invented because the question of causality is difficult and one commonly assumes that completing the process tends to support good outcomes. That assumption can always be questioned. There are historical examples of both unreasonable resistance to sound process measures, (such as the objections raised in the nineteenth century to hand washing in obstetrical care) and retention of poor procedures (such as the rules requiring chest X rays of all patients on admission, which remained long after rates of lung disease had declined below the capabilities of X-ray detection). A good hospital reviews the validity of its process measures routinely and discards those that are no longer necessary.

Characteristics of Quality Measures. How one treats data on quality depends heavily upon one's assumptions about the data's reliability and validity. If one thought the scoring was totally reliable and valid, the only remaining question would be the achievement level—what score, or what percent of attributes, was acceptable. "Your job is to produce 98 units satisfactory to the user a day" is a complete statement of both output and quality expectation. But suppose an inspector is substituted for the user, and the inspector only approximates the user's judgment. Further suppose that, because the product involves patient care rather than inanimate objects, it is unreasonable to ask for 98 units each day; one therefore modifies expectations to an *average* of 98 units which pass the inspector per day. The quality assessment question has been translated to a statistical one: "Given that today N units passed the inspector, what is the probability that the average of 98 satisfactory units per day will be achieved?" That is the question encountered in most hospital activity.

Handling the realistic question, in which the quality assessment is neither perfectly valid nor reliable and patient care depends on factors outside the control of the activity, requires statistical approaches. The simplest solution is to set standards well below the range of variability. Thus one might believe that the inspector is right at least three-quarters of the time and that only 5 percent of the patients are so different that the standard cannot be achieved. Then the expectation becomes "at least 69 units passed (98 $\times$ .75 $\times$ .95) by the inspector each day." This solution is cheap and common in hospitals.

Other approaches use more sophisticated statistical techniques. The exact approach will depend upon whether an attributes or variables measure is used. The statistics themselves are found in texts on statistical quality control.[8] For an attributes measure, the result will be a statement of probability that the expectation was achieved, given the sample data (that is, that the sample was not unlike the universe that forms the basis for the expectation). For a variables measure, the results will include this information plus information showing the variability of performance on the individual units: the range, or variability, of scores for the universe represented in the sample and the probability that variability differs from a preset expectation.

While the more complex statistical concepts may seem esoteric, they permit a much closer control for a given expenditure on quality measurement. Their most important characteristic is that they incorporate past improvements into the report. If an improved technique is discovered, the statistical reports will adjust to it. Analysis of the reports will allow a new, more rigorous expectation to be set. Instead of "anything over 69 good units is okay," statistical approaches will encourage steady improvement. For this reason, statistical quality control has been widespread in for-profit endeavors for many years. It will become a key tool in the improvement of hospital quality as computers make data collection less costly and data interpretation, including the statistical calculations, routine.

Examples of Quality Measures. The following are examples of measures of quality:

— Mortality and complication rates are attributes ratio measures of overall quality outcomes. The rates are created by dividing number of patients dying or with complications by the appropriate number of patients at risk. Success rates, such as "percent of hernia repairs without recurrence," are also possible. They are commonly but selectively used. Although their ultimate validity is obvious, their validity for individual units or activities is highly questionable. The patient may have died for any number of reasons outside the reasonable control of the unit.

— Percent of patients receiving a specified test or treatment is an attributes process ratio measure. It is necessary to specify both the numerator and the denominator carefully to attain validity and reliability; for example, "percent of surgical patients receiving one and only one unit of blood" or "percent of patients with elevated blood pressure discharged without diagnosis of hypertension."

— Meals returned to the kitchen is an attributes outcomes measure treated as a nominal count, presumably because it is expected to be low. Were it larger, it could be treated as a percent or rate, using "meals served" as the denominator.

— Incidents, that is, unexpected, undesirable events that may reflect badly upon the hospital, are also an attributes outcomes measure treated as a nominal count. Incidents can happen to patients, visitors, employees, or doctors. The number is so vague that a denominator is indeterminate; therefore there is no true incident rate. There are two problems with this measure, even though incidents are not unusual. First, an incident is hard to define, so the number reported is unreliable. Second, since people reporting incidents are likely to be criticized, they may be tempted not to report, further reducing reliability. Validity of this measure is hard to assess, but it is generally thought to be helpful in risk management as a tool to focus corrective action.

— Nursing quality score is a variables process measure constructed by having a trained inspector review the record or the condition of a patient, or both, and produce a score or percentage of compliance, which is an interval scale, for each patient reviewed. Similar scores have been constructed for many hospital activities.

— Laboratory unknown values is a variables outcomes measure of validity for laboratory tests, where a blind sample of known composition is analyzed. The difference between reported value and actual is a ratio scale.

— Laboratory control statistics are variables outcomes measures of the reliability of laboratory tests, used routinely to maintain laboratory quality. (Concepts of statistical quality control have been used longer and more extensively in clinical laboratories than anywhere else in the hospital.)

Measures of Resources

Resources involve goods, services, and funds. Measures of cost, revenue, and profit are involved in the cycle in which hospitals acquire, use, and replenish their resources. The resources, or inputs, consumed by an activity are measured in two ways—real volume, as in labor-hours, hours of physical facility, or counts of consumable supplies; and cost, the estimated dollars required to purchase or replace real resources consumed. Cost is a function of price and volume of real resources. Other issues, such as quality of resources and cost of resource acquisition, are sometimes important.

Many activities are expected to enhance resources by generating revenue. Other activities are so remote from any actual patient transaction that accounting revenue is impractical or impossible. In accounting terms, these are *overhead* or *indirect cost* activities. For revenue-producing activities, expectations can be established for costs, revenue, and profit. Profit, the difference between revenue and cost, is an essential requirement, even for not-for-profit hospitals, if the enterprise is expected to continue.

Cost and Resource Consumption Measures

Kinds of Cost and Resource Consumption Measures. Real resource consumption is frequently categorized as labor, supplies, or facilities and equipment. Supplies are not reused or have a short life. Facilities and equipment generally have a life greater than one year. Measurement of real consumption is usually limited to easily identified resources, typically:

— *Labor.* Real labor is usually measured in hours of personnel time by class or skill level. It is useful in understanding productivity but also in identifying skill mixes for planning and quality control purposes.

— *Supplies.* Physical counts of major or important supplies are used to control productivity.

— *Physical facilities.* General physical plant is usually measured by the square foot, and specialized areas or machines are measured by hours of availability. Real physical measures are usually incorporated in occupancy or load factor efficiency calculations. Because the quantities of physical resources are relatively static, the measures have little use on their own.

In addition to consumption measures, measures of resource availability and resource quality are frequently maintained. The classic measure of availability is inventory. Real inventories are kept as well as dollar inventories and are used to assure continuity of necessary supplies. By analogy, personnel and physician files describe the human resources available to the hospital. Long-range plans frequently address the recruitment needs necessary to maintain human resources. Finally, resource acquisition activities such as purchasing or employee relations can be considered cybernetic processes themselves. Their outputs are the numbers of persons and items required, but more attention is paid to the quality of these activities, measured by employee and employer satisfaction. Turnover, absenteeism, and grievance statistics are measures of the quality of the human resources system.

The following are measures of resource cost:

— *Labor.* Labor costs are derived by multiplying labor hours times price of labor (wages). Prices are often monitored separately, particularly for premium time, such as overtime. Costs of employment benefits are also monitored separately to make it possible for both the human resources system and the line supervisor to be held accountable.

— *Supplies.* The cost of supplies consumed always includes purchase price and physical volume. Departments maintaining substantial inventory (usually food service, central supply, laundry, radiology, anesthesiology, and pharmacy) can also be held responsible for inventory costs, including the loss of interest on working capital. The major inventory of the finance system is money itself. The finance system is accountable for the cost of money (borrowing) and the earnings on available money (lending).

— *Physical facilities.* Two measures of the cost of plant and equipment are commonly used. One, depreciation, usually does not include the time value of money. The other, rent or imputed rent, does, and therefore is theoretically preferable. Much of the weakness of the depreciation measure can be overcome by setting careful expectations.

— *Other.* A variety of nonlabor, nonsupplies resources is used in hospital activities, such as licenses, insurance, consultations, and telephone services. Physical measures for these are rarely meaningful, but costs are readily available and commonly used for monitoring.

Characteristics of Resource Consumption Measures. Resource consumption measures are collected by the finance system and are among the most accurate in the hospital. By far the largest share of hospital costs is for labor. Reporting of labor used is prompt, usually occurring within a week after each two-week pay period. Modern computer systems permit both physical and cost measures to be reported for each worker in an activity and for aggregates of workers by wage group, work group, and shift. Hours may be divided into those worked and not worked, with special items such as overtime segregated for better control. Separation of wages and nonwage benefits is routine. Counts and costs of supplies are also readily available, as are costs of other resources. Thus cost control is one of the most advanced cybernetic systems in hospitals.

The actual labor usage of hospitals is highly dynamic. Stochastic and cyclical demand, part-time personnel, shift and weekend coverage, and varying patterns of absenteeism combine to make staffing even relatively simple units surprisingly challenging. Control is achieved by reducing variation in demand and adjusting the availability of labor (that is, by scheduling both patient and worker) and by developing sophisticated budgets. The budget to control labor costs in a patient service unit may specify several dozen expectations, one for each shift, day of the week, wage group, and level of demand. The finance system supports monitoring and control through the budget and reports of actual achievement. (The details of the budgeting, patient scheduling, and employee scheduling systems are discussed in later chapters.)

Fixed and *variable* are two extremes on a continuum of resource availability. They are usually used to establish two arbitrary categories into which resources can be placed. A third category, *semivariable,* is also used. Distinguishing which category is applicable is an early step in building a resource control system. Variable resources are those which can be consumed when needed. Fixed resources are those which are consumed whether demand is present or not. Semivariables are consumed in lumps. An expenditure must be committed if demand is present at a certain level, even though the commitment will serve a much larger demand.

Buildings, equipment, insurance premiums, and the like are fixed costs. A commitment must be made in advance, and the resource cannot be adjusted to actual demand. Supplies are an almost perfect variable cost. Aside from some relatively small inventory costs, no cost is incurred until the supply is actually used. If demand is low today, the supply is kept for tomorrow. Labor can be in any of the three classes. Certain employees, usually supervisors, are needed even if there is no demand. Other employees must be added if demand is expected to exceed a certain level. When employees must be added in relatively substantial increments (as, for example, hiring a second, temporary physical therapist when demand exceeds what one can serve) labor is a semivariable cost. This is the condition for most clinical work units. Occasionally labor can be hired only when needed, through part-time contracts, overtime, or contract labor services. Then it is a nearly perfect variable cost.

Even under the most flexible arrangements, sufficient labor must be hired in advance of the service to meet the full expected demand. Thus scheduling systems that balance demand and labor and that forecast labor requirements enough in advance to adjust the work force are the key to labor efficiency. A careful balance of full-time, part-time, and overtime personnel and cross-training to permit reassignment are also important for labor cost management.

A fixed resource cannot be adjusted at all. Any improvement in its efficiency must come through changing or scheduling demand. If demand is below capacity, efficiency is low and cost is high. Cost is also high if demand is stochastic and emergency; sufficient resource must be available to meet peak demand, but average demand will be lower. These conditions of built-in inefficiency and high cost are present in many hospital activities. Delivery rooms and coronary care units are examples . It is important to note that not only the physical resources, but also the specially trained personnel are likely to be fixed costs.

Management must identify expectations and costs as fixed, semivariable, and variable; forecast demand; and establish the resources required at each level of demand. If resources are routinely adjusted to varying demand, flexible budgeting is required. Similarly, monitoring reports must show variation in demand as well as in costs, and they must show the portion of cost variation attributable to change in demand.

One immediate lesson from the identification of fixed and variable resources is the importance of understanding, forecasting, and scheduling demand. Eliminating peaks in demand improves efficiency and cost of both fixed and variable resources. Scheduling demand makes personnel scheduling systems less complicated and more reliable. Forecasting demand allows a larger share of resources to be treated as variable. In improving the efficiency of hospitals, demand management —forecasts and scheduling systems—is as important as resource management.

In the long run, of course, all resources are variable. The definition of variable, therefore, depends upon time. The longer it takes to change the quantity of resources being consumed, the less variable the resource is. *In terms of cybernetic systems, a resource is variable if the quantity can be controlled to any extent within the ability of the manager to foresee changes in demand.* Under this rule, overtime and supplies are almost always variable resources, part-time personnel are usually manageable as variable resources, full-time personnel are sometimes variable resources, and physical plant is rarely a variable resource.

Examples of Resource Consumption Measures. The following are examples of measures of resource consumption:

— Typist hours, physical measure of variable labor

— Typist wages, cost measure of variable labor

— Registered nurse (RN) hours, physical measure of variable or semivariable labor

— RN overtime, cost measure of variable labor

— RN benefits, cost measure of fixed labor

— Head nurse wages, cost measure of fixed labor

— Equipment rental, cost measure of semivariable or fixed equipment

— Building lease, cost measure of fixed equipment

— Number of pieces of equipment, physical measure of fixed equipment

— Supplies, cost measure of variable supplies

Resource Conservation Measures: Revenue, Price and Profit

Exchange theory suggests that resource consumption control, or cost control, is not enough. Any successful service must exchange its activity for sufficient new resources to continue. These exchanges generate revenue, which is used to purchase more resources, and provide profit to expand or reinvest. Many hospital activities are held accountable for resource conservation, that is, for specified revenue and profits.

Kinds of Resource Conservation Measures. Services are sold for a price, and the aggregate of all sales constitutes *revenue.* Revenue is a function of two elements, output and price.

Price is theoretically the value of a specific exchange. In concept, it is set by a free market which forces the seller to set an expected price but to accept the market's result. Historically these concepts have been far from the reality of hospitals. Many hospital transactions are purchased in large blocks, such as an entire admission or even an annual contract for necessary services. Also, buyers of hospital services often have insurance, which is designed to protect them from the price of specific transactions. Competition has forced hospitals to respond to block purchases, resulting in more meaningful prices.

Price guidelines are set in well-managed hospitals by the finance system (chapter 8). Well-managed hospitals are moving to establish the final prices in negotiations with the primary monitors of the various units or activities. When these prices are combined with expected demand, it is possible to generate revenue expectations and, finally, profit expectations. These expectations can be compared against various exchange needs. However, as noted below, not all activities can be sold to the outside world for an identifiable price.

Costs of hospital activities that have no sales to the outside world are traditionally treated as overhead and transferred to activities that do sell their services. Under this scheme, revenue and profit considerations are centralized, and activities of overhead departments, particularly human resources and plant systems, are insulated from competitive market forces. Well-managed hospitals are moving to the establishment of *artificial revenue* or *imputed revenue,* for units that cannot sell directly to the public. In order to do this, an expected **transfer price** is established by complex cost accounting. Wherever possible, the transfer price should be compared against market prices. Each department receiving service is charged at its transfer price, as though the transaction were with an outside unit.

Profit is defined as the excess of revenue over costs. It is essential that for-profit organizations earn profits, and goals are usually set for returns based in large part on market conditions and the degree of risk involved. Not-for-profit organizations must also earn profits or receive charitable donations if they are to survive. An organization with zero profits has no growth capacity, no funds for charity care, no protection against risk or unexpected losses, and no protection against inflation. If it encounters any of these conditions, it will soon be unable to pay its bills. It either goes bankrupt or becomes dependent upon charity.

Using automated cost-accounting technology, it is possible to carry transfer pricing and profit calculations to very small units of the hospital. Actual profit expectations will differ with the unit involved. Frequently the governance function is viewed as analogous to a holding company. It receives profits from "subsidiaries" and, after deducting its own costs, must achieve the net profit necessary to continue operation. Multihospital systems account costs and revenues in exactly this way.

Characteristics of Resource Conservation Measures. Until the advent of competition in health care delivery, hospitals tended to put little emphasis upon expectations for prices and profits. Under competition, price is a key factor in attracting market share. Therefore setting the expected price becomes a key financial decision. The well-run hospital establishes expected prices on the basis of careful forecasts of market conditions. It then sets levels of cost and efficiency that permit it to operate on satisfactory levels of profit and quality.

Examples of Resource Conservation Measures. The following are examples of measures of resource conservation. The first four are revenue measures and the last four, profit measures.

1. Room, board, and daily care—These represent the sum of aggregate charges posted for each patient-day of care, covering any service not specifically charged, and constituting nearly 50 percent of inpatient revenues.

2. Drugs—Drugs are one of several supplies revenues. They can be subdivided into revenue for goods sold and revenue for administration or service.

3. Adjusted revenue—Because many payers do not pay charges, the posted revenues of hospitals are often not valid. This situation is handled by a series of revenue adjustments, usually set for each contract or source of revenue (Blue Cross, HMO, Medicare, and so on). It is noteworthy that the adjustment usually applies to several categories of revenue, such as both drugs and room, board and daily care, but not to all revenues within the category. Thus the adjusted revenue can be reported back to the pharmacy or the nursing department only with great difficulty.

4. Net revenue—This is a measure of actual cash receipts rather than postings. It includes both adjustments and allowances for bad debts.

5. Gross profit—This measure is frequently used for intermediate product units; it includes few or no overhead costs.

6. Net profit—This measure is used for aggregates of profit for higher organizational units with more overhead cost attribution. Several levels of net profit can often be identified.

Notes

1. Walton M. Hancock, "Dynamics of Hospital Operational Control Systems," in *Cost Control in Hospitals,* ed. J. R. Griffith, Walton M. Hancock, and Fred C. Munson (Ann Arbor, MI: Health Administration Press, 1976), pp. 129–49.

2. D. E. Singer, et al., "Rationing Intensive Care—Physician Responses to a Resource Shortage," *New England Journal of Medicine* 309 (1983): 1155–60.

3. W. A. Knaus, E. A. Draper, and D. P. Wagner, "The Use of Intensive Care New Research Initiatives and Their Application for National Health Policy," *Milbank Memorial Fund Quarterly* 61 (Fall 1983): 561–83.

4. R. C. Jelinek, "An Operational Analysis of the Patient Care Function," *Inquiry quiry* 6 (June 1969): 53–58.

5. Walton M. Hancock, *Admission Scheduling and Control System* (Ann Arbor, MI: AUPHA Press, 1983).

6. Avedis Donabedian, Explorations in Quality Assessment and Monitoring, vol. 1, *The Definition of Quality and Approaches to its Assessment* (Ann Arbor, MI: Health Administration Press, 1980).

7. Mindel C. Ships, "Approaches to Quality of Hospital Care," *Public Health Reports* 9 (1955): 877–86.

8. D. C. Montgomery, *Introduction to Statistical Quality Control* (New York: Wiley, 1985).

4

Foundations of the Hospital Organization

The idea that emerges from the definition of the community hospital (chapter 1), open systems concepts of responsiveness to community needs and desires represented by the views of external and member exchange partners (chapter 2), and consensus on expectations that can be achieved by small work groups (chapter 3) is both philosophically appealing and reasonably realistic as a description of actual well-managed hospitals. There is little dispute that well-run hospitals are flexible in their approach to the use of resources, they do carefully consider the desires of both external exchange partners and members, and they expend much of their energy on the development of consensus regarding expectations. One implication of these theories is that there will be great diversity among well-managed hospitals. To the extent that community needs and attitudes differ, well-managed hospitals will differ. That ability to respond to local variations is a valuable, possibly an essential, attribute of a democratic and capitalistic society. A second implication of this set of theories is that well-managed hospitals are constantly changing in response to dynamic external conditions. While a condition of equilibrium or homeostasis may be the goal, it can never be the reality for an institution embedded in a society whose economic needs, demographic structure, and technological capability are constantly changing. The well-managed hospital should be perceived as a state of becoming, rather than a state of being.

Despite these forces toward and advantages of diversity, there must be some shared attributes of well-managed hospitals, that is, those which are successfully tracking the changing needs of their local communities and being rewarded for it with resources and prestige. This chapter attempts to identify those common elements, finding them in three areas:

1. *Ethical values*—Well-managed hospitals share a commitment to the value and dignity of each human life and to a number of ethical positions which flow from that commitment.

2. *Structure of the organization*—The uniqueness of health care dictates common systems of organization, focusing on the optimal use of several levels of professional skill. The common parts of hospital organization are the five systems previously identified: governance, finance, clinical, human resources, and plant. The clinical system is central in well-managed hospitals, and it is the function with the greatest structural similarities across hospitals.

3. *Processes of organization design*—Although the actual organizations within the five systems are not the same in all well-managed hospitals, there is a common process by which well-managed hospitals design these structures.

Ethical Values

For hospitals, success requires responding to customer demands for service and economy, and meeting the demands necessary to recruit and retain members, chiefly doctors and employees. (Barnard notes that in a democratic society there is a mutual commitment rather than a superior-subordinate one. No worker can be ordered without his or her acceptance of the order.[1]) The three goals of service, economy, and member needs are potentially contradictory. Well-managed hospitals begin with ethical concepts that avoid or minimize these contradictions.

— Underlying all values of the well-managed hospital is a love of human life and dignity, which is expressed as a willingness to give service and to respect each individual's rights and desires.

— Quality of service is taken as primary and inviolate. The well-run hospital satisfies all reasonable expectations of quality and requires adequate quality as the immutable foundation of any activity it undertakes.

— Service and quality are closely related concepts. Both are multidimensional and must be viewed as including access, satisfaction, continuity, comprehensiveness, prevention, and compliance, as well as the narrow technical issues of accurate diagnosis and treatment.[2] Since all of the dimensions of service and quality are important to the patient, the well-managed hospital attempts to consider them all in its mission, plans, and expectations.

— Quality defined in this broad manner is inherently economical. Improvement in quality is as likely to improve economy as to reduce it. Members of the organization are expected to search for improvements in meeting customer needs rather than for narrower aims that simply trade some goals for others.

— Members are expected to understand the importance of improvements in both service and economy and to derive part of their work satisfaction from identifying and achieving them. Recruitment and incentives for members reinforce the shared ethical values of the organization. That is to say, well-managed hospitals seek and encourage members who agree with their ethical position. They avoid and discourage those who disagree, particularly those who are unable to express love and respect for individual dignity.

— Love and respect extend to members as well. Each member is accepted as an individual and is respected for his or her contribution. The well-managed hospital rewards loyal service and dedication to these values. A broad spectrum of incentives is used, including encouragement, praise, and recognition, as well as promotion and tangible compensation. Sanctions are used rarely, in cases where the individual's behavior threatens the quality of care or the continued effectiveness of the work group.

Organization Structure

One implication of the ethical values common to well-managed hospitals is dedication to the importance of clinical activities. Well-managed hospitals have improved and extended these services at good levels of quality for many years. As open systems theory would predict, they have been rewarded for it by substantial increases in the resources available to them. With the growth in resources has come a growth in complexity. Activities that were once the part-time tasks of a single individual now require entire sections of a much larger organization.

By the 1980s, the process of stimulus and response to exchange opportunities had resulted in the five major systems, which are subdivided into 50 or more specialized work units in even moderate-sized hospitals. A review of these parts and their approximate date of origin shows not only what the modern hospital is, but reveals much about how it came to be.

Governance

The following are governance functions:

1. *Trustee or governing board*—The board is an old and essential part of hospitals, whose role has evolved toward boundary spanning, identification of exchange opportunities, and strategic planning of the organization's response. Emphasis has moved away from direct financial contribution and the contribution of specialized skills, although many examples of these still occur.

2. *Executive*—This function has emerged gradually since 1930. The title "president and chief executive officer" became relatively common in the 1970s. The number and kinds of executive personnel grew with the prominence of the office. Several dozen people now work in the executive office of well-managed hospitals, supporting the needs of the governance system.

3. *Medical staff organization*—Although the functions of the medical staff are clinical, the nature of the contract between medical staff members and the organization as a whole is a critical governance activity. It began to emerge as such when the open staffs of the early twentieth century gave way to the closed staff of the 1930s and the privileged staff of the 1970s and 1980s. Quality reviews enforced by the JCAH were made increasingly rigorous through the postwar decades. Utilization review, that is, peer concern over the quantity of service ordered, was first mentioned in the late 1950s, became widespread in the early 1970s, and increased strikingly in importance in the 1980s. The complexity of medical staff organization grew steadily with these trends. Staff leadership was almost exclusively volunteer in community hospitals until the 1970s, when employed staff leadership became more popular.

4. *Planning and marketing*—Well-managed hospitals began rudimentary planning in the 1950s, but the concepts were not widespread until the 1970s, when planning was stimulated by federal legislation resulting from concerns over cost and equitable access to health care. Marketing, a concept that subsumes planning and extends beyond it, received great impetus in the 1980s, as pressures for cost control caused revenues to be threatened. Well-managed hospitals use the concept of marketing to assess, evaluate, influence, and respond to exchange

opportunities. A more aggressive strategic planning stance developed with the marketing concept and will continue in the foreseeable future.

5. *Public relations and fund raising*—Formal efforts emerged around 1940 and grew slowly but steadily. Many hospitals paid more attention to the function around 1980. Promotion, an activity that is part of marketing, includes both advertising and public relations. The broadest concept of these activities, involving all considerations of the way the institution is perceived by its exchange partners, is just beginning to be understood and implemented.

6. *Information management*—Information arises from the activities of three major systems, finance, clinical, and governance. Contributions from these three sources developed at unequal rates, but by the 1980s well-managed hospitals had perceived the importance and interrelation of the three. Although few hospitals have formally identified information management as a governance rather than a finance function, the nature of their needs suggests that they will.

Finance

The use of private insurance and fee-for-service payment for hospital care has led to a greatly enlarged finance system, compared to those in other advanced nations. The spread of private health insurance (paying either cost or charges, depending on location and kind of insurance) and government health insurance (paying costs) stimulated first an increased accounting capability and later a vastly improved financial analysis capability. Computer technology expanded with increased demand from the payment sources, encouraging the strong growth of the finance function. Fund accounting, emphasizing the proper use of donated money, was dominant until the 1960s. Financial accounting, emphasizing accurate identification of costs, charges, and revenue, became central with the growth of outside payment. Last to be added was an emphasis on financial planning. This arose with the use of borrowed funds, which grew throughout the 1970s and early 1980s in response to the stimulus of widespread and generous insurance.

The following are controllership or accounting functions:

1. *Patient accounting*—Patient charges, or bills, generate much of the hospital's revenue. Patient accounting has been present throughout the century, grew rapidly from 1945 to 1970, and has continued steady growth since.

2. *Internal and external financial audit*—Audits are concerned with protecting owners' assets. Very little attention was paid to auditing until after the passage of Medicare, which demanded external auditing as a basic protection of public funds. Internal audits arose from the need to meet external standards and may be expected to continue to expand in the new environment of cost control.

3. *Payroll and accounts payable*—These routine business accounts have been present throughout the century, but the increase in value of items purchased and the increases in both wages and nonsalary benefits prompted substantial growth, particularly between 1970 and 1980. Newer systems emphasize cost control by providing more specific and timely data.

4. *Cost accounting*—Efforts to determine accurate costs of treatment provided started with the use of costs to determine revenue at the close of World War II, but they remained simplistic until 1967, when Medicare adopted a cost-based reimbursement system. Cost accounting is expected to become even more important in the coming decades.

The following are functions of financial analysis:

1. *Management of capital sources*—Long-term debt became an important source of capital for hospitals in the 1970s; it was supported by extended insurance coverage and the availability of tax-exempt bonds. In the 1980s, joint ventures and for-profit capital subsidiaries introduced the use of equity finance, and the development of multihospital organizations expanded the financial management obligations.

2. *Budgeting and capital budgeting*—Careful projections of expenditures did not become routine in hospitals until the 1970s. Well-managed hospitals began to use budgets derived from careful assessment of the economic exchange environment, the hospital's long-range plan, and its long-range fiscal plan in the early 1980s. These budgets establish mutually agreed-upon expectations for future expenditures at the level of the responsibility center. Relatively short term capital budgets are used similarly, to set priorities for new programs and capital equipment. These two activities are essential elements of cost control and can be expected to grow in importance and sophistication throughout the 1980s.

3. *Financial planning*—Sophisticated financial planning controls the use of borrowed and equity capital as well as the growth of expenditures and pricing strategies. Financial planning became

more elaborate as the payment mechanisms of insurers became more complex, borrowing and equity sources became more widely used, and the exchange environment became more demanding. It is a major component of strategic planning, lending reality to what would otherwise be mainly wishes and dreams.

Clinical Care

Exponential growth in medical specialties, nursing specialties, other clinical professions, treatments, and diagnostic procedures can be traced throughout the century. Three major groups of clinical activity have emerged: medical staff, those making the central treatment decisions and undertaking surgery; nursing; and clinical support services.

Medical Care

The medical encounter, which occurs when a patient contacts a doctor or one of a few similar practitioners, is the central event in the health care process. In the encounter, the doctor identifies a series of patient needs for diagnosis and treatment. These needs, translated into orders for services, stimulate most hospital activities. Almost all demand for inpatient or outpatient hospital services results from them.

The issues of quality and economy involve the encounter, the orders, and their fulfillment. The major outcomes of care are determined by three elements of the encounter:

1. How valid the set of needs identified is
2. How well those needs are carried out, including both professional and patient perceptions of validity
3. How satisfied the patient is with the elements of the encounter and the resulting services

Any hospital that aspires to be well managed must assure that medical encounters for its patients are done well across all three of these dimensions. Yet medical encounters are often highly individualized, intimate, and anxiety producing. Society gives physicians significant and unique prerogatives to carry these encounters out. The privacy and flexibility they demand prohibits the normal organizational approach to quality control, which emphasizes uniformity and direct oversight.

This dilemma gives rise to unique contracts between the physician and the organization that supports her or him. The one that is most common in hospitals involves the granting of annually renewed **privileges,** rights to perform certain kinds of care in the hospital. The extent of privileges is determined by professional peers, based upon the doctor's education and past performance. (Other organizations, such as HMOs or clinics, which employ or contract with physicians, develop similar structures.)

The medical staff organization conducts peer review, evaluating the credentials of applicants and annually reviewing the performance of physicians with privileges. It also fulfills several other functions supporting the quality of care. The number and importance of these functions have been growing for several decades. Representation of doctors' needs is an old but continuing function. Management of privileges has grown steadily more complex in the last 50 years; in fact, annual review of privileges was begun only recently. Recruitment of physicians as a coordinated activity is also recent. The development of consensus on methods of care, expressed as protocols that guide economy and quality, appears likely to become a fourth critical contribution of the medical staff. In addition to these four functions relating to the patient encounter, medical staffs provide education to their members and to other health professions.

The system of peer review normally stops short of direct supervision or direct observation of the medical encounter. It relies upon self-supervision by each physician with privileges. In order to assure the quality of the medical encounter, the well-managed hospital must attract doctors who are both well trained and well motivated, that is, who can be trusted to complete medical encounters well. This, in turn, requires the successful completion of all the medical staff functions.

The most common financial arrangement for medical staff members is a fee-for-service contract between the doctor and the patient, without direct involvement of the hospital. However. the form of association between the doctor and the hospital has been changing steadily. At present, about 25 percent of doctors are employed in hospitals, excluding doctors in training. The balance are independent practitioners who are paid directly by patients or their insurers; these doctors are increasingly entering into financial arrangements with the hospital or with the hospital and a third party. It is likely that multiple and hybrid forms will continue. The growth of HMOs and prospective payment contracts will stimulate more complex financial arrangements at the expense of traditional fee-for-service payment. This book assumes a model called the **conjoint medical staff,** a flexible and pluralistic relationship between doctors and the hospital that assumes increasingly close ties.

Clinical Support Services

The services which physicians and others order as a result of medical encounters are provided by numerous health care professions, including several medical specialties. Many of these have employment relationships with the community hospital. Nursing, the oldest and largest of the clinical services, was often the source of the first members of the newer professions. The others were once called *ancillary services* but now fill too important a role in diagnosis and treatment for that label. They provide the components of health care, the intermediate products that collectively support the physician's plan for diagnosis and treatment.

Each of the clinical support services has a set of specific functions arising from its unique technology or skills, but there are several generic functions as well. All must control the processes and outcomes of their intermediate product. Quality of service, including the physician's perception of quality, is essential. In addition, the support services are responsible for several management functions, including patient scheduling, personnel logistics, planning, budget development, and cost control for the intermediate product.

Nursing

The nurse's contribution to patient care rivals the physician's in both inpatient and outpatient settings. It is defined by the concept of homeostasis, helping the patient to achieve a maximally effective interchange with his or her environment. This concept encompasses not only the traditional nursing activities, but a broad range of preventive and educational services as well. The nursing care plan arising from the concept of homeostasis is also important in lowering the final product cost.

Nursing emphasizes the development and maintenance of the comprehensive care plan in addition to functions that resemble those of the other clinical support services. Nursing is responsible for its own quality and monitors the quality of several other services in order to ensure patient and physician satisfaction. It must manage its own work force, the largest in the hospital, support a variety of logistical services for the patient, and assist the governance system with planning advice.

Human Resources

Several factors have spurred the growth of the human resources function beyond what is necessary to support other activities. The number of hospital employees has grown to about three per occupied bed, from fewer than two 30 years ago. In addition, hospitals employ more professionally skilled individuals, who tend to be recruited from regional or national rather than local markets. The number of such skills has increased as well. Unionization has become important in some regions. Both federal and state workforce regulation have become more complex, and hospital exemptions have been removed. The human resources function includes the following activities:

1. *Recruitment and work force planning*—National markets, recurring shortages, increased labor costs, and federal equal opportunity provisions changed recruitment from a casual, local event to a regional or national one. Advanced planning of personnel needs was accelerated in the 1980s by concern over the cost of additional personnel and the need for humane policies of work force reduction.

2. *Work force support*—Large, expensive, specialized work forces demand certain maintenance activities, such as training and orientation, counselling, and promotion and termination interviewing. These have been centralized slowly in hospitals, but they now take place largely in human resources departments rather than the clinical units.

3. *Compensation*—Improved financing for hospital care, competition for employees, regulation of wages and hours, and collective bargaining have improved the once notoriously low salaries of hospital workers. Employment benefits also expanded and now constitute about 10 percent of hospital expenditures. These benefits—vacations, sick leave, health insurance, retirement pensions, and life insurance constitute a minimum package—all require administration. Federal employment law governing wages and hours, overtime, working conditions, affirmative action for disadvantaged groups, and collective bargaining rights apply to hospitals receiving payment under Medicare. State laws deal with many of the same subjects but also cover unemployment compensation and workers' compensation. Finally, many hospitals in the Northeast and some in other parts of the country have union contracts. The American Federation of State, County, and Municipal Employees and the 1199 Union of Hospital and Health Care Workers are numerically important. Some hospitals negotiate with up to six different unions, some of them representing house officers and nurses.

Plant

Historically, each section of the hospital managed its own environmental needs, with the exception of such simple common areas as roof, corridors, and lawn. In medieval hospitals, housekeeping, food, and laundry were done on individual wards. Centralization of these activities began in the nineteenth century, when low-cost electricity and steam power became available. The combination made it cost-effective to operate plumbing and heating systems, and later kitchens, laundries, and sterilization services. The following are elements of the plant, supplies, and maintenance function:

1. *Operation of buildings, utilities, and equipment*—In the 1950s, the use of general air conditioning and devices posing radiation hazards expanded greatly. Infection control and energy conservation became routine. Automobile parking became an essential service. Each development added to the complexity of the environmental systems. The result is that the power supply of the modern hospital is a sophisticated technical achievement in itself. Communications and computing equipment began major developments in the 1970s which appear likely to continue for some years. The proliferation of complex equipment forced specialization among repair services, with the most complex technical tasks frequently contracted to outside companies. All of this growth made careful planning and control of the use of space essential.

2. *Housekeeping and environmental safety*—Housekeeping became increasingly mechanized as wage increases justified substituting capital for labor. It is an important element in infection control. Patients, employees, and guests must be protected from environmental hazards by a routine surveillance function.

3. *Work force, patient, and visitor support services*—Hospitals provide food, various amenities, and communication services to members, patients, and guests. All but the smallest hospitals have trained security forces, and some inner-city institutions have what amounts to a small police force protecting property, patients, and personnel.

4. *Materials management*—Centralized materials management functions are relatively recent in hospital organizations. Many aspects of obtaining supplies were left to the using unit even in the 1980s, but standardization, competitive bid solicitation, and collective purchasing had grown steadily. Cost concerns accelerated their growth in the 1980s.

The Process of Organization Design

The environment of U.S. hospitals changed radically between 1980 and 1985, but the impact of that change on organization structure is not yet known. The most successful hospitals will be those that can identify and implement the changes most satisfactorily to the American people. It is likely that hospital organization in the next decade will face as much change as it did at the peak of the post-Medicare years. Well-run hospitals therefore will be those that can manage a high rate of organizational change effectively.

The Criterion for Organization Design

Success for hospitals requires both correct assessment of community desires and effective response to them. Pressures from the outside environment affect much of the hospital organization, and a successful organization is one that responds effectively to those pressures. Some tasks are assigned by licensure laws and others by educational programs. For example, the roles of many professionals in hospitals are determined by professional practice acts. Educational programs are constructed to follow the acts; thus, even if a hospital wanted to reassign certain tasks, its personnel would not know how to carry out their new duties. Organization design is also influenced by the marketplace, including reimbursement mechanisms. A hospital operating in an affluent community or under generous reimbursement may have a different organization than one in a poorer environment. Design also depends upon technology. The growth of laboratory medicine caused the creation of a new organizational unit, the clinical laboratory, which in 100 years has grown to be the second largest department in the hospital. Computers are expected to have an important effect on organization.

To respond correctly, the hospital must coordinate the efforts of several hundred or thousand people. This begins by assigning every member of the organization to either a work group or a supervisory position. The work groups and their arrangement under various levels of supervisors creates what is called a **bureaucratic organization.** The term was coined by researchers to describe a form of human endeavor where groups of individuals bring different skills to bear on a single objective in accordance with a formal structure of authority and responsibility. The formal structure generates the familiar pyramidal shape of organization charts. Most of the economic activity of modern society is carried out by means of bureaucratic organizations (as is most religious, artistic, and social activity: the Catholic Church, the New York Philharmonic Orchestra, and the Boy Scouts of America are bureaucratic organizations). All hospitals are bureaucratic organizations.[3]

Bureaucratic organizations permit individuals to contribute to an overall objective that is larger than the sum of their individual efforts. They use specialization to enhance the individual's contribution and coordination to make the whole responsive. Coordination begins with small groups and continues with the supervisory structure. The purpose of bureaucratic structure is to facilitate responsiveness, and the two keys to responsiveness are supporting the small groups and building coordination. No hospital is ever totally successful at the effort; the well-managed hospital is more responsive, and its responsiveness underpins its success.

Components of Organization

Although many people think of the pyramidal chart as describing an organization, reality is substantially more complicated. To have an effective understanding of a hospital organization, one must recognize that it has at least three broad dimensions: a formal hierarchy, represented by the pyramid; a set of formal collateral activities, or boundary spanning;[4] and informal networks, which are generated by members of the organization acting as individuals rather than through their formal authority.

The Hierarchy of Accountability. The bureaucratic organization of hospitals identifies the roles and tasks that must be accomplished, assigns them to individuals and groups, and establishes a network of communications. The network is based upon the concept of **accountability,** the notion that the organization can rely upon the individual to fulfill a specific, prearranged expectation. Just as every worker is assigned to a work group, every member of the organization should have a clear position in the accountability hierarchy.

Mintzberg notes that, in addition to the accountability hierarchy, the parts of the pyramid all have boundary-spanning activities with each other and often with the external environment. In addition, he notes that some of the accountability hierarchies serve the central purpose of the organization and are traditionally called line units, while others serve technical and support activities, sometimes called staff units, and still others constitute the strategic apex.[5] Mintzberg's models fit manufacturing better than hospitals, but it might be said that the finance group is a technical activity, and certainly the human resources and plant management groups are support activities.

Even though a work group is in a support section or is dedicated to boundary spanning, it is still in the accountability hierarchy and reports to the chief executive. Like every other work group in the well-run hospital, it has specific and often quantitative expectations for each of the closed system parameters. Assignment of accountability includes mutual understanding of the expectation, assignment and acceptance of the authority necessary to carry it out, and designation of a communication route for reporting both difficulties and performance.

The accountability hierarchy creates a form of contract between superior and subordinate components of the organization and to a large extent between the two individuals which implement it. This contract holding both parties responsible for prearranged expectations is the essence of the formal hierarchical organization. The relationship is enforced by the traditions of bureaucratic organization; by the information flows which report performance on the closed system parameters; by the authorities over expectations, appointment of individuals, and distribution of rewards; and finally, but perhaps most important, by the ability of the superior to meet the work place needs of the subordinate.

Informal Organizations. All groups of people working together develop informal organizations. They consist of the network of communications the members establish for their own desires. The informal organizations of hospitals are exceptionally important. Hospitals must give great latitude to doctors and nurses dealing directly with patients because patients' needs vary. The three-shift operation is another factor encouraging informal organization. The night crew is almost certain to encounter situations in which it must devise its own answers. Although it is usually impossible to describe the informal structure in detail, the best formal organizations not only recognize their informal shadows, but are designed to exploit their strengths and to overcome their weaknesses. One useful perspective is that the formal organization strengthens the informal one and does what the informal one cannot.

The Collateral Organization. In addition to a formal hierarchical structure, hospitals make heavy use of collaborative communications and clearances among units in different hierarchies. Such devices are used to accomplish daily work and to understand and communicate perceptions about the outside environment. These activities comprise the **collateral organization.** The collateral organization can be understood as a network of committees and work groups providing cross-communication and linking middle managers at several different levels. Members shift collateral relationships much more often than hierarchical ones, and collateral activities rarely have direct authority. The well-managed hospital uses collateral organization to build consensus about exchange opportunities and to coordinate expectations. Committee work can be time-consuming for middle managers, however, and in extreme cases may impair the hospital's function. The well-designed hospital attempts to move the consensus as quickly as possible into the formal accountability hierarchy, where quantitative expectations can be negotiated to encourage efficient responses.

The *code team,* a multidisciplinary group assisting in cases of cardiac arrest, is a dramatic example of a collateral organization. The discharge planning committee, which coordinates the efforts of nursing, medicine, and social service, is another. The oldest is the surgical team, with members from nursing, surgery, and anesthesia. The principal function of these activities internally is to integrate members of different accountability hierarchies.

Collateral activities addressing exchange issues from the external environment are frequently longer lasting and more complex. Many planning and expectation-setting activities demand the collaboration of several work groups. Attaining appropriate levels of patient care quality and satisfaction requires both in-depth technical knowledge and an understanding of customer needs. Competing opportunities for exchanges must frequently be evaluated jointly, in light of overall external needs. Well-run hospitals meet this broader need through collateral units such as the planning committee and the joint medical staff–board conference committee at the governance level. At lower levels, structures such as the pharmacy committee and the medical records committee pool technological knowledge from several areas and make decisions affecting productivity and quality.

It is impossible to dispense with the collateral organization. The dynamic nature of the environment and the variability of patient needs call for collateral activities. Control of the collateral organization can be a problem, however. Performance is improved if the collateral organization has specific expectations about its functions and reporting. Thus a well-managed collateral organization is kept relatively small, given explicit charges, supported with adequate data, monitored closely, and expected to reach conclusions on explicit schedules.

Decisions Establishing the Organization Design

The hospital organization is designed through three interrelated actions:

1. Specifying the tasks and the accountability for each small work group
2. Establishing the reporting and supervisory responsibilities of middle management, which constitutes the accountability hierarchy
3. Building collateral relationships between hierarchies, thereby allowing them to coordinate and integrate their expectations toward a common goal

The process of coordination and integration depends upon the participation of individuals and groups. One of the proven ways to gain participation is to seek it habitually in all important organizational decisions. Since the design of the organization is one important decision, it is not surprising that much of the design of the accountability hierarchy is determined by the collateral organization. The executive office stimulates and guides the participation of a variety of people in an ongoing process of designing and amending both the accountability hierarchy and the collateral organization itself.

Organization Design as a Process of Collaboration

The responsibility for successful organization design falls more heavily on the executive office than on any other unit of the organization. The governing board is rarely involved in the design process, although it sometimes approves the final plan. The executive office controls the design process and its outcome.

Good executives encourage broad participation from others in the organization. Design decisions require much detailed information that the executive office is not likely to possess. On the other hand, breadth of vision and an understanding of relationships among hospital activities are important to successful organization design. It is unlikely that individuals in the clinical, financial, human resources, or plant systems will have sufficient perspective to make wise design decisions unaided. Because of the importance of the task and the value of experience, organization design is a frequent activity for the chief operating officer and his or her immediate deputies. A critical part of that activity is deciding who else will participate in the design decision at hand.

A second critical function of the executive is control of the rate of change. There are always some arguments for fixing the organization. Too much change is confusing, expensive, and fails to take advantage of learning and experience to improve performance. Too little, however, leads to insularity of viewpoint and unresolved adjustments to technological and economic changes. Identifying the correct pace of change for the organization is the responsibility of the executive.

Good practice requires that the members of the organization participate in the design of the parts that relate to their own functions. Doctors should participate in the design of the medical staff and its reporting hierarchy, food service managers, the food service, and so on. Design begins conceptually with identification of all the tasks and activities that must be performed. These are then grouped around common factors, usually equipment, training, time, or geography. Much of the success of the well-managed hospital arises from the close fit that emerges from years of effort in specifying these groupings and the resulting interfaces. The process of organization design specifies in advance the nature of this growth by structuring the flow of information.

Deliberate efforts must be made to identify, discuss, and resolve conflicts and omissions of responsibilities that arise in the design process. It is the job of the executive office to assemble all the various viewpoints, hear their views, and establish formal hierarchies that will improve integration among groups.

Defining Responsibility Centers

A responsibility center (RC) is a small group of workers and one first-level manager. A nursing station crew with its head nurse or a housekeeping crew with its foreman are typical examples. The managers are the primary monitors from the closed system model and are called **responsibility center managers** (RCMs). Even a modest hospital will have upwards of 50 RCs, with several RCs in each large department. Very large hospitals have over 100.

Criteria for Design. The design criteria for each responsibility center are:

1. *To assign every necessary task to a single RC*—Tasks assigned to more than one RC or to no RC are not accountable.

2. *To assign related tasks to the same RC*—If related tasks are assigned to different RCs, problems of continuity and coordination may arise.

3. *To assign tasks requiring similar skills to the same RC*—A work group and a manager with a common background can communicate with each other more easily.

4. *To limit each RC to a reasonable span of control*—The RCM must be able to maintain control of the activity by direct observation, to carry out the principle of no surprises (see chapter 3). Direct observation imposes geographic, temporal, and size limit on RCs.

Dealing with Conflicting Criteria. Typically hospitals have an RC for each nursing floor, or unit. They divide a large department in a single geographic location into RCs on the basis of technical function (for example, the laboratory is divided into chemistry, hematology, bacteriology, and histology RCs). They may organize a 24-hour service, such as security, into shifts. They divide a dispersed activity like housekeeping geographically in order to maintain a reasonable span of control. Laundries and operating rooms are organized around equipment—wash wheels and irons, heart pumps and lasers.

For a great many important hospital activities, the criteria for design are in conflict, and their parameters (tasks, relationships, skills, and span) cannot all be optimized at once. There are frequently two geographic units with similar functions, or two functions in the same geographic area, or two skills required for the same function. Many large hospitals have several laboratories. Emergency rooms require almost every clinical profession, plus housekeeping and other plant services. Nursing, medicine, and social service contribute to the function of discharge planning. Even the task assignment of the nursing unit RC is slightly ambiguous, because housekeeping, dietary, several diagnostic and treatment services, and medical staff are all important to the function of the nursing unit.

In every case where these conflicts arise, trade-offs must be selected to resolve them. As a result, there is no perfect list of RCs for a hospital, and, because conditions change, there is no permanent solution. Rather, well-run hospitals consider the next two steps of organization design—setting the reporting hierarchy of middle management and building collateral communications—as ways of overcoming the weaknesses of a specific set of RCs. When the RC design process is properly done, it generates three results:

1. It specifies the RCs and the RCMs.

2. It identifies the trade-offs, or departures from criteria, arising from that particular solution.

3. It suggests hierarchical relationships and collateral relationships that will optimize these trade-offs.

Another way to say this is that there are always three avenues to organizational improvement—changing the RCs, revising the middle management structure, and strengthening collateral relationships.

Responsibility Centers for the Medical Staff. Traditionally, medical practice has been left to the authority and responsibility of the individual physicians who are privileged to practice. In effect, each doctor is his or her own RC and RCM, but the closed system parameters have been only partially and ambiguously specified. More or less formal allegiances based on medical specialty have grouped doctors, but the mechanisms for accountability have also remained limited and ambiguous. The result is that an accountability hierarchy is only beginning to emerge in the very best hospitals. There are important arguments for allowing the attending physician freedom to exercise professional judgment on the patient's behalf. If done badly, specification of the activities of professionals can be more damaging than total freedom. The issues underlying the medical decision process, discussed in chapter

11, are complex, and successful medical designs will continue to recognize the importance of the individual practitioner's on-the-scene judgment.

Despite the importance of individual judgment, the trend has been toward organizing physicians into work groups and increasingly specifying closed system parameters. Several developments have eroded the tradition of completely individualized medical practice. As discussed in chapter 10, a new model of medical staff organization, the conjoint staff has emerged. Under the concept of the conjoint staff, work groups of physicians who share similar patient and disease populations are likely. These work groups have leaders, who increasingly take on responsibility for quality and appropriateness of medical care. As they do, their parallels to the traditional responsibility center and RCM become clearer. Competition for groups of patients that pay on a capitation basis is the strongest force among several supporting this trend. The emergence of explicit and annual expectations for specialty groups under HMO practice may come quite quickly in large well-run hospitals.

The absence of a well-understood hierarchy for physicians throws all communication with doctors into the collateral organization, contributing to the burdens of a relatively weak part of the organization.

Issues in Middle Management Design

In the formal accountability hierarchy, each responsibility center manager reports to a supercontroller. The levels of supercontrollers between the RC and the executive constitute middle management. The sole function of middle management is to facilitate the effective performance of the RCs. Middle managers are accountable upward for adherence to agreed-upon expectations and downward for resolving issues their subordinates cannot. (That is to say, middle managers have an explicit obligation to respond to their subordinates as well as to their superiors.) They communicate expectations downward and subordinates' views upward. They must ensure that each of their RCs receives the resources it needs and meets the demands for service anticipated in the expectations.

Middle managers also constitute much of the collateral organization. The questions referred to them by the RCs are such that they must communicate across reporting hierarchies as well as within them. Meeting the expectations for the RCs reporting to them will usually be a matter of improving the fit of inputs, outputs, and demands with those of other units. Hospital managers are usually professionally trained people with unique insights into the trends of specific technology. Thus, their views are also important to issues of environmental assessment.

The nature of the responsibility center design suggests the difficulty of the middle manager's role. If each small work unit were ideally designed, with all related tasks within it, no other RC performing similar duties, and no patients presenting unusual problems, middle management would be a small cadre of experts working on planning, budgeting, and recruitment for occasional RCM vacancies. In reality, middle management is a group numbering from a few dozen to a few hundred people attacking the problems arising daily from the RCs. In poorly designed hospitals they are so consumed by these issues that they have no time for planning, budgeting, or recruitment. There is a Catch-22 involved: middle managers are overworked, so there is a temptation to add more middle managers; but the reason middle managers are overworked is that they have many problems of communication and coordination. Adding more middle managers increases the size and complexity of the collateral organization. It simply intensifies the communication problem without necessarily improving productivity or quality.

Effective design of the collateral organization is an ongoing problem. Well-run hospitals have been improving the collateral organization by establishing timetables of repetitive activities, formally reiterating certain common themes and objectives, and specifying the charges and procedures of collateral activities. Well-managed hospitals now commonly rely upon:

— Formal mission statements amplified in sufficient detail to provide guidelines on major interests or directions.

— Long-range plans for services, personnel, and capital requirements amplifying the mission statement and establishing timelines for specific events.

— An annual and multiannual cycle of environmental assessment and revision of the mission and plan.

— Grouping and annual review of specific proposals for capital expenditures and new program requests.

— An annual review of the closed system parameter expectations for each responsibility center (although this review began as a cost-oriented budget, it is spreading to demand, output, efficiency, quality, and resource conservation as a comprehensive and integrated set).

— Recruitment protocols guiding the selection of key individuals.

The current initiative among leading hospitals appears to be strengthening the planning, scheduling, and coordinating of clinical matters by improving the accountability hierarchy within the medical staff. This will transfer much activity from the collateral to the hierarchical organization, over a period of several years. As progress is made, the burdens of the collateral organization can be minimized by such tactics as the following:

— Developing precise and complete expectations within the accountability hierarchy to clarify coordination needs.

— Encouraging a variety of specific ad hoc collateral communications, including formal and informal, grouped and individual.

— Strengthening the medical staff organization and recognizing the interdependence of medicine, nursing, and clinical support services.

— Supplying information systems and capable staff support to middle management to encourage full analysis of facts and to clarify requirements for collateral discussions.

— Increasing outcomes-oriented incentives to stimulate flexibility and acceptance of innovative solutions.

— Using the executive group to focus, coordinate, and set priorities for agendas.

Forms of Middle Management Structure

Middle management structure includes both an accountability hierarchy and a collateral organization, although, because of the complexity, the collateral organization is almost never shown on organization charts. Charts also tend to show single lines of accountability when actually there are more. Three major approaches to the accountability hierarchy have been used: conventional pyramidal organization, matrix organization, and functional organization. Most hospitals are a blend of the three, with the conventional form dominating. Well-run hospitals appear to succeed not so much because they have picked a specific structure as because they identify and correct problems as they arise from the structure they have selected.

The executive office is the only place in the organization that can resolve the problems of middle management design. It has three basic options. First, it may reconsider RC activities. Second, it may devise variations of conventional, matrix, and functional middle management structures. Third, it may develop the system of collateral communication to overcome apparent weaknesses. Sensitivity to these options is a critical part of the executive role. The third option, yet another committee, is too often pursued when the first or the second should be.

Conventional Organization. Hospitals have traditionally emphasized similar skills or professional knowledge in establishing the hierarchy of middle management. The result is an organization like that shown in figure 4.1.

For many years it was common to indicate the medical staff as a separate and distinct organization. A variety of reporting relationships was used, many of them deliberately ambiguous about how the medical staff, executive office, and governing board shared responsibilities.[6] There was also a tendency to treat the medical staff organization as a parliamentary body representing the wishes of the staff majority rather than responding to the exchange needs of the organization. As noted above, thinking has moved steadily away from this view, and apparently will continue to do so. Although many persons are concerned with the need to protect the physician's independent authority in patient care, there is room for well-planned collective action without endangering, and possibly enhancing, the independent physician's contribution. Consistent with the discussion of conjoint staff in chapter 10, figure 4.1 shows a medical staff hierarchy reporting to the administrator directly but otherwise similar to that of nursing or finance. This reflects the modern environment. It is noteworthy that many doctors are now employed as RCMs and middle managers in clinical support organizations. Their obligations in these roles are no different from others'. Issues of quality and appropriateness of care involving the medical staff organization might best be addressed by a variant of the conventional organization, one emphasizing intermediate and final products, as discussed below.

The conventional organization has one great strength and a number of annoying but not disabling weaknesses. Its strength is that many of the hierarchical chains—all of nursing and the clinical support services and financial system, for example—have strong professional content. This allows them to use the professional knowledge, skills, and socialization of personnel to define activities and maintain control over them. Research, education, and innovation tend to follow the same organizational lines. As a result, a new practice can be adopted quickly unless it crosses hierarchical lines. Laws of licensure and standards of practice used in malpractice trials dictate the roles of certain professionals and certain traditional hierarchies.

Conversely, the conventional organization makes each hierarchy responsive to a separate professional organization. Competition sometimes develops among professions, and all of them, not just medicine, have a tendency to concern themselves with professional objectives rather than hospital objectives or exchange needs. They all pressure the hospital to give them equal recognition regardless of their relative contributions. This results in many short hierarchies, such as physical ther-

Figure 4.1

Functional Organization Design

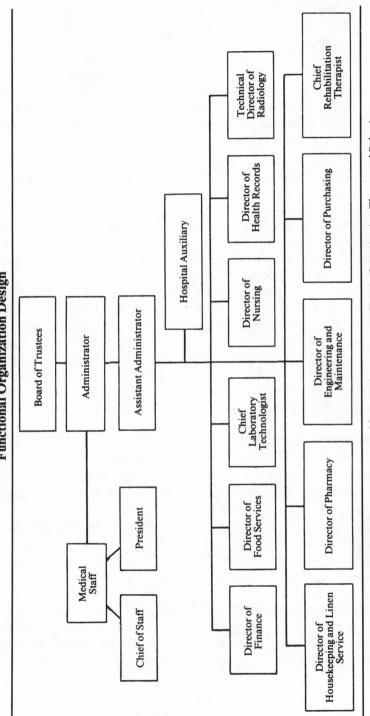

Source: Stephen M. Shortell and Arnold D. Kaluzny, eds., *Health Care Management: A Text in Organization Theory and Behavior* (New York: Wiley, 1983), p. 304.

apy or medical records, and a few long and complex ones, such as nursing or laboratory. As a result, some RCMs report directly to the executive office, while others are insulated by several layers of middle management. More important, middle managers on the same level have vastly different hierarchies reporting to them. The tendency of the professions to proliferate, driven by the increasing specialization of science, has increased the weaknesses of the conventional organization. There are more professions, more hierarchies, and more concerns about the weakness of the conventional organization in 1980 than there were in 1960.

Under the conventional model, the hierarchical organization does not enhance collateral communication among the professions. The executive group must continually stimulate the collateral organization. Informal communications among individuals treating the same patient (for example, among a doctor, nurse, pharmacist, and social worker about the care of one patient) tend to die out as the organization becomes larger. Deliberate efforts to support the informal organization often become necessary. The 1980s version of the conventional organization is supplemented by a great variety of collateral committees, task forces, work groups, networks, and affiliations, all aimed at integrating the various hierarchies effectively. Examples include discharge planning committees, ethics committees, operating room committees, planning teams and task forces, budget committees, and recruitment committees. There are usually a number of ad hoc committees and work groups as well.

Extending Accountability to the Medical Staff. In recent years, as the need for quality, economy, and appropriateness of care has increased, a variant on the conventional organization has emerged. This establishes a medical staff hierarchy divided into scientifically-oriented specialties as responsibility centers. Each specialty is responsible for the cost and quality of the final product or episode of care. The specialty's accountability lies predominantly in what component services, or intermediate product services, are selected to provide diagnosis and treatment. In effect, the members of the specialty buy the units—tests, drugs, days of care—but have no control over the costs of producing the intermediate services. The intermediate producers, on the other hand, have little or no control over the quantities of services ordered, but can be held responsible for the cost and quality of each unit produced. This approach to organization design tends to continue the traditional separation of medicine from other professions. Difficulties that remain to be dealt with include:

— Defining the final product requires identifying ways in which patients can be meaningfully grouped. Some consensus pattern of care, or patient group protocol (see chapter 11), must be developed for each important group.

— Nursing, the largest intermediate service, has substantial control over both costs and quality of the final product. It is unclear how to incorporate the nursing view into patient group protocol.

— The other large, intermediate producers also affect quantities and costs, although to a lesser extent.

— Not all patients fit the scientific structure of medical specialization. Important groups of cancer and heart disease patients are treated by both surgical and nonsurgical specialists, for example.

The scheme also requires sophisticated information processing to measure both intermediate and final product parameters. It has the great virtue of assigning responsibility for cost and quality to medical responsibility centers.

The Matrix Organization. One alternative to the conventional organization is the matrix organization, so called because many RCMs and middle managers have explicit, permanent, dual reporting responsibilities.[7] Figure 4.2 shows such an organization. The matrix organization is difficult to draw in detail because the dual reporting relationships are so complex. From the perspective of the RCM, the existence of the dual responsibility is clear, although its implementation may be obscure. The housekeeping supervisor in the surgical suite, for instance, would report to both the head of the housekeeping department and the supervisor of operating room nurses. The head nurse in intensive care would report both to the supervisor for surgical nursing and to the doctor in charge of intensive care. Matrix organizations around final product protocols have been suggested, presumably with the dominant medical specialty being accountable in some part.[8]

The practical effect of the matrix organization is to emphasize the most important of the collateral relationships by making them permanent and adding them to the conventional reporting relationships. It has intuitive appeal as a description of hospital organization because many RCMs have a subordinate relationship to another profession in addition to their hierarchical one. As the examples in the preceding paragraph suggest, these relationships are frequently with a clinical organization such as nursing or medicine as well as with the administrative organization shown in the accountability hierarchy. Under the conven-

Figure 4.2
Matrix Organization Design

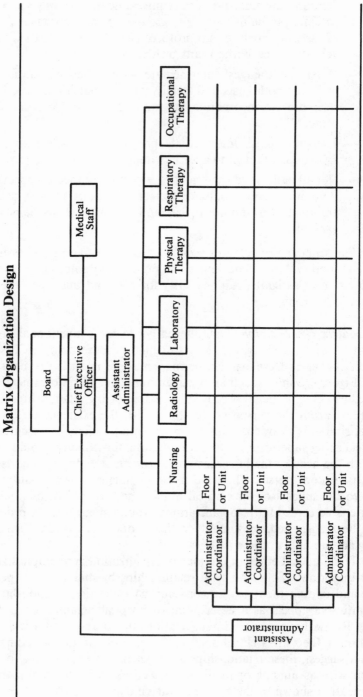

Adapted from: Stephen M. Shortell and Arnold D. Kaluzny, eds., *Health Care Management: A Text in Organization Theory and Behavior* (New York: Wiley, 1983), p. 307.

tional organization, such obligations can be overlooked, even though the result impairs quality of care. Matrix organization makes the most important obligation outside the RCM's own profession or trade explicit.

Despite its initial appeal, the matrix organization has not had widespread success,[9] for two reasons. First, although the communications difficulties of the conventional organization frequently involve several professions or hierarchies, it is impractical to consider more than a dual reporting matrix. Thus, many of the problems of the conventional organization remain. Second, and more serious, the dual reporting structure can easily deteriorate into a competitive relationship among three people, the RCM and his or her two supercontrollers. Three-person relationships are notoriously unstable in general, and those in hospital matrix organizations are exacerbated by conflicts in professional and status relationships (for example, among a head nurse specializing in intensive care, a doctor with the same specialty, and a nursing supervisor whose specialty is surgical nursing.)[10]

Functional Organization. Hospitals frequently create separate conventional organizations for various functions, the most common being for all or part of the outpatient service. (Under functional organization, for example, the director of inpatient nursing would have no direct relationship to or responsibility for outpatient nursing.) Functional organization is also useful for geographically separate or largely self-contained units. Among inpatient activities, pediatric, obstetric, psychiatric, and long-term care units are most often considered for functional organization.

The functionally organized unit is frequently organized conventionally within itself. Some such units border on being totally separate organizations, but more commonly, they are partially self-sufficient and rely on collateral communications to receive services from conventionally organized departments. For example, the long-term care unit may have full nursing, housekeeping, and dietary services but rely on the larger organization for all other clinical and plant services.

The main problem of small, functionally organized units is ensuring effective response from their conventionally organized support services. When the functionally organized unit is geographically remote or an infrequent user of the support service, the problem is aggravated. The best known solution is to place the relationship on a quasi-external basis. In the classic case of prewar General Motors, the parts suppliers and car brands were functional divisions that "sold" to each other on an imputed price basis, with each division accountable for a profit from sales.[11] So far, hospitals have not adopted an organization in which component units can "buy" services from each other. The model holds promise, however, as the medical staff hierarchy is strengthened and the final product–intermediate product concept is implemented.

The most common variant of functional organization now in place is the multihospital system. Under for-profit versions of the system, individual hospitals or other provider units tend to be self-contained except for their planning, strategic governance, and finance functions. Not-for-profit multihospital systems have tended to decentralize even the governance function, centralizing only some elements of strategic planning and finance.[12] At present, multihospital systems are best understood as several separate hospital organizations with certain limited functions centralized; however, the trend is clearly toward more centralization.

A new variant of the functional organization has emerged from The Johns Hopkins Hospital, which assigns complete management authority and responsibility to physician chiefs who also chair departments in the medical school. This explicitly establishes the hierarchy for medical staff organization on the basis of medical specialty. The prewar General Motors conditions have been reasonably well met: in particular, doctors are responsible for resources—cost, efficiency, and revenue —as well as quality of care. In the constrained revenue situation that exists at Hopkins, they must seek efficiencies and profits to support technological advances and expansions of care. The management team of the hospital argues that their organization has done so more successfully than a conventional organization would have.[13]

The functional organization seems to hold promise for the distant future in community hospitals. There is much to be said for organizing accountability around identifiable groups of patient care needs, but this model, like its predecessors has inherent difficulties. It is noticeably easier to apply to a medical school hospital, where the hierarchical organization of medicine by specialty already exists, than it would be for a typical community hospital. It requires full-time medical managers, a situation that is outside the tradition of most hospitals and politically demanding. Very few doctors are trained for such a role, either by education or experience. The model also requires a sophisticated cost-finding system to calculate the necessary imputed prices.

Multihospital Systems

The affiliation of individual hospitals into groups and superorganizations, sometimes called **horizontal integration,** began only 15 years ago, but it has evolved rapidly. It is estimated that 40 percent of all community hospitals had such an affiliation in 1985. The nature of the affiliation ranges from simple contracts for services to elaborate ownership structures involving several corporate layers combining both for-profit and not-for-profit charters. The impact is similarly diverse, but in general, hospitals that are part of even the most centralized system still look much like their independent competitors. They have better resources in governance, finance, training, information systems, and recruitment which they are still learning to exploit but which have already given them significant advantages. The greatest contributions of the multihospital system seem to be in resources rather than in structure.

In general, well-run hospitals and multihospital systems recognize that there are legal, financial, marketing, and organizational dimensions to integration and that it is desirable to address each one separately. Some may be centralized while others are not. Under this philosophy, the organizational questions are driven by management needs rather than by theories.

The most obvious organizational influences of multihospital systems are in the governance function. For-profit hospitals have a trustee or director function, but it is likely to be at the corporate office rather than in the local community. Not-for-profit organizations use their corporate offices to guide local boards; they provide expanded environmental assessment, enhanced financial planning information, and suggestions for procedural questions. Increasingly, they are reserving certain decisions for themselves: final approval of long-range plans, annual budgets, and the selection and compensation of the chief executive officer are often centralized.

The future is likely to bring more centralization: services that can be purchased from the parent company more effectively than they can be provided by the local unit will disappear from local sites. These are likely to be such easily transported services as finance, information systems, human resources, plant maintenance, and laundry. Laboratory service is the obvious candidate among clinical services.

In addition to the integration of hospitals into multihospital systems, outreach to new kinds of services, particularly supporting the aged and the mentally ill, is common, and hospitals are making new, more formal affiliations with their physicians. These expansions, often called **vertical integration,** are supported by joint ventures, partnerships, subsidiary corporate structures, and holding companies, as are the multihospital systems. (Several multihospital systems are involved in both horizontal and vertical integration.) Vertically integrated units are obvious candidates for functional organization.

Many common communication and accountability tasks must be performed in health care delivery. As a result, most health care institutions look like hospitals organizationally. The names of the components often differ more than the functions, and the profile of services offered is far more distinctive than the nature of the hierarchical and collateral structures. This is likely to remain true in more integrated horizontal organizations in the future. There may be many labels and much expedient variation but similar underlying structures. All operating health care units must have a medical staff, a laboratory, and a laundry; even if the function is geographically remote, it must fill local needs for the unit to thrive. In fact, geographic remoteness becomes less and less important with advanced technology. It is organizational remoteness, even in the simplest, smallest health care provider, that is fatal: it signals the failure of accountability for quality, productivity, and patient service.

Using the Organization to Improve Productivity and Quality

Well-run hospitals improve. Their service capability expands as their members learn from experience. Exchange theory suggests that these gains will be divided among productivity, quantity, quality, and scope of service in proportion to the rewards offered by the outside environment. Recent history supports the theory. Between 1960 and 1980, hospitals recognized the public's willingness, despite loud protestations to the contrary, to spend money for increased quantity and scope of services. Hospitals spent what they were offered. In well-managed hospitals, real gains in productivity were made, but they were converted to expanded services, more amenities, and higher quality. Exchange demand shifted in the early 1980s toward economy and productivity. When the marketplace or the regulatory environment demands, costs can be significantly reduced through the same efforts that produced expansion. The well-managed hospitals that properly sensed and responded to their environment in earlier years will do so now. As they do so, they will find that substantial strength already exists within their organization.

The new environment has not abandoned quality or expansion, particularly for technology. It has, however, generally rebalanced its expectations, placing a much heavier emphasis on economy than ever before. To gain economy without reducing service is the essence of productivity, so the successful hospital must now divert more of its efforts toward improving productivity. A hospital seeking to do this undertakes a series of steps.

First, it reevaluates strategic elements:

— The hospital assesses the magnitude and permanence of the new public concern. (In general, the concern appears likely to endure for the foreseeable future. The magnitude differs substantially among communities, with some making only negligible changes.)

— Constraints and guidelines suggested by the hospital's mission are evaluated and incorporated into a revised mission. These often include assessment of potentially desirable affiliations, acquisitions, and mergers; identification of the needs of loyal physicians; programs to protect the employment and rights of workers; and religious and other concerns unique to the particular institution.

— The governing board and the collateral organization revise the long-range plan (see chapters 5 and 10) to reflect new exchange needs. The finance system revises the long-range financial plan (see chapters 5 and 8) to be consistent with the long-range plan.

Second, it educates members of the organization to the new environment and the hospital's response. (Specific, quantified goals are often helpful in educating members).

Third, it reviews the accountability hierarchy and the information systems with an eye to improving them:

— The hierarchy is checked to see that each work group complies as nearly as possible with the criteria above and that clear lines of accountability extend to the strategic level.

— The information systems for reporting cost and quality of performance are adjusted to conform exactly to the accountability hierarchy. Reporting schedules are shortened, and reports are redesigned to emphasize critical departures from expectations.

— Quantitative goals or guidelines are established on hospital-wide measures of performance to guide the budget process (see chapter 8). It is important that these be set at levels consistent with external demands and the long-range plans. If the environment is strongly HMO-oriented, these will be in terms of annual cost per beneficiary per year. If it is oriented to per-case care (for example, DRGs), the measures will be per case. Rarely will an intermediate measure like cost per unit of service suffice.

— The system for setting improved expectations (basically the annual budget development) is reviewed. Attention is paid to improving background information available to RCMs, procedures for establishing expectations at the RCM level, the number and kinds of expectations set, and the response of upper management.

— Budget discussions are expanded to expectations regarding demand, quality, and revenue as well as cost.

— Upper and middle management accountabilities are reviewed and clarified. In particular, middle management obligations to RCMs are emphasized, and redundant levels of middle management are identified and removed.

Fourth, it undertakes a similar review of the collateral organization:

— Unproductive committees are eliminated. Many well-run hospitals make all but legally required committees ad hoc, and give them specific termination dates. Calling such committees "task forces" or "working groups" emphasizes their temporary or flexible character.

— Committees with overlapping functions are combined.

— The hospital establishes a productivity improvement program appropriate in extent and duration to the concern. A permanent shift requires a response of indefinite duration and the program must be established as a support service in the hierarchical organization rather than the collateral one.

— The charges and membership of remaining committees are adjusted. The new charge emphasizes productivity and, if possible, offers a quantitative goal and appropriate measures. The new membership reflects all parts of the accountability hierarchy routinely affected by the committee action.

— Committee procedures are improved to require specific agendas and minutes documenting progress. Responsibility for following procedures is explicitly assigned to middle or upper management.

— Committees are encouraged to consult with nonmembers affected by proposed actions.

— Information systems supporting committees are strengthened to provide data on relevant questions.

Finally, it systematically reviews both tangible and intangible incentives:

— Supervisory training is expanded, and emphasis is placed on providing clear expectations, effective tools and methods, and prompt response to employee needs and questions (see chapter 14).

— Employee training and orientation are expanded, with attention to promoting doctor, patient, and visitor satisfaction (see chapter 14).

— Opportunities are created for personal and public recognition of above average performance.

— The importance of removing intangible disincentives, particularly any nonresponsiveness on the part of upper management, is stressed to upper management, trustees, and physician leadership.

— Retrospective salary recognition for performance improvement is established for RCMs and middle managers.

— Rewards of money and promotion not related to improved performance are diminished or removed. This includes discontinuing routine annual pay increases and cost-of-living adjustments, usually substituting performance-related incentives. When indicated, wages can actually be reduced.

— Physicians' rewards are identified and established. Initial rewards are often only tokens, but well-run hospitals are rapidly rewarding performance with access to capital for clinical and support services. Joint ventures and other income-sharing schemes are being explored.

The hospital that carries out these steps effectively, other things being equal, will systematically improve productivity for many years to come. In general, a cycle is begun. In it, RCMs achieve savings within their centers and in the process identify improvements that require collateral action. Thus committee agenda setting moves from top management to lower management as the program matures. Early gains are relatively small in well-run hospitals and may actually be exceeded by the costs of setting up the program. As the program continues to develop, more and more complex and far-reaching topics come under scrutiny. As an illustration, the impact of a well-designed program on a small RC, such as electrocardiography, might proceed as follows (the time required for each round would be a function of environmental pressure; rounds could certainly overlap, but the energy required would be greater):

1. In round one, the RC is established and the RCM becomes familiar with budget and quality measures. Necessary revisions in the information system are made to provide these measures. The RCM reduces costs of supplies and miscellaneous other costs and in the process begins a dialogue with physicians using the service. The distinctions implicit in measuring cost per electrocardiogram (EKG), EKG cost per discharge, and EKG cost per beneficiary-year are grasped, and rewards are passed out.

2. In round two, attention moves to labor costs, and internal steps are taken to reduce them. Policies regarding workers' rights will be tested. The RCM will recognize the importance of managing demand (discussed in chapter 12) and will turn to a committee for assistance in scheduling it and eliminating inappropriate demand. The information system will have to be strengthened to meet the needs of demand management. Rewards for the RCM will be both tangible and intangible, and tangible rewards will be growing. The question of rewards for cooperating physicians will surface and will require study by a different committee.

3. In round three, a medical committee will identify new approaches to EKG selection in final product protocols (chapter 11); this will result in a significant drop in demand. The RCM will be forced to make further reductions in the work force. Revisions of the reporting hierarchy are likely. Rewards for the RCM continue, and physician rewards are established.

4. In round four, such issues as the possibility of capturing larger market shares in EKG, competitive pricing, requirements for specialist interpretation, and fees for interpretation will come under study by the committee. Reward emphasis will have to move from EKGs per se toward hospitalwide performance, because so many people are involved in the success.

5. In the following years, study will broaden to areas of cardiac disease generally; prevention and reduction of risk will be important. The reward system will incorporate both hospital and doctor performance and may be extended to the workers as well as to managers and doctors.

Many of the problems raised by such a productivity improvement program are discussed in detail in the following chapters. Solutions to these problems, as well as answers to the questions of hospital organization, lie in the mastery of the governance, finance, clinical, human resources, and plant systems.

Notes

1. C. I. Barnard, *The Functions of the Executive,* (Cambridge, MA: Harvard University Press, 1938).

2. Avedis Donabedian, Explorations in Quality Assessment and Monitoring, vol. 1, *The Definition of Quality and Approaches to Its Assessment* (Ann Arbor, MI: Health Administration Press, 1980).

3. George F. Wieland, *Improving Health Care Management: Organization Development and Organization Change* (Ann Arbor, MI: Health Administration

Press, 1981); Stephen M. Shortell and Arnold D. Kaluzny, *Health Care Management: A Text in Organization Theory and Behavior* (New York: Wiley, 1983).

4. J. D. Thompson, *Organizations in Action* (New York: McGraw-Hill, 1967).

5. Henry Mintzberg, *The Structuring of Organizations,* (Englewood Cliffs, NJ: Prentice-Hall, 1979), pp. 18–34.

6. E. Johnson, "Revisiting the Wobbly Three-Legged Stool," *Health Care Management Review 4* (Summer 1979): 15–22.

7. Duncan Neuhauser, "The Hospital as a Matrix Organization," *Hospital Administration* 17 (Fall 1972): 8–25.

8. L. F. McMahon, Jr., et al., "Hospital Matrix Management in DRG-Based Prospective Payment," *Hospital & Health Services Administration* 31 (January-February 1986): 62–74.

9. L. R. Burns, Matrix Management in Hospitals: Patterns and Developments, unpublished.

10. L. F. McMahon, Jr., et al., "Hospital Matrix."

11. Alfred P. Sloan, Jr., *My Life With General Motors* (New York: Doubleday, 1972).

12. Sisters of Mercy Health Corporation, *Integrated Governance and Management Process, Conceptual Design* (Farmington Hills, MI: SMHC, 1980).

13. Robert M. Heyssel, et al., "Decentralized Management in a Teaching Hospital," *New England Journal of Medicine* 310 (1984): 1477–80.

Suggested Readings

Goldberg, A. J. *Hospital Departmental Profiles.* Chicago: American Hospital Association, 1982.

Mintzberg, H. *The Structuring of Organizations.* Englewood Cliffs, NJ: Prentice-Hall, 1979.

Shortell, S. M., and Kaluzny, A. D. *Health Care Management: A Text in Organization Theory and Behavior.* New York: Wiley, 1983.

The Governance and Finance Systems

Introduction to Part II

The governance function is best understood as an interface between the demands of the external world and the operation of the internal organization. Its purpose is to perceive and select exchange opportunities, establish frameworks to support exchange relationships, and direct the remaining systems so that both explicit and implicit exchanges are carried out. Governance is accountable to the outside world, to owners, creditors, the government, and others. It has all the responsibilities any corporation has, along with legal and moral responsibility for the medical staff and the quality and appropriateness of care.

As a result of its responsibilities, the governance system has authority over the other four systems. It is in itself a small hierarchical organization but one that has many staff elements, particularly factfinding and analysis. As one progresses down the governance organization, breadth of authority diminishes rapidly. While the governing board and the chief executive have total authority, the lowest levels of governance have authority only for a few departments or activities. There is a strong tendency to focus outward, on the environment, at the top; and inward, on the balance of the organization, at the bottom.

The question, "What would happen if there were no governance system in a hospital?" is an interesting way of visualizing what these people do. Members of other systems often look on the governance system as redundant or even a hindrance; they assume it could be dispensed with or greatly reduced in size without serious harm. A well-run hospital can dispense with its governance system for about six months, but after that obvious and serious deficiencies will develop. In a few more months, the survival of the institution might be in question: the outside exchange partners might be threatening to cancel their relationships. Blue Cross and Medicare contracts, accreditation, licensure, and ability to incur debt might be in danger. The best doctors and the most discerning patients might be going elsewhere. Employees might be leaving, or the best candidates failing to join the hospital. All of these dangers are related: deterioration in one area is soon transmitted to another.

One brief definition of the job of the governance system is "to make the other four systems look good." When difficult problems emerge in the other systems, particularly if they emerge in two or more, correction usually requires action by the governance system.

The modern community hospital's governance system undertakes several essential activities. While each activity is represented by an organizational unit in large hospitals, the activities are combined in smaller hospitals.

— *The Governing Board.* Chapter 5 deals with the governing board, which, in the sense of an outside overseer of the organization, is universal among community hospitals and has existed since the earliest times. Its function is complicated, but its goal is simple: the governing board exists to fulfill a trust to the owners. In not-for-profit hospitals that trust is the community and involves protecting and using the resources of the hospital in the best possible way for the community's benefit. In for-profit community hospitals the trust is to earn stockholders a fair return on invested capital. In both cases, the board is responsible for acceptable quality of medical care. Because of its trust, the board is the ultimate authority.

— *The Executive Office.* Chapter 6 discusses the executive, which is given authority by the trustees to operate the institution and to carry out the surveillance process by which the hospital develops its exchange relationships. All but the smallest hospitals have full-time executives. Increasing corporate hospital responsibility for quality and economy is requiring broader executive responsibility for clinical affairs. Increasing complexity and competition are increasing the executive's obligation to manage all the governance functions for the board.

— *Planning and Marketing for Community Hospitals.* Chapter 7 examines the role of planning and marketing in the light of increasingly complex exchange relationships. A formal plan for assessing the environment several years into the future is considered essential to good management. Analysis and selection of markets are often required for survival. Planning and marketing are staff units charged with both recognition of trends and development of proposals for meeting them. Marketing includes public relations, advertising, and fund raising. The active solicitation of gifts from individuals, foundations, and corporations is a major function in this area. Most large hospitals have units devoted to maintaining the hospital's favorable position with various external groups.

— *The Finance System.* Chapter 8 addresses the activities of the finance system; because there already exist major works on financial management per se, this chapter emphasizes critical questions of interface.

— *Hospital Information Services.* Chapter 9 is concerned with information management, which is becoming increasingly important as a governance function because of the rapidly growing, centralized, and overlapping need for data and the equally vigorous improvement in computer capability. The largest sources of data are the finance subsystems and the medical records system.

The top executives of the clinical system have essential responsibilities in the governance system as well as in their own organizations. Leaders of medicine, nursing, and clinical support services participate actively in policy formulation, representing the views and conveying the specialized knowledge of their subordinates to the board, and vice versa. Their dual roles are characteristic of all middle management and are essential in linking the elements of the organization to a central mission.

5

The Governing Board

Because their responsibilities are so important and because most people have only infrequent contact with them, governing boards tend to be surrounded with mystery. In fact, however, they are units of bureaucratic organization and are more similar to than different from the other units. They are committees by design—individual board members have no authority per se—and they are subject to all the usual problems of committees. Like the simplest manufacturing unit, the governing board can be described in terms of its purposes, functions, membership, and internal organization and the measures by which its performance is judged. I will use that five-part paradigm in describing all parts of the hospital. Chapter 5 and many following chapters also include discussion of some more complex, less settled issues where leading hospitals demonstrate their excellence.

Society has established, through law and tradition, two basic criteria for the actions of governing boards, including hospital governing boards. The first is that the yardstick of action is **prudence** and **reasonableness** rather than the looser one of well-intentioned or the stronger one of successful. Board members should be careful, thoughtful, and judicious in decision making. They need not always be right. The second is that the board members hold a position of **trust** for the owners. They must not take unfair advantage of their membership and must to the best of their ability direct their actions to the benefit of the whole ownership. In for-profit corporations, this means avoiding situations that give special advantage to some owners, particularly the directors themselves. In not-for-profit corporations, this means the board members must attempt to reflect the needs of all individuals in the community who depend upon the institution for care.

Purpose

The basic purpose of the governing board has already been stated: the board is accountable to the owners and must attempt to identify and carry out their wishes as effectively as possible. Two long and relatively clear traditions, one for-profit and the other not-for-profit, amplify this deceptively simple statement. It is fair to say that the differences between the two forms of organization are clearer at the governing board level than anywhere else.

In the for-profit tradition, the focus is upon maximizing profit. Board members, usually called directors, are compensated for their efforts and are usually given strong financial incentives for success. Subject to legal restrictions designed to protect the owners, directors may choose to maximize profit in either the long or the short run. They should select among opportunities for expansion on the basis of the profit expected. They may sell all or part of the assets whenever that is the most profitable course of action. They may discontinue all parts of the business and liquidate the assets when profit can be enhanced by investment in some other area or activity.

In the not-for-profit tradition, the owners are the members of the community served. Although this is a less precise concept, it is assumed that assets should be protected, although not necessarily enhanced through profit making, and used for the health care needs of the community. The governing board members are called *trustees,* reflecting their acceptance of the assets in trust for the community. They are rarely compensated except for out-of-pocket expenses. It is illegal and unethical for them to benefit financially as individuals. They should expand in directions that best fulfill community health care needs. They may sell assets or discontinue services only when these are no longer necessary, and there are important legal barriers to their liquidating or transferring the entire assets of the hospital.

The responsibilities that the governing board assumes must always be met, but surprisingly many hospitals have no governing board as such. These are hospitals owned by larger units, such as churches, government agencies, universities, and multihospital systems. A committee or group (rarely an individual) in the larger organization performs the essential board functions in such a situation. As a generalization, the more the responsible group is organized like, and thinks of itself as, a governing board, the more successful this solution will be.

Some multihospital systems have divided the governing board's responsibilities between a local board and the central corporation. Such forms of divided responsibility are still evolving, but there appear to be two keys to their success: total clarity and completeness in the division of responsibility. No board function may be omitted or left ambiguously to both groups.[1]

Functions

In both legal and organization theory, responsibility can never be completely delegated. Thus one statement of the governing board's responsibilities is that the board is responsible for everything that goes on in the hospital, as well as things that did not go on but might reasonably have. Under this theory, whether a hospital has an advanced perinatal treatment center or no obstetrics unit at all, the board is responsible for the decision and its consequences. Whether an employee or doctor wins worldwide acclaim or works impaired by drugs, the board is responsible. Whether the organization thrives or fails, the board is responsible. In fundamental and inescapable ways, these statements are true. No one active in hospitals should ever forget the ultimate, all-inclusive responsibility of the governing board.

On the other hand, the all-inclusive viewpoint seems to contradict the foundation of bureaucratic organization, which is to subdivide tasks to allow for many participants and to gain the benefits of specialization. While the board may be responsible for delivering babies safely, the plain fact is that most board members know nothing about delivering babies. This dilemma can be resolved by looking at responsibility as a multidimensional concept and finding those elements which can be done best by each participant. Then the list of functions of the governing board is the list of things it can do best. With the governing board and many other units, the list of functions begins with those activities *only* it can do.

Many writers have tried to list unique or appropriate board functions. Their lists reflect the diversity of opinion across the nation, the developments of thinking over time, and the subtlety of the question. Several common themes have emerged, however, and there is now little or no disagreement about the following list[2] of essential functions:

1. Appoint the chief executive.
2. Establish the long-range plan.
3. Approve the annual budget.
4. Appoint members of the medical staff.
5. Monitor performance against plans and budgets.

In addition, most analysts feel that board members function as resources for the organization, although they have different perspectives on the nature of these resources. (The question is discussed later in this chapter.)

Appoint the Chief Executive

Most members of governing boards have only limited time for the hospital. The typical board member has a full-time occupation and volunteers his or her services to the hospital. She or he will serve only a few years and will be replaced by someone else. Board decisions are made by committee, whereas implementation requires an individual. All of these factors—the competing obligations of board members, the lack of continuity, and the need for an individual to implement the will of the majority—demand an executive. Rarely, if ever, can the executive's job be done by volunteers. Thus in all but the very smallest hospitals, there is a full-time paid executive. It has become fashionable to refer to this person as the **chief executive officer** (CEO). In the largest hospitals, there is an executive office consisting of the CEO and up to several dozen deputies and support staff.

The functions of the CEO are developed in detail in chapter 6. They are far-reaching and critical, making the selection of the CEO an extraordinarily demanding board decision. In summary, the CEO selects and supervises all other employees of the hospitals, coordinates the design and operation of the governance system and the other four systems, and represents the board internally and externally. Although appointment of the medical staff is made directly by the board, the CEO makes critical contributions, as will be described below. The CEO is literally the agent for the board and in important senses is the servant of the board. The CEO acts for the board in all emergencies and countless small, unforeseen events, where he or she must divine and do what the board would have wanted. The CEO generates almost all the internal facts the board sees and influences what external facts are brought to the board's attention. Finally, the CEO is often the only person in the community professionally trained in health care delivery. That training covers technical questions of need, demand, finance, quality, efficiency, law, and government regulation that are not included in the training of doctors, lawyers, or business persons. As such, the CEO is the sole routine source of information in this complex and rapidly changing area.

Appointing the chief executive is actually a two-part function: it involves the selection of the CEO and the development and maintenance of a sound working relationship later.

Selecting the CEO. Many persons would say selecting the CEO is the most important decision a board will make, principally because of the impact the CEO has on other board decisions. The decision is also exceptionally difficult. It involves judging the future skills of individuals, always a hazardous undertaking. It is made without the assistance of a CEO, whereas other decisions have the benefit of her or his counsel. It is made infrequently, and the people who make it may never have selected a CEO before.

How does a board make such a difficult decision? The best way is to follow with extra thoroughness and care the rules that improve all high-level personnel decisions. There should be a description of duties and responsibilities, even though for this job they are ambiguous. The job description should be translated into selection criteria identifying the desired skills and attributes of the individual. The priority or importance of these criteria and the ways in which these skills will be measured in specific applicants should be specified.

The job description should include typical CEO functions (see chapter 6), but it should also be tailored to the long-range plan, because the plan identifies directions the board believes are important. Selection criteria are derived from the available personnel pool (also discussed in chapter 6) and the needs developed in the long-range plan. Sometimes the board is seeking a CEO because it is dissatisfied with the long-range plan, so a key part of the new CEO's job would be to develop a plan. The criteria in such a case would emphasize planning skill.

A wide-ranging search for applicants should be undertaken. Large hospitals usually search nationally, or over large regions. "The best possible training and experience" is now preferred as a criterion over "knowledge of local customs." For most U.S. hospitals, the law requires not only equal opportunity on the basis of race, age, sex, and handicap, but affirmative action in seeking candidates disadvantaged on those grounds. An unbiased procedure relying on the judgment of several people should be used to select among the applicants. Formal reporting of independent opinions is often sought, both to encourage conformation to the selection criteria and to avoid bias. The interviews and activities used to acquaint the board with the candidates must also be used to acquaint the candidates with the job opportunity and convince them to accept it if offered.

Given the rigor and complexity of these procedures, it is not surprising that many boards fail to follow them completely. To the extent that they fail, they rely on good luck to find the executive they need. Increasing numbers of boards have found that using consultants trained in executive recruitment is effective. Consultants have substantial experience with the process, knowledge of how to complete the procedures efficiently, objectivity regarding local history, and familiarity with candidates and their demands. They lack knowledge of local needs. Like any other group of people they differ in skill and motivation, but their record can be assessed by talking to previous clients. Evaluating consultants is easier by far than evaluating executives.

Board-CEO Relationship. One way to minimize the difficulties and risk of CEO selection is to keep a sound relationship with the current CEO. While this is obviously a complex matter, there are four guidelines for improving the effectiveness and prolonging the tenure of CEOs. Not surprisingly, these are similar to the guidelines for all participants in bureaucratic organizations.

— *Actions, procedures, and assignment of responsibility should be consistent.* The governance structure of even a small hospital involves a dozen or more people and relates frequently to perhaps 100 others. Written records, formal procedures, and adherence to consistent traditions are necessary for such a large group to work effectively together. The bylaws of the board specify these procedures, and well-run hospitals adhere to their bylaws in order to gain predictability. Many people become impatient with such formality. A hospital can establish a deliberate tradition of informality, but only within certain formal constraints.

— *The board and the chief executive should agree upon short-term (usually one-year) goals and expectations and should review progress toward them at the end of the period.* The expectations for the CEO are more ambiguous than those for others in the organization, and they are also more subject to unexpected outside influences. They must occasionally be revised radically in midcourse. Even in extreme cases, however, it is far easier to evaluate the accomplishments of the CEO when the desired directions have been established in advance. The expectations for the CEO are related to the goals of the institution as a whole. They emerge from other activities of the governing board, particularly establishing the long-range plan and approving the annual budget.

— *The board and the CEO should have a mutual understanding of the employment contract.* There is always a contract between the board and the chief executive. The formality of that contract depends upon the situation, but more formal, written contracts have become popular in recent years.[3] The contract should specify any departures from the usual duties of the CEO, mechanisms for review of performance, and compensation and ways in which it can be changed. It also should state the procedures for terminating the relationship, including appropriate protection for both the hospital and the CEO. Properly performed, the hospital CEO's job is now and always has been a high-risk one.[4] Thus even handshake agreements should include appropriate protection if the CEO must leave the institution.

— *Compensation should be based upon market conditions and contain incentives for effective performance.* As a general rule, the only fair and reasonable guideline for designing a compensation package is the marketplace, that is, what the institution would have to pay a similarly prepared person and what the person could earn in similar employment elsewhere. This statement is true for all employees, but particularly for CEOs. The high visibility of the CEO in the community and her or his relatively high income tempt unsophisticated board members to use other criteria, but these are likely to encounter difficulty. The value or contribution of a CEO to the hospital is almost impossible to determine. Comparison to other personnel in the hospital is therefore problematic. No matter how much others earn, if a similar position would pay more elsewhere, the executive is underpaid; if his or her pay is higher than anyone else would offer, the community's money is being wasted. The marketplace used to determine pay should be the same one used in the selection procedure. For almost all large hospitals, and for increasing numbers of small hospitals, this is the national market for people trained and experienced in hospital management.

Compensation includes payments in addition to salary that frequently are unique to the CEO. A compensation package can consist of a salary, the employment benefits offered to all employees, special benefits offered the chief executive, the terms under which bonuses and merit increases will be paid, an agreement on the disposition of any incidental income the CEO might earn as a result of related professional activity, and an agreement on both voluntary and involuntary termination compensation. Special benefits usually exploit both the mutual interests of the hospital and of the CEO and the income tax laws. Many different items can be included, such as payment of housing, transportation, education, association and club membership costs, and deferred income provisions. Bonuses and achievement incentives are more common in for-profit hospitals, but they are spreading among not-for-profit institutions. Annual reviews and merit increases are now routine, even where no prearranged bonus has been established. In the review the CEO is rewarded for his or her efforts toward the agreed-upon goals, the amount determined by board members who consider the overall success of the institution and the contribution of others as well.

Establish the Mission and Long-Range Plan

Modern corporations work by a process of goal setting, assessment, adjustment, and achievement. They repeat this process many times and in many ways, striving for three ideal conditions:

— The goals of the organization as a whole are those which the larger society will appreciate and reward.

— There is for each unit of the organization a readily visible goal that is consistent with the goals of the organization as a whole.

— The process of assessment and adjustment is carried out in a way that maximizes achievement.

No organization ever achieves the ideal. Good organizations are competitive on all three conditions, and those which fail significantly on one or more of the ideals tend to pass from the scene. Success requires frequent attention. Organizations that do well spend more time communicating and coordinating goals among units, and more thought and effort determining what society will appreciate. They assess and adjust more frequently at all levels. It is the weaker organizations that treat the goal-defining process as busy work, or irrelevancy. Goal defining in the well-run hospital begins with the establishment of the mission, continues through the amplification of the mission into a long-range plan, further develops and tests the reality of the plan with a carefully developed financial plan, and uses the two plans to guide annual budgeting exercises, which establish all the closed systems parameters for individual work units. The board is involved at both the beginning and the end of this process, but the well-managed hospital focuses the board's attention on the initial steps of mission setting and long-range planning in order to improve the consistency and efficiency of the process.

Setting the Mission Statement. The first step toward these ideals is the identification of an explicit mission for the hospital. Responsibility for the mission statement rests almost exclusively with the governing board and superior organizations in multihospital systems. The mission is only infrequently changed. It is developed from the functional definition of the hospital as a community resource by specifying more exactly the community served and the scope of activity. Mission statements distinguish one hospital from another, and the quality of the mission statement is a hallmark of good management. Too broad a mission makes planning decisions difficult and potentially inconsistent. A more serious problem is that it can dilute limited resources to the point where no job is done well. Too narrow a mission can cause the hospital to overlook important community needs and opportunities. These usually are met by the competition, which may then supplant the original institution in other areas as well.

The mission statement should specify three things:

1. *Community*—What geographic, demographic, religious, or financial group is to be served? Under free choice of physician and hospital, the hospital often indicates an offer or an intent to serve a community. The measure of how well it actually serves that community is represented by its market share. A broad statement would be, "All the citizens of XYZ County and those who seek our care from elsewhere." A narrow statement would be, "All children (or some other limited population) who live in XYZ County."

2. *Service*—Clinical services almost always include acute inpatient care and at least some outpatient care. They are increasingly being extended to more outpatient activity, mental and substance abuse programs, chronic care, and prevention and health education. Hospitals are also extending their services beyond health-related issues to include residential care and social services, particularly for the aged. Some hospitals identify specialized missions or services such as teaching and research. Individual hospitals are usually constrained either by resources or market size from undertaking a comprehensive set of services. Multi-institutional systems operating over broad markets generally have the most comprehensive mission statements.

   A comprehensive service mission, representative of a well-run large hospital in a moderate to large city, might be, "Acute inpatient care that falls within the scope of all established medical specialties and multiple sites for primary care." Although this is in itself an extensive mission, large hospitals are now adding substance abuse programs, outpatient mental health, home and hospice care, and occasionally nonhealth services for the aged.

   A narrow statement, typical of the only hospital in a small community, would be, "Acute inpatient care for diseases routinely encountered and for procedures routinely undertaken by primary care physicians and general and orthopedic surgeons, with referral arrangements for diseases requiring more specialized physicians, facilities, and support personnel; ambulatory services for emergency and surgery; and assistance to private primary care physicians." More of these hospitals are also providing long-term care in nursing homes, and are expanding their missions toward nonhealth services for the aged.

3. *Financing*—Financial constraints should be explicitly stated. Breadth of mission is determined by the amount of unfunded or underfunded work the institution is willing to undertake, and it is often wise to set that amount annually. Thus a broad mission would be, "Provide services to the paying public at the lowest price consistent with long-term financial needs and provide charity care to the identified community to the extent resources permit. Precise allowances for financial need and charitable care will be established annually by the board of trustees." A narrow mission might be, "Services will be priced competitively but must earn the return on equity required by market conditions. Service will be offered to all those who can demonstrate sufficient resources."

Obviously the process of setting the mission is complex and political. A good mission-setting procedure is based upon an accurate and comprehensive view of the desires of the exchange environment and the interests of **stakeholders,** that is, those exchange partners whose views are sufficiently important to directly affect the hospital's success. The unique responsibility of directors or trustees is to pick, from all the possible things the organization might do, those that society will appreciate and reward most. The perspective they bring to the task is more that of an outsider than an insider. They rely on the CEO and the planning staff to amplify their insights into exchange needs and to describe what the organization needs to achieve potential goals. In the end, the trustees must balance what is wanted with what is practical.

Contributing to Long-Range Planning. In the well-managed hospital, the mission statement becomes the touchstone for judging the competing opportunities uncovered by a dynamic enterprise. As the planning process proceeds through more and more specific expectations in the long-range plan, fiscal plan, and budgets, the contributions of executive staff and line management, including the medical staff, increase and those of the board concentrate on maintaining consistency and responding to short-term changes in the environment.

Planning decisions are best approached by developing several scenarios. It is seductive but dangerous to focus on a single scenario, design ways to implement it, and evaluate the difficulty and rewards.

Developing multiple scenarios involves technical rather than policy questions and should be left to planning staffs or consultants. At the level of the long-range plan, scenarios can be quite abstract and ambiguous. Although one part of the long-range plan is a statement of specific, agreed-upon activities to implement the mission, an equally important aspect evaluates potential **strategic opportunities.** These generally involve quantum shifts in service capabilities or market share, usually by interaction with competitors or by very large scale capital investments. Mergers, acquisitions, and joint ventures are generally strategic opportunities. Like the more unilateral proposals for future activities, strategic opportunities require careful evaluation. Since they often are triggered by events external to the hospital, and since they often require rapid decisions, the governing board of the well-run hospital quietly but thoroughly evaluates the more probable strategic scenarios in advance and is therefore prepared for prompt action when required.

Virtually the entire management group contributes to the planning cycle. The chief executive, the chief financial officer, clinical leader, and a staff of the governance system dedicated to planning and marketing make especially important contributions. The processes by which these contributions are made are described in detail in chapters 7 and 8; the contributions of the individual systems are described in their respective chapters.

Approve the Annual Budget

The budget is the final step through which the mission and the long-range plan are translated into reality. Like the long-range plan, the budget is a detailed, complicated construction that requires substantial staff work and several months to complete. (The details of preparing the annual budget are described in chapter 8, because in most hospitals they are coordinated by the finance group.) The board is involved at two critical points in the budget development. At the outset, board committees are deeply involved in establishing guidelines for the budget. At the conclusion, board committees make the final choices among competing opportunities, and the board as a whole approves the finished budget. Final approval may be anticlimactic; a well-managed budget process conforms to the guidelines and settles the questions before the full board's approval.

All the plans of a well-managed hospital are implemented through its annual budgets, which specify in advance the resources to be expended and the results expected. The budget includes both operating and capital expenditures. In the best hospitals it is being broadened to incorporate the full array of closed system parameters discussed in chapter 3, including demand, efficiency, quality, revenue, and profit, as well as costs and outputs. The role of the board, implemented mainly through its planning and finance committees, is to provide general short-term guidelines and to check the final proposal for consistency with mission and plan. Since the procedures through which the budget is developed stress the mission and plan as well as the guidelines, inconsistency is rare. There will be, however, important decisions among strongly defended alternatives which the board must resolve as the community's or stockholder's agent.

Budget Guidelines. The budget requires effort by almost every member of the well-run hospital. To coordinate such widespread activity, the board sets desirable levels of key financial indicators, called **budget guidelines:**

1. The total expenditures of the hospital, including total employment and compensation of employees
2. The pricing structure, and with it both the total revenue of the hospital and the amount to be paid out-of-pocket by local citizens
3. The surplus, or contribution to owners' equity, determined by items 1 and 2
4. The expenditure on new programs, plant, and capital equipment, and with these much of the cost increases that will occur in future years
5. The amount of indebtedness to be incurred

Trustee Roles in the Budget Process. Quality, scope of service, and cost are determined by the annual budget. For example, hours of operation affects access to care; number and type of staff affect waiting time; expenditures on supplies and maintenance affect amenities offered; and investments in education, capital equipment, and information systems affect the technical quality of many aspects of care. Well-run hospitals use the budget exercise as a way of eliminating conflicts between quality and productivity—the board's insistence on basic levels of quality forces management to seek innovations, which often improve both quality and productivity.

In addition to these considerations, there are important people-oriented concerns. The annual budget is also the point at which the subgoals and specific targets of the many parts of the hospital are clarified, coordinated, and communicated to members of the organization. The exercise is therefore the primary vehicle not only for implementing the long-range plan, but also for communicating it to all members of the organization and hearing from them their views on the difficulties and opportunities it might present.

Specific, focused, two-way communication is an attribute of all well-run hospitals, and budget discussions are the most important avenue for such communication. If the budget does not reflect the views of team members, it can destroy the concept of a team. Communication between the board and other members of the hospital occurs principally at the upper levels, with board members rarely talking directly to lower-level supervisors. Yet persons on every level can appreciate the interconnection between the long-range goals and the activities proposed for the coming year and can enter their comments on how those activities affect their specific area of expertise. The board provides leadership by example. It encourages comment from executives and makes it clear that the views of even the lowest ranking members are thoughtfully evaluated.

The effective trustee or director approaches annual budget decisions with five questions in mind:

— How well does the budget proposal reflect the mission and long-range goals?
— How well does the budget incorporate basic standards of quality?
— How appropriate are the specifics of the budget to the needs and desires of the community?
— Has the process of developing the budget fulfilled the need for two-way communication at all levels?
— Has any new information affecting the long-range plan emerged?

Appoint Members of the Medical Staff

The fourth essential duty of the governing board is unique to hospitals. The governing board is responsible for appointing the members of the medical staff and is legally liable for failing to exercise due care, whether on behalf of the patients and the community or on behalf of physicians desiring to use the hospital. Although other kinds of organizations employ professionals, community hospitals generally allow doctors to use hospital resources while billing patients independently, thereby establishing a contract that is to the community's advantage as well as the doctors'. Members of the medical staff are granted the privilege of using the hospital (as defined in chapter 10), and the board must manage the granting of privileges in the owners' interest without unnecessarily impairing the rights of doctors.

The uniqueness of this privileges tradition and the social status accorded doctors combine to make this responsibility the most obscure of the board's five. All of the others have clear analogies in business and government and as a result are within the experience of many sophisticated Americans. Activities like the granting of privileges are rare. Admitting lawyers to the bar and granting professors tenure in universities are useful parallels, but they are limited and not many people know much about them. To the surprise of most lay people, medical staff organization is not formally taught in medical school. Thus new doctors arrive at the tradition almost as ignorant as new board members.

The systems for granting privileges are described in chapter 10. There are five specific points at which the board acts on medical staff recommendations. First is the approval of medical staff bylaws. Medical staffs govern themselves, but the trustees, in approving the bylaws, set the rules for self-governance. Second is the approval of the medical staff recruitment plan, a part of the long-range plan which indicates how many doctors in each specialty the hospital is prepared to admit to privileges. Third is the annual appointment of each doctor to privileges to use the hospital for certain specific kinds of cases. Fourth is the selection of the individuals who will implement the process of medical staff governance. Fifth is the establishment of mechanisms for communication between members of the medical staff and the board.

Underlying all five are some basic facts that heighten their importance. First, the hospital is not owned by doctors; rather it is an expensive capital resource made available to them by the owners in return for either profit or community health care. The board has an obligation to see that the owners receive fair value for the use of the resource. The courts have interpreted that obligation to include limiting privileges to the competence of each doctor. Second, very few doctors can survive economically without hospital privileges. Most would find their income severely reduced if they could not admit and care for patients in the hospital. To deny a doctor privileges is to invite him or her to leave the community. Third, a shortage of doctors in a community can be as serious as giving privileges beyond a safe level of competence. Access to a doctor with the proper specialization is as important to quality as the ability of the doctor. Fourth, many specialties require expensive capital and trained support personnel. If community demand is low, costs will mount drastically, and lack of practice will impair quality. Fifth, all doctors stand to lose income if there are too many doctors in a specialty. In short, the matter of medical staff privileges involves a sensitive balance of quality and economic interests.

Despite the difficulties these facts suggest, effective systems can be designed and operated in such a way that doctors, administrators, and board members enjoy a mutually rewarding relationship. Not surprisingly, these systems recognize the complexity of the issue, emphasize frequent, candid communication, build upon their own history and tradition, and assume the good intentions of all parties. That is to say, successful medical staff relationships have the same foundations as any other successful human relationship.

The key to medical staff organization is the concept of peer review. Since only doctors can effectively evaluate the technical services of doctors, medical staffs are obligated to review each other's performance and tell the board whether acceptable quality is being maintained. Doctors originated the concept of peer review, and have implemented and improved it over the years. Much of the collective wisdom of peer review is embodied in the publications of the Joint Commission on Accreditation of Hospitals.[5]

Approval of Medical Staff Bylaws. In each hospital, the procedures of peer review and medical staff governance are written into bylaws. These documents have substantial legal importance. Most lawyers believe that sound, well-implemented bylaws are the best protection against litigation, either for malpractice or for unjustifiable denial of privileges. Bylaws must be revised regularly, with advice of counsel, and approved by majorities of both the medical staff and the board. The CEO frequently serves as coordinator and resource for the maintenance of the bylaws and is the board's authority on the issues involved. The CEO should have a detailed understanding of the usual contents of bylaws and the implications for the hospital of various alternative provisions. Board members should rely on the CEO and legal counsel to deal with most of the issues involved. The better the process of revision, however, the more likely it is to raise issues that will require board action.

Although bylaws are procedural rather than substantive documents, certain procedural issues have profound substantive content, and the trustee relies primarily upon the chief executive and the medical staff leadership to identify these issues and their implications. Such issues arise frequently in questions of departmentalization, which indicates the groupings and the levels that must undertake peer review; membership and medical staff committees addressing quality and efficiency of care; methods of selecting and compensating medical staff leadership; and medical staff participation in planning and governance activities, including staff representation on the governing board. In each of these matters, trustees should solicit the advice of medical staff members and their chief executive but should reach an independent decision, one that best represents the needs of the owners. Risk management and the use of quantitative data to assess quality and appropriateness of care are emerging as critical issues in medical staff management. The authority of the executive to collect and report these measures should be stated in the bylaws.

Approval of Medical Staff Recruitment Plan. One of the areas most likely to distinguish the well-managed hospital is sophisticated medical staff planning and recruitment. Well-managed hospitals decide the appropriate numbers and specialties of doctors to be given privileges based on careful forecasts of community demand. The **medical staff recruitment plan** is a fundamental element of the long-range plan because it establishes both the size of the medical staff and the services the hospital must provide. Each medical specialty requires certain kinds and quantities of hospital support services, and, conversely, most hospital services require certain specialties on the medical staff. Each service must attract sufficient volume to support its fixed costs at a price the community can afford. Each individual doctor must have enough work to maintain his or her skills, and the group must generate enough demand upon support personnel that they too remain proficient.

The plan is normally developed by the planning staff, with extensive consultation from the medical staff. It is submitted to the governing board for approval along with the general plan, but because of its central position it usually receives individual attention. The medical staff should not approve the plan, because that action might constitute a potential antitrust violation: the doctors can be voting collectively to restrain entry of other doctors into the local community.

Trustees must weigh four questions in adopting the plan:

— Whether sufficient volume will exist to maintain skill levels of doctors and support personnel

— Whether the estimated cost of the proposed service is consistent with community desires (specialized health services being rarely unavailable)

— Whether the proposed service is consistent with others offered by the hospital

— Whether the community's funds can better be spent on some other objective, whether in health care or some other areas

Once the plan is adopted, it guides the recruitment efforts of the medical staff and the executive. Although there appear to be adequate numbers of physicians entering practice, the best doctors can always choose where they will go. Thus the best hospitals always recruit, recognizing that the first step to effective medical staff relations and to quality of medical care is to attract good doctors who are sympathetic with the hospital's goals and method of operation. Being competitive in recruitment usually requires significant financial investment. Doctors are financially assisted in a variety of ways at various times in their careers. Funds for this support become part of the budget and are approved as part of the recruitment plan.

Annual Appointment of Physicians. Good practice now limits the appointment of each physician to a 12-month term. Rather than being automatic, reappointment requires a positive action. The bylaws establish both the criteria for and the process of annual appointment to privileges. In all cases, final responsibility for the appointment rests with the board of trustees. Annual appointment follows a review of all areas of contribution to the hospital's goals, but the emphasis is on the quality of care given individual patients. Community hospitals, except for government hospitals, are not required to appoint or reappoint any physician. (Hospitals owned by governments must appoint any licensed physician but may restrict privileges to areas of demonstrated competence.) All hospitals are required to follow due process in the granting of privileges, however. In addition to fair and reasonable procedures, *due process* means four things:

1. Adherence to the hospital's own bylaws
2. Assurance of adequate supporting facilities and trained personnel
3. Avoidance of discrimination based upon race, age, sex, or (in most cases) religion
4. Avoidance of restraint of trade

Well-run hospitals generally make a probationary or restricted privilege appointment of qualified physicians and move them to clinically appropriate privileges as soon as they have demonstrated their ability. Permanent status should reflect a long-term commitment on the part of both the hospital and the doctor. Most physician reappointments are unchallenged. In these cases, the principal role of the board is to assure adherence to the bylaws. The chief executive is usually held accountable for this assurance. There are several cases, however, in which board review must address more substantive issues.

— *Appeals.* Most bylaws require the governing board to hear appeals of staff members dissatisfied with their privileges.

— *Quality of care.* The board must, under its obligations to the community, deny privileges recommended by the medical staff if basic standards of quality are not being met. These cases are typically brought to the board's attention by surveyors from the JCAH, the board's chief executive, or concerned individuals on the medical staff.

— *Availability of service.* The board must not grant privileges for specialties or kinds of patient care which are not adequately supported by other clinical resources. The number of doctors in each specialty and the kinds of privileges must be consistent with the medical recruitment plan, the long-range plan, and the annual budget.

The well-run hospital makes every effort to avoid cases requiring substantive board review. When they occur, they are expensive and difficult for the hospital as a whole. They also raise the personal liability of the trustees. Clearly, effective privileges review procedures in the medical staff and effective planning for the hospital as a whole and for medical staff recruitment help prevent such cases. Trustees of well-run hospitals can normally expect their executive and the medical staff leadership to have minimized the occurrence of appeals and case-by-case considerations of quality and service.

Appointment of Medical Staff Leadership. The medical staff organization of even a small hospital has committees for peer review, education, and representation. These committees are also the major channels of communication between the medical staff, nursing staff, and other clinical services about issues of clinical policy, issues ranging from levels of training for nursing and other personnel, to the drugs kept in inventory, to methods of dealing consistently with informed patient consent to treatment. Many of these committees also comment on aspects of the long-range plan and the budget. They constitute part of both the accountability hierarchy and the collateral organization, as defined in chapter 4.

Each committee requires a chair and a secretary. Although one person can fill both roles, there are advantages to having two people, and possibly also a vice-chair. The quality of the work these people do directly affects results. Good leaders set agendas, prepare individual members for meetings, encourage compromise and mutual understanding, introduce fresh ideas, discourage frivolous behavior, and keep good records. The effectiveness of the medical staff structure thus depends upon the skills of the individuals in leadership positions.

Medical staff leaders also play an increasingly direct role in assessment and control of quality. Through risk management, utilization review, and outcomes quality concerns, sophisticated information systems are being developed. One role of staff leaders, for which they may be held accountable, is the setting and achieving of expectations on these measures.

At the same time, the medical staff organization can be viewed as a collective bargaining organization for doctors. From that perspective, the best leader may be the person who understands the doctors' viewpoint best. Thus members of the medical staff and the board may disagree not only on the specific people who should lead, but also on the criteria for leadership. In practice, successful hospitals resolve this disagreement in two ways. They seek people who meet both criteria (and there are usually many), and they identify other opportunities for representation of and communication with the medical staff, as discussed below. Boards of successful hospitals have steadily increased their influence in selecting medical staff leadership within this framework: many key clinical leaders are appointed by the board, serve at the board's pleasure rather than for a fixed term, and are employed by the hospital for this service. Boards of well-managed hospitals enter actively into the final stages of selecting medical staff leadership, relying on the CEO to ensure that well-qualified nominees arise from the medical staff.

Communication with the Medical Staff. Good bylaws consistently applied and reasonable leadership are indispensable to sound relations between medical staff and governing board. Yet the successful hospital does not limit its communication with medical staff to quality of care and clinical issues. It also ensures that the economic and related concerns of its doctors are heard. This is usually accomplished by involving doctors in the "business" decisions of the hospital, particularly the long-range plan and the portions of the budget dealing with capital equipment and new programs. Chapter 10 describes an emerging form of medical staff that strengthens both the involvement and the accountability of members.

In the mid 1980s the list of issues requiring close communication is longer than usual, but some such list will always exist. Board members will have to resolve the conflicts that list represents. If they yield too much to the doctors' perspective, the cost of care may mount and quality of care may suffer. If they demand too much of the doctors, shortages of doctors may result and, ironically, quality may suffer. While answers to complicated questions do not come easily, successful boards do follow some useful rules. They make sure doctors understand both what the current issues are and how new ones can be raised. They encourage flexibility and innovation in dealing with issues. They strive to be fair and even-handed. They gain consistency by relying on their own long-range plan. They forestall many disputes by involving doctors in some of their activities: developing the mission, appointing the CEO, approving the budget, and monitoring progress.

Monitor Performance Against Plans and Budgets

The board is responsible for performance as well as planning, so it must monitor events in the hospital. It its first four duties are carried out effectively, however, monitoring becomes a very small part of its activities. The board compares actual events to the established expectations and considers deviations, if any, in the light of changing expectations. All other matters are left to the CEO.

The goal is never to reach the point where the deviations are unacceptable. If they are, a major failure has occurred. The board is then obligated to identify clearly what has gone wrong and why. There are only four general reasons why, although several of them may occur at once:

1. There has been a major change in the environment. Such changes are usually widespread and affect many hospitals or other enterprises.

2. The long-range plan, the annual budget, or the medical staff bylaws are inconsistent with current community needs.

3. The processes by which these documents are communicated and implemented have failed.

4. The board has altered its perceptions of either the hospital's goals or its own role in implementing them.

Usually a painstaking reexamination must begin with the long-range plan. The question of retaining the CEO should usually be examined. When changes in board perceptions are suspected, board membership, orientation procedures, and organization need review. In all cases, the demands upon board members' time mount drastically.

Resource Functions of the Governing Board

The five major functions listed above are by no means the only possible ones. The list can be lengthened by subdividing these five. It also can be lengthened by including functions that some hospitals leave to the executive, such as public relations and fundraising. Board members frequently want to help the hospital, therefore a list of what they actually do is much longer than a list of what they must do.

Another way the list is lengthened is by adopting a different perspective on the board's role. If board members are viewed as resources for the hospital as well as decision makers and representatives of the community, three functions must be added to the initial list. Although each of the additional functions has merit and many board members perform them well, they have to be ranked as less important than the five decision-making functions. Among the three, board members as influentials is probably the most important.

Board Members as Influentials. One resource function stems from exchange theory, which holds that the board represents access to resources the hospital must acquire in order to succeed. Thus, board members must know people who can give large sums of money, have entry to political offices where the hospital can be helped or hurt, and be able to speak for the hospital at other centers of community power, such as the boards of major employers. In short, board members are influential people who use their influence to help the hospital achieve its mission.

Board Members as Spokespersons and Donors. Board members are expected to exhibit loyalty to their organization and to speak well of it whenever possible. In that sense, all board members participate in public relations. Some individuals are so well known that the use of their names is in itself an endorsement; thus their first service to the hospital is simply the lending of their names. Similarly, some board members can afford to make major gifts to the hospital. There is an old, largely vanished tradition that board members provide the major charitable support for the hospital.

Board Members as Specialists. A slightly different theory of board decision making holds that board members are selected for their particular skills—in law, finance, medicine, and so on. Such people are expected to contribute their professional perspectives to board deliberations rather than or in addition to a general understanding of community needs and values and broad experience making complex decisions.

Difficulties with Resource Perspectives of Board Responsibility. The three resource-oriented functions obviously have merit. Many board members are selected because they can contribute in one or more of these ways. The resource perspective raises some potential difficulties, however, if it is allowed to substitute for or replace the orginal list of functions.

The theoretical case against substitution is simple: the decision-making functions of board members are not fulfilled. However, it is possible for nearly all the decision-making functions to be performed by the management staff, including physician leaders. A few well-run hospitals and many for-profit corporations operate very successfully this way. Some insider consensus of doctors and executives sets the long-range plan, adopts the budget, establishes and supervises peer review, and even appoints the chief executive. The insider-based board, in general and in hospital applications, can be criticized for its lack of insight into the long-term needs of its exchange partners. Because of the complexity and sensitivity of their services, hospitals are particularly vulnerable to the dangers posed by lack of such insight. Thus a board of donors and influentials alone, lacking the input of outside views, may overlook hidden perils.

A more likely difficulty of decision making by insiders is lack of consensus. Internal teams have, by design, diverse viewpoints. When conflict exists, it frequently takes a third party to resolve it. That third party is de facto the board. A similar situation exists when the CEO post becomes vacant. The group which selects the successor is the board de facto. While exceptions can be found, even successful ones, the board members of most organizations must be prepared to fulfill their general obligations.

The case against adding the resource-oriented functions to the decision-making ones is clear-cut. The time required of trustees goes up as the list of functions is expanded. Hospitals would be forced to seek a wealthy, influential volunteer who was knowledgeable about his or her community, experienced in making difficult decisions, skilled in an important profession, and interested in the job. Such a demanding list of criteria would result in very small boards because few persons would meet all of them. An important consideration in selecting board responsibilities is to keep the job within limits that make it attractive. Impracticality has already driven "wealthy" from the list; few board members now contribute large amounts of their own funds. "Skilled" is clearly the next to go. All the necessary skills can be purchased, and there are important benefits to hiring consultants outright rather than confusing consultant and board roles. "Influential" remains an important attribute and should be considered when choosing board members.

Selecting Members

The capability of the board of directors or trustees may be the central factor in a hospital's success or failure. Well-qualified boards tend to make sounder decisions, and they encounter less difficulty when they present their case to others in the community. They attract well-qualified hospital executives and doctors, as well as other well-qualified board members. The success of boards depends more on the combined skills of a team than on the star qualities of one or two individuals. Thus success feeds upon itself. The issue of board membership is a continuing search for qualified, interested members, followed by ongoing programs to help those members make the biggest possible contribution. This section discusses selection criteria, selection processes, education, and support for hospital boards. It also addresses three special issues of membership: conflicts of interest for board members, supplements to boards to increase community representation, and roles for doctors and CEOs on boards.

Criteria for Membership

Skill and Character. The first criterion for board membership should be ability to carry out the five functions of the governing board described above. If the board is well chosen by this criterion, the community will have a hospital closely tailored to its needs and wants. Without question, such excellent hospitals exist. Their doctors and managers are capable, and their board members bring to each meeting good judgment based upon an acute sense of the directions the community as a whole would feel were appropriate. What characteristics predict these critical skills?

— *Familiarity with the community.* The *raison d'être* of community boards is their ability to relate hospital decisions to local conditions. This means insight into how much money the community should pay for hospital care, how to recruit professionals to the community, how to attract volunteers and donations, how to make community members feel comfortable in their hospital, and how to influence local opinion and leadership. Most communities are comprised of many different groups whose views on these questions differ. A board can accommodate differing viewpoints both by having representatives of different groups as members and by having members whose grasp includes the diversity of the community. Desirable board members are those whose understandings transcend their own sex, race, and social group. (See the discussion of the representation criterion, below.)

— *Familiarity with business decisions.* Most board decisions are multimillion-dollar commitments. They are measured and described in business terms. Hospitals are part of the commerce of the community and therefore must communicate in the common languages of accounting, business law, finance, and marketing. Techniques for evaluating decisions use these languages and incorporate increasingly sophisticated forecasting and statistical analyses. The hospital board room, like other board rooms, is a place where technical language is frequently used to communicate complex concepts. Thus board members need to be familiar with the languages and styles used to make these decisions. There is also an emotional component to multimillion-dollar decisions. Although concepts from household management are important, and householders can make excellent board members, moving from hundred-dollar decisions to million-dollar decisions takes some practice. Both for familiarity with the languages and for psychological preparation, previous experience at decision making is important.

— *A record of success.* Candid managers will confess that selecting people for any job is difficult, and selecting them for jobs like board membership is exceptionally risky. The best predictor of success is a record of success. More important than experience or formal education is how well the person has done on similar assignments. This indicator is important after the individual has joined the board, as well. Effective members should be promoted to higher board offices. Reliance on achievement is also a way of overcoming biases in board membership. Becoming familiar with the community and with business decisions takes both time and access to opportunity, so boards selected solely on those criteria will be heavily middle-class and middle-aged. The success criterion opens the door to the young and the poor, who have proven their ability to join governing boards.

— *Reputation.* The general reputation or character of an individual is important in two senses. First, like the record of success, it is an indication of what the individual will do in the future. Second, it serves to enhance the credibility of the individual. A person with a reputation for probity frequently gains influence because of that reputation. What she or he says is received more positively. Boards have a legal obligation for prudence. The appointment of people whose reputation is suspect could be construed as imprudent.

Representation. By law and tradition, the community hospital is an institution for persons of all races, creeds, and incomes. Most Americans seem to disapprove of "two classes of hospital care." Federal law prohibits hospitals receiving Medicare funds from excluding people on the basis of sex, age, ethnic origin, or handicap. There is less agreement that the way to get a successful "one-class" hospital is to have representation from all the identifiable constituencies that make up the community. However, some people believe a good board would have representation from the poor, from important ethnic groups in the community, from labor as well as management, and so forth. The concept of representation can be extended to include hospital employees, doctors, religious bodies involved in ownership, and other groups.

There are appealing arguments for a representation criterion. It is impolitic to disagree with representation from groups that have supplied most of the resources for the hospital. Representation was embodied conceptually in national health planning laws. Many people support the political argument that only a member of a certain constituency can understand truly how the hospital treats that group. And constituencies are usually pleased by recognition at the board level.

Several caveats must be attached to the representation criterion. Most important is that a representative who lacks the necessary skills and character is unlikely to help either his or her constituency or the community at large. Second in importance, the board acts *by* consensus *for* the community as a whole. A board composed of representatives of each sex, ethnic group, and socioeconomic group could easily fail because the individuals could not integrate their constituencies' views to a reasonable whole. The concept of representation tends to foster adversarial positions and compromise instead of consensus—and the compromise process may be inferior to consensus. Third is the problem of tokenism. A seat on a board, particularly a single seat, does not necessarily mean influence in the decisions. Finally, the appointment itself changes the individual. The lessons of the board room are not available to his or her constituents, and over a period of time, the board member loses the view for which he or she was selected. Cooptation and tokenism can be deliberate adversarial strategies to diminish a group's influence.

Diverse viewpoints from the community are usually helpful. There are individuals from all walks of life who can appreciate the needs of others as well as they can articulate their own and who are willing to join in an effort to maximize the common good.

Affirmative action, that is, ensuring that competent individuals are not excluded from board membership, is encouraged under the law and seems likely to make hospitals more successful. A balance can best be struck if two points are kept in mind:

1. Board members are appointed as individuals. They should be competent to serve in their own right, regardless of their position in the community.

2. Board members act on behalf of the community as a whole. This does not rule out special considerations of groups with unusual wants or needs, but it places those considerations in a context—they are appropriate to the extent that they improve the community as a whole.

Representation on the board is not the sole vehicle for assuring that the hospital is responsive to special needs. Many planning and marketing techniques can do so. The board may survey or establish other direct communications with special groups. Finally, and perhaps most important, surveys of patient and visitor satisfaction can be routinely incorporated into the quality assessment. Both the clinical system and the plant system should use satisfaction surveys routinely.

Influence. If the viewpoint that board members can influence the hospital's access to resources is valid, then board members should be selected on the basis of their influence. There is evidence that hospitals which can gain support from various parts of their communities do better than hospitals which cannot.[6] What is missing is evidence that successful hospitals have such difficulty gaining access to resources that they need to select board members on the basis of influence. Successful hospitals may have influence because they are successful, that is, because they have provided services that the community needs and wants. In that case, the most influential board members are those who can carry out the general responsibilities of trusteeship, and selection should be based upon that ability. It is also true that able people tend to be influential people. In sum, although influence enhances the attractiveness of otherwise qualified candidates and the possibility of occasional appointments to gain specific influence must be borne in mind, heavy emphasis on an influence criterion does not seem warranted.

Selection Processes

Selecting board members involves issues of eligibility, terms, offices, committees, and the size of the board as well as the actual choice of individuals. Officers and committee chairpersons have more power than individual members, so their selection is equally important.

Appointment to Membership and Office. The most common board structure for community hospitals is the *self-perpetuating.* Other methods include election by stockholders, the prescribed procedure in stock corporations, and election by members of the corporation, who sometimes are simply interested members of the community. Boards of government hospitals are frequently appointed by supporting jurisdictions or, rarely, through popular vote. Boards of community hospitals in multihospital systems, where they are formally designated, are usually appointed by the parent corporation, sometimes with local nomination or advice. The board elects its own officers and its successors. In addition to the officers, there are a number of committee members and chairs to be appointed, a job usually left to the incoming chair.

Role of the Nominating Committee. Nominees are usually asked beforehand if they will serve. On most boards and similar social structures, truly contested elections and overt campaigning are rare. Many hospitals nominate only one slate for boards and board offices. Although formal provisions for write-in candidates and nominations from the floor exist, they are rarely utilized and usually fail when they are. The existence of these provisions and the fact that they can be successfully used in times of extraordinary need is an important safeguard in the corporate structure. However, in the normal course of events, selection occurs in the nominating committee. The committee often proposes not only board members, but also corporate and board officers and occasionally chairs of standing committees.

The nominating committee is usually a standing committee with membership at least partially determined by the bylaws. It is common to put former officers on the nominating committee. Such a strategy emphasizes continuation of the status quo in the organization, so organizations wishing fresh ideas broaden nominating committee membership and charge it with searching more widely for nominees. It is typically in the confidential discussions of the nominating committee that individuals are suggested or overlooked, compared against criteria, and accepted or rejected. This makes the nominating committee one of the most powerful groups in an organization. Sophisticated leaders generally seek membership in it, or at least a voice in it. A key test of power in an organization is, "Who nominates the nominating committee?"

Size, Eligibility, and Length of Terms. The number of nominations to be made each year is a function of the number of board members and the length of their terms. The number of new members nominated depends upon these factors and also upon the rules of eligibility. There is little consensus on these issues. Board sizes range from a handful to a hundred, although between 10 and 20 members is probably most common. Terms are generally three or four years, and there are usually limits on the number of terms which can be served successively. Lengthy terms or unlimited renewal of terms can lead to stagnation—and it is difficult for the nominating committee to pass over a faithful member who wants to serve another term unless the rules forbid it. Too-short terms reduce the experience of officers as well as members. (It is possible to allow officers to extend their service beyond the normal limits.) Inexperienced officers rely more heavily on the CEO, thereby increasing his or her power, but the entire board is more prone to error because of its inexperience.

If there are 15 members, three-year terms, and a two-term limit, there will be five nominations each year, but many of these will be proforma nominations for second terms. Only two or three new people will be added in most years. The median experience of board members will be about three years. (Some members will not serve two terms, of course.)

In addition to a length-of-service eligibility limit, many hospitals have eligibility clauses related to the owning corporation. For-profit boards can require stock ownership. Church-sponsored hospitals, even when they are operated as secular community institutions, can require that board members be from the religious group. Some government and voluntary not-for-profit hospitals require residence in the political jurisdiction for board membership. Other eligibility clauses include phrases like "good moral character," although so much judgment is implied that they are more selection than eligibility criteria.

Education and Support for Board Members

Successful hospitals have both formal and informal programs for the education of board members. Even if new members meet the selection criteria perfectly, there are several unique aspects of hospital management in general that they should be taught. There are also issues unique to the particular institution. While new members should bring fresh perspectives, they should not operate in ignorance of history.

Formal programs are limited principally by the time available to incoming members. They include tours, introductions to key personnel, conveyance of written documents and texts, and planned conversations and presentations. A typical list of subjects is shown in figure 5.1.

To be effective, formal programs for board members should follow certain rules. Brevity is essential. Small segments should be scheduled for each specific topic. Most important, the member should be a participant. Questions should be encouraged, the style should be conversational, and the discussion should be extended over several sessions.

Most of the education board members receive is on-the-job. Well-organized boards make committee appointments carefully, allowing new members to become acquainted with the organization in less demanding assignments. They fill chairs with experienced members. They use chairs and hospital executives to help members learn as they serve. The three critical committees, executive, finance, and long-range planning, should be composed of the more seasoned board members, and their chairs should be members nearing the end of service. The nominating committee is frequently the last service of a board member.

Special Issues

Three issues of board membership have become prominent in many communities. They are issues on which there is room for substantial difference of opinion, but in each case a national consensus appears to be emerging. The latter two, doctor and CEO membership on boards, are philosophically related to the first, conflict of interest, but are more potent politically in most communities.

Figure 5.1

Outline for Orientation of Trustees

Mission, Role, and History of Community Hospitals
Difference between for-profit, not-for-profit, and government ownership
What hospitals give to the community
How Hospitals Are Financed
Operating funds
Private insurance
Government insurance
Uninsured patients
Charity care
Capital funds
Donations
Use of earned surplus
Sources of long-term debt
Hospital-Physician Relations
Nature of contract between doctors and hospitals
Concept of peer review
Trustee responsibilities for the medical staff
Approving bylaws
Annual appointments
Maintaining communication with the medical staff
Need for communication
Why communication should go through channels
Duties of Trustees
Appoint the CEO
Approve the long-range plan
Approve the annual budget
Appoint the medical staff
Monitor performance
Legal Issues in Trusteeship
Trustee liability
Trustee compensation
Conflict of interest

Conflict of Interest. The law and society assume that members of governing boards are serving on behalf of owners and that they should not serve when their personal interests conflict with the owners'. Conceptually, this is clear enough. A member of one for-profit board would not serve another company competing for the same markets. Someone who sold one competing product would not be trusted to act for the buyer. In practice, difficulties crop up quickly. The local banker meets all other criteria for board membership—should the community deny the bank the profits of the hospital account, or deny itself the benefit of the banker's volunteered service? The mayor's wife is knowledgeable, popular, and successful. It happens that she and her husband own a tract of land critical to the hospital's future expansion. Should she be invited to serve on the board? Unfortunately, the criteria for board membership make it likely that situations analogous to these will arise frequently. It is hard to find people who meet the skill, character, and influence criteria but have not also become involved in activities that eventually will conflict. Most board members will themselves have analogous conflicts. They would tend to invite these individuals to serve.

The problem assumes a slightly different dimension when considered from the perspective of those who want broader constituency representation on hospital boards. The banks and the powerful are represented too well, and the poor and the disadvantaged are overlooked, they feel. One way to advance their cause is to argue that people serving on boards should be free of identifiable conflict. They would say the banker and the mayor's wife should not serve on the board. At its heart, this is often a special-interest position, the special interest being the poor or some other identifiable group.

The problem of conflict of interest is not unique to hospitals. It is inherent in any governance structure, and it cannot be permanently resolved in a democratic society. (Totalitarian structures resolve it by giving the rulers special rights.) Most communities find practical solutions on a case-by-case basis, judging whether the benefits to the community outweigh the possible cost of self-interest. Guidelines like the following help:

— Potential conflicts of interest should be recognized at the outset, for example at nomination or at the formation of a committee. Major, recurring conflicts should be listed in formal documents.

— It is the moral obligation of each individual to search for and declare his or her conflicts and also to comment on any conflicts of others that are not publicly declared.

— It is the privilege of any member to challenge or question unmentioned possible conflicts. Observing this privilege includes protecting the challenger from retribution.

— Individuals are normally excluded from participating in actions that involve their conflicting interests. For example, the banker would not participate in selecting the hospital's bank, or in reviewing the bank's services; a landowner would not vote on the purchase of comparable land.

— Exceptions may be made with the consent of the majority and within the limits of the law (government hospitals are more frequently limited by legal restrictions). Exceptions are presumably made to benefit the community. For example, a landowner might serve on the long-range planning committee, particularly if a majority of the board thought the owner might be persuaded to donate the property to the hospital.

— Individuals with such extensive conflicts that their service to the hospital would be impaired are not appointed.

CEO Membership. Because their principal livelihood is from employment at the hospital, most CEOs have fundamental conflicts of interest in serving on the board. The conflict is particularly apparent when possibilities for merger or closure of the institution are considered. It also occurs when other employees or doctors present grievances against the CEO. Although less obvious, the CEO can influence the board by controlling the information it receives, (including the minutes) and by her or his role in suggesting the agenda.

Despite this, there has been a steady trend toward appointing CEOs to the board and even toward giving them prominent offices, such as chair of the executive committee or president of the corporation. The justification for this lies in the same rule governing other conflicts, that the community's potential benefit exceeds its potential loss. The arguments commonly used are the following:

— The structure that combines the office of president and CEO is part of what is called in hospital jargon the *corporate model*. This model is commonplace in industry and works well there. The president and CEO is always a voting member of the governing board.

— In an increasingly complex world, volunteer and part-time board members are not as well qualified as the CEO, who is both full-time and professionally trained.

— Status as an officer of the corporation is necessary if the CEO is to represent the hospital effectively to employees, doctors, patients, and the outside world.

— The CEO needs the influence or authority of the expanded title in order to act on the community's behalf. Other board members can still carry out their five decision-making functions on behalf of the owners, and the potential dangers to the community can be effectively monitored.

The case is not proven, but it certainly is popular. Competitive pressures of various kinds develop when some hospitals take a step of this kind and others do not. Further, there is little or no evidence of negative results: it appears that competent non-CEO board members can monitor the hospital's performance effectively whether the CEO is on the board or not.

Physician Membership. Physicians practicing at the hospital also have clear conflicts of interest. The national consensus, however, is even clearer for physician than for CEO board membership; in fact, the JCAH has recommended it. The arguments generally cited in support of physician membership involve representation:

— The board needs to hear the viewpoint of doctors.

— Doctors need to know their views are being expressed.

— It is wrong to exclude doctors who are otherwise qualified for board membership.

It is sometimes argued that the board needs the expertise of doctors (their knowledge, as opposed to their viewpoint). This argument is irrelevant, because a board can and does invite any experts it requires into its deliberations.

As in other cases of special-interest representation, a hospital may face serious competitive pressures if it does not appoint doctors to its board. Also, there is no clear evidence of harm to the thousands of hospitals that have made such appointments. In many cases, seats are set aside for doctors and nominations are solicited from the medical staff. It is not uncommon for the medical staff to elect its representatives to the board. Usually only a few seats are available to doctors, however.

The question of doctor membership on hospital boards is essentially resolved, but the resolution leaves behind some new problems. All of the general caveats about representation apply here. Most seriously, one or two doctors cannot reasonably represent the view of all doctors on important issues. They are not technically knowledgeable outside their own specialties, and their economic and political views are influenced by their specialties as well. Family practitioners and primary care doctors generally earn more of their income outside the hospital than surgeons, are paid less overall, collect less from health insurance and more from patients directly, and are paid more on the basis of day-to-day services than on episodes of illness. It is unlikely that a surgeon would effectively represent a family practitioner on important board issues, or that any family practitioner would feel reassured being represented by a surgeon.

In short, the placing of one or two doctors on a board in no way fulfills the responsibility of the board to communicate with the medical staff. Other mechanisms must still be found to ensure communication across the broad spectrum of medical skills and interests.

Supplementing Board Membership

A board can use any adjunct or supplementary group it wishes. Most boards use consultants for specialized knowledge, but the better ones also use committees, work groups, and task forces to obtain opinions from the community. Groups to assist in meeting the needs of minority constituencies, committees to expand physician input into key decisions, and task forces to explore major issues of mission and future direction are common examples. In addition to these special-purpose groups, many boards appoint nonmembers to standing committees.

Taking steps to involve outsiders has three important advantages:

1. It expands the opportunities for hearing diverse views, meeting some of the objections raised by advocates of representative board membership.
2. It allows the board to make clear the hospital's needs and opportunities, and in so doing build public understanding and consensus.
3. It provides an opportunity for future board members to gain experience and familiarity with the issues.

Supplementary groups are completely legal so long as the final authority and responsibility of the board are kept clear. They can be as formal or informal, permanent or temporary, specialized or general as desired. Their flexibility is another important advantage. Thoughtful use of such groups seems to be a key to success for hospitals.

Organization of the Board

Committee Model

The most widely accepted governing board organization, particularly in not-for-profit hospitals, is the committee model. It is popular among government hospitals, and seems to have had its origin in parliamentary or congressional government. It balances the wisdom of incorporating many viewpoints from the community against the practical limits on individual trustees' time. A group of board members may focus upon a set of related topics such as facilities planning, medical staff relations, or finance. (Although committees can be as small as a single individual, such a practice is rare.) In the process of their deliberations, they may use a variety of communication devices to garner a broad spectrum of views which they then condense into a report and a recommendation to the board as a whole. The final action of the board can be pro forma if committee discussion has been thorough and conclusive.

Deciding what committees exist, who is on them, and what issues will be referred to them, is a key source of influence. In the traditional version of the committee model, that privilege is reserved to the chair of the board of trustees, with the consent of the board as a whole. The CEO and her or his staff frequently advise the chair and gain influence by providing staff assistance to the committees.

The committee model has several strengths. The use of committees and subcommittees allows the hospital to involve as many individuals outside the board as desired in each kind of decision. The limited time of board members is enhanced by delegating specific tasks. The limited scope provides training for beginners. Delegation allows large numbers of individuals to evaluate proposals and small groups to focus on designing the review process and making the final decision.

The most serious weakness of the committee model is its lack of speed. Many issues must go through several committees. If the logical sequence of the committee discussions is the same as the scheduled order of the meetings, the issue can be handled promptly. Unfortunately, if delays arise or the meeting sequences are not convenient, multiple committee review can consume several months of time. A second weakness is that some members of the board as a whole may be impelled to repeat the work of the committee. To the extent that this occurs, the process becomes dangerously inefficient.

Corporate Model

An alternative theory of organization is referred to as the **corporate model.** The corporate model apparently springs from the prevailing styles of large industrial and commercial corporations. It is more prevalent among for-profit hospitals, but interest in it has been growing in all hospitals. The CEO rather than the chairman of the board decides what issues will be on the agenda, subject to board approval, and structures committees and subcommittees as he or she thinks appropriate. The CEO may ask board members or subordinates, or both, to serve on specific committees. Assignment of an issue to a single individual is more prevalent under the corporate model. Reports to the board are channelled through the CEO and are frequently presented in the form of recommendations. The executive is often empowered to implement much of the result, simply reporting actions to the board for its information.

The strength of this model is speed and flexibility. Although the board may assert itself in committee design and may overrule any specific action, it rarely finds this necessary. The results of analysis and committee work are accepted, and the attention of the board moves to more fundamental and obscure issues, advising the CEO on emerging and future issues of importance.

In the extreme, the corporate model denies the need to involve the community directly in the decisions of the hospital. Advocates of the model do not believe community opinion is irrelevant, just that community involvement in decisions is less important than professional execution. They note that community and customer views are better represented by surveys, complaints, and market share than by the speculations of board members. They point out the increasing complexity of decisions and the need for technical skills to analyze alternatives.

Blended Model

Well-managed hospitals have been evolving toward the corporate model, for several reasons. Increasing technical complexity has forced boards into more global and abstract decisions. The role of staff in preparing and analyzing alternatives has grown. The authority of line managers has steadily increased. If anything, these trends are accelerating. On the other hand, it is not difficult to blend the committee and corporate approaches, and the best hospitals seem to succeed because they do this effectively. A **blended model** has the following characteristics:

— The board has several standing committees which are used to review proposals and gain insight into differing viewpoints. In general these committees parallel the major responsibilities of the board. There is a planning committee, a finance and budgeting committee, and a committee on medical staff relations. An executive committee is responsible for monitoring and oversight and works closely with the CEO.

— The board has the right to create ad hoc committees and usually has several at work on timely issues. Ad hoc committees may report to the board as a whole, but they more commonly report to standing committees. Particularly complex questions go through several committees.

— The CEO and her or his staff are responsible for environmental assessment and surveillance, for analysis and development of proposals, for background knowledge, and for understanding the needs of the community. They are principally responsible for identifying issues. If an issue is not identified in time for appropriate action, the CEO may be criticized. (Under the committee model, no specific individual is accountable for failing to identify an issue.)

— The amount and intensity of debate decline as proposals take shape and are referred to higher-level committees. Staff are used extensively, both to gather facts on disputed issues and to negotiate or eliminate conflicts. (Meetings of the full board can be reduced to formalities, if desired.)

— Any issue can be delegated to the CEO to pursue, with authority either extended to implementation or limited to recommending solutions to the board.

— Responsibility for monitoring the flow of activity can be assigned either to the executive committee, strengthening the role of the board, or to the CEO, strengthening the executive. Proposals and opportunities requiring decisions must be ranked according to their importance. The most critical can be assigned more board involvement; the less critical are given entirely to the CEO.

The flexibility and power of the blended model are appealing. The model can utilize the volunteered contributions and the diverse viewpoints of the citizens of the community to the full extent of their interests and skills. At the same time, it assigns clear responsibility for the operation of the system, first to the executive committee to set and monitor the agenda, and second to the CEO to identify issues. (The board as a whole can serve as the executive committee, if desired.) With thoughtful management of the agenda, the blended model can closely resemble a committee model with expanded CEO responsibilities. If circumstances require, it can be moved closer to the corporate model: in the extreme, only formal approval of plans, budgets, and bylaws and the selection of the CEO need the direct attention of the board.

Measures of Board Effectiveness

Organizational performance must be measured in relation to realities rather than ideals. Thus the essential question in assessing the board's performance is whether owners' wants have been filled as well as other realistic alternatives would permit. The board's functions clearly imply that it is an interface between the hospital and its exchange partners. Pursuing the notions of realistic achievement and interface leads one to suggest that there might be two basic categories for measuring board performance. The first, analogous to outcomes, consists of measures of how well the community identified in the mission was satisfied. The second, analogous to process, consists of evidence on how well the organization performed in meeting its own expectations. Measurement problems within the community satisfaction category are much more severe, but the measures are more fundamental. Measures in the achievement category are the same as those used for the evaluation of the chief executive and the components of the organization, but the board has failed in its role as interface if the agreed-upon expectations are not routinely achieved. For example, initial failure on a typical closed system expectation such as labor cost or process to quality falls somewhere within the accountability hierarchy. Repeated failure is likely to be traceable to the governing board.

Measures of Community Satisfaction

The board is to a large extent self-governing. Other than financial audits and inspection by licensing and accrediting agencies, there is no routine surveillance. It is therefore incumbent upon the board to have a rigorous program of self-assessment. The central theme of this self-assessment is the extent to which community wants have been satisfied. The basic measure of satisfaction is the willingness of doctors and patients to use the institution at a price that recovers the full economic costs of service. These two components, willingness and cost recovery, are measurable. It can be said that the institution, and therefore its governing board, was successful when the percentage of people in the community seeking service either increased or remained at a satisfactorily high number and when all costs of doing business, including an appropriate level of profit, were met. The two key measures are *market share* and *profitability.*

Direct measures of market share and profitability are outcome measures of governing board and organization performance. However, they are relatively slow-moving and as a result are poor indicators of potential improvement. The wise board, therefore, supplements them with more responsive measures. Measures underlying market share directly assess access and the satisfaction of major exchange partners—customers, third parties buying on customers' behalf, and members. Measures underlying profitability assess price acceptability, competitors' prices, costs, and financial stability.

The measures that can be developed by expanding the concepts of market share and profitability are shown in figure 5.2. Data on market share and community costs per capita are difficult to come by because they require information on the activity of other providers. Other measures of figure 5.2 are readily available from the information systems of well-managed hospitals.

It is desirable for governing boards to set expectations for themselves on their performance. An annual report on the measures, including historic trends, would provide a basis for setting expectations. The process is likely to be more rigorous and more effective if an effort is made to quantify improvements anticipated in the coming year. Well-managed hospitals undertake such reviews with increasingly thorough staff preparation and increasingly specific expectations. Properly, such a

Figure 5.2

Indicators of Governing Board Performance

Profitability
Pricing
  Price comparability to competing institutions
  Price acceptability to third-party purchasers
  Price acceptability to patients
Costs
  Comparative costs per episode of service (per discharge, per visit)
    Current values for this hospital and competing hospitals
    Percent change from preceding year
  Community costs per capita (costs per community member for hospital
    care
    Current values for this community and similar communities
    Percent change from preceding year
Profitability
  Bond rating
  Debt-equity ratio
  Funds available for capital and new programs
Access
Changes in size and scope of service of this hospital and competing hospitals
Patient Satisfaction
Hospital market share
  By community group (age, economic, ethnic, and so on)
  By kind of service (inpatient, outpatient, long-term, and so on)
Satisfaction surveys (issues of costs, access, amenities, quality)
  Current patients
  Potential patients (community residents)
Donor Satisfaction
Responses to fund drives
  Wealthy individual donors
  Corporate donors
  Community fund drives
Physician Satisfaction
Number of doctors terminating privileges
  Transferring to other hospital
  Leaving community or retiring
Number of doctors newly privileged in community
  This hospital
  Only at other hospitals
Satisfaction reported by physicians
  Formal surveys
  Informal surveys
  Complaints received
Employee Satisfaction
Vacancy statistics
Turnover, grievance, and absenteeism statistics
Employee satisfaction surveys

review is done at the start of the hospital's annual budget cycle. Introspective review of this information and information from environmental surveillance identifies necessary revisions to the mission and long-range plan and identifies the general goals guiding the hospital's budget activity.

Measures of Achievement of Closed System Expectations

Measures of community satisfaction lack diagnostic content; they reflect what has happened but give little insight into why it happens or how to change it. A study of the closed system performance frequently suggests opportunities for improvement.

The search for measures of effectiveness of the governing board begins with the measures used as goals by the operating units of the hospital. Under the theories of management outlined in chapter 3, each unit of the hospital should be accountable to a superior unit, with quantitative expectations and routine reports of progress. This accountability hierarchy ends at the board. A great many such measures are generated in the modern hospital. Despite efforts to limit the amount of information from the monitoring function, too much information is a more pressing danger than too little. The burden can be kept manageable by adopting the same rules for reporting used elsewhere in the organization:

— Reports should focus on aggregate measures, subordinating or removing components appropriate to lower levels of the organization.

— Every measure reported should have an established expectation, tolerance limits of variation from the expectation, and highlighting if actual variance exceeds the limits.

— Most measures should be handled well below the board level. Unsatisfactory deviations from expectations should reach the board only rarely.

— Reports should be organized according to the major objectives of successful operations. Responsibility for preparing the report should be assigned to units of the governance and financial systems. The following major topics can be summarized in a few pages each:

  • Financial position
  • Revenue and cost
  • Clinical quality and appropriateness review
  • Service volumes and environmental changes

- Progress reports on ad hoc committees and ongoing projects

Preparation of these reports is discussed in the appropriate chapters. Most expectations used in the reports should be set as part of the annual budget. Expectations for the progress reports are set when the charge is written. Expectations for environmental changes are forecasts, and attention must be drawn to situations in which the environment did not behave as predicted.

In well-run hospitals, it is rare for these reports to be anything but confirmations of planned progress. Even when deviation occurs, sound management requires that the responsible executive have at least one period to correct it. Boards of well-run hospitals spend most of their time gathering and sharing intelligence about the community. The energy of well-managed hospitals is devoted to setting expectations rather than monitoring achievement—in other words, to planning rather than fixing.

A well-managed board reports on the progress of its own deliberations. That is, the charge of every board committee contains an expectation as to schedule and progress reports. Reports of achievement against this timetable are usually most relevant for the chair and chief executive but should be available for discussion by others if necessary.

Encouraging Effective Performance

Strategies for a Well-Managed Governing Board

Governing board service in any bureaucratic organization is difficult. The board's role as an interface, sorting and ranking the complex information from the external environment and the conflicting views of the exchange partners, and its responsibility for the most critical questions of the organization create a demanding situation. In hospitals, the relationship to the medical staff increases the difficulty. There appear to be two important strategies to help governing boards improve their performance. The first is an orderly timetable of events, and the second is reliance upon the chief executive or, in some cases, the chief executive plus some or all members of the executive committee. The role of these individuals is to pay extra attention to matters of process and board performance.

An Orderly Timetable. Boards generally meet quarterly or monthly, and their activities should be synchronized with the annual budget process. Many predictable events precede the adoption of the budget, and the well-managed hospital can therefore expect an annual cycle to its board meetings. If the budget is adopted in the last quarter of the fiscal year, board activities by quarter will follow this pattern:

— Quarter 1, receipt of the annual report; environmental assessment, review of the mission statement, review of corporate position, and developments in strategic opportunities; consideration of amendments to the long-range plan; amendment of the long-range fiscal plan reflecting changes in the environment and in the plan.

— Quarter 2, establishment of budget guidelines for the forthcoming fiscal year, pursuant to specific items arising from quarter 1 activities, and response to issues raised by management and medical staff.

— Quarter 3, attention to issues arising from the external environment.

— Quarter 4, approval of the annual budget and selection of new members and officers.

Given that some matters will always require additional time and that much of the work of the board must be done in subcommittees, this schedule constitutes a moderate demand on board members. Focusing on planning and expectations not only makes board membership feasible for busy people, it also moves the board into the proper leadership position. In reality, unexpected events often disrupt this timetable. It presumes, for example, that the chief executive will not be replaced during the year and that external opportunities occur neatly in the third quarter. Even if it is honored more in the breach than in the observance, the timetable is still useful. It schedules the necessary reports and debates that must take place in the internal organization. It reduces the danger of taking piecemeal or unilateral action on opportunities that should be studied in the context of a long-range plan or strategy. Finally, by concentrating the budget decisions in a single quarter, it imposes a discipline on management and the medical staff which is likely to be constructive.

Role of the Chief Executive. Because board membership is usually voluntary and board members have other important obligations, it is important to have someone charged with continuing attention to the processes of board management. Normally this is the chief executive, although in small institutions it may be the chair, aided by one or two key members. All board members have an obligation to identify issues arising from their personal experience and constituencies. They can and should rely on the chief executive and his or her small group of assistants to see that everything possible is done to make it easy for them to fulfill these obligations.

The board should expect CEO assistance in procedural areas. A good CEO anticipates all board issues and is prepared, particularly in the following areas:

— Review of the membership of the board, advice on its improvement, facts about possible candidates, and suggestions of individuals for the nominating committee

— Advice to the chair on a development program for each individual and accessibility to all board members for specific questions

— Advice on the committee structure, including both standing and ad hoc committees, and on the use of nonboard members

— Specific recommendations for committee charges and timetables

— Environmental surveillance and suggestion of issues needing attention

— Concise but complete position papers identifying issues and providing factual background on them

— Willingness to accept the corporate model responsibilities of the CEO, including acting in lieu of the board and resolving issues referred by the board in a manner consistent with the board's intentions

All of this can be summarized in the statement, "One role of the CEO is to make the board look good." When the board looks bad, the CEO is automatically implicated. If the problem is severe, the CEO frequently is discharged.

Failures of Governance and Their Prevention

Well-managed hospitals encourage board performance by pursuing the timetables and procedural matters identified in the preceding section and by foreseeing and forestalling difficulties. Despite their best efforts, they occasionally encounter problems; less well run organizations tend to encounter the same kinds of problems more frequently and in more serious forms. There are no easy solutions, but several common causes of these failures can be identified.

— Membership failures:
  • *Representation.* The views of the board drift toward some groups in the community, such as the current medical staff

and board members, or families under age 65, or families with health insurance. Adequate management must represent all the legitimate owners and meet the needs of a sufficient market to permit efficient operation.

- *Judgment.* Because of excessive turnover or poor selection, board members lack the knowledge and experience for their roles.
- *Motivation.* From lack of training or poor selection, board members fail to recognize the seriousness of the decisions.
- *Attendance.* From unrealistic assessment of time commitments, board members, particularly committee chairs, are absent from key meetings.

— Structural failures:

- *Overcentralization.* Because there are too few committees or some committees are ineffective, power becomes concentrated in a small group within the larger body.
- *Overdelegation.* Too many committees debating each question involves so many people that peripheral views get excessive attention and decisions are no longer made expeditiously.
- *Individualism.* Board members forget that their authority derives only from consensus and that they serve all owners rather than a special-interest group. (When board members act as individuals, they automatically become executives; conflict with the appointed executive is an immediate danger.)

— Process failures:

- *Identification of issues.* Critical trends are not identified quickly enough to deal with them satisfactorily. It is the chief executive's obligation to identify critical issues, but a badly managed board can ignore the executive's warning. Board members are also able to identify issues, and the well-managed hospital encourages them to do so.
- *Inadequate staff preparation.* The CEO and executive staff fail to present concise, complete descriptions of problems and analysis of facts.
- *Poor control of agenda.* Ineffective management of agendas omits key viewpoints, fails to specify the opinions solicited, or allows committees to delay projects by inaction or by spending excessive time on less critical functions.

- *Repetition.* The board recapitulates debates and decisions of subcommittees unnecessarily.

Well-managed hospitals devote considerable attention to preventing these kinds of problems and to containing them when they occur. Troublefree performance is an ideal, achieved only by rigorous attention from the chief executive and the board leadership. The various difficulties and their corrections are interrelated. If motivation is weak, an extra effort to clarify the question and present the background concisely may help. If a standing committee has exercised questionable judgment, an ad hoc supplement may be in order. If recapitulation of debate has no other benefit than to ease the pain of defeat for a major constituency, it may be the right action.

Notes

1. Sisters of Mercy Health Corporation, *Integrated Governance and Management Process, Conceptual Design* (Farmington Hills, MI: SMHC, 1980).
2. Anthony R. Kovner, "Improving the Effectiveness of Hospital Governing Boards," *Frontiers of Health Services Management* 2 (August 1985): 4–33. See also commentaries by Robert F. Allison, Robert M. Cunningham, Jr., and Douglas S. Peters.
3. Witt Associates Inc., *Contracts for Health Care Executives* (Oak Brook, IL: Witt, 1984).
4. David M. Kinzer, "Turnover of Hospital Chief Executive Officers: A Hospital Association Perspective," *Hospital & Health Services Administration* 27 (May-June 1982): 11–33.
5. Joint Commission on Accreditation of Hospitals, *Accreditation Manual for Hospitals* (Chicago: JCAH, 1985).
6. Ivan Belknap and John Steinle, *The Community and Its Hospitals* (Syracuse, NY: Syracuse University Press, 1963).

Suggested Readings

Kovner, A. R. "Improving the Effectiveness of Hospital Governing Boards." *Frontiers of Health Services Management* 2 (August 1985): 4–33. See also in that issue commentaries by R. F. Allison, R. M. Cunningham, Jr., and D. S. Peters.

Shortell, S. M. and Kaluzny, A. D. *Health Care Management: A Text in Organization Theory and Behavior.* New York: Wiley, 1983. See especially L. R. Burns and S. W. Becker, "Leadership and Decision-Making," pp. 128–66, and R. D. Luke and B. Kurowski, "Strategic Management," pp. 461–84.

6

The Executive Office

The executive office complements the governing board and with the leaders of the other three systems constitutes the governance system. At the broadest level, the executive office is related to every activity of the hospital, since it must support the other parts of the governance system in order to carry out its direct responsibilities. The executive office is led by the chief executive officer. Much of the activity of the office is oriented toward completion of the functions assigned to the chief executive, and the office acquires considerable influence through its central position.

The functions of the CEO and the executive office are an inescapable part of any bureaucratic organization. The CEO is appointed by the governing board and selects her or his direct subordinates, including the chief operating officer (COO) and the chief financial officer (CFO), usually with advice from other governance leaders. The executive function may be contracted to an outside management firm, but the contract usually designates that the CEO be acceptable to the governing board. In very small hospitals, the job of CEO can be part-time; in these cases, it is usually held by someone who is also director of nursing or financial officer. Rarely, and usually ineffectively, executive functions are performed by volunteer board officers formally designated for the task. Most commonly, the executive function is directed by the CEO and carried out by a group of full-time employees organized into several activities.

Purpose

Most broadly, the purpose of the executive office is to implement the decisions of the board and to assist the board in making decisions. The executive office is responsible for all information and other support formally supplied to the board, for all implementation of board decisions, and for important relationships with the medical staff. It is also responsible for a number of outreach and boundary-spanning functions, such as public relations, government relations, and fund raising. The executive office has three jobs: it maintains effective commerce downward from the board to other systems, upward from those systems to the board, and outward to the external world. Effective commerce in this context must include whatever steps are necessary to fulfill exchange relationships supporting the hospital. Messages must be conveyed in both directions: intelligence, or environmental assessment, must report changing needs, and agreements must bring necessary resources.

There are two conflicting stereotypes that may confuse persons trying to understand what executives do. One is that the executive is a communications facilitator, bringing people together to discuss their problems. While this stereotype is an excellent start, it is incomplete. Discussion is not enough. Action must result, and it must be effective in terms of the exchange relationships. Executive responsibilities do not end until effective action occurs. The other stereotype is that the executive is the chief decision maker. In reality, decisions of great importance are made at every level of the hospital; the executive office makes no more decisions than other groups. The character of executive decisions is different, however, because these decisions frequently deal with very long-range issues.

The success of the executive function lies in decisions understood, implemented, and broadly accepted in the hospital, even though many people outside the executive office participated in making the decisions. It lies in changes foreseen far enough in advance to allow a smooth transition—crises avoided rather than crises resolved. The best hospital executives become almost invisible. So smoothly does the organization respond to the pressures of the outside world that the hand of the executive office in the response is noticed by only the most observant.

The purpose of the executive office sounds much simpler than it is. The subtlety and complexity of its contributions become clearer in the following review of functions, organization, personnel, performance measurement, and special opportunities and problems.

Figure 6.1

Functions of the Executive Office

Functions Supporting External and Board Relations
  Planning and marketing
  Public relations and fund raising
  Relations with other organizations
  Staff support for the governing board
  Managing the annual budget activity
Functions Supporting the Internal Organization
  Recruiting supervisory management
  Organization design
  Managing the information system
  Monitoring operations
  Maintaining the hospital disaster plan
Functions Supporting the Medical Staff
  Assisting in planning and recruitment
  Negotiating contracts
  Providing staff support
  Assessing attitudes and needs
  Risk management and surveillance of quality and utilization
  Acting in emergencies

Functions

The executive function in bureaucratic organizations has proven quite difficult to describe, although many texts have striven to make it clear (see, for example, the suggested readings at the end of this chapter). The unlimited scope of executive responsibilities is a major source of the difficulty: the executive can be held responsible by the board for almost anything the board chooses. A second source of difficulty is the collaborative nature of executive behavior. Rarely is anything done by the executive office alone; often members of several other units participate.

Admitting the difficulties, the need for communication and coordination demands that the general functions of the executive office be clear to other members of the organization and to the outside world. The responsibility for effective commerce upward, downward, and outward can be expanded into more specific functions, but it should be understood that in reality these functions are overlapping and blurred. Rarely does an executive do only one thing, for one group, or for one purpose. The functions discussed in this chapter and summarized in figure 6.1 constitute a description of the major areas to which the executive office contributes. It describes the kinds of things the executive office should do—that is, what an outsider, a doctor, an employee, or a board member should expect from the executive office. Most of these activities are dealt with in other sections of the book. The discussion here is limited to comments specifically about executive responsibilities.

Functions Supporting External and Board Relations

The executive office is staff to the governing board, and it carries out or assists with most of the contacts that represent the hospital to the outside world. These are vital strategic activities determining future mission, resources, constituencies, and, ultimately, survival. The chief executive acquires information and other resources through these contacts and negotiations, and they become one of the important sources of his or her influence.

Planning and Marketing. All large hospitals have (or have access to through multihospital systems) planning and marketing sections for environmental assessment, suggestions regarding the hospital's mission, development of the long-range plan and long-range fiscal plan for board approval, and identification, development, and coordination of specific proposals to implement the plans. In many hospitals, the planning and marketing section is also responsible for public relations, fund raising, and promotion. These functions are extensive and are developed in detail in chapter 7.

The governing board generally resolves planning and marketing decisions, at least to the extent of setting the general direction. Members of the executive office are frequently responsible for translating broad directions into specific expectations, acquiring the necessary resources, revising the organization structure, and other activities involved in implementing the board's decisions. They interact closely with the financing system, which retains direct accountability for long-term finance.

The chief executive makes important contributions to the success of planning and marketing. In the well-run hospital, he or she usually concentrates on the following four areas:

1. *Designing the planning and marketing system,* including defining the role of the planning unit, recruiting planning personnel, and coordinating that unit with other parts of the hospital.

2. *Setting the hospital mission,* particularly providing the governing board with a mature perspective on various possibilities.

3. *Providing counsel to the board,* aiding them in evaluating specific proposals.

4. *Sponsoring strategic proposals,* particularly those involving mergers, acquisitions, or joint ventures and those whose scope exceeds the normal activities of any one individual in the organization.

Public Relations and Fund Raising. The CEO and members of the executive staff are normally the public spokespersons for the hospital. They routinely present the hospital's mission, achievements, and needs to the community through speeches, meetings, and interviews. They also identify and establish communications with key individuals in the community—political leaders, business leaders, major donors, and important figures in religious, charitable, and cultural activities. Often the most successful individual relationships are established with potential leaders in each of these activities.

Funds for expanding hospital activities come from loans and gifts as well as past operations. The newer forms of corporate structure involve equity capital (stock and partnership agreements) as well. The CEO is generally expected to present the case for major new capital from any of these sources. Success frequently depends upon earlier general communication and individual relationships.

Larger hospitals appoint professional staff for public relations and fund raising. This staff is part of the executive office. Although it handles routine communications and relations with the news media and provides essential support for fund raising, it does not eliminate the need for direct participation of the CEO and other ranking officers.

Relations with Other Organizations. Most well-run hospitals now have relations with other corporations through holding companies, partnerships, or membership in multihospital systems. Communication with these bodies is frequently delegated to the departments directly involved, but the establishment, review, and revision of those relations is the function of the executive, usually subject to board review and approval. (Corporate bylaws generally require board action on any contracts that are over a certain size or that transfer major components of the directors' trust obligations. Contracts affecting ownership usually require the owners' approval, although trustees may be the only accessible body for voluntary community hospitals.)

When the hospital is owned by a multihospital system, the executive is frequently accountable to the system as well as to the local board. Even in not-for-profit chains, the executive is often hired by the corporate office and is expected to confer regularly with it on important executive functions. The central corporation often provides direct assistance with these functions and sometimes must approve the local board's recommendation.

Most states have regulatory activities of various kinds, and all community hospitals maintain voluntary accreditation by the JCAH or the American Association of Osteopathic Hospitals. Contact with these agencies may be delegated, but it is always coordinated by the executive.

Staff Support for the Governing Board. The CEO is the agent of the governing board in most transactions except her or his own appointment and evaluation. All of the support activity required by the board should be supplied through the CEO except the external financial audit and the hiring of consultants for evaluating or replacing the CEO. Providing these services is another important source of influence. Commonly the chief financial officer and several others in the executive group also spend significant amounts of time supporting the board.

In well-run hospitals, the CEO is in frequent, informal contact with board officers. The CEO always surveys the performance of board members individually and as a group, and suggests both new member nominations and committee assignments. He or she periodically reviews board bylaws and suggests revisions when appropriate. The CEO also supervises the following activities, which support the board functions described in chapter 5:

— Providing formal and informal training for each member

— Suggesting and transmitting the charge for most committees

— Suggesting the agenda of the board and its committees

— Preparing full documentation and recommendations for each item on the agenda

— Offering an oral briefing on each topic

— Preparing the minutes of board and committee meetings

— Communicating and implementing the board's decisions

When this job is properly done, each board committee consists of well-selected people, properly oriented. It meets on an agenda known well in advance, related to a specific charge, with both written and oral briefing, and with an executive recommendation. Minutes, communication, and implementation of action are automatic from the board member's perspective.

In addition to these formal responsibilities, the CEO accepts a professional commitment for the long-term operation of the hospital in the best interests of the community it serves. The CEO's obligation in this regard is stronger than outside board members' for two reasons. First, the CEO is employed principally, and often solely, to do the job. Most board members are volunteers whose own jobs occasionally take priority. Second, the CEO is usually the only board-level person with professional training in health care management. Understanding the role of the hospital in society, the contribution of health care to health, the programs of health care finance, the design of hospital systems and procedures, and the legal concerns unique to health care and tax-exempt organizations is included in such professional training. It is missing from the training of others, whether they be professionals in the law, clinical services, or business.

Managing the Annual Budget Activity. The well-run hospital relies increasingly on expectation setting, rather than expectation achievement, to improve. As described in chapter 4, virtually all the members of the hospital will be involved in expectation setting for most of the major parameters of the closed system model: demand, resources, output, quality, and productivity. By the time new expectations are set, they are fully understood and supported in such a way that they will almost always be achieved. Then the organization can reward achievement rather than correcting failure and can provide positive incentives for further improvement.

Although the budget began as an effort to establish resource requirements, costs, and revenues, it is becoming a general review of all aspects of performance for the next year. It tends to occupy about half the year for middle and upper management, the other half being devoted to identifying and designing improvements. As competition raises sharper questions about quality and appropriateness of medical care, the medical staff is being increasingly drawn into the budget cycle. (Details are described in chapters 11 through 15, with an overview from the finance system's perspective in chapter 8 and from the board's perspective in chapter 5.)

The process for establishing the operating budget and the new programs and capital budget is usually iterated two or three times in order to find the most attractive solution. Extensive collaboration of all line and staff units is required. Board involvement should be limited to the beginning of the process, when key operating parameters are agreed upon, and the end, when the best capital, new program, and operating solutions are adopted as expectations for the coming year. In particularly difficult situations, it may be necessary to solicit advice from the board in the interim, but excessive board involvement is evidence of a poorly running process.

The role of the executive is to coordinate the activities so that clear, realistic, and timely decisions are made. The following major steps involve the executive:

1. *Briefing for initial budget decisions*—In the well-managed hospital, the annual budget process is stimulated by an environmental assessment and followed by review and modification of the long-range plan and the long-range fiscal plan. The executive not only prepares factual analysis and commentary on these issues, but also makes a deliberate effort to involve key medical staff and management personnel. Specifically:

   a. The executive notifies the medical staff of the upcoming budget activity, with particular reference to cost and resource constraints, capital investment, and new programs allowances considered.

   b. The executive reviews the importance of the budget, the kinds of issues to be addressed, the procedures which should be followed, the timetable, and sources of assistance with all lower levels of management.

2. *Recommending levels for key budget parameters*—A hospital's annual budget has four related parameters:

   a. Percent change in expenditures for previously authorized programs

   b. Amount to be expended on new programs and capital equipment

   c. Percentage change in price, expressed as an overall average or as a percentage of change per discharge and per outpatient visit

   d. Net profit

   In addition, the executive should draw the board's attention to any potential environmental factors that might affect the forecasts. When these parameters are set, both the hospital's operating situation for the coming year and the cost that the community will bear are established. The executive recommends a value for each parameter to the board, usually the finance and the executive committees. Modification is likely, and the executive must identify what implications each change has for the balance of the parameters. The chief operating officer and chief financial officer generally lead the presentation.

3. *Developing and ranking a list of desirable new programs and capital investments:*

   a. Ideas for new programs, capital replacement, and capital expansion are identified by responsibility center managers and department heads and are developed with assistance from the planning and marketing section (see chapter 7).

    b. Proposals are then ranked within each department and section, and are later ranked by representatives of the medical staff. These rankings are compiled by the executive, and the recommendations of the CEO, COO, and CFO are attached.

    c. The proposals are submitted to the board, along with the various rankings and summary comments, for final ranking and funding.

4. *Developing the operating budget proposal*—The executive briefs medical staff leaders and employee supervisors on the process of developing the operating budget and explains how to coordinate several iterations of it. In each iteration:

    a. Each of the departments and responsibility centers of the hospital sets expectations for quality, demand, resources, costs, and prices.

    b. The finance section compiles the totals of these and compares them to the budget guidelines (chapter 8).

    c. The executive and finance groups identify potential difficulties, implications of the new programs and capital requests, and opportunities for further improvement; they then either return the budgets to the line managers or recommend the budgets to the board.

5. *Presenting a budget recommendation*—The executive is responsible for the final recommendation of the operating and new programs and capital budgets to the governing board. Under normal circumstances, the recommended operating budget must be consistent with the board's guidelines on budget parameters, and the new programs and capital budget would be consistent with the long-range plan. The executive should identify where serious constraints, risks, and objections to the recommendations lie and should discuss the implications of changes in budget parameters.

Functions Supporting the Internal Organization

Recruiting Supervisory Management. The CEO is normally responsible for management recruitment, retention, and training. Much of this responsibility is delegated through the other systems. Board advice is commonly sought for the chief operating officer, and board approval is required for medical staff appointments and the chief financial officer (see chapters 5 and 8). Recruitment and retention of all supervisory personnel is a matter of offering rewarding jobs, competitive salaries, and opportunities for professional growth. Good chief executives use the recruitment, promotion, and annual review intervals as ways of establishing a style of management and encouraging its continuity throughout the organization. Well-run hospitals generally have a style of participation, candor, fairness, and adherence to procedures which places them in a position to make key decisions before the need for them is critical. These elements of style are usually personified by the chief executive and emphasized by her or him as desirable behavior for subordinates.

Organization Design. The first executive concern is the design of the clinical system. This large group includes three-quarters of the people in the hospital, generates all the revenue, and provides all the care. The executive, financial, human resources, and plant systems must be organized to complement the clinical organization.

Both the collateral organization and the accountability hierarchy require the attention of the executive. As indicated in chapter 4, organization design is very much a collaborative process, one led rather than done by the executive. Within this context, the executive makes several contributions:

— *Specifying the process of organization change.* Process decisions would include the objective or opportunity, the timing, the length of debate, and the group to be approached initially for comment. The executive has several avenues for introducing innovations. Reports, position papers, and consultants can be used to document the need for change.

— *Establishing a style of openness and candor.* The CEO and the executive staff must express their commitment to candor frequently in words, reward it when appropriate, and make a scrupulous effort to avoid punishing it. Otherwise, members of the organization will hesitate to bring out their most serious concerns and their most innovative ideas.

— *Guiding and encouraging discussion.* The executive is often the only part of the organization that would feel comfortable raising issues that address functional organization, drastic revision of the accountability hierarchy, or matrix approaches. Some conflicts between members of the organization may require executive intervention. Placing initial discussions on distant and neutral ground, such as a retreat provides, can diminish the importance of status relationships and historical difficulties between the participants. Processes that deliberately conceal the authorship of ideas, such as the nominal group technique or Delphi approach, are also useful.[1]

— *Adopting and implementing revisions.* Organizational changes are usually approved by the CEO rather than the board. Notification of the individuals involved and implementation of the changes, including revision of the information systems, are the responsibility of the executive.

— *Reporting the revisions.* Organizational changes must be reported to the board, outside agencies, doctors, and patients, as well as to members of the organization.

Managing the Information System. The information system is increasingly important as a vehicle for guiding the expectations of the accountability hierarchy and supporting the deliberations of the collateral organization. The distribution of information reinforces the accountability hierarchy as well. Although most information systems in hospitals have been in the finance and medical records departments, the increased importance of nonfinancial data and the need for integrated data have encouraged leading hospitals to move the function to the executive office. Present systems focus primarily on accounting, but support for medicine and the clinical services, planning and marketing, and human resources is being developed rapidly. The expanded functions of the information system and related issues are discussed in chapter 9.

Monitoring Operations. Monitoring tends to be more important on lower levels of the organization. An organization either achieves control through the managers of its responsibility centers or it fails to achieve control. When problems occur, the first-line manager must be given the opportunity to correct them; higher levels react only after she or he fails. The executive office and middle management make three contributions to control:

1. Designing and operating the information system
2. Establishing and administering the incentives for control
3. Assisting with control problems that stem from sources outside the authority of the responsibility center manager or lower-level supervisor.

Maintaining the Hospital Disaster Plan. Providing care during civil disaster is an important and respected function of community hospitals. When disaster strikes, people turn instinctively to the hospital. Victims are brought by rescue vehicles, in private cars, or by other means. Even a large emergency service can face 20 times its normal peak load with very little warning. Word of disaster spreads quickly, particularly under the stimulus of television and radio. The hospital may be inundated with visitors, families, and well-meaning volunteers in addition to the sick and injured.

Warning, medical needs, and severity of injuries differ greatly, depending on the disaster. The most common disasters are storms and large-scale accidents such as fires and mass transport crashes. It is fortunate that in many cases the larger the number of injured, the lower the percentage of very serious or fatal injuries. Few if any hospitals make any serious effort to deal with military attack, although response to terrorism and civil disorder is increasingly relevant.

(Nuclear warfare is well beyond the response capability of any hospital directly involved. The term "last epidemic" is horrifyingly appropriate. Not only would there be incalculable numbers of injured persons, but the hospital could expect total loss of its medical supplies. Providing care to survivors would be more a Samaritan than a medical matter. Famine and untreatable infectious disease would kill a large fraction of people who survived the initial attack.)

Response requires a detailed plan that must be rehearsed periodically to comply with JCAH regulations.[2] The design of the plan is a major project requiring the coordinated efforts of all hospital management except members of the finance system.[3] The elements of the response include:

— Rapid assembly of clinical and other personnel
— Reassignment of tasks, space, and equipment
— Establishment of supplementary telephone and radio communication
— Triage of arriving injured
— Provision of information to press, television, and volunteers

Functions Supporting the Medical Staff

In virtually all community hospitals, the chief executive is accountable for the proper operation of the medical staff organization. This complex and essential part of the hospital is described in detail in chapter 10. Although medical staff organizations are becoming larger and more formal, with employed staff to assist them, the executive units of well-run hospitals spend substantial time on medical staff matters. Among their more important functions:

— *Assisting in planning and recruitment.* The well-run hospital has a long-range medical staff recruitment plan for expansion and replacement of its membership and pursues it actively to ensure the highest possible quality of doctors (see chapters 5 and 10).

— *Negotiating contracts.* Formal employment contracts with attending physicians are increasingly common in well-run hospitals. The executive is directly involved in these negotiations as the agent of the hospital.

— *Providing staff support.* The executive supports the medical staff organization in ways directly analogous to the support it provides trustees. It suggests charges, membership and agendas for committees, and provides briefings, documentation, and minutes.

— *Assessing attitudes and needs.* Both formal and informal communication with the medical staff is necessary, and the executive acts as the board's spokesperson and representative. Formal surveys of staff satisfaction are increasingly common. Informal communications are still more important; most CEOs and COOs of well-run hospitals deliberately position themselves to hear staff comments. As one successful executive said, "I try to stop by the staff lounge about three times a week."

— *Risk management and surveillance of quality and utilization.* Surveillance of quality and utilization is the central function of peer review. It consumes the largest amount of medical staff time and requires a correspondingly large investment of executive time. It is carried out by a large number of committees under a variety of names (for example, tissue, medical care, death, complications, infection, and utilization review).

The executive function in surveillance is operation of the information system, including statistical and other techniques to improve the efficiency of search by the committees. The tasks involved are increasingly being grouped under a function called risk management. In addition, because committee minutes are important legal and accreditation records, executives routinely provide them. This combination of responsibilities means that in well-run hospitals there is a representative of the executive office present at every meeting of the review committees. Usually the rank of the executive depends upon the importance of the committee.

— *Acting in emergencies.* The CEO and COO of well-run hospitals are obligated to enforce the bylaws of the hospital and the medical staff in any emergency during which medical staff officers are not available. In extreme situations, such as obvious physical or emotional impairment of a physician, they must suspend medical privileges and find another doctor for the patients involved.

Selecting Executive Personnel

Large hospitals now have several levels of executives. Chief executives lead a team, promoting or hiring individuals as they mature. Clearly the quality of the team is a major determinant of the well-managed hospital's success. Since it also determines the experience of future CEOs, it may be critical to the long-term success of community hospitals in general. Issues in the selection and development of that team are the subject of this section. The experience and skill required are discussed from the perspective of a superior seeking a subordinate executive. The same perspective should be useful to a younger executive planning a career.

Career Ladders for Hospital Executives

A career in hospital management should pose continuing professional challenges, from entry (usually between the ages of 25 and 35) to mature achievement (just before retirement). Like other management careers, it should present an opportunity for continuous growth and for personal and psychological rewards at all levels. Financial rewards should reflect the increasing skill and contribution of the individual, with major increases in compensation reserved for those few who wish to be and are capable of being successful CEOs.

An executive ready to undertake the position of CEO of a large hospital should have accumulated a substantial list of varied and successful hospital management experiences. As hospital management becomes more complex, the value of directly relevant experience and education is likely to be proven even more clearly.

Those seeking a manager want the skills that are the distillate of successful experience, but these are harder to appraise. Experience and skill can be amplified to provide a useful profile for selecting an individual health care executive. Experience includes entry education; continuing education; decision support, especially in information systems, planning, marketing, board, and medical staff; organization design; and directing successful units or corporations. Skills include technical areas such as construction or finance, leadership and human relations, decision making, and ethics, emotional strength, and commitment.

Executives' Experiences

Experiences are listed on the applicant's record, but to understand them fully often requires interviews with both references and the applicant. Those executives who aspire to be CEO of a major institution should acquire a significant amount of experience in each of the areas below.

Entry Education. Graduate education is increasingly the norm for all but the lowest levels of executive activity. Although exceptional individuals occasionally arrive through other routes, successful completion of graduate education is evidence of general intellectual ability, energy, and perseverance. High class standing or a degree from a particularly competitive school is usually a predictor of future success.

The kind of graduate education influences the knowledge and skills acquired. Clinical education and legal education emphasize skills other than management, and the knowledge they impart is only partly relevant to health care. Finance, marketing, organizational design, and human relations are topics dealt with only in management-oriented graduate programs. A factual and analytic review of the health care system is generally available only in health care administration programs. The odds for a young person seeking a career in health management favor the person with graduate education in health care management at the most selective school he or she can get into. For the individual who possesses other graduate education, an alternate strategy would be to replace missing skills by experience and missing knowledge by continuing education.

Successful managers have arisen with all kinds of education, and without it. The executive seeking junior staff must weigh formal education against other criteria.

Decision-Oriented Experience. Hospitals recruiting executives should seek a wide variety of experience as well as a record of increasingly demanding responsibility. One way of viewing an applicant's record of experience is to consider it in terms of decision-oriented and implementation-oriented experience. These concepts provide a more meaningful dichotomy than most, for several reasons. They suggest the inseparability, complementarity, and equality of the two classes. They hint at the mind-set and skill requirements involved in executive performance.

Decision-oriented experience relates to the processes by which the organization sets its expectations, from environmental surveillance, planning, and marketing analyses to supporting board, medical staff, and middle management. Beginners often do fact-finding and preliminary work on budgets and long-range plans. These exercises are particularly fruitful because they show the range of possibilities and restrictions of the organization so well. They also are not sensitive; the inevitable beginners' mistakes will almost certainly be caught in subsequent reviews.

More seasoned executives move to activities closer to final decisions: negotiating expectations with middle management and primary monitors, ranking new program activities, developing plans to implement broad goals, specifying information requirements, and designing systems to produce them. Mature executives, often CEOs, address the most sensitive and difficult decisions: weighing the importance and permanence of environmental changes, setting profit requirements and price increases, and resolving serious disputes. As the executive progresses, the cost of error mounts, but so do his or her skills, wisdom, and emotional maturity.

Implementation-Oriented Experience. Implementation experience focuses more clearly on leadership skills, the ability to convince others and to gain their cooperation. It is equal in importance to decision-making skill, although in specific positions one or the other may dominate. The skills involved transcend human relations, although they require effective interpersonal skills. Leadership skills also transcend the old line-staff dichotomy; they are perhaps easier to learn without the mantle of authority conferred by line hierarchies. In the hospital world, where little gets done without a team, implementation is getting things done through a team, and implementation experience is learning how to make it happen.

Little is known about the development of leadership. Leaders sometimes emerge and sometimes are annointed; neither method is infallible. What does seem reliable is that both decision-making and implementation skills are apparent early in most leaders and that they are improved by practice. Leadership experience for hospital executives can appropriately begin before the professional career, with college activities, for example, and can include experience outside the hospital if time permits. Smaller voluntary organizations, local government, and charitable fund drives are common examples. So are state and national professional organizations.

In the hospital, leadership skills are developed by supervisory experience and other practice in getting things done. For CEO-level skills, the composition of the group led is probably more important than its size. Opportunities to lead groups containing doctors and other extensively educated individuals, and opportunities to lead groups of leaders, such as trustee groups, are valuable. It is important to understand that several jobs traditionally labelled "staff"—especially consulting, planning, and board and medical staff support—can include all of the experience opportunities of line positions, except that of routine supervision of large numbers of people. Certainly good staff work exercises both decision-making and implementation skills.

Continuing Education. Formal continuing education has three roles in an executive career: remedial, complementary, and supplementary. Remedial functions address oversights in previous formal education. Evening studies, weekend programs, extended summer conferences, and study on one's own can do much to overcome the lack of entry education. The most able and conscientious students can compensate completely for this lack, but it requires continued effort for a long time.

Complementary education is often factual knowledge of new developments. If skills are developed, the focus is on solving rather than identifying problems. The most common examples are factual presentations on various new contracts and regulations. New analytic techniques can also be conveyed this way—making long-range forecasts, using discounted cash flows, or installing patient-scheduling systems, for example. Complementary education seems to do better with decision-oriented techniques than implementation skills. Complementary education must be self-contained and appropriate to any of several devices, from books and electronic media to one- or two-day conferences. Study on one's own is, and should be, by far the most common vehicle for complementary education. The American College of Healthcare Executives, the leading professional organization for hospital managers, has developed an extensive series of conferences supplemented by audiovisual and print materials for individual study.

Supplementary education is the least common of the three forms. It includes additional formal degrees and programs designed to broaden perspectives beyond the normal professional limits. Study of the health care systems of other nations is relatively popular. Some universities offer summer courses in the liberal arts. Religious studies are important supplementary education. Some executives read literature, history, biography, and philosophy. Broader perspectives are useful in evaluating the changes in the environment and the opportunities they imply. They are also useful in coping with the frustrations inherent in management. Among executives fully qualified in professional knowledge and skill, they distinguish the exceptional from the adequate.

Executives' Skills

Honest assessment of one's skills is a powerful tool. In addition, profiles of skills provide evidence for promotion, although they fall short of answering the critical question, "How well will this individual do in the future?" Some suggestion of the answer may come from interviews and references, but these cannot be relied upon for a definitive answer. Reliability is improved by a clear list of the skills desired. Four classes of executive skills are described here.

Technical Skills. Most technical skills are acquired through formal education and developed through practice. Some technical skills are specifically managerial—for example, bond marketing, construction planning, human resources management, and fund raising. Many activities of middle management require such skills. Unfortunately, technical skills are often not transferable, and they are irrelevant to many critical questions facing CEOs and COOs. Even the jobs of medical director and nursing director have only modest technical content; they are filled by people possessing the professional degree as much from tradition as from day-to-day requirements. The CFO is the highest ranking executive job requiring extensive technical skills.

A fruitful approach to learning the technical skills required of executives is to gain ability to communicate in several important technical fields. Perhaps the best approach is to learn how to handle complex issues requiring coordination of several technical skills. An important test of chief executive skill is such coordination.

Leadership and Human Relations Skills. Leadership skill is developed exclusively through experience, and it is difficult to test. Very capable executives incorporate diverse viewpoints so skillfully that the origins of the resulting decisions are obscure to all but the most sophisticated observers. A list of experiences provides only a rough guide to the real abilities of the individual. An extended working relationship with the executive is the best known way to assess leadership skill. Commentary from a variety of references is second best. One test of a leader is how well her or his decisions are accepted and respected by those who wanted another outcome. If possible, therefore, opinions should be sought from hostile and disappointed references.

Decision-Making Skills. The quality of past decisions speaks loudly. If they were successful decisions, more success can usually be predicted. How an executive reaches decisions is important. Autocratic styles, particularly styles that include neither the thinking nor the feelings of others, are destructive of the fabric of well-run hospitals.

Character: Ethics, Emotional Strength, and Commitment. The ethical commitment of health care executives is as important as that of physicians—and is as easy to state. It is to run an organization in which each patient is treated as the executive would wish to be treated were he or she similarly afflicted, each employee is offered competitive compensation and an opportunity to grow, and the community as a whole is provided the optimal choices for its health care system. High executive offices in hospitals are taxing, stressful jobs worth the compensation and respect they command. There are a great many ways to do less than one's best. Success requires not only professional skill and experience, but also emotional strength and ethical commitment. The temptation to avoid potentially painful decisions is always present and is sometimes encouraged by the governing board. Some of the ways an executive can fail the hospital are very difficult to detect. Others, like alcoholism and stress-related disease, are more evident—and more tragic. In the last resort, one must rely on the character of the individual. Evidence of character is available only through references or extended contact.

It is probably true that character can be strengthened. Ability to handle stress can be improved by practice at increasing levels. Multi-million-dollar decisions are less stressful with practice, beginning with thousand-dollar decisions. A stable and balanced life-style seems predictive of strength of character. Stability means that all personal needs are fulfilled in reasonable ways; balance means the executive has interests beyond the job. An executive's character can be assessed by interviews and references, but only within the bounds of respect for individual privacy. Inquiry within those bounds is desirable. Evidence of good character and ability to withstand stress is an imperfect predictor, but an executive who has given such evidence in the past is preferable to one who has not. The community is entitled to hold health care executives to higher than average standards because of the risks involved.

Organization of the Executive Office

The executive office is small relative to other units of the hospital. In small hospitals it may be only one or two people; even in large hospitals the office accounts for only about 5 percent of total payroll costs. Despite its size, it presents several important design problems, principally because of its role in integrating the other four systems and the complexities of supporting the governing board. This section presents representative examples of executive office organization and accountability of key executives, with special attention to the accountability of the CEO and the COO.

Typical Executive Office Designs

Organization charts for executive units depict reality poorly, largely because they show only the accountability hierarchy, while many activities take place in the collateral organization. Figure 6.2 shows a progressive organization for a moderately large hospital. Executive system designs must include not only the executive office but also the relationship to the vice-presidents or chiefs of the other four major systems. These individuals are as important in the governance and executive activities as they are in their own systems. Smaller institutions tend to collapse functions under fewer headings, but they should not eliminate them from the written record of assignments. In the smallest hospitals, all responsibilities for clinical systems coordination, finance, information systems, human resources, and planning and marketing may be consolidated under one (busy) individual, but it should be clear to all that this individual has each of these responsibilities.

The key problem in designing executive organizations is how to bring a very large number of activities together into decision-making groups that are effective both in size and in representation. This problem is not particularly well solved by figure 6.2, nor is it clear that any best solution exists. The most promising concept appears to give equal weight to three components of the clinical system: medicine, nursing, and other support services. Reality tends to fall short of theory on three counts. First, the medical staff is only beginning to mature as a bureaucratic accountability hierarchy. Second, nursing has not assumed the stature indicated in figure 6.2. Third, the disparity among clinical support services and their traditional independence causes them to be individually treated as equal partners, even at the vice-presidential level. These issues are discussed in more detail in chapters 10, 12, and 13.

Alternate forms are easy to visualize. Information services, fund raising, and public relations can be handled in various ways. Clinical services can be combined under one executive. Figure 6.3 shows a more traditional form, which adds a vice-president for clinical affairs, who would be responsible for the medical staff, clinical support services, and nursing; eliminates the COO; and centralizes information services, human resources, and plant under a single vice-president.

The alternatives for executive organization appear to have their greatest impact on the expectation-setting capability of the institution. A key committee charged with developing the budget, for example, might consist, under figure 6.2, of the chief operating officer (chair), the chief financial officer, the vice-president for planning and marketing, and the vice-presidents of each of the five services. This group of eight is probably manageable, but the three clinical vice-presidents will have to coordinate activities carefully with their many subordinates. Some of these matters would be brought to the committee for resolution. Under figure 6.3, one officer would be responsible for achieving clinical coordination, and the CEO would have to chair the committee. (A very large hospital might insert a COO over the clinical and plant managers.) The advantages of figure 6.3 are cohesiveness and speed in decision making at the top executive level. Those of figure 6.2 are of broader input, more thorough integration, and a stronger voice for clinical issues. Given the demands being made upon hospitals in the competitive environment, the figure 6.2 forms are likely to become more common.

It appears that many hospitals have even less concise organizations than appear in the figures. Several clinical support services may report individually to chief operating officers, and the role of the medical staff may be ambiguous. These organizations face severe difficulties

Figure 6.2

Emerging Organization of the Executive Office

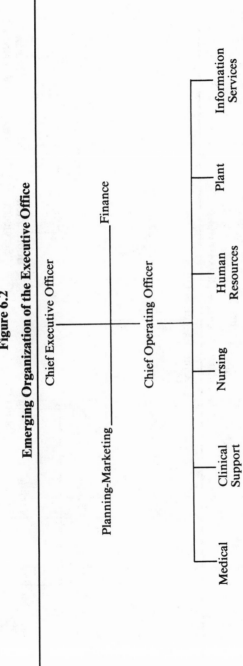

Figure 6.3
Alternative Executive Organization

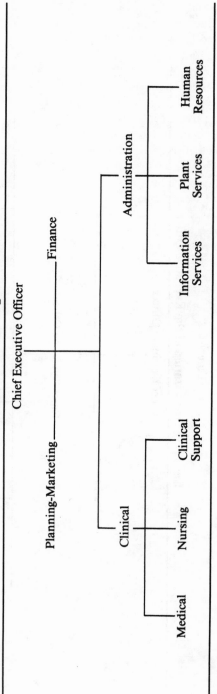

in establishing and implementing expectations for high-quality yet inexpensive care. Such care requires close coordination among the clinical units, and the collateral organization of committees and task forces cannot do the job efficiently without rational, unambiguous hierarchies.

Responsibilities of Executive Officers

The chief executive officer and chief operating officer are responsible for integrating operations and assessing the environment. Under the corporate model discussed in chapter 5, one or both of them may be given dual titles and voting positions on the board of trustees in recognition of this responsibility. Titles such as "president and chief executive officer" or "executive vice-president and chief operating officer" are increasingly common. Clinical vice-presidents represent what is traditionally called the line of organizations. They are responsible for meeting the needs of their subordinates, monitoring their technical area of expertise, and maintaining the exchange relationships necessary to support a professional work force. The staff vice-presidents for planning and finance are more concerned with external activities. The vice-president for planning and marketing is frequently responsible not only for environmental surveillance, but also for environmental manipulation through public relations and promotion. The CFO has specific obligations directly to the governing board, particularly for the preparation and implementation of the long-range fiscal plan.

Unique Responsibilities of the Chief Operating Officer. In well-run hospitals, the chief operating officer is responsible for total cost (resource consumption) and revenue (resource conservation) expectations, for acceptable quality of care, and for quality of work life. She or he is accountable for any failure of structure or process in medical staff organization, clinical care, recruitment, collective bargaining, nonfinancial records, and plant safety. In short, the COO, by virtue of hierarchical accountability, must meet most of the operating expectations. Clearly, these are met by working through subordinates.

In addition to these obligations, the COO will want to provide active guidance to planning and marketing and finance, the only two units not under her or his direct control. It is increasingly important for the COO to monitor the information system. (The CFO has similar obligations.) The COO will pay careful attention to recruitment of key personnel and will participate directly in the recruitment of executive personnel other than the CEO. He or she will coordinate all issues of organizational design and will stimulate collateral communications to supplement the inevitable design weaknesses. Finally, the COO will want to play the central role in both the design and the administration of compensation and reward systems. Not only does rewarding follow logically from her or his role in directing and controlling, it also provides an opportunity to increase the loyalty of subordinates.

Unique Responsibilities of the Chief Executive Officer. The chief executive officer is accountable for the success of the chief operating officer, of the planning and marketing function, and, in most organizations, of the chief financial officer. In addition, the CEO must deal with the external environment, relate to the governing board, and provide leadership.

It is through the success of the COO that the CEO ensures the successful operation of the hospital. An effective CEO does little directing or controlling personally. The directing she or he undertakes is at the most strategic level, such as proposals for initial budget targets, strategies for major union negotiations, evaluation of corporate restructuring, and stimulation of task forces to study new ideas. The meaning, implications, and importance of major directions should be explained to the organization at large by the CEO, but the process of expanding the ideas into specific expectations is left to the rest of management to carry out, under the supervision of the COO.

There are several reasons why the CEO should maintain direct supervision of planning and marketing. His or her external orientation calls for a close liaison. The focus of the board in well-run organizations is heavily on planning decisions, and the planning and marketing staff can provide direct support through the CEO. Finally, the most successful new plans and products require the broadest and most imaginative search of the environment. All other organizational homes for planning and marketing limit its perspective. They also reduce contact with the governing board and chief executive, who have the broadest exposure to the outside and usually the most experience. Limited perspective—the opportunity not seen and therefore not pursued—is undoubtedly the greatest risk of planning and marketing in a turbulent environment.

In some hospitals, the chief financial officer reports directly to the governing board, through the treasurer of the corporation. It is probably more common for the CFO to report to both the CEO and the treasurer, via the finance committee of the board. Lower CFO reporting levels are rare, both because they do not provide adequate protection of assets and because the financial officer plays a major role in many planning decisions. The theory of internal control of assets suggests strongly that operating personnel not have access to the accounting system; placing the CFO on a higher level reduces by one step the opportunities for collusion below the ownership level. More important, however, is the need for the closest possible collaboration between the major direction-setting activities and finance. Failure to understand the financial ramifications of planning decisions can be a fatal error, and failure to orchestrate the flow of large sums can be exorbitantly costly. The CEO gains an independent view of the functioning of the organization and direct advice on the financial implications of plans by having the CFO report to her or him.

The CEO is usually the spokesperson for the hospital, representing it in regional and state associations and to the other organizations and forces in the community. These activities develop exchange relationships and are therefore critical to the well-run hospital. The accessibility of a hospital spokesperson to the business clubs, charitable organizations, financial leaders, and political representatives of a community determines whether they will feel free to share their views about hospital operation. When they lose that freedom, the stage has been set for actions not in the hospital's interest. There are many avenues for such action, including aiding competing institutions, denying access to funds or real estate resources, and taking restrictive political steps. Influential people must feel comfortable communicating with the governing board (often by being members) or with the executive. In well-run hospitals, they are comfortable with both.

For hospitals that are part of a multihospital system, the CEO is the first point of contact with the larger organization. As these systems become more sophisticated, contacts are being developed at several levels in the organization. Certainly the negotiation of contracts specifying privileges and responsibilities between subsidiaries and parent or between partner organizations must involve the chief executive.

Successful chief executives always play an active role in the affairs of the governing board, whether or not they have voting rights. They monitor the agenda, making sure it is complete but not inefficient. They provide full factual support for all agenda items, almost always including a recommendation. They brief the chairs of the major committees on likely debate and its management. They maintain profiles of board members, suggest new board members, and provide criteria for selection. They guide orientation and training programs. They identify promising members and develop them through committee assignments. They make themselves available for informal discussion at the instigation of members, and they facilitate direct communication with their own subordinates and those of the other systems of the hospital. Many of these duties cannot be delegated, but the most effective CEOs find ways to use board members and lower executives in these activities, both to save themselves time and to increase training opportunities.

For the CEO of the well-run hospital, communications with the COO, CFO, the planning and marketing unit, and even the board are merely resources for the larger job, which is providing leadership. Leadership combines the ability to identify winning ideas with the ability to maintain an environment in which they will flourish. It increases the enthusiasm and receptivity to innovation and promotes the vigor with which tasks are carried out. Because of this, it influences the level of risk that a hospital may safely assume. A vigorous, self-confident organization can take selective risks and count on its ability to protect itself from serious loss. A poorly run one cannot.

Leadership also involves representing the increasing body of knowledge possessed by health care executives. The consequences of actions are not always what they seem: clinical innovations that appear to save lives can decrease survival in certain circumstances. Programs that seem irrelevant can improve life for a large sector of the community. Highly touted solutions are occasionally proven failures, fraudulently or foolishly advocated by special interests. And programs that are sometimes ineffective can be highly effective in the right combinations and with the right management. A board considering medical staff recommendations on new technology, the appropriateness and selection of reimbursement contracts, the development of preventive care or outreach programs, cost reduction, or the revision of health insurance benefits should expect its chief executive to be competent in these matters.

The best CEOs seem to achieve leadership in a three-phase process. First, they establish themselves and then their subordinates as respected sources of problem solving. That is, they make the bureaucratic organization responsive to its employees, doctors, trustees, and patients. This improves the performance of the hospital, but equally important, it raises the confidence of its members and its exchange partners. Second, the CEO works to open and expand conversations about the hospital so all ideas can be discussed; he or she puts a premium on useful innovations. This climate results from candor and objectivity, virtues that are themselves achieved by effective staff support and information systems. It also results from a CEO who reflects credit for progress on others. Third, the CEO uses the momentum of growing confidence and achievement to explore external threats to and opportunities for the organization—issues too frightening to debate openly in poorly run hospitals—in ways that allow innovative and rewarding responses. The CEO's sound relationship with the board and personal focus on external issues are essential to completing this process.

Measuring Executive Performance

It is important that no one in the hospital organization be exempt from the process of expectation setting and achievement review. There should be explicit expectations, reviews, and rewards for all executives, from the CEO to the beginning assistant. The process should be quantitative wherever possible. An effort should be made to make the review process fair, and it must relate to the long-term survival of the hospital. Applying the survival criterion to executive performance, it is clear that measurement should address both open systems and closed system considerations.

Open Systems Assessment of Executive Performance

The higher the rank of the executive, the greater importance should be placed upon open systems evaluation. At the CEO level, open systems could be considered more important than current operations represented by the closed system measures. The chief planner might have almost all of his or her evaluation based on an open systems assessment. The most precise possible expectations should be formulated for these activities, although much evaluation will inevitably be subjective.

The goals of open systems activity are easy enough to state—they are to identify trends in the environment, relate them to influential groups which have or might have important exchange relationships with the hospital, and specify the implications in terms of current or future exchanges. In most hospitals, they can be applied to specific areas of concern, divided among several people with separate accountabilities, and used as a basis for specific expectations. For example, the vice-president for human resources would probably track trends in nonprofessional labor, union activities, and employment conditions. She or he would then prepare an annual report indicating what wage and personnel policies should be changed in response. The CEO might review trends in the community power structure, relate these to trustee membership, and suggest names to the nominating committee.

There seem to be four approaches to assessment of open systems performance: standards based on structure or process; prior agreements on the expectations; and two outcomes measures, informed users' opinions and market share. The outcomes measures are increasingly accessible and increasingly important. Market share may, in fact, be the single most important measure of performance for not-for-profit hospitals, although it must be judged in the light of long-term financial stability.

Use of Structural and Process Standards. One approach to assessing open systems expectations is subjective judgment of the structure or process used to arrive at the decision rather than the content of the decision itself. This approach assumes that good results will accrue from correct processes, an assumption that is not wholly justified. Statements describing professional quality of work can be found for such areas as planning, community relations, advertising, information systems, and law. A series of questions or criteria can be developed to indicate acceptable practice in these areas. The usual standard is prevailing practice, although higher ones can be imposed with advance agreement. General criteria are set out in the JCAH sections on planning[4] and in the AHA's *Program for Institutional Effectiveness Review.*[5] More specific criteria can be found in textbooks on planning and marketing. There are few published commentaries on the CEO's obligations to represent the hospital, to maintain contact with influential persons in the community, and to assist in board selection and development.[6] Whatever criteria are used, there should be full understanding about them at the outset. Review of performance against criteria is generally a face-to-face talk. Occasionally, a consultant can be used to gain an independent professional opinion or even to provide remedial counselling. More often, the task falls to the immediate supervisor, or, in the case of the CEO, to a committee of the board.[7]

Prior Agreement on Expected Achievements. Another approach is agreement in advance between the executive and the reviewer as to the accomplishments, documents, or projects to be completed within the period. This technique, often called **management by objective** (MBO), is particularly suited to difficult and ambiguous work. It involves a more or less formal contract between the worker and his or her superior on what is to be accomplished and, in some cases, how. Management by objectives is a useful approach, but is subject to a number of weaknesses. Quite the opposite of structural standards, it tends to specify outcomes, what is or will be done, not how well it is done. Setting the objectives can become an end in itself. In practice, there is a strong tendency to keep the objectives too vague to be useful. Objectives are difficult to adapt to changing conditions. Once set, they may excuse the omission of important steps that were not foreseen in the negotiation but were indicated by subsequent work.

Despite its weaknesses, MBO seems to be a useful supplement to process criteria, particularly for relatively short term, specific tasks unique to the hospital's environment. Thus "Move to establish productive communications with XYZ Company" is probably fruitful, while "Develop a plan for an HMO" or "Improve relations with the media" are dubious. (The first lacks any clear specification in terms of existing environment or scope of planning activity; the second is simply vague.)

User Evaluation of Service. One outcomes approach that is useful for evaluating both open and closed systems performance is to ask the user or customer to comment. In some cases, the user or customer is the superior or another person in the organizational hierarchy. Within the executive group, the customer is usually the doctor or the patient.

Formal surveys of customer satisfaction are becoming increasingly popular. They follow specific protocols and sampling routines and provide considerable planning data as well as an overall assessment of the attractiveness of the institution.

A few hospitals routinely survey influential persons in the community, using standard questions and a structured but open-ended approach. The results of such a survey not only identify what important exchange partners are seeking, they also measure executive performance. In a more restricted sense, the contribution of lower-level executives, such as the information services manager, can be assessed by internal review of other supervisors' opinions about the department's work. The most influential member of the hospital is the doctor. Informal medical staff surveys are commonplace; formal ones are being done more frequently.

Surveys are not without their difficulties. Rigorous design and administration are essential to unbiased responses. Questions must be checked for bias, surveyors trained, and samples, or selection of respondents, carefully checked. Weighting multiple questions on different topics is difficult. Cost is roughly $25 per sample point, and a sample of 500 or more is usually necessary.[8] Cost can be minimized by designing a survey that has a variety of uses in the hospital.

Measures of Market Share. There are three approaches to measuring market share. All require explicit prior definition of the service community. For most voluntary hospitals, the community is measured geographically and the market is measured in terms of the number of persons living in the geographic area.

1. Household surveys can yield a market share by tallying responses to such questions as "If you needed a hospital, which one would be your first choice?"

2. Market share can be estimated from comprehensive measures of a community's actual discharges or emergency room visits. Special techniques are necessary to deal with migration, both persons who leave the community for hospitalization elsewhere and persons from elsewhere who come in.

3. For hospitals which market predominantly through HMOs or specialized insurance networks, market share may be estimated from the percentage of the population enrolled in the insurance plan. Although this approach is currently useful only in a few closed-panel insurance situations, it will become more useful as the number of HMOs and other selective contract devices expands.

Under conditions of free choice, market share is an important, realistic test of customer opinion. Thus it is increasingly common to set specific expectations for it in places where it can be measured. Several states now have statewide in-hospital data collection systems that permit direct calculation of market share. Using such documents as the Medicare cost reports, and the AHA *Guide to Hospitals,* at least rudimentary measures of market share can be constructed. These tend to be one to two years out of date. Market share measures tend to be relatively stable, with large changes accompanying acquisitions, closures, and relocations; however, it is possible for a well-run hospital to systematically expand its share, at least slowly, by paying more attention to promotion and customer satisfaction.

Closed System Measures of Executive Performance

There are five major categories of executive performance measures, and countless specific measures, within the closed system alone, namely:

1. *Demand (market and volume) measures*—True demand and market share estimates are generally open system considerations; however, measures and trends of volume of major service aggregates such as inpatient discharges by service, outpatient care, or ambulatory surgery are the starting point for all closed system demand and output expectations. There are potentially several dozen measures. Higher executive ranks are responsible for large groups. The groups cannot be aggregated easily.

2. *Cost measures*—These can be aggregated easily in accordance with the hierarchical structure. At each executive level there is one total cost for which an expectation can be set.

3. *Efficiency measures*—Comprehensive measures of hospital efficiency focus upon global applications of the output-input ratio, such as "inpatient cost per discharge" and "outpatient cost per visit." Measures can be aggregated on the basis of expectations, such as "expected cost–actual cost" or "percent of times efficiency equaled or exceeded expectations." These constitute the most sensitive possible efficiency measures for the executive and are most useful in exceptionally well-managed institutions. These hospitals so often achieve expectations that the best evaluation simply focuses upon exceptions.

4. *Quality measures*—Community pressure is forcing hospitals to rely increasingly on outcomes measures of quality, both of health care and of the general satisfaction of exchange needs.

Thus a typical list might be "zero defects for licensure and accreditation inspections; physician, employee, and patient satisfaction scores in excess of expectations; recruitment and retention measures in excess of expectations; morbidity and mortality measures below expectations." More or less univariate measures can be established within each of these groups, but aggregation is not desirable.

5. *Resource conservation measures*—Expectations for revenue and profit arise from the budgeting system and are easily aggregated at each level of executive performance. While improvements are actually achieved via volume, cost, and pricing, the measures are so central to long-term survival that it is wise to identify them as explicitly as possible. For human resources and plant systems executives, this means a process of transfer pricing, described in chapters 14 and 15. The highest levels of the organization can be judged only by the strength of their subordinates' performance. That is, the chief operating officer is accountable for achieving the revenue and profit expectations. The financial officer, executive office, chief executive, and planning vice-president make substantial contributions, but in ways that can only be identified subjectively and retrospectively.

Executive Evaluation Process

Given the competing importance of so many open and closed system measures of executive performance, the central question in evaluating a specific executive is weighting multiple and conflicting measures. Within the major categories, multiple measures can often be aggregated or eliminated, as suggested in chapter 3; however, the problem of evaluating the executive when performance is improving in some categories and deteriorating in others remains serious. A first step is the establishment of expectations for each measure. This permits a single measure for each category if a percent of expectations achieved is established. Such an approach assumes arbitrarily, or at least in advance, that a failure in one element bears a specific relationship to a failure in another (one-to-one, unless a weighting scheme is used.) Not only may this not be true, it may be impossible to determine the degree to which it is true until after the evaluation period is ended. Thus well-run hospitals tend to avoid excessively mechanical evaluations of executives in favor of retrospective judgments. Often a small panel of board officers and the three top executives guide the evaluation of the executive office; afterwards, the board panel evaluates the three remaining executives. Self-evaluation is an important adjunct of this activity. The evaluation can be used for incentive payment. Although the evaluation logically should precede the setting of the next period's expectations, this is rarely practical; it therefore tends to precede the second following period.

Encouraging Effective Performance

The attitude of the executive group in well-run hospitals seems to be different from that of the executive group in other hospitals. The CEO, COO, and first two or three ranks of associates are more positive, more helpful, more open, and more encouraging in their relations with the other systems, while at the same time they are more effective. They achieve this deceptively uncritical state because they have worked harder on the structure and process of management. They criticize less because there is more to praise, but there is more to praise because the executives have established a system that helps people do well.

The issues an organization deals with come and go rather quickly. The organization makes appropriate responses and thrives, or inappropriate ones and declines. However important the issues of today, they will be replaced by others tomorrow. It is the structure for dealing with this stream of transient issues that is the constant and the key to success. Although the executives of well-run hospitals are always deeply involved in the issues of the day, it is their ability to focus upon the underlying structure and improve it that makes them exceptional. Using the issues themselves as opportunities, they work tirelessly to achieve certain characteristics of structure. These criteria are never fully met, but the continuous effort to do so brings the organization closer to the ideal. Some of the criteria of excellence are discussed below.

Timing the Organization's Response

Ideally, an organization should perceive each new external or exchange demand far enough in advance to respond to it as it is articulated. As a result, the organization is rarely surprised or unprepared, and its members are relieved of the stresses that constitute one of the major negative aspects of work.

Farsightedness may be the single most important characteristic of well-managed hospitals. It results from extensive environmental surveillance and prompt resolution of conflicts. Most other desirable characteristics are eroded quickly under crisis management. A hospital with problems must generally concentrate on environmental surveillance and education of important decision makers and stake holders to regain its necessary farsightedness. The hospital that is farsighted can afford the time to educate, debate, and innovate in formulating its response.

One key role of the CEO and the executive office is in managing this process.

Management Style

Six elements of style that are repeatedly cited as important in organizational literature are predictability, candor, responsiveness, persuasiveness, conflict resolution, and participation.

— *Predictability.* Much of the success of a hospital organization depends upon teamwork, and teamwork depends upon knowing the role of others. Thus an organization which handles similar decisions in similar ways and follows predictable cycles of behavior reduces stress and enhances the contribution of its members. So important is this element that it is sometimes better to be predictably wrong than erratically right on the responsiveness and participative aspects of style.

— *Candor.* There is an ever-present temptation in organizations to tell people what they want to hear rather than the truth. Unfortunately, they all want to hear something different, and the practical result of lack of candor is chaos. The withholding of information is as self-defeating as overt distortion, and many poor managers do it, whether accidentally or deliberately. Ignorance leads first to guesswork and surprises and shortly thereafter to suspicions and paranoia. It is characteristic of well-managed hospitals that one can easily find what one wants to know and rely on what one hears. Good executives encourage this characteristic by personal action, repeated reference to its importance, and reward for its practice.

— *Responsiveness.* One obligation of management is to respond to subordinates' questions and concerns. It is clear that, the more effectively the superior responds, the greater the productivity and performance of the subordinate will be.

— *Persuasiveness.* An ability to articulate objectives, describe potential rewards, explain how difficulties can be overcome, and inspire confidence is a valuable tool in building consensus and motivation. The impact is enhanced by predictability, candor, and responsiveness. It is often based less on rhetoric than on a thorough understanding of both people and concepts, backed by a record of success.

— *Conflict resolution.* Closely related to responsiveness is the ability to resolve conflicts in ways that are both predictable and reasonable. Predictability applies both to the method of con-

flict resolution and the result. Understanding the likely outcome tends to minimize the conflicts. "Reasonable" is a better
criterion than "fair," because the conflict should be resolved in
the organization's favor rather than an individual's.

— *Participation.* Generally speaking, an organization that solicits
the opinion of its members, both formally and informally, as a
matter of course will do better than one that discourages member participation. This is especially true in hospitals, where the
constant variation in patient need places a great many decisions at the bedside or at lower levels of the organization.

Design of the Organization

As noted in chapter 4, the executive has critical roles in designing the
organization. Well-run hospitals achieve designs that are simple and
easily understood. Simplicity is usually achieved by limiting the collateral organization and keeping the accountability hierarchy as short as
possible. General understanding of the organization must be promoted
by communication and education. Reliability of the organization is a
specific form of predictability.

Well-designed organizations have another characteristic, one that
is somewhat difficult to describe. Although they are kept as simple and
as clear as possible, they are designed and operated in ways that encourage frequent informal cross-communication. For example, they try to
associate activities that require integration in ways that promote informal conversation among their managers.

Functioning of the Organization

The accountability hierarchy works better under the following circumstances:

— There are clear and complete expectations for each level; they
have been developed with member participation and, with
reasonable effort, are within the capability of the unit.

— Within these expectations, the unit has high autonomy to
achieve; flexibility and originality are encouraged.

— The higher levels of the organization are responsive and supply
appropriate resources.

— The collateral organization and other elements of the hierarchy
provide support for setting and achieving the expectations; that
is, education, information systems, and staff assistance are
available when required.

— There is a measurement system comparing achievement to expectation, a record of success, and a reward for success.

The collateral organization works best when it is smallest and least taxed, that is, when the accountability hierarchy carries out as many functions as possible. In addition, performance of the collateral organization is enhanced when:

— The collateral organization relies more on ad hoc than on standing committees. Ad hoc committees have preset expiration dates, which allows their contributions to be reviewed without implied criticism of their membership.

— Members are selected carefully, and consultant status is assigned to persons who have limited interests. Consultants can be given minutes and encouraged to come only when invited or when they see a topic in their particular area.

— Attention is paid to writing the charge and providing the factual base for all committees. The executive office should help clarify the charge, set time limits on ad hoc committees, and facilitate fact finding.

— Executives participate in all committees to assist the chairperson with agenda setting, membership selection, and agenda management, and to assure that a written record is made and brought to the attention of interested persons not on the committee.

Motivation. Well-run hospitals motivate their members through individual professional and personal goals established in light of the exchange demands of the external environment. They attempt to make the exchange requirements clear to each member, and let the outside environment guide the member's thinking. They avoid relying on authority and minimize the role of the governing board and executive group. They recognize that success itself is a great motivator and therefore strive to keep expectations within reasonable reach of every member.

Executives in well-run organizations appear deceptively passive. They let the external world and the individual members build the motivation and devote their attention to the communication of differing viewpoints, timely management of the decision structure, and careful attention to consistent application of the mission.

Incentives and Rewards. Good management is its own intangible reward. The sense of a job well done accompanies a successful project or the achievement of the year's expectations. Executives influence these accomplishments; their activities make committees and middle managers look better to outsiders and participants. Exceptional executives always share praise and usually absorb blame. They also incorporate recognition into the culture of the organization.

Both tangible and intangible rewards reinforce desired behavior. Intangible rewards include praise and public recognition. Having an opportunity to get these from sources other than superiors is important. Well-run hospitals have an air of mutual respect among their middle managers that is carefully fostered by executives.

Tangible rewards include salaries, bonuses, and promotions. Well-run hospitals appear to use retrospective evaluation at the time of annual performance and compensation review. As noted, it is important to establish in advance the concept of rewards, the expectations, and the method of evaluation. The actual evaluation and the amount of tangible reward can then be set retrospectively. Prospective commitments to amounts of bonuses and incentive pay should be avoided. The variability of the work makes equitable prearranged systems expensive, and in some areas almost infeasible. Retrospective awards are much easier to administer and can accomplish many of the same purposes. Cost-of-living adjustments and scale adjustments in salary, if any, should be kept strictly separate from rewards for merit. Hospitals are increasingly moving away from cost-of-living adjustments, focusing all increases on merit. There is some experimentation with the use of bonuses, which can be granted annually without inflating the fixed salary commitment. The record of rewards for merit becomes part of the consideration for promotion.

Notes

1. Andre Delbecq, *Group Techniques for Program Planning* (Glenview, IL: Scott, Foresman, 1975).

2. Joint Commission on Accreditation of Hospitals, *Manual of Hospital Accreditation* (Chicago: JCAH, reissued periodically).

3. G. L. Stanley, *Hospital Safety and Disaster Policy and Procedure Manual* (Manon, IL: Hospital Physician & Consulting Service, 1977); American Health Research Institute, *Disasters & Disaster Planning: Medical Analysis Index* (Annandale, VA: ABBE Publishing Association, 1985).

4. Joint Commission on Accreditation of Hospitals, *Accreditation Manual for Hospitals* (Chicago: JCAH, 1985), pp. 59–78.

5. American Hospital Association, *Program for Institutional Effectiveness Review* (Chicago: AHA, 1980).

6. The Foundation of the American College of Healthcare Executives, *Evaluating the Performance of the Hospital Chief Executive Officer* (Chicago: ACHE, 1984).

7. K. A. Dumbaugh, "The Evaluation of Performance in the Management of Health Care Organizations," in A. R. Kovner and D. Neuhauser, ed., *Health Services Management, Readings and Commentary,* 2d ed. (Ann Arbor, MI: Health Administration Press, 1983), pp. 121–140.

8. Ann H. Walker and Joseph D. Restuccia, "Obtaining Information on Patient Satisfaction with Hospital Care: Mail Versus Telephone," *Health Services Research* 19 (1984): 291–306.

Suggested Readings

Kovner, A. R., and Neuhauser, D. *Health Services Management: Readings and Commentary,* 2d ed. Ann Arbor, MI: Health Administration Press, 1983, especially pp. 21–113.

Shortell, S. M. and Kaluzny, A. D. *Health Care Management: A Text in Organization Theory and Behavior.* New York: Wiley, 1983, especially pp. 1–202.

7

Planning and Marketing for Community Hospitals

Planning and marketing constitute the organization's basic response to its environment. Excellent planning and marketing not only leads to rewarding exchanges and a mutually satisfactory relationship between the hospital and its community, but also encourages timely, responsive, consistent, and even-handed process for dealing with many potentially conflicting interests. Planning and marketing activities involve the entire governance structure and many others in the hospital as well.

Well-run hospitals understand the environment, test and modify it by their own communications and activities, and respond to it—all before the exchange demands become critical. Such timing is called **proactive.** It emphasizes foresight, and places the thinking of management ahead or in the future compared to the present. Because success requires that the institution be accepted by its environment, good planning is always **market-oriented,** or community-oriented; that is, it identifies the interests of the community and searches for ways the hospital can meet them. In the search, exchanges with the hospital's members—its employees, medical staff, and volunteers—are carefully considered. If community and member interests diverge, the well-run hospital relies on the ability of its members to change in response to community needs.

Planning and marketing are such extensive activities that it is difficult to develop uniform definitions of them. Different authors use different, sometimes conflicting terminology. To minimize the risk of adding to the confusion, I will define as few terms as possible in this chapter. In particular, I make little distinction between planning and marketing. **Planning and marketing** jointly identify the set of support activities usually undertaken by the governance system. **Planning** refers to the more generic activity involving decisions about the future made by all members of the organization. I avoid using the term **marketing** because of the sharp distinction between its technical and common usage. (To professional managers, marketing incorporates all of what is described here as planning and marketing; in common usage, as it might be understood by doctors, nurses, and some trustees, it generally implies promotional or advertising activity.)

Most hospitals have a planning-marketing section of the executive system which is formally accountable for the activities that support long-range and strategic decisions. Planning and marketing's product, or output, is both a long-range plan embodying the decisions ratified by the governing board, and a process for reaching decisions about long-term investments. Both the process and the plan are present in well-managed hospitals, and they are derived by expanding the following nine steps:

1. *Surveillance,* an ongoing search for exchange threats and opportunities both inside and outside the hospital.

2. *Mission development,* a deliberate selection of community (or market), service, and finance capability embodying the hospital's broadest and longest range objectives. The mission has an indefinite life and is revised as infrequently as possible.

3. *Development of long-range plans,* articulation of more detailed intentions and quantitative forecasts; these include major expansions and contractions of services and are coordinated with fiscal plans. Most plans have a horizon of about five years and are revised every year or two.

4. *Development of strategic options,* exploration and negotiation of major acquisitions, mergers, and revisions of service. These activities frequently depend on situations outside the institution's direct control. They are rarely planned in the sense that nonstrategic proposals are and sometimes must be conducted in confidence.

5. *Development of programmatic proposals,* preparation and review of detailed expectations for internally developed investment proposals that are competing for a place in the long-range plan or capital budget.

6. *Selection,* an explicit choice between developed strategic options and programmatic proposals, competing against each other and the status quo. The selection process begins as low in

the organization as possible and progresses to final action by the governing board.

7. *Implementation,* the commitment of resources to approved proposals; this involves incorporating funding into capital budgets and incorporating both funding and expectations into operating budgets.

8. *Promotion,* advertising and other activities to promote desired outcomes by influencing patient or community behavior.

9. *Evaluation,* the review of actual achievements against expectations.

This chapter focuses on what the CEO and governing board should expect from a formally designated planning and marketing activity; that is, it attempts to specify the functions the planning and marketing unit must perform to support proactive, market-oriented planning.

Purpose

The purpose of planning is to optimize the hospital's future exchange relationships. This purpose encompasses almost any decision concerning the hospital which is outside current operations. Only the word *future* distinguishes this purpose from the purpose of the entire governance system. It includes analysis of future community needs and interests, response to external threats and opportunities, design and promotion of new programs, assembly and recruitment of necessary resources, and securing of required permits and certificates. Compounding planning's broad scope, the subtlety of the concepts that lie behind the word *optimize* makes planning one of the most fascinating activities in hospital management.

Optimization implies the best possible achievement of some good or benefit through decisions allocating scarce resources. One optimizes the benefits of a specific activity relative to its costs, but in the final analysis, both benefits and costs are in the eye of the beholder. Especially for the not-for-profit hospital, a key part of the planning process is understanding and reaching consensus on the benefits to be achieved. For the well-run hospital, this understanding is embodied in the mission, a statement of the preferred good or benefit couched in terms of community, service, and finance (see chapter 5). The wisdom of a hospital's mission is measured by its viability and consistency. The missions of well-run hospitals reflect practical goals likely to be rewarded by their surrounding community. They provide a guide which is used routinely and consistently to make resource allocation decisions.

The first and most simplistic interpretation of optimizing is "to select those projects which have the greatest ratio of benefits to costs, and implement them." The costs and benefits are conceived mostly within the proposal or opportunity at hand. Conceptually, one finds a project, evaluates it in terms of the hospital's mission, and, if the benefits are enough greater than the costs, proceeds. Practically, it is almost never so simple. Neither the benefits nor the costs are easy to measure. They are even less easy to evaluate, that is, to compare against one another and against other projects. Once measured, two formidable questions remain: "How much is a health care benefit worth in terms of other kinds of opportunities?" and "Given that the future is always uncertain, how do I deal with the risk that my forecasts are incorrect?"

Whenever a given proposal is accepted, a decision is made about the last two questions, that the risk is tolerable and that the likely cost-benefit ratio is greater than that of any other opportunity. If it is rejected, the opposite decision is reached, other opportunities are more attractive, even those that have not been explicitly identified. The well-run hospital makes these decisions in such a way that even with complete hindsight it would change few of them. The purpose of planning-marketing can be expanded as:

— To improve the exchange relationship of the hospital to its environment by discovering, analyzing, and evaluating both the events of the environment and the opportunities of the hospital

— To review the hospital's mission in light of the environment and to indicate alternative missions to the governing board

— To identify opportunities optimizing the exchange relationship

— To promote a response by patients, members, and the community consistent with the selected opportunities

— To assist in the development and implementation of selected opportunities

Functions

Planning-marketing functions are closely related to its purpose. These functions are interrelated, which suggests that good management might spread its resources equally over all of them. The sequential nature of the planning-marketing process suggests otherwise, however. If one wishes to enhance the effectiveness of planning-marketing, one usually improves the surveillance function. The result is to increase the extent and quality of understanding and to increase potential opportunities, creating demand for improvement in the other functions.

Surveillance

Surveillance is the sensory function of the hospital organization. It identifies all changes in the environment, including both threats and opportunities. It also identifies the perspectives of others in the community on these changes, with particular attention to those of other care agencies, patients, doctors, and employees (or customers, competitors, and members of the hospital). All members of governance are responsible for surveillance. Trustees bear a particular responsibility. Excellent CEOs and chief planners often devote substantial personal time to the activity. Surveillance can occasionally lead to mission revision. Revising the mission is clearly a governing board responsibility (see chapter 5), but the planning-marketing unit checks the mission annually and suggests any necessary revisions.

Environmental Assessment. Those aspects of surveillance which require detailed factual and quantitative analysis or which are easier with prior experience are delegated to planning-marketing; they are embodied in the function called **environmental assessment**. Because all planning decisions require substantial lead time, forecasting is essential. As much as possible should be quantified, but the appeal of numbers should not overshadow the importance of changes in unmeasurable topics, particularly attitudes, beliefs, and technology. Good environmental assessment takes into account the following:

— *Community demographics and economics.* The size and age distribution of the community should be forecast quantitatively, usually relying on other primary sources. Trends in employment characteristics, health insurance coverage, and the percentage of persons in the community living in poverty are important predictors of health care expenditure and payment source; they should be forecast quantitatively. Type of health insurance has proven important. Plans discouraging the use of services are effective for purchasing groups and may spill over to more conventional insurance plans.

— *Consumer and purchaser attitudes.* Trends in total purchases of health care, selection of form or site of care, and market share should be described and quantified if data can be obtained at a reasonable cost. Particular attention should be paid to the attitudes of unions, employers, and governments, whose decisions affect large groups of individual consumers. While state and national trends are of interest, the view of local groups on key matters such as service, debt, price, and amenities should predominate. Communities vary substantially within a single state. Household surveys are a useful, although expensive, vehicle for assessing attitudes and behavior, and their popularity is growing rapidly.

— *Trends in clinical practice.* Technology and the attitudes of practitioners and patients interact to create demands for new services and new modes of delivery. (In the 1980s, for example, patients began to prefer outpatient over inpatient care. At the same time, technology supported rapid growth in organ transplantation.) While clinical trends are difficult to forecast quantitatively, describing them improves decision making.

— *Role of other providers.* Success can result from avoidance, competition or collaboration modes of interacting with other providers. Well-managed hospitals select the best mode based on careful analysis, and often use all three modes simultaneously. The choice requires careful identification of what each provider can do better than others. Service-specific market shares are one measure of achievement. Trends in market shares reflect success and failure. Surveys and data from the past are the sources for market share information. Since the data are often kept secret, quantitative forecasts are not always available. Subjective observations should be included in their absence. The optimal position of the hospital in the future marketplace depends heavily on this assessment.

— *Member attitudes and capabilities.* While any human resource can be obtained by training or recruitment, the starting point is the current member group. Therefore, even in a market-oriented hospital, trends in the skills and attitudes of current employees, physicians, and volunteers are important background to planning decisions. Formal surveys are frequently used, but additional insights can be gained by informal discussion.

— *Forecasts of demand.* The knowledge gained through assessments of the preceding must be translated into quantitative demand for discharges, patient-days, outpatient visits, and emergency visits. Aggregate forecasts of these six demand measures are included in the environmental assessment and the budget guidelines. They are frequently used to forecast demands for more specific services. All forecasts should include both an expectation and a range of probable values. Conditions applicable to these forecasts, such as the kind of patient expected or the events that might shift demand upward or downward, should be included. Supporting these forecasts with a discussion of dynamics avoids excessive detail, yet provides a basis for later forecast of any specific service desired.

Planning and marketing should be held accountable for a thorough survey of all of these elements every three to five years, and for a written annual review highlighting important trends and developments. It should also be accountable for reporting and, where possible, integrating insights or beliefs regarding future trends offered by other members of governance.

Issues in Quality of Environmental Assessment. Despite its use of statistical techniques and, occasionally, sophisticated data, environmental assessment remains basically a test of good judgment. The most serious dangers are bias and omission. Unfortunately, these may occur unintentionally and go unrecognized. To avoid these dangers, the best hospitals emphasize two principles.

The first is that surveillance must be concerned primarily with the marketplace rather than the views of corporation members. While it is true that a successful organization must make some exchanges with its members if it is to thrive, members other than owners must generally subjugate their views to customers. If surveillance is pursued in the order described above, the goal of market orientation is facilitated. In the four P's mnemonic of marketing—product, price, place, and promotion —surveillance identifies the most promising products, establishes a realistic price (actually, the total cost the customer is willing to bear for the product), and defines the proper place (the segment of the market reached and issues of style, location, and amenities that make the product more attractive to the customer). The knowledge gained from surveillance is critical to designing promotion.

The second principle is that surveillance be broad. No risk is as great as the risk of the unnoticed idea. The missed trend away from an old product or service, the overlooked interest in a new one, the too-narrow perception of capability—these underlie many wrong investments and the demise of entire industries. The speed with which opportunities are identified is important, because early identification permits the longest possible debate and preparation for the response. There is a danger of too rapid response, of elevating a transient variation to the status of a permanent shift. Yet, perversely, this danger often arises from incomplete surveillance. The transient fad is more likely to be identified as such when one's knowledge is broad. Thorough surveillance opens opportunities for revision and compromise, that might otherwise be overlooked.

Revising the Mission

Because the mission represents the most central desire of all the owners and because it is the benchmark for all subsequent planning decisions, it should be as permanent as possible. But in a dynamic environment, even the most carefully set mission may lose its relevance. Suburban flight, for example, has left many institutions behind. Tuberculosis, once a major, contagious, and untreatable disease calling for Samaritan effort, has been almost eliminated by technological advances. When such a situation arises, the hospital must revise its mission. Well-run hospitals identify such needs well in advance, through environmental surveillance. They probably contemplate mission revision far more often than they actually revise, since it is wise to consider many scenarios that in the end do not materialize. Given the mission's central role of setting values and directing the optimization process, it is important to deal decisively with possible changes. Each year's environmental surveillance is reviewed for mission consequences by a small group of leaders, who usually act individually until an important opportunity for revision is identified. The chief of planning and marketing, the CEO, the CFO, and governing board officers are the persons responsible for this review. The possible changes that arise are often combinations of three factors:

— Market data reflect a changing receptiveness to the established mission
— Review of unmet needs suggests an opportunity to expand the mission
— Review of roles of other providers reveals collaborative or acquisitive opportunities

Actual revisions of mission require formal board action. The planning-marketing staff marshalls the arguments for and against, and suggests appropriate wording.

Maintaining the Long-Range Plan

The long-range plan of a well-managed hospital serves three purposes:

1. It expands upon the mission statement with necessary goals, forecasts, and decisions that are both more detailed and more likely to require revision
2. It provides a standard for the development of the long-range fiscal plan and for the evaluation of various strategic and programmatic proposals
3. It is the focus of a management process or dialogue that builds broad understanding and consensus on the hospital's future direction

Something considerably more complicated than a single document is necessary to serve these purposes. One can conceptualize the long-range plan in three parts: a book, a library, and a process. The "book" is the document usually referred to as the long-range plan, serving the purpose of expanding the mission by specifying the broad outlines of the major actions the hospital intends. The "library" is the detailed files supporting each one of these projects. In very large projects, like replacement of a complete facility, the library grows to rooms full of plans and documentation. The "process" is the ongoing activity of collecting, disseminating, testing, and evaluating possibilities for the future.

The Long-Range Plan as a Document. The mission, environmental surveillance, and previous planning decisions are incorporated in a specific document called the **strategic plan.** The plan for a well-run hospital includes the following:

— The mission statement, expanded to include quantitative expectations about:

   • Geographic and other appropriate definitions of the community to be served

   • Major kinds of services to be offered

   • Financial needs of the institution

— Forecasts of the community in terms relevant to mission-implementing decisions. In general, these are derived from the environmental assessment, cover five years, and identify potential directions of change for a second five years. They include:

   • Age, sex, health insurance, and income characteristics of the community

   • Community demand for major service groups

   • Market shares by institution for major service groups

   • Demand at this hospital for major service groups by year

— Major changes in services—additions, deletions, expansions, or contractions—intended by the governing board, and the timing and extent of commitment to each

— Identification of major competing organizations by service, with their current size and announced intentions

— Identification of major uncertainties, identifiable risks of failure to achieve mission, and unmet community demand

— Summary of the major elements of the long-range fiscal plan (chapter 8), usually indicating annual net revenues, net surplus, and capital investment levels

Well-run hospitals emphasize brevity in the long-range plan. Even for a large and complicated enterprise, the plan above can be summarized in six relatively short chapters (mission, forecasts, commitments, competition, needs, and finances). The document does not describe processes supporting planning or detail methods for addressing unmet needs. It includes only the final forecasts, with ranges or estimates of uncertainty. Alternative scenarios are rarely presented, and alternative solutions and arguments supporting proposed actions are omitted. Forecasts beyond five years are included only when such commitments as major construction projects require them. All of these matters are addressed in the planning process, but to allow proper focus on the plan itself, supporting material is supplied in separate documents.

Certain elements of the long-range plan may be kept confidential. These generally include all cases in which knowledge of the hospital's interest would deleteriously affect achievement of the hospital's goals. The hospital's interest in a piece of real estate often increases its price, for example. Mergers, acquisitions, and entry into new markets can be hurt by untimely public recognition.

The Long-Range Plan as a Process. All well-run hospitals now have long-range plans; their current planning efforts, therefore, are addressed to revision, rather than preparation de novo. Well-run hospitals raise the question of revision annually. If a major environmental change occurs, the hospital should not wait to revise its plan. A routine annual review, revising as necessary and extending the plan an additional year with each review, protects the hospital in a dynamic environment. The effort involved in achieving a good plan requires several years. Even where the current process and document are judged seriously inadequate, annual revisions should usually stress the most critical improvements rather than an entirely new plan. The extent of the review effort is conditioned more by the perceived need than by a specific calendar.

The planning-marketing unit is responsible for drafting a revised plan along with the annual environmental assessment. The required forecasts are part of the assessment. Commitments are documented in the board minutes, and planning-marketing is responsible for a concise, current summary. Competition, needs, and finances are the critical parts of strategic planning. They are normally developed through several iterations by a small group of top management led by the CEO, using board advice on an informal basis. The mission, the environmental assessment, and the opinions of medical staff, other members, and influential persons in the community provide guidelines for this group, and its best effort is reported to the planning committee of the board for discussion and approval by the full board.

Fulfilling these responsibilities is a major part of planning-marketing activities. It is pursued intensively for several months each year and intermittently throughout the year. The process is ideally one of dialogue. Individual and group views are exchanged and incorporated into the draft. In the process, broad political support is built for the final document. When the process is well managed, acceptance of the environmental assessment stimulates consensus on the plan; external need drives organizational response.

Pursuing Strategic Opportunities

Given a mission, a plan, and annual surveillance, a hospital must still respond to its changing environment. Much of that response should be encouraged from within. Managers at all levels will see opportunities to revise, replace, expand, and contract their programs. Many of these programmatic revisions will require capital; most will alter the long-range plan at least slightly. They will usually be limited in their impact to part of a system, however. A different kind of response arises from the outside or affects so many parts of the existing hospital that only members of the governance system would be able to formulate it. It is called strategic because of its external origin and broad implications.

Strategic versus Programmatic Responses. Although one can think of examples overlapping the rough categories of programmatic and strategic responses, it is easier to understand the efforts involved by considering them in two groups.

Strategic responses are those which reposition the hospital in its environment. They usually have several of the following characteristics:

— They are stimulated by and often dependent upon specific events outside the hospital itself.

— Their timing is frequently dictated by these outside events.

— They involve large sectors or all of the institution.

— They require major redirections of the mission.

— They change the ownership or require restructuring of the governance system.

— They make a major change in the contracts between the hospital and its medical staff.

Programmatic proposals are more numerous than strategic responses and generally more modest, although they may grow to strategic dimensions.

— They usually arise from the units or departments within the hospital.

— They tend to affect only the nominating department or a few others.

— They are evaluated in light of the existing mission and long-range plan.

This distinction permits radically different procedures for handling proposals, recognizing differences not only in the effect and source of initiatives, but also in their timing and the hospital's freedom to speed or delay response.

Examples of strategic responses include:

— Additions or closures of major services, such as ambulatory care, psychiatry, substance abuse, obstetrics, and long-term care

— Expansions or replacements of major services, such as replacement of the inpatient facilities or the construction of satellites

— New organizational relationships, such as risk sharing with the medical staff, joint HMO or PPO contracts, or formal referral arrangements

— Affiliations, acquisitions, or major joint service agreements with other institutions

— Mergers, sales, or changes of ownership

The typical hospital will face many strategic issues in the coming decades—even the most remote rural institution will face several. Urban institutions will offer management contracts, long-term care needs will surface, and medical staff relationships must remain competitive with the rest of the world. Larger hospitals will face medical staff reorganizations and major service revisions as well as offers from other corporations for contracts, mergers, and affiliations.

Handling Strategic Opportunities. Strategic opportunities have a number of potentially troublesome characteristics. They tend to be unique, so experience is not directly applicable. The timetable by which they arise and must be evaluated is usually outside the hospital's control. Even though wise management can foresee many general possibilities, specific offers are good for limited periods or the environment changes to foreclose the option. They often involve sums of money several times the normal operating and capital budgets. They imply disruption of the lives of many members of the hospital organization. They may require secrecy, because premature public knowledge would substantially change the nature of the transaction. And, they are usually irreversible.

In short, strategic opportunities generally require high-risk decisions that test the governance structure and the skills of its leaders like no other activity. The uniqueness of each opportunity makes rules impractical, but there are some characteristics common to successful responses:

— Effective surveillance of competitors' activity can alert the hospital to many opportunities. Who is growing, failing, buying, selling, or approaching a critical organizational juncture can usually be detected in advance.

— A well-written mission statement, long-range plan, fiscal plan, and the history of discussion surrounding them provide the criteria for evaluating most strategic opportunities. Many such opportunities can be predicted some years in advance. The general issues can be debated as revisions to the mission rather than as specific options. For example, expansion into a new clinical service should be discussed as a mission revision first, and only later as a proposal for acquisition or construction of a facility.

— Well-run hospitals assemble a response team for each specific strategic opportunity. The team is as small as possible, and its membership emphasizes maturity in business decisions. The CEO is usually team leader, although a senior board officer occasionally assumes this role. Planning-marketing staff and finance staff make up the work force. Trusted senior physicians should be included. Outside consultants are frequently useful, particularly in situations without parallels in the hospital's history.

— Opportunities are evaluated against long-term cost-benefit criteria, where benefits are derived from goals previously stated in the mission.

— Opportunities are analyzed consistent with their benefits. Given the high risks involved, opportunities that involve only small or short-term benefits are dismissed quickly or redirected as programmatic. Newly discovered big gains are viewed sceptically. The unexpected chance to serve new markets at great benefit is ephemeral; well-run hospitals decline such opportunities, confident that if they were real they would have been foreseen.

— Response teams may be accountable only to the executive committee or senior governance officers until the project has undergone initial review. This arrangement preserves confidentiality where that is necessary. It also introduces all the dangers associated with secrecy, including opportunities for improper personal gain, but formal action always requires governing board approval, with the result that secrecy can at best be temporary. The costs of secrecy are such that well-run hospitals formalize and reveal strategic options as quickly as possible.

Developing and Evaluating Programmatic Proposals

Programmatic proposals also respond to approaching threats and opportunities. These may be revealed by the formal surveillance of planning-marketing or by the perceptiveness of line management. Line management in the well-run hospital monitors its own activities, particularly the technology associated with its professional area. Many proposals below the strategic level come from line sources. The well-managed hospital encourages proposals, because they reflect an alert, flexible work attitude and because they provide an opportunity for recognition of praiseworthy performance. An abundant supply of programmatic proposals minimizes the danger that the best solution will be overlooked.

If the first review step is an inexpensive but effective test against reality, unpromising ideas can be abandoned quickly. The remaining set of programmatic proposals must be evaluated thoroughly, involving significant time, effort, and cost. The evaluation method places great responsibility on line management, which must implement the proposal if it is accepted and achieve the benefits claimed. In most situations, planning-marketing provides assistance to line managers to assure a thorough, accurate, but persuasive presentation.

A good system for handling programmatic proposals is as follows:

1. The planning-marketing section is responsible for broad communication of exchange opportunities via environmental assessment and distribution of appropriate sections of the mission and long-range plan.

2. A supportive management environment encourages line supervisors to look within their own areas for imaginative ideas.

3. Individuals and informal line groups develop ideas in terms of their closed system parameters, but in a subjective, nonquantitative, inexpensive way.

4. The most promising of these ideas win the support of line superiors and are relayed to the planning-marketing department, where they are recorded as proposals. A planning staff mem-

ber is assigned to the project. He or she and the line advocate comprise a line-staff team for initial formal development.

5. Using a set of equations like those shown in figure 7.1, the line-staff team develops more precise costs and benefits. Depending on the magnitude of the proposal, this step may include several additional reviews by line and planning groups. The proposal may be integrated with others and a larger team created. A member from finance is usually added to large projects. The completed proposal must be fully specified in terms of the closed system parameters, including detailed procedures for the activity and all resources required.

6. Annually, completed proposals are grouped by hospital system and ranked by system management teams. The larger systems may have several rounds of internal ranking. A programmatic proposal in the laboratory would be ranked against other laboratory proposals, then other clinical support service proposals, and finally other clinical proposals before it left the clinical system. Even within the line systems, proposals are judged in light of the hospital's mission, environmental assessment, and long-range plan. The fate of low-ranking proposals becomes increasingly clear; they are often withdrawn by mutual consent. (The proposals withdrawn are often reworked; the impact of competitive review improves them.)

7. Ranked lists of proposals from the system groups are integrated into a single list by a larger committee that includes representatives from all the principal systems and often trustees from the planning and finance committees. The ranking of the integrated list continues to be based on mission, environment, and plan.

8. The integrated, ranked list of proposals becomes the annual capital budget request.

9. The governing board acts upon the individual elements of the capital budget request, authorizing expenditure, conditional expenditure, deferral, or rejection. This action is part of the annual budget approval. Projects are normally approved in rank order. The total amount of funds to be committed is decided at this point, based not only on mission, environment, and plan, but also on financial considerations.

10. Detailed implementation plans and schedules for approved proposals are developed by the line-staff team. A project manager is appointed and held accountable for conformance to both plans and schedules. Progress is usually monitored by an

Figure 7.1

Issues in Evaluating a Programmatic Proposal

The assistance provided by the planning-marketing department to line supervisors considering programmatic proposals begins with a thorough checklist of the issues likely to be involved. There is no perfect list, but a schema such as the one below tends to reveal the important questions in an order which identifies those most likely to be disabling early, when the idea can easily be modified, deferred, or abandoned.

Mission and Plan
What is the relationship of this proposal to the hospital's mission?
How does it enhance or improve the current long-range plan?
Benefit
In the most specific terms possible, what does this project contribute to health care? If possible, state
  The nature of the contribution, the probability of success, and the associated risk for each individual who benefits
  The kinds and numbers of persons who benefit.
If the hospital were unable to adopt the proposal, what would be the implication? Are there alternative sources of care? What costs are associated with using these sources?
If the proposal contributes to some additional or secondary objectives, what is the value of these contributions?
Market and Demand
What size and segment of the hospital's community will this proposal serve?
What fraction of this group is likely to seek care at this hospital?
What is the trend in the size of this group and its tendency to seek care here? How will the proposal affect this trend?
To what extent is the demand dependent upon insurance or finance incentives? What is the likely trend for these provisions?
What impact will the proposal have on the hospital's general market share or on other specific services?
What implications does the project have for the recruitment of physicians and other key health care personnel?
What response or initiatives does this proposal suggest for competing hospitals or health care sources?
What are the promotional requirements of the proposal?   *Continued*

appropriate line manager, with the aid of the line-staff team. The planning staff is responsible for all outside negotiations for permits and approvals. Special teams are usually assembled when negotiations with competitors are involved.

11. Unfunded proposals are returned to the line systems, which can resubmit them the next year, improve them, or abandon them.

These steps are easier to describe than to follow in the real world; processes described here as discrete are really continuous and inter-

Figure 7.1 Continued

Costs and Resources
What are the marginal operating and capital costs of the proposal, including start-up costs and possible revenue losses from other services?
Are there cost implications for other services or overhead activities?
Are there special or critical resource requirements?
Are there identifiable opportunity costs associated with the proposal, or with other proposals or opportunities facilitated by this proposal?
Are there other intangible elements (positive or negative) associated with this proposal?

Finance
What are the capital requirements, project life, and finance costs associated with the proposal?
What are the competitive price and anticipated net revenue?
How much uncertainty is associated with the demand forecast, and how sensitive is the cost-benefit ratio to fluctuations in demand?
What are the insurance or finance sources of revenue, and what implications do these sources raise?
What is the net cash flow associated with the proposal over its life, and the discounted value of that flow?

Other factors
What opportunities are there to enhance this proposal or others by combining them?
Are there any specific risks or benefits associated with the proposal which are not identified elsewhere?
Does the proposal suggest a strategic opportunity, such as a joint venture or the purchase or sale of a major service?

Timing, Implementation, and Evaluation
What are the elements on the critical path of the installation process, and how long will each take?
What are the problems or advantages associated with deferring or speeding up the implementation?
What are the anticipated changes in the operating budget of the units accountable for the proposal? What changes are required in supporting units?

---

twined. The basic structure has several important advantages. Its iterative, expanding approach to evaluation and its insistence on competitively ranked recommendations promote efficiency. The integrated line and staff roles encourage thorough competitive review and limit expensive governing board time without diminishing board influence. Broad hospital, employee, and medical staff participation promotes development of realistic expectations, but also enhances a sense of involvement. Finally, the development of specific implementation plans and schedules smooths the process of change.

Assisting in the Development of Proposals. The planning-marketing staff helps the line managers to articulate benefits in light of the hospital plan and mission, to specify the market as precisely as possible, and to forecast demand. Planning-marketing also provides the protocol for developing proposals uniformly, in order to permit fair competitive evaluation. Planning-marketing should help articulate costs and benefits and make each proposal as competitive as possible. The issues listed in figure 7.1 are designed to prompt thorough review of costs and benefits.

A completed proposal must state expectations for all the parameters of the closed system model, including the procedures for the proposed activity or service. Early rounds of review will demonstrate that the necessary resources and procedures are available, that demand is present, and that adequate quality can be maintained. Later evaluation and competitive ranking will be based upon output, cost, benefit, and risk. Even using an iterative evaluation process that relies first on crude estimates, it is necessary to begin by specifying how the product or service envisioned will be provided. Once procedures are described, it is possible to forecast the output, cost, and benefit parameters. Risk is associated with the forecasts themselves. Additional elements of the closed system model, chiefly quality and efficiency, can be considered in every proposal but developed into quantitative expectations only where necessary.

Preparing the proposal, particularly in its later, more precise stages, requires collaboration of many units of the hospital. Demand is forecast from planning-marketing surveys. Considering the need and availability of specific resources usually requires assistance from the human resources and plant systems. Health care benefits are often derived from scientific literature and clinical opinion. Revenue or profit benefits require careful analysis of pricing and service contracts. The marginal costs used in evaluation are rarely available from routine accounting data and must often be developed through special studies. All future costs and revenues should be discounted to a common time so they can be compared. Determining risks and ranges for expectations requires experience and statistical skills. Planning staff should be prepared to carry out many of the specific calculations. Their role is to coordinate the process, collect the necessary knowledge efficiently, and make sure appropriate technical procedures are followed.

The key to effective assistance is to encourage iterative evaluation aimed at identifying promising ideas early. Although each element of the closed system model must be considered, the rigor and precision of each expectation should be reduced in the early stage of proposal development. This technique allows the well-run hospital to consider many proposals and to select the best from a large pool. Iterative evaluation requires a willingness to work with imprecise estimates and an ability to make sound initial judgments. The longer and more completely a proposal is considered, the more is invested in it. A proposal abandoned after much work represents a hidden cost that can be avoided by good initial judgment.

Communication, Promotion, and Coordination

Building consensus is often underrated as part of an effective planning process. Debate and disagreement are useful and important in the early stages of planning, but as decisions become firmer, agreement should extend well beyond a simple majority. Large numbers of people, including customers, must agree with planning decisions if implementation of them is to succeed. Even after a project is accepted or rejected, an influential group that continues to oppose the decision can be disruptive to future planning activities.

In the well-run hospital, the planning-marketing executive is accountable for minimizing dissent by communicating with all those who might hold an opinion. Communication takes several forms. It includes issues of both content and process. It often extends to negotiation when influential parties are involved, sometimes jointly by the CEO and other members of the governance system. Advertising and public relations are increasingly used to reach large groups.

The following activities comprise the communication, promotion, and coordination function.

Recommend and Implement Planning Processes. The process by which the long-range plans, strategic opportunities, and programmatic proposals are developed and evaluated is in itself a mechanism of communication and consensus building. Well-designed and well-implemented processes promote candid discussions, identification of differing opinions, and the resolution of differences. Confidence that process will be followed consistently diffuses antagonism and promotes resolution. To achieve a sound, constructive process requires both detailed procedural steps and philosophical positions specified in advance and interpreted for specific projects. The normal timing and participation for environmental assessment, mission review, and long-range plan revision are well known in the well-managed hospital. Procedures for strategic review are clearly identified, and a policy of necessary secrecy is articulated. (It is better to define a specific domain of confidential action than to have members infer what that domain is.) Review of planning procedures themselves should be widespread, promoting understanding. Final approval is a policy matter for the governing board. Once procedures are developed, the planning-marketing unit is accountable for implementing them.

Disseminate Appropriate Portions of the Long-Range Plan. The plan and the mission statement constitute the major policy statement on direction for the organization. They are the principal guides for both strategic and programmatic decisions. As such, they should be broadly shared among members and friends of the organization, so that all have similar criteria for assessing new ideas. While it may be necessary to conceal some parts of the plan for competitive reasons, the plan should generally be used to initiate the consensus-building process. Concealing the plan may protect a hospital from its competitors, but it is just as likely to confuse members and friends.

Maintain Public Information and Public Relations Functions. The twentieth century has seen a major expansion of the public's right to know. Hospital planning is particularly subject to this trend because regulations require disclosure well in advance of action. The well-run hospital must respond affirmatively to this trend, using the obligation to inform the public as an opportunity to promote broader consensus. Public information should be coordinated with advertising. Both may deliberately promote use of hospital services.

Public information on planning projects is one of several sources from which people derive a positive image of the hospital. Maintaining this image is the purpose of public relations activity. All members of the hospital are involved in public relations; the governing board and the CEO are accountable for the entire image. Specific accountability for public information and promotion should be assigned within the governance system, and planning-marketing has strong claims to the assignment.

Manage Advertising and Promotion. Direct efforts to influence buying decisions, member attitude, and public image are new to hospitals, but the change appears to be permanent. Promotion is a small component of marketing, but an integral one. Each approved strategic or programmatic proposal should have a section dealing with promotion. The eventual form of hospital advertising and promotion remains to be determined. Advertising in particular has become a highly technical area, although it does not yet appear that the sophisticated technology used in general consumer advertising has been fully transferred to the health care arena. The relative merits of promoting to the doctor as the patient's agent versus promoting directly to the patient have not been worked out.

The planning-marketing function of well-managed hospitals is being rapidly expanded to include accountability for a comprehensive promotional program. At present, this appears to include the establishment of a service contract with a reputable advertising agency. In the future, it may involve employment of an advertising or promotional specialist as a member of the planning-marketing unit.

Three important factors will govern promotion. Stimulating demand in general may run counter to community pressure for economy, leading the governing board to curtail certain forms of promotion. Second, efforts to gain a larger share of the market may be no more than protection from the promotional efforts of others. The impact of all hospitals' advertising may be very similar to the impact of no advertising. Third, it remains true that most hospital services are dependent on volume. The unit cost of a service is lower if the volume is high. The combination of these three factors defines the role of promotion. It should help the hospital maintain its share of the market, sustain adequate volume for all services, and speed the introduction of new services, particularly when these will reduce cost.

Advertising can be considered a closed system activity whose parameters are at least partially quantified. In well-run hospitals it is a specific cost center, with a budget including expectations about cost, outcomes, quality, and efficiency. Generally speaking, advertising has two outputs or goals—the increase of demand, or market share, and the improvement of owner satisfaction. Both of these are measurable by surveys, and market share is often measurable by the behavior of patients and doctors. It is difficult, however, to associate specific changes with specific promotional activities, particularly when the hospital's competitors are also advertising. The cost of advertising is relatively straightforward. Efficiency is generally assessed in terms of the number of persons reached for a given expenditure, because the ultimate statistic, the number of people influenced by the communication, is inaccessible.

Quality of advertising might best be judged in the context of the fundamental goals of the owners: Samaritanism, private health, public health, economy, and community development (see chapter 2). An admirable advertising activity is one that promotes not only the effective and efficient use of medical care, but the desirability of maintaining health and preventing illness. An image of the hospital as contributing to the quality of life of the community is certainly advantageous. The well-managed hospital begins its promotional campaign by making real contributions to these goals. Its promotional efforts reveal reality and never mislead the hospital's exchange partners.

Defend the Hospital Before Regulatory Bodies. As a result of national laws enacted in 1966 and 1974, many states require **certificates of need** for new services and construction or renovation. State approval of construction as a requirement for reimbursement by Medicare is more uniform; no new capital cost can be recovered from Medicare unless section 1122 approval is obtained. These laws are enforced with varying degrees of vigor, and their importance is diminishing. They apply to all hospitals, so the regulatory body enforcing them, usually a health systems agency, can become an important competitive arena when two or more hospitals desire the same service.

Success at the HSA depends upon timing, well-designed and attractive services, technically well-prepared proposals, and the views of influential persons in the community. One individual should be accountable for the management of HSA relations. The planning-marketing executive, or, in very large hospitals, a deputy, is the best informed person, although the task is sometimes retained by the CEO. Strategies for dealing with HSAs and certificates of need vary. The influence of these laws on long-range hospital plans is arguable, but many predict it will decline. Most well-run hospitals have developed strategies and tactics for gaining the approval of all or nearly all their important options and proposals.

In some communities there are voluntary or other regulatory bodies, and in most cities, hospital construction requires zoning board approval, construction permits, or both. These negotiations are clearly the responsibility of planning-marketing.

Assist in Negotiations with Competing or Collaborating Organizations.
Planning-marketing staff are frequently involved in strategic opportunities. As noted above, strategic responses should be based on thorough, ongoing surveillance of institutions with related or potentially related missions. This surveillance frequently includes considerable direct communication. The planning-marketing staff is often involved in these dialogues.

There is a long-standing tradition that community hospitals should collaborate with one another, principally because they share a common obligation to the same community and because such collaboration appears to be more economical. However, in the era of unlimited financial support and significant subsidization for growth, the tradition was exceptionally difficult to implement. In the newer, more restrictive and more competitive environment, collaboration appears, ironically, to be more successful, even as competition is more common.

Even bitterly competing hospitals tend to communicate frequently. Trustees, medical staff leaders, executives, and planners are often involved in dialogue. The hospital situation appears to be similar to more traditionally competitive industries; both secrecy and communication are used constantly. The antitrust implications of dialogue between competitors are difficult to describe. The law on per se violations is clear: conversations between competitors cannot include collusion to set prices, divide or establish markets, or exclude other competitors. Such actions are criminal, and individuals have been prosecuted for them. On the other hand, exploration of merger or shared service possibilities is neither a criminal nor a civil violation of the act if it can be defended as being in the public interest. A practical suggestion is that dialogue is necessary, but that the per se topics should be avoided in action, implication, and intent.

One way to increase market share is to provide joint marketing of selected services. Such activities are not automatically proscribed by antitrust laws. Similarly, both winners and losers—for different reasons —under competitive pressures are motivated to seek mergers and affiliations. The actual negotiation of these arrangements is usually reserved to the CEO and selected members of the governing board, but the planning-marketing executive is a member of the well-run hospital's strategic response teams, and planning-marketing data are the appropriate bases for many of the decisions. The planning-marketing executive is frequently the appropriate emissary.

Personnel and Organization

Personnel Requirements

Even a large hospital will employ only a handful of people in its planning activity. Other members of the governance system, particularly the CEO and CFO, will have important planning functions, and outside consultants are often used. The well-run hospital has at least one designated, professionally prepared planning executive to give continuity and coordination to its planning-marketing program. Very small hospitals must assign planning-marketing responsibilities directly to the chief executive or one deputy. Hospitals that do not hold a single executive accountable have difficulty completing the functions in an orderly and timely manner, thus losing opportunities to respond to the market. A small professional staff supporting the executive is not uncommon and can often be justified by reduced expenditures for outside consultants.

Multihospital systems frequently centralize some aspects of planning to improve the technical skills of personnel, to provide economies of scale, and to ensure consistency when appropriate. On the other hand, health care remains a locally generated and locally delivered product. A major advantage of not-for-profit multihospital systems is their ability to tailor their response to differing local situations. Many leading not-for-profit chains deliberately retain local planning-marketing staffs, at least in each of their geographical communities. One of the key questions in design of the multihospital system is the question of who may negotiate mergers or joint agreements.

Professional Skills of Planning-Marketing Executives. Effective institutional planning requires an ability to build consensus by negotiation, together with mastery of a growing body of professional knowledge and skill. Professional requirements include techniques for analysis, knowledge of health care administration, and understanding of community and individual opinion formation. Analytic techniques should include practical skills in cost accounting, present value analysis, statistics, and forecasting. The nature of hospitals requires detailed knowledge of the dynamics of health care: current status and trends in health insurance, government financial programs, health personnel availability, health care technology, sources of capital funds, the role of regulatory bodies, and prevention of disease. Finally, the planning executive must understand community power structures and decision processes, methods of information dissemination, and the uses of advertising and public relations.

Most of the professional subject matter is covered in an accredited master's degree program in health care administration. A graduate degree in business also covers many of the topics, although with important omissions in specifics of the health care field. A competent individual with a degree in either of these fields can improve his or her skill through continuing education and reading. The combination of both business and health administration degrees is increasingly relevant and becoming more popular.

Negotiating skills are learned by practice. Certainly the mature planning-marketing executive should be able to conduct fruitful meetings, identify and assist in the resolution of disputes, and present information clearly and convincingly, both orally and in writing. Beginners must learn those skills by observation and supervised experience, although community and extramural collegiate activities are useful.

Planning-marketing personnel are recruited in national markets. Deputies and beginners are often selected from among recent graduates. Planning-marketing executives are promoted from within, attracted from consulting firms, or hired from other hospitals. Although experience and maturity are important, it is not uncommon to rely upon the experience of the CEO to overcome immaturity in the planning unit. The centrality, breadth of scope, and requirements for planning-marketing suggest it as an excellent background for CEOs and COOs.

Outside Consultants. The variety and extent of skills required in planning-marketing make it a fruitful area for the use of consultants. Many activities of planning-marketing can be assigned to outside firms. These include:

— *Surveillance,* demographic and economic forecasts, trends in technology and personnel availability, evaluation of future plant and equipment needs, consumer demand and market surveys, and surveys of competitors' behavior.

— *Strategic responses,* investigation of competitors' interests and positions, evaluation of expansion and acquisition options, advice on entering new markets or offering new services, and experience in strategic procedures and negotiations.

— *Proposal development and evaluation,* suggestions for new products and services, feasibility and cost-benefit analyses, and design of response evaluation protocol.

— *Communication and promotion,* promotional campaign design and completion, advertising design and layout, and general public relations assistance.

The possible uses of outside consultants are so extensive that specifying what they *cannot* do may be the easiest way to identify their contribution. Consultants cannot replace the judgment of either operating personnel or governing board members, and, of course, they cannot and do not accept accountability for the mission, long-range plan objectives, or selection of specific programs. Thus any consultant's recommendation must be carefully and fully evaluated by those responsible for the institution. Consultants cannot provide the continuity of an ongoing executive presence.

Consultants can specialize in understanding demographic, economic, and underlying attitudinal trends; act as extra hands; impart technical skills for specialized responses; bring knowledge of what others facing the same problem are doing; and mediate entrenched conflicts over the nature of the mission, the objectives, or a specific response.

The keys to successful use of consultants are as follows:

1. The assignment should be clearly specified in terms of process, timing, and result. As a general rule, the clearer the assignment and the more details of the work specified in advance, the better the chances for success. It is occasionally wise to use consultants to gain fresh insights into vague, ill-defined problems, but such use should be limited to very short-term assignments.

2. To be cost-effective, topics assigned to consultants should require skills or quantities of effort not available locally. Using consultants as neutral third parties is essentially correcting a failure of the local process, and this should not occur often.

3. Consultant firms should be selected on the basis of relevant prior experience. In the absence of direct experience with a consultant, opinions of other clients should be solicited before any major assignment is made.

4. Consultant activities should be carefully monitored against the specifications throughout the project. This job is often assigned to the planning-marketing executive.

Organization

Most planning units in U.S. hospitals are so small that there is little internal organization. A division into each of the six functions suggests itself, but a better approach might be to hold deputy planner-marketers accountable for specifics along the lines of surveillance, mission, and strategic options; programmatic proposal selection, evaluation, and implementation; and public relations and promotion. A functional view is to attach planning-marketing individuals to major clinical units, and certainly individuals should be responsible for maintaining relations between planning-marketing and medicine, nursing, major clinical support units, and outpatient care. This suggests that a practical organization of a planning unit follows matrix organization principles, with each deputy of the planning-marketing executive accountable for a functional area and relations with specific line units.

The supervision of consultants should also be explicitly assigned to individuals, with accountability running through the planning-marketing executive. Failure to identify a point of contact slows the consultants and adds to their costs, and defeats the possibility of continuous monitoring during the contract period.

Many hospitals prefer to make public relations and promotion a separate staff activity within the governance unit. One should be aware of issues of span of control in the governance activity; a group of several staff units each reporting to the CEO may or may not be more effective. Assignment to the planning-marketing executive enhances the planner's responsibility for accurate market assessment and reduces recriminations between promotion and planning when demand forecasts turn out to be unrealistic. Similarly, this structure minimizes the distance between surveillance and public relations, two activities that are synergistic.

Well-run hospitals keep planning-marketing activities very close to the CEO and the governing board. Split reporting of planning-marketing functions, some to the CEO and some to the COO, may cause some aspects to get less attention than they should. Assignment of planning-marketing to the COO risks an undesirably short term focus and may result in insufficient attention to strategic options and community needs. Assignment of planning-marketing to the CFO increases the dominance of the financial aspect of decisions; in the long run, responsiveness to community need should determine the decisions more than financial implications for the hospital.

Measuring Performance

The planning-marketing activity, like every other part of the well-run hospital, should have established, short-term expectations and regular reporting of achievement against these. Although the complexity and ambiguity of the task are great, some implementation of closed system management principles remains essential. Expectations should be set for demand, output and quality, resource consumption and resource conservation, and for the scope of the planning-marketing activity. These should be as quantitative and objective as possible. It is possible to assess many of the necessary expectations by using a combination of outcomes and process measures. Those important expectations not qualifiable at even a process level must be covered by discussion and agreement. The expectations should be set at the time of the annual budget and monitored monthly thereafter. The surveillance and long-range planning functions of the planning-marketing department in themselves generate considerable information. Much of this is now quantified in the well-managed hospital. In particular, the planning-marketing activity generates estimates of market share from hospitalization behavior and from customer surveys. Surveys of patients and doctors provide evidence on customer and member satisfaction. Social, demographic, and economic information describe the community identified in the mission. The planning process establishes desirable expectations on all of these measures that are under hospital control; the planning-marketing unit generally establishes forecasts for all those that are not under hospital control.

The first measure of planning-marketing performance, therefore, is the extent to which forecasts were accurate and expectations were achieved. Unfortunately, multiple factors contribute to those results. Evaluating the adequacy of the planning-marketing activity must obviously be subjective. When forecasts are wide of the mark, the cause should be apparent. Consistent departure from expectations, either by underachievement or overachievement, is cause for concern.

The evaluation of planning-marketing is inevitably bound up with that of the chief executive. The ultimate judgment, that the hospital is or is not positioned where it should be in the community, is based upon environmental surveillance but is the governing board's function.

Demand Measures

Viewed from an outcomes perspective, the measure of demand is market share, but this must be evaluated in light of acceptable levels of quality, economy, finance, and community need. Assessment of unmet need is important. Market share, or percentage of the total community need met at the hospital, is central; because so much of the efficiency of hospitals depends on maintaining adequate volume to cover fixed costs, ability to meet market share expectations is usually the key to financial performance and growth.

The demand for planning-marketing can also be viewed as the amount of service expected by other hospital units. Demand can be assessed by the quantities of routine reports, special reports or projects, promotional campaigns, committee meetings and assignments, and other activities anticipated during the forthcoming year. These items can rarely be fully quantified, and the dimensions are not additive. In addition, planning-marketing plays an important standby role, which cannot be foreseen. As a result, demand expectations are best described in a memorandum of understanding and left unquantified.

Output Measures

It is also difficult to specify expectations for planning-marketing output, although there are exceptions for certain parts of the total activity. Reach and frequency of advertising campaigns may be specified, as may number of public presentations; however, these are only partial contributions to the real goal. As a result, few hospitals rely on quantitative output expectations; instead, they emphasize an understanding of the kinds of service requests anticipated and agreement on the quality, including the timeliness, of services with which the demand will be filled.

Because of the difficulties of quantifying output, efficiency has little meaning in planning-marketing. The term is occasionally confused with promptness, which is a dimension of quality. Advertising efficiency, cost per contact, can be addressed, but it is a relatively small part of overall evaluation.

Quality Measures

Quality of work includes outcomes measures on how accurate, timely, and effective the work was and process measures on the methods and approaches used. Unfortunately, the more important the work, the less likely it is that accuracy and effectiveness can be judged in a year or less. The difficulties of measurement and of isolating the contribution of planning-marketing to the results suggest strongly that these measures must be considered subjectively, as a major element of planning-marketing assessment. Often, evaluation must be limited to a few events that are complete and self-contained enough to yield lessons for the future. These "anecdotes" may still be enough for beneficial review and evaluation.

Outcomes Measures

Outcomes measures include the accuracy of forecasts of exogenous events, the achievement of expected values for cost, revenues and demand from newly planned operations, the rate of acceptance of proposals by outside review bodies and influentials, and improvements in attitudes of specific exchange partners. The relationship between the result and the planning-marketing activity is often tenuous. Good results can accrue after bad planning and vice versa. Thus outcomes measures should not be the sole basis for quality assessment; however, to omit them is to lose sight of the fundamentals of organizational success. Only those hospitals which achieve good results from these activities succeed.

A well-run hospital will have expectations concerning and routine measurement of at least the following:

— Variations from annual forecasts of major measures of market share and demand for service

— Achievement of market share and demand increases anticipated from advertising campaigns

— Rates of growth of demand and revenue for new services implemented, compared with forecasts from programmatic proposals

— Comparisons of actual implementation costs with expectations stated in programmatic proposals

— Comparisons of actual operating costs and profit with expectations stated in programmatic proposals

— Comparisons of implementation timetables with programmatic proposal expectations

— Percentage of applications successfully submitted to regulatory and planning bodies

— Fund-raising success, in dollars and percentage of potential contributors, for specific projects and general campaigns

— Attitudes of community partners toward specific hospital programs and overall acceptance, with particular attention to influentials

— Attitudes of patients and families toward the hospital

— Attitudes of members toward specific hospital programs and overall acceptance

— Timely recognition of opportunities and potential problems

— Timely completion of projects relative to community and market needs and opportunities

A final consideration in outcomes assessment is the development of the hospital as a whole. The long-range financial plan, discussed in chapter 8, provides general guidelines for growth or shrinkage of demand by area or service. While countless forces contribute to realizing these forecasts, at least a subjective recognition of the contribution of planning-marketing is useful.

Process Measures. In addition, planning-marketing should be evaluated periodically on structure and process. Measures include:

— Satisfaction of members and committees working directly with planning-marketing
— Attitudes of other members of management and medical staff toward the planning-marketing activity
— Evaluation of work by outside consultants
— Compliance with JCAH criteria
— Customer acceptance of advertising
— Counts of media insertions and recognition

Resource Consumption

The planning-marketing activity should have an explicit budget like any other unit in the hospital. Because of the difficulties of measuring demand, the budget should be fixed rather than flexible. Expenditures for outside consultants and for advertising are likely to be major items, in addition to personnel costs. The budget should be considered in light of agreed-upon demand expectations and the desirability of quality improvements.

Resource Conservation

The planning-marketing activity has no direct revenue or profit. It can be evaluated on revenue from specific programmatic projects, as noted. Successful advertising activity may generate new demand and new revenue. Given the relatively high fixed cost for most clinical services, these gains may be highly profitable for the hospital. It is probably better to evaluate planning-marketing on the most direct measure, that is, changes in market share, than on the more remote, profits. It is also possible to specify a strategic objective—that the unit must identify and develop several appropriate new sources of revenue that will yield a certain total revenue or profit by a certain time. Such an objective is probably more appropriate to a five-year horizon than to an annual one, but it could be included in the hospital's long-range plan and used to support more specific annual expectations.

The difficulty with general revenue or profit expectations is more in their application than in their philosophical acceptability. Actual achievement should be compared judiciously against expectations, with due regard to exigencies that could not reasonably have been foreseen and to the dangers that arise from excessive zeal in pursuit of short-term profits. When this warning is ignored, there is serious danger of destructive outcomes. It must be recognized that the purpose of planning-marketing is not to contribute to profits, but rather to facilitate the hospital's successful adjustment to a complex and sensitive web of relationships. If the warning is heeded, an expectation that the unit will contribute to general profits serves well to focus planning-marketing activities.

Management Issues

Success in planning-marketing occurs when the hospital is led into fruitful endeavors. Failure comes in two ways, when weaker ventures are selected and when better ones are overlooked. From that perspective, a formal planning-marketing activity must justify its existence by being faster and more thorough: it must uncover the obscure and move promptly on the obvious. From one viewpoint, planning is an intelligence activity, uncovering hidden risks and overlooked opportunities. From another, it is a service to expedite a decision-making process. The conventional model for success emphasizes surveillance, mission setting, and long-range planning as the background and guide to decisions that must be made on strategic opportunities and programmatic proposals. Experience with this model has revealed some areas where special attention is useful. The issues are reviewed in four groups:

1. Technical foundations within the planning-marketing unit

2. Integrating promotional activity

3. Techniques for orderly review of programmatic proposals

4. Premises for evaluating opportunities and proposals in not-for-profit hospitals

Technical Foundations

Successful planning-marketing units seem to excel in four technical areas: (1) they take extra pains to guard against oversights, (2) they use the most objective forecasts they can obtain, (3) they are rigorous in their evaluation of costs and benefits, and (4) they follow procedures that deliberately use comparison and competition to debate the best course of action.

Guarding Against Oversight. The first step in avoiding overlooking the best ideas is in recognizing the danger of doing so. Most planning and forecasting is done by extrapolating from past history, often assuming *ceteris paribus,* or other things being equal. No other approach is practical or prudent as a mainstay of a planning-marketing unit, or a governance activity generally. Truly radical departures are rare; the past is usually prologue to the present and most change does occur incrementally. Thus most of the time this approach is both the least expensive and the most likely to be correct. Success lies in discovering those few cases in which the future will depart radically from the past. There are several ways to check for this possibility:

— Radical change often occurs at different times in different places. A check of conditions elsewhere may show trends not yet evident in the local community.

— Radical change usually arises from individuals with different views from the rest of the group, sometimes to the point of being outcasts. Careful study of the opinions of critics of the status quo can suggest practical improvements upon *ceteris paribus.*

— Imagination can be prompted by deliberately trying to think the unthinkable. The most successful planners deliberately insert a step in each forecasting or planning exercise which asks two questions:

  • What could occur that would make this forecast totally wrong?

  • Is there any other scenario, however improbable, that would be significantly more attractive than this one, and what might make such a scenario more probable?

— An environment in which ideas can be openly expressed promotes discovery of the rare radical departure. Many successful institutions promote such an environment by periodically inviting consultants and speakers known for their unconventional views; making sure that those who express unusual views are protected from personal insult or injury, such as losing promotions or salary increases; and opening their plans to widespread debate and discussion, with the intention of finding conflicting views and evaluating them.

Using Objective Forecasts. Subjective forecasts, those prepared intuitively by people working in the hospital, can be very accurate for periods of less than two years, if they are carefully prepared. Their accuracy deteriorates rapidly over longer terms and in unfamiliar applications.

Successful hospitals take pains to find independent sources of forecasts, to use several different sources, and to use rigorously unbiased methods to describe the future and to evaluate opportunities for response. Such coldblooded realism improves planning in two ways: it reveals projects based on fantasy soon enough to avoid them, and it develops a climate of credibility in which the surviving proposals can be effectively evaluated.

To develop successful plans, exogenous factors influencing demand must be forecast as accurately as possible. These include community population, age structure of the population, birth rate, income, insurance coverage, and the need for goods and services other than health care. Most of these are forecast by several independent sources, and well-run hospitals use these forecasts rather than their own. They discard predictions by groups with vested interests (such as the local power companies and the Chamber of Commerce), and use the remaining ones to project both an expectation and a range of possibilities. They then explore costs and benefits of proposed responses across the range, rather than simply for the expected value.

Using Cost-Benefit Measures Effectively. The costs and benefits of many different proposals must be assessed quickly and inexpensively. The iterative evaluation described above is one step toward this goal. Some others that well-run hospitals adopt include:

— Adhering to a formal protocol that prompts recognition of obscure costs and hidden risks. The protocol should strongly encourage investigation of several areas known to be overlooked in less rigorous approaches:

  • Costs of borrowing or leasing
  • Costs of obsolescence, or unduly optimistic estimates of project life
  • Opportunity costs in committing irreplaceable resources
  • Overhead costs or burdens on other units
  • Promotional costs and the implications of competition for limited demand
  • Intangible costs, including possible political repercussions, member dissatisfaction, and malpractice liability

— Searching for combinations of projects which increase the attractiveness of both. Often a project that is too costly if undertaken on its own is valuable when it is included in a package with others. Renovations, for example, create conditions in which many previously impractical revisions become cost-effective. They also represent windows in time. When the renovation is complete, projects overlooked may be forever lost. The well-run hospital sees more possible combinations because it looks for them.

— Encouraging complete identification and description of benefits which cannot be assigned precise dollar valuation. Most benefits, particularly those related to health, are difficult to evaluate and impossible to measure in dollar terms. They can be identified and described, and the number of people likely to receive them can be forecast. These estimates are much less expensive than imprecise dollar estimates and probably as useful.

— Requiring ranges of possible outcomes as well as the most likely outcomes, and full exploration of risk and the implications of less desirable possibilities.

— Using staff experts, individuals from other hospital systems, and outside consultants to enhance the accuracy of cost and benefit estimates. Physicians, industrial engineers, purchasing agents, finance department staff, and plant department staff can improve the reliability and the credibility of estimates. Outside consultants bring objectivity and greater experience to bear.

— Using examples from other hospitals. The most convincing evidence of accurate cost-benefit estimates is the existence of a smoothly operating example elsewhere. Few hospitals have the resources to pioneer; those that do, do so in only a few areas. Many poorly run hospitals are trapped by delusions of uniqueness or unrealistic visions of leadership.

Maintaining Objectivity in the Evaluation Process. Objectivity and realism must extend beyond the exogenous forecasts and the development of cost-benefit measures to the entire process of response evaluation and selection. There are natural human tendencies not only to overstate the ratio of benefits to costs, but also to distort it in favor of one's personal desires. The well-run hospital must use systems for evaluating response that minimize both these risks. The following are specific steps:

— Use line-staff teams to develop projects, because their dual contribution tends to reduce bias.

— Group programmatic proposals together with an annual timetable tied to the budget cycle, and start comparative review as far down the accountability hierarchy as possible, even within a single responsibility center, should it have two proposals to compare in a single cycle.

— Provide sequential review against broadening competition and at higher levels of the accountability hierarchy. (Among other virtues, this tends to uncover hidden drawbacks in projects before large financial or emotional commitments have been made to them.)

— Keep a broadly representative membership on the planning committee or the capital budget committee. The committee that makes the final recommendation to the board frequently must weigh several expensive, strongly advocated projects, each of which has considerable merit. Faith in and credibility of this committee are essential to continued generation of proposals.

— Encourage candid discussion of proposals by minimizing the negative consequences of honesty. There are large differences in rank and power in a hospital. Influential people must visibly respect the opinions of individuals who are less powerful. Power should not be rewarded in the planning process. Helpful techniques for encouraging candor include:

- Adhering to the established protocol for all proposals
- Selecting planning committee members so that powerful people are balanced against one another rather than against groups of less powerful people
- Chairing meetings competently, so that all can be heard
- Using outside consultants to counterbalance local experts
- Instructing or sanctioning individuals who endanger the process of development and evaluation

Integrating Promotional Activity

Until the 1980s, little was said about marketing in connection with hospitals. The notion that professional wisdom was superior to consumers' wishes in health care prevailed throughout most of the century, thus planning was a professional or technocratic endeavor rather than a market-oriented one. The shortage of health care resources facilitated technocratic planning, in effect permitting professionals to decide which patients they would accept. Advertising and promotion were considered unethical, partly because they imply patient or customer selection rather than professional selection and partly because the American Medical Association (AMA) and most other professional societies viewed them as contrary to the best attitudes of professionalism.

The professional view was significantly diminished by a general loss of faith in technology and a national shift to consumerism which began in the late 1960s. Doctors' objections to advertising were over-ruled on antitrust grounds in 1980.[1] Recognition of surplus hospital and medical resources, declining markets, and the competitive environment of the 1980s spelled the end of the older views.

There is no question that hospitals must respond to the public, finding out what specific customers want, what price they will pay, and what products the hospital can emphasize to create its own *niche,* or unique advantage, in the market. This concept of market responsive-ness, or customer orientation, is the principal difference between the concept of planning-marketing as opposed to the older concept of plan-ning. Marketing not only uses planning techniques to define three of its four P's, product, place, and price, it is philosophically meaningless in the absence of a mission and an objective. The old-style planning with-out marketing cannot succeed in a competitive environment.

Advertising and promotion, the fourth P, are the most obvious differences between the new concepts and the old. They are often delib-erate efforts to convert customers to a more favorable view of a specific institution. Despite the antitrust ruling, many health care people remain uncomfortable about the ethics of promotion. It appears that advertis-ing and promotion are necessary in a market-oriented environment. They clarify the exact contribution of medical and hospital services and help customers to make informed choices in health care, as in other ac-tivities. The use of communications media to make the customer aware of preventive health care, price advantages, extended hours, new loca-tions, and the availability of specialized services is likely to be benefi-cial. While advertising unnecessary services, procedures of questionable merit, and forms of care that increase costs to the individual or to soci-ety is a danger of the new policy, it must be considered in light of the disadvantages of the old professionally oriented, technocratic system, in which shortages prevailed and some customers were inevitably incon-venienced by them or by lack of responsiveness. Thus the question of the general ethics of advertising and promotion tends to break down. It is less a question of overall benefit than of particular benefit, and less a question of whether to advertise than how.

The well-run hospital of the future will use promotion and adver-tising of all kinds to stimulate demand for its services. It must do this in order to survive in an environment of surplus, where less adept hos-pitals will certainly advertise and probably set lower standards for their advertising. The true ethical question is one of mission and scope of service rather than advertising. The well-run hospital will rarely offer a service it hesitates to advertise. A service that cannot be widely known to the hospital's public is suspect in itself.

Advertising should be efficient, effective, and totally consistent with the hospital's mission and objectives. To achieve this state, it is necessary to use competent professionals to design campaigns and to establish clear expectations for the usual closed system parameters. The output of advertising is increase in demand, or loss of demand forestalled, although process measures such as "number of individuals reached" and "frequency of exposure" are commonly used. The efficiency is a ratio of demand gained to dollars spent. Quality has more to do with truth and effectiveness of communication than with aesthetics. The importance of the message goes beyond the specific campaign. Each contact also carries an impression of the hospital and may be effectively used to influence attitudes and behavior toward health. Thus a set of expectations for an advertising unit of planning-marketing might state the topic of each anticipated campaign, reach and frequency of contacts, message content, impact on demand by service, scores on effectiveness of communication, and total cost.

Techniques for Orderly Review of Expedited Proposals

Strategic opportunities must frequently be evaluated expediently, without the luxury of competitive comparison. Even among programmatic proposals there frequently arise matters which disrupt the orderly timetable described above; for example, advantages may result from linking proposals together, emergencies arise, oversights are discovered, or new managers demand attention for a proposal.

The well-run hospital may be slightly less subject to these vagaries than other hospitals, but it can better provide an expedited response without making mistakes or destroying the process. There are several keys to accomplishing this:

— The line-staff team is always formed. Without it, the planning committee is at the mercy of the judgment of a single, biased individual.

— The mission and long-range plan are sufficiently clear and detailed to be used as criteria for both strategic and programmatic opportunities.

— Any project accepted for expedited attention must have obvious compelling benefits. A project without such benefits should be slowed down and studied until its justification is clear.

— Despite the expediency, accurate cost estimates are developed. Carelessness in this area can have devastating results in cost overruns or even infeasible projects.

— Timetables for implementation are also protected and are developed carefully. Because of the trouble they can prevent, it actually saves time to think these timetables through than omit them.

— Effort is made to keep continuity and experience on the planning committee so an expedient proposal can be considered by people familiar with recent decisions and able to compare the project to others accepted or rejected.

— Managers are encouraged to understand the values of process and to avoid requesting expedient handling. In particular, the expedited route is never allowed to become a way of escaping competitive review. To do this, the committee and the board must be willing to accept the costs of deferring otherwise worthy projects because they unnecessarily depart from the usual process.

Evaluating Opportunities and Proposals in Not-for-Profit Hospitals

It sometimes happens that the same opportunity, or a very similar one, is attractive to one hospital but not another. Ruling out error and assuming that both hospitals are well run, considerations other than the opportunity itself must lead to this result. There are five elements of planning-marketing decisions that are independent of the individual proposal or opportunity and related to the basic values or beliefs of the decision makers:

1. Time horizon used for decision making
2. Willingness to accept risk
3. Willingness to assume debt
4. Value placed on unique, ambiguous assets
5. Relative importance of various community groups

Most decision makers, and well-managed boards and committees, have positions on these elements. Such positions can be called **valuation premises.** Each of them involves a set of trade-offs in which certain proposals will face diminished chances of acceptance, while others will face enhanced chances. The trade-offs are by definition intangible (that is, impractical to measure in dollar terms in most situations) and, like other issues of value, they are implicitly decided by any action taken, even an action to defer or delay. A hospital's typical profile on the valuation premises, reflected in its actual decisions, constitutes its *style.*

Implicit Pricing. *Implicit pricing* is a key part of the concept of valuation premises. When a decision is made to select one of two specific proposals which differ on one of these five premises, a value is implicitly set on that premise. Perhaps the easiest trade-off to understand is the time horizon, and it can be used to illustrate the phenomenon of implicit pricing. The impact of time on value is explicitly addressed in finance through discounting techniques, but the rate at which one discounts the future remains problematic. A high discount rate puts little weight on remote future events; no discount weighs them equal to the present. If there are two proposals which differ only in the size of the benefit and the delay before the benefit is received, the extent to which either proposal is favored measures the implicit value assigned the discount rate. If the early proposal yields one unit of benefit now and the later yields two units five years from now, those choosing the later project discount the future at a rate of less than 15 percent per year (two units at year 5 are worth one unit now). Those favoring the early proposal discount at a greater rate (two units at year 5 are worth less than one unit now). Thus any vote on the proposal implies a discount rate and a perspective on the future.

Each of the other four valuation premises is similarly evaluated when it is part of a specific decision. In the real world, each proposal is likely to contain all the valuation premises in varying degrees. Because of the impact of implicit pricing on a series of real proposals, any real hospital establishes a position, or style, on these five valuation premises. Styles are difficult to describe. They are often labelled "conservative" or "radical," but with several premises a one-dimensional scale is obviously inadequate.

The relationship between style and success is not clear, but both extreme and inconsistent styles can endanger the institution. An extremely conservative style, favoring no risk, no debt, a very short horizon, retention of the old, and responding mainly to a like-thinking oligarchy, is dangerous; however, so is one that dismisses the past, speculates heavily on the future, disregards risk, and is willing to incur large debt. Wisdom lies in some harder-to-identify middle course. It also lies in consistency. One can succeed as a consistent (but not extreme) radical or conservative more easily than by vacillating or being indecisive. The well-run hospital makes a deliberate effort at consistency, by identifying and discussing the premises repeatedly. It therefore has a stronger consensus, greater uniformity of application, and the advantage of being able to act more quickly on specific opportunities.

Time Horizon Used for Decision Making. The benefits of specific proposals are inevitably linked to the motivations for operating hospitals, classified in chapter 2 as Samaritanism, personal health, public health, community economic good, and health care economy. Most of these have long time horizons, but it can be argued that Samaritanism, public health, and possibly health care economy, which are concerned directly with the well-being of the group as much as the individual, have the longest horizons, in the sense that only a small fraction of the total benefit is recovered in the short term. Time horizons vary within the motivations as well. Preventive personal health care, like public health, tends to have long horizons. Preventive care for young children, for example, produces large benefits 20 to 50 years later. High-tech care and care of the dying tend to produce much shorter range benefits. Thus a short-term style will emphasize motivations for high-tech personal health care and community economic benefits (such as employment), and will select proposals whose benefits lie in those motivations.

Costs also differ in their time implications. Many costs tend to appear only in the long run, particularly the replacement of space and highly specialized personnel. Opportunity costs are more insidious. The major market orientation of a hospital, for example, toward the suburb rather than the city, toward high-tech curing rather than prevention and caring, toward fee-for-service rather than capitation, carry with them large and irreversible opportunity costs. As resources are committed by constructing facilities and adopting at least implied contracts with physicians, the hospital must inevitably foreclose on some directions and bias toward others.

There is no universally correct time horizon, because what is correct depends on time and place. There is no long-term future if short-term imperatives are ignored. Totally ignoring long-term implications reduces short-term decisions to meaninglessness. Even survival of the institution should be a step toward some long-term purpose. Thus the question of time horizon becomes one of who will set it and how. In the well-run hospital, it is set by the planning committee of the governing board, balancing various interests but giving heavy weight to community needs. In well-managed hospitals, the merits of longer or shorter horizons are frequently considered, developing consistency of action and fostering adaptation to change.

Risk. A second valuation premise involves how much risk is acceptable for the hospital. In an oversimplified example, two projects are proposed. One may save thousands of lives if it works, but no one can estimate the chances that it will work. The other is virtually certain to save 200 lives. If both cost exactly the same, and only one can be adopted, which should the hospital choose? At some level of risk—say one chance in three, or one chance in two—most decision makers would opt for the riskier opportunity. At only one chance in five that the riskier project will succeed, the certain project will probably be selected without much disagreement. There is an underlying bias for prudence, expressed in the law and tradition of management, which in this example would favor the more certain opportunity. Yet prudence itself must be defined. Time and place determine what is acceptable risk. A research hospital might accept much higher levels of risk than a community hospital, for example, and hospitals in a wealthy nation would take more risk than those in a poor one.

In real hospitals, the odds are never so well known, costs are never exactly the same, and projects are rarely in direct competition. A series of specific decisions sets acceptable levels of risk. These should be considered for consistency and compared to the other valuation premises. Generally, low tolerance of risk (sometimes called *risk aversion)* is consistent with a preference for short time horizons and high liquidity and has no clear relationship to how assets are valued or the relative importance of various exchange partners.

Liquidity. Third is the issue of liquidity and borrowing, which is inseparably related to risk. Resources in their liquid form are usually invested in readily salable instruments earning a tangible return. On the other hand, strategic and programmatic proposals almost always have some opportunity cost. A decision to wait, or to remain liquid, is a decision that the benefits of the project do not overcome the loss of flexibility. It implies that a better, as yet unforeseen, opportunity will arise. A decision to spend is the opposite, and a decision to borrow, which itself carries a tangible cost, is a decision that the value of the project exceeds the cost of borrowing. The tangible costs and benefits of borrowing are handled by competent technical analysis. What complicates the decision is that the cost of borrowing has intangible costs that apply to all projects rather than to any specific opportunity. Borrowing reduces the future ability of the hospital to borrow and thus its ability to respond to unforeseen trouble. That is to say, the opportunity cost of borrowing is increased risk.

It is also important to understand the relationship of liquidity to expansion and to economical health care. Borrowing permits rapid expansion, which for hospitals means increased costs to the community. A strong motivation for economy discourages borrowing, but strong motivations for high technology and convenience in personal health care and for community economic benefits encourage borrowing. The cost of borrowing, and to a certain extent the risk, is set by the interest rate. The hospital may add to the interest rate the intangible cost of borrowing, or preference for liquidity, sometimes called the *hurdle rate.* Hospitals that prefer liquidity generally set a high hurdle rate: they expect any successful proposal to repay not only the interest, but also the hurdle. The result is that fewer projects are accepted; those that are tend to have short-term benefits and lower risks.

Unique and Ambiguous Assets. Assets, or resources, have a precise definition in accounting, but not necessarily in the real world. The hospital's achievement of a certain mission, such as care of the poor, is an asset to the community that never appears on any balance sheet. There are accepted techniques for establishing tangible values for many long-term assets, even one as ephemeral as goodwill. Generally, these involve what the organization would sell the asset for, what an outsider would buy it for, or what the asset can earn for the organization. Establishing these three estimates and resolving the differences among them is often difficult, but some consensus is usually possible.

There are assets and resources for which these techniques simply cannot be made to work, however. One empirical problem involves the **opportunity cost** of earnings, or benefits foregone. Opportunity cost is the cost of committing a resource and thereby eliminating it from other potential uses or opportunities. The clearest example is in land and space, because each lot or place is to some extent unique. If the hospital uses one of four entrances for the emergency room, it may not be able to use it effectively for other services. Then other services must be located elsewhere at some continuing expense, or the hospital must reduce its total program. These expenses, or the cost of foregoing part of the program, are the opportunity cost of the emergency room location. Obviously, the true opportunity cost is the cost of the most expensive services foregone or disadvantaged. The first step to an empirical estimate of opportunity cost is recognition of the full scope of activities potentially benefiting from the desired location. Often one can conceptualize a tangible value for the opportunity cost even if the problems of estimating it are so complex that the answer is left in intangible form. One might say, for example, that the cost was equivalent to that of setting up a new service down the street.

Beyond the empirical difficulty, there are important philosophical problems. Suppose that there is no practical way to set up services down the street, and, further, that some of the services disadvantaged are considered part of the hospital's religious or political mission. (The value of a mission can rarely be established empirically.) Now, when the decision is made for or against the emergency room, it implicitly prices the disadvantaged portion of the mission. There are many more such questions than one would at first think. What, for example, is the value of affiliation with a medical school or a religious organization? What is the importance of remaining in a certain location, such as a downtown site near the homes of poor patients and unskilled workers? How much is it appropriate to spend on aesthetics, such as a statue or a traditional building? (The Johns Hopkins Hospital has kept its nineteenth-century entrance with the large marble statue of Christ and the famous dome over it at very high cost. How can one decide whether the cost is worthwhile? One cannot, except by voting yes or no on the specific proposal. Those who vote to save the entrance consider tradition, visible expression of a Samaritan commitment, and aesthetics more important than the benefits which might have accrued from alternative uses of the space and funds.)

Relative Importance of Community Groups. The values selected by implicit pricing ultimately reflect the individuals who made the decisions. Thus the final valuation premise is the relative weight placed on different perspectives within the community. There are many classifications of the community that can be used. The consumer-provider dichotomy of planning law is an important but simplistic one. Whether decision makers are poor or rich, influential or not, religious or secular, male or female, or white or black also influences the final values placed on the premises. Wisdom, however, appears more important than affiliation. The wise decision maker not only transcends her or his self-interest and background, she or he recognizes the need for compromise and the importance of understanding specifics in order to compromise effectively. One characteristic of well-run hospitals is that they recognize when special interests are important and accommodate them in specific, rather than general, terms.

The subtleties of the question begin to emerge if one considers the issue of market versus internal orientation. Here clearly is one potential trade-off, because hospital members and the larger community may have legitimately conflicting interests. Optimization will call for finding that balance which maximizes the totality of interests met, emphasizing those of the community. If too much is conceded to the members, some community goals may not be achieved, and the community may demand replacement of the members; if too little, the members may leave, strike, or otherwise resist. Conflicts often result in failure to achieve either member or community goals. A hospital through its planning-marketing decisions, inevitably places itself on the community versus member continuum. That is, it implicitly prices the values of the decision makers on questions such as the importance of hospital employment and the attractiveness of the community to other commerce.

Members versus community is only one of several trade-offs between exchange partners. In not-for-profit hospitals, trustees accommodate competing groups' interests in some way that continues to optimize the good of the whole. The classic illustration is the donation of something most constituencies do not want—inconveniently located land for a facility, or a service of special interest to the donor but not really needed by the community. When the donor is very influential, few wish to argue with him or her. The question which must be answered is, "Is the influence of this donor sufficient to overcome the drawbacks of this project?" The question becomes multifaceted, involving the interests of many different groups. Consistently good judgment on this question, quite independent of the individual projects being considered, is the hallmark of the exceptional hospital.

The consistency, wisdom and good judgment that distinguish the well-run hospital are fostered by finding planning committee members who have shown it in the past. Finally, major decisions of this complexity must go to the governing board, whose members determine the success and whose preferences determine the direction of the well-run hospital.

Ultimately, the values placed on the five premises have to do with who makes the decision. The membership of the governing board is the most central consideration in planning-marketing, because the well-run hospital will refer its toughest valuation decisions to that level. The predisposition of that group, toward short- or long-term, high- or low-risk, greater or less liquidity, and for or against certain missions and values, will determine the eventual shape of the hospital.

Notes

1. American Medical Association v. Federal Trade Commission, 638 F.2d 443 (2d Cir. 1980).

Suggested Readings

Kimberly, J. R., and Zajac, E. J. "Strategic Adaptation in Health Care Organizations: Implications for Theory and Research." *Medical Care Review* 42 (1985): 267–302.

Kotler, P. *Marketing for Non-profit Organizations.* 2d ed. Englewood Cliffs, NJ: Prentice-Hall, 1982.

Kropp, F., and Greenberg, J. A. *Strategic Analysis for Hospital Management.* Germantown, MD: Aspen, 1984.

MacStravic, R. S. *Forecasting Use of Health Services.* Germantown, MD: Aspen, 1984.

Shortell, S. M., Morrison, E. M., and Robbins, S. "Strategy Making in Health Care Organizations: A Framework and Agenda for Research." *Medical Care Review* 42 (1985): 219–266.

8

The Finance System

The finance system of the modern bureaucratic organization controls all the assets, collects all the revenue, arranges all the funding, settles all the financial obligations, and makes a major contribution to information collection and cost control. It is headed by a professional with training in accounting and finance who is usually the second or third most powerful person in the organization. The modern hospital is no different, although it arrived at this state only in the last 15 years, about 40 years behind its industrial counterparts.

Because of the importance and visibility of financial management it is subject to much study, regulation, and standardization. Comprehensive texts describe the overall operation of the system. Laws, regulations, contracts, and standard practice guides control what is done in countless specific situations. Much of this goes on without any assistance from the governance system, effectively monitored by the processes themselves and by a unique characteristic of the financial system, the annual outside audit. The audit itself, almost always conducted by one of a few national firms, is a major force toward standardization. It is not necessary to review here the aspects of financial management controlled by these elaborate devices.[1] The focus of this chapter is upon the issues that require attention from the governance system.

The governance concerns with finance are those issues where finance interacts directly with other systems, principally strategic planning, provision of capital, budgeting, monitoring and reporting, and expectations for the performance of the financial system itself. Although this list is only slightly shorter than the full list of finance system functions, I emphasize within them the parts most relevant to the other systems of the hospital. The chapter outline follows the usual pattern of purpose and function, personnel and organization, performance measures, and management issues.

Purpose

The purposes of the finance system are to support the enterprise by

1. Recording and reporting transactions that change the value of the firm
2. Guarding assets and resources against theft, waste, or loss
3. Assisting operations in setting and achieving cost and revenue expectations
4. Assisting governance in short- and long-term planning
5. Arranging the funding to implement governance decisions

These five purposes are accomplished through two general functions—controllership, incorporating the first three, and financial management, incorporating the last two. The activities supporting these functions are shown in figure 8.1. Although the list is lengthy and complex, most of the activities can be easily associated with one or two of the five purposes.

Controllership Functions

Accounting

Accounting represents a direct obligation to the owners, to conduct, record, and report all transactions affecting the value of the firm. It relies heavily on the principle of division of tasks between two or more individuals, minimizing the opportunity for defalcation. In practice, it is common to assign responsibility for authorizing the transaction (a payment or a charge) to line managers and responsibility for collecting or disbursing funds to accounting personnel. As a result, accounting personnel are involved in most areas of the hospital and by far the largest fraction of finance system employees is involved in accounting.

Revenue Accounting. Revenue accounting is a complex function that supplies, directly or indirectly, almost all the hospital's financial resources. Donations and income from sources other than operations are

Figure 8.1

Activities of the Financial System

Controllership
Accounting
　Revenue and collection
　　Patient accounts
　　Third-party billing
　　Patient billing
　　Cashiering
　　Collections
　Expenditures
　　Payroll
　　Payables
　　General ledger
　Disclosure
　　Owners and directors
　　Private third parties
　　Government agencies
　Asset protection
　　Program for asset protection
　　Internal audit
　　External audit
　　Management letter
　　Conflict of interest
　Budgeting and reporting
　　Budgeting
　　Pricing
　　Reporting
　　Cost accounting
Financial Management
　Financial planning
　Securing long-term funding
　Managing short-term assets and funding

---

also financial resources, but they are a small part of the total in most hospitals. Borrowing, the final source of funds, requires revenue to assure the lender of repayment.

The following are the major components of revenue accounting:

— *Patient accounts receivable.* Charges made to patients or their third parties for care generate most of the hospital's earned revenue. Charges are posted to individual **patient ledgers**. The sum of all posted charges is called **gross revenue**.

— *Revenue adjustments.* Revenue accounting must accommodate the complexities of real payments from third parties and individuals. Many insurance companies and government agencies pay amounts different from the posted charges, and, of course, some patients cannot or do not pay for care and are treated as charity patients or bad debts. These discrepancies are accounted as revenue adjustments. **Net revenue** is the income actually received, as opposed to what is initially posted; it is equal to gross revenue minus adjustments.

Insurance companies and third-party payers have often insisted on discounts, rebates, and special accounting procedures. Recent developments have included a nationally promulgated price structure for Medicare, the **prospective payment system** (PPS), and various kinds of price offerings by private buyers, including capitation (HMO), other risk sharing, and discounts or rebates. The noncapitated offers vary widely but are usually referred to as preferred provider organizations. Each such contract accepted creates a new set of adjustments and has complex effects upon net revenue. The negotiation of these contracts is frequently a responsibility of the CEO because the contracts have clinical as well as financial aspects. Finance is always deeply involved in the negotiations. It is accountable for major aspects of the agreements, including the accuracy of expectations regarding net revenue and regarding profit within given assumptions about volume and costs.

— *Collections and cashiering.* The revenue function includes the collection of cash. Significant efforts must be made to assure that third parties and individuals pay promptly and fully. The hospital's property must be protected against both theft and embezzlement by carefully designed systems.

Revenue accounting is almost universal in the United States. Only some prepaid capitation plans and some government hospitals do not maintain patient ledgers. Community hospitals have been rapidly expanding their revenue accounting. Much of the growth is stimulated by the need for information and cost control rather than by requirements of financial control. Accounting detailed individual charges for each service or supply is expensive, but it provides extensive, reliable, patient-specific data on the quantities of services rendered. These data can be used in clinical marketing and cost control. Modern computer programs for receivables accounting permit virtually limitless specification of the patient ledger; they also support a clinical abstract containing summaries of diagnosis and treatment. The computerized file of patient charges has emerged as the principal source of data for achieving clinical economy and quality control. It is used both historically and concurrently in clinical review systems, and it supports the analysis for long-range planning, strategic decisions, and new program proposals.

Expenditures Accounting. Accounting for expenditures serves a similar dual role. It controls and reports the disbursement of funds and simultaneously generates basic information on costs. Thus the payroll system generates both paychecks and data on labor costs; the accounts payable system pays for purchased goods and services and generates data on cost of supplies.

General Ledger. Some financial transactions are internal rather than external exchanges and deal with resources that last considerably longer than one budget or financial cycle. These are called **general ledger transactions.** General ledger entries adjust inventories, assign capital costs through depreciation, and recognize other long-term transactions. General ledger transactions must be recognized in order to generate accurate financial reports, and they, too, contain essential management information.

Disclosure of Financial Information

Three main reports have become standard for hospitals and most other nongovernmental enterprises. They are the position statement, or balance sheet; the income, or profit and loss statement; and the statement of sources and uses of funds. These summarize the financial activities and situation of the hospital in a form now almost universal in the business world. It is important that each governing board member read and understand these three documents. They are usually issued monthly or quarterly to the board and monthly to the CEO. Each year the board receives the audited, final versions of these statements. They constitute the record of the board's own financial management and the discharge of its obligation to exercise fiscal prudence. The audited annual statements are the basis for most of the hospital's financial communication with the outside world.

Audited income and position statements must be reported to the federal government as a condition of participation in Medicare. Once filed, they are accessible under the Freedom of Information Act. Several states now require public release of financial reports as well. Hospitals issuing bonds on public markets are also required to reveal standard financial information. As a result, many hospitals choose to publish their financial reports as part of their program of community relations. Most other private and all governmental activities are required to make such disclosures to the public, so nondisclosure by the hospital can arouse suspicion. Governing boards, however, have some flexibility in reporting, stemming from their ability to form foundations and other corporations separate from the general hospital. Hospitals owned by multihospital systems, both for-profit and not-for-profit, are not required to disclose their financial information directly; the obligation is on the parent corporation.

Protection of Assets

The hospital as a corporate entity is required to maintain control of all its properties for its owners. The governing board and members of management are responsible for prudent protection of assets, including avoidance of inurement.

Inurement. Inurement is the diversion of funds to persons in governance or management as a result of their position of trust. Not-for-profit structure requires that no individual benefit from service to the corporation beyond any stipulated salary or compensation. For-profit structure has an analogous protection against exploitation of stockholders by directors. Under these rules, directors, managers, or trustees may not engage in business which allows them to derive financial advantage from their governing board role. Neither can doctors or lower-level managers, but such examples are less frequent. The corporation is not enjoined from doing business with a board member, if such business and board membership are in the owners' interests. Thus the key word is "advantage."

To protect against inurement, the hospital must establish, and the CFO must enforce, policies that reduce financial conflict of interest. These policies have two parts. First, every governing board member and officer is required to file an annual disclosure statement identifying all their financial interests and potentially conflicting commitments, including membership on other voluntary boards. Second, members are expected to divorce themselves from any specific decision or action which involves their interests or conflicting affiliations. Well-run hospitals achieve this by making the point well in advance of any specific application and by selecting members who understand both the law and the ethics.

Physical Assets. Generally, the protection of the physical assets is considered part of the function of the plant system, assigned to security, maintenance, and materials management. Prudent purchasing practices are included in the responsibilities of materials management. The risk of misappropriation of assets is probably greater than the risks of physical theft or destruction, however, and the finance system is responsible for prudent protection against it. The finance system is also responsible for the physical protection of cash, securities, and receivables, and for assuring that plant and equipment were used as anticipated. The major risks it guards against are

— Unjustified free or unbilled service to patients
— Embezzlement of cash in the collections process
— Bribes and kickbacks in purchasing arrangements
— Supervision of financial conflicts of interest among governing board members and officers
— Diversion or theft of supplies and equipment
— Falsified employment and hours
— Purchase of supplies or equipment without appropriate authorization

Program for Protecting Assets. All hospitals face continuing real losses of assets, and acceptable performance requires continuing diligence. Most well-run hospitals find that control of assets can safely be delegated to the finance system with only brief annual review. This is because a sound and well-understood program has been developed for the purpose; it has four parts:

1. Detailed, written procedures govern the handling of the various assets and transactions. These procedures rely primarily on the division of functions between two or more individuals and the routine reporting of checks and balances to protect assets.

2. Adequate written records and accounting systems document the actual use of assets.

3. Adherence to risk control procedures and documentation requirements is monitored through a small group of internal auditors, who usually report directly to the CFO.

4. Annual outside audits verify both adherence to procedure and validity of reported outcome.

The governing board's role is to select the outside auditors, receive their report and review it carefully, and take action to correct any deficiencies noted. For obvious reasons, the report goes directly to the governing board. These activities are usually delegated to the finance committee, but never further. Thus the auditors are free to comment upon the CEO and CFO as well as others. Their comments are included in a document called the **management letter**, which accompanies their audited financial reports. Well-run hospitals have little trouble with this system. The expectation for the management letter is "no deficiencies," and it is usually achieved. The success of this system means that governance groups and CFOs of well-run hospitals need spend little time on asset protection activity, despite its complexity and importance.

Budgeting

The contributions of controllership that distinguish the well-run hospital are its support of budgeting and its monitoring of performance. The functions of accounting and asset protection are done well as a matter of course. Budgeting and reporting deal with expectation setting and achievement, the basic engine for competitive operation. At present, leading hospitals are expanding the annual budget process to include expectations on virtually all elements of the closed system parameters. Reporting to responsibility center managers is being strengthened by improving the reliability and specificity of cost reports, adding quality and revenue reports, and providing historic data on the new measures to support expectation setting.

The finance system provides the cost and revenue data and sometimes assists with other measures. A section of the finance system, the budget office, generally coordinates budget development. The development and approval process is usually called budgeting; the monitoring process includes cost accounting and reporting. The two parts are actually intertwined.

Budget Components. The usual hospital budget is a full, detailed description of expected financial transactions, by accounting period, for an entire year. Because it takes time to develop, the forecast must cover about 18 months into the future. Some well-run hospitals budget a second or even a third year in preliminary terms as part of their yearly budget cycle. The review of future expectations is useful to them in making smooth progress toward their financial goals.

The major parts of the annual budget include the operating budgets and the financial budgets. The *operating budgets*, in turn, are made up of the following:

— *Expenditures budget*, that is, costs incurred by reporting period, responsibility center, and functional account (for example, labor, supplies, equipment). Successive "roll ups," or aggregates, summarize larger sections of the organization paralleling the accountability hierarchy.

— *Revenue budget*, that is, gross revenues for each revenue center, with aggregates. Well-run hospitals are currently expanding their capability to reckon adjustments and net revenue at this level of detail. They are developing transfer pricing and revenue proxies for services sold to other units rather than to the patient.

The *financial budgets* are composed of the following:

— *Cash flow budget*, estimates of cash income and outgo by period, used by finance in cash and liability management.

— *Capital and new programs budget*, lists of capital expenditures and new or significantly revised programs, with their implications for the operating and cash budgets by period and responsibility center.

Forecasts of volume of activity are the starting point for developing the budget and are incorporated in the final result. Important price decisions are incorporated in the revenue budget. Prices are based principally on competitive, or market, forces, but they include consideration of cost expectations from the expenditure budget, volume forecasts, and needs developed in the long-range financial plan. The capital budget includes all anticipated expenditures for facilities and equipment, as well as sources of funds for them. It is increasingly common to consider new programs and revisions of services as part of the capital budget, even though new programs involve revenue and operating costs as well as capital. This permits initial consideration of a status quo operating budget and more rigorous evaluation of both components.

Budgets and Closed System Parameters. The budgets specify expectations in enough detail to serve as an unambiguous guide to the RCM in managing activity; for each month of the coming fiscal year, expectations for labor hours and costs by pay class, major expenditures for other resources, and revenue by major category of payer are stated. Reports parallel the budget in their detail, permitting prompt identification of variances.

The major sources of budget expectations, along closed system parameters, are as follows:

— *Demand*, from volume forecasts developed first by the budget office for major activity measures, and then refined for each unit by line personnel; modified by actions taken on new programs and capital.

— *Resource consumption (costs)*, from estimates of physical requirements developed first by the RCM, priced by the budget office, and included in the expense budget; subject to intensive review within the line hierarchy and usually a binding constraint on total increase for the entire hospital. Resource consumption is also modified by new programs and capital actions.

— *Resource conservation (revenue)*, gross estimated from forecasts of output and prices for those units providing directly charged services and net from analysis of adjustments, when available.

Many units have not been identified as revenue centers in the past, even though some, like nursing and dietary, could easily be isolated from more general charges. Those that "sell" only to other RCs have historically been treated as overhead. It is possible to establish prices for both these situations, and well-run hospitals are moving to do this. Either real or imputed prices give the buyer incentives to avoid overuse of the good or service, and an earned "profit" is a measure of achievement for the seller.

— *Output*, derived from the volume forecast by the RCM and subject to review by the accountability hierarchy. Many outputs in a hospital are demands on some other unit and as a result must be carefully coordinated.

— *Efficiency*, calculated by the budget office from input and output. It is often compared to internal and external standards or norms and used to validate or modify resource consumption expectations.

— *Quality*, measured separately from the financial and accounting systems, but clearly involved in budget decisions. Well-run hospitals are moving to increase the measurement of quality and to incorporate it explicitly in the annual budget negotiations.

Budget Development and Approval. The expense and revenue parts of the budget are developed simultaneously in iterative stages marked by the transfer of packages of information. The package concept allows the budget office to route information to the correct location, permitting many different teams in the hospital to work at once. Figure 8.2 shows the major steps, although the process is usually more complex than the figure indicates. Details and procedures for hospital budgeting are described elsewhere.[2] As a general rule, there is a specific information package for each RCM at each step, although later rounds of revision tend to focus on only a few unresolved areas.

The revenue budget is developed from volume forecasts, prices, and price adjustments. Much of the effort is carried out by employees in finance. Pricing is becoming an increasingly market-driven issue in hospitals. The correct price depends upon the market and determines the cost at which the hospital must produce. Until recently, the opposite was true: prices were driven by costs. With the change has come increasing line involvement in pricing decisions, both to gain line insights into market behavior and competition and to hold line units accountable for contributions to profit. Preparation of transfer prices for imputing revenue to units serving only other RCs is also principally an

Figure 8.2

Major Steps in Developing Operations Budgets

1. **Review of Plans and Financial Resources**
   Establishes budget guidelines
   Volume forecasts on major activities
   Limits on change in operating expense
   Profit requirements
   Reiterates relevant policy on quality, human resources, operations
2. **Preparation of Information Packages**
   Provides instructions, forms, and timetables to responsibility center managers
   Provides more detailed forecasts and historical and comparative information relevant to RCs and departmental groupings
3. **Preparation of Decision Packages**
   Records initial agreements at departmental and RC level on volume, physical resource, and prices
   Evaluated by budget office in dollar costs, revenue, and profit
   Forms basis for subsequent rounds of negotiation
4. **Reiterations of Step 3 To Improve Compliance with Guidelines from Step 1**
   Incorporate new programs and capital projects
   Accommodate late changes in external environment
5. **Recommendation of Final Budget to Board**
6. **Distribution of Copies of Approved Budget and Implementation**

accounting responsibility. Both cost analysis and market surveys are required. (See discussion in chapters 14 and 15, where these units are most common.)

The capital budget is developed initially from the ranked list of individual proposals (as discussed in chapter 7). The budget itself consists of those proposals funded by the board, considering its capital needs and resources as reflected in the long-range plan and long-range financial plan. Often the finance committee simplifies the capital and new program budget process by specifying a hurdle rate related to its estimates of the expense of borrowing. This serves to remove less deserving proposals more quickly.

The following are guidelines for a well-run budget process:

— The parts of the budget must constitute an integral whole. The planned activities must be consistent
   • With each other
   • With the long-range plan
   • With the long-range financial plan
   • With the annual environmental survey

— Well-run hospitals achieve consistency by developing budget guidelines at the outset. These include

- Forecasts of major activity aggregates
- A limit on increase in total cost
- A minimum acceptable return from operations

— A separately developed and approved budget for capital expenses and new programs is a critical element. It simplifies the dialogue for the expense budget and

- Permits ad hoc debate on the relative value of programs
- Allows the approval of new programs and even replacement capital to be adjusted quickly as conditions change
- Encourages deletion proposals for obsolete or uneconomical programs
- Permits the use of new programs as rewards for achieving cost and efficiency goals

— A presumption that the normal condition is improvement in efficiency is helpful. One can presume that, if nothing else changed, an RC could redo last year's work with slightly fewer resources because its people would have the advantage of practice. This suggests that any increase in resource consumption requires some justification. The usual justifications are increased volume, increased complexity of tasks, and new services. In addition to placing new services in a separately justified budget, well-run hospitals often rule out volume and complexity changes in initial budget discussions, focusing on a *ceteris paribus* improvement in efficiency. Subsequently, justifications can be offered for volume and task changes.

— The quality of data and the preparation of information by the budget office are important contributions to success, measured both by time to completion and usefulness of result. These should be improved from year to year, building upon past work.

— The budget process should be made more rigorous over time. A hospital using an expense budget for the first time is well advised to limit its attention to elementary concepts, assuming a stable environment. Even though the marketplace may in fact be highly variable, it is pointless to address variation until basic concepts of control are accepted. A well-run hospital with many years' budgeting experience will accommodate fluctuating demand, fixed, variable, and semivariable expenses, efficiency and quality standards, transfer prices, and possibly alternative profit scenarios. It also would have extended the detail of its reporting, both by type of resource and number of RCs. Similar growth in sophistication would occur in the capital and new programs budget.

— The dialogue within general management encourages acceptance of the expectations by having RCMs participate in their development. The effectiveness of the dialogue is more important than issues of data quality or process sophistication. When an effective dialogue exists, quality and sophistication often improve as a result. Without effective dialogue, there is a constant danger of having the RCMs adopt an adversarial or destructive approach to the budget.[3]

— The best budget development process is a lengthy and sometimes heated dialogue among all elements of management. Although it is time-consuming, it can replace many other less organized and less rewarding discussions.

Reporting and Control

Several kinds of cost and revenue details are reported to other systems by finance, including reports on budget performance, cost studies, and special analyses.

Reports to the Accountability Hierarchy. The controller provides monthly reports to general management, from the RCM to the governing board, to assist them in achieving expectations. The design, content, and delivery of these reports are a major part of the controller's job. The reports should

— Correspond exactly to the expectations set in budgets, both in definition and time. (A common error is to report accrued rather than actual data for calendar months, creating a noticeable distortion because of varying numbers of weekend days. One solution is to avoid accruals; another to use a 13-month year.)

— Be delivered promptly, within a few days of actual events.

— Be clearly and usefully presented. (A common problem is excess information, confusing the control purpose of the report with an archival one. Line managers who request a copy of the archive should receive it, but the control report focuses on material elements.)

— Present both physical and dollar measures on labor and other major costs.

— Be available to each person in the formal organization for his or her exact area of accountability.

— Condense information so that it is both automatically summarized from lower hierarchies and presented with equal economy at all levels. (This means that the COO's report is about the same length as a typical RCM's. It usually follows very similar design.)

— Emphasize financially important variation so that major problems can be identified quickly.

— Use flexible budgeting to show whether cost variation is attributable to demand or efficiency. (This step had been achieved only by the most sophisticated hospitals in 1985.)

Reports on "Product" Costs. Hospital responsibility centers tend to prepare individual services, such as a laboratory test or an administration of a drug. Patients, of course, are interested less in these individual products than in the combined package of care. Increasing emphasis on economy has led to closer attention and more need for control of the package of care, which is identified in this book as the *final product.* Final products are more conceptual than concrete, but the Social Security Administration has identified 468 DRGs as specific final products and has established a price for each. Cost control requires that the hospital provide care to the average patient in the group at a cost close to or below the DRG price. Since the cost of the final product must be calculated by counting up the intermediate products and multiplying each of them by its unit cost, a new step and a new cost-reporting activity has been added by the introduction of DRGs. Other insurers and governmental payment agencies are following Social Security's lead. As a result, the well-managed hospital must develop a reporting system for final product costs. A well-designed system would accommodate several approaches to defining the final product, including, eventually, episodes of outpatient as well as inpatient care.

The accounting for final product cost requires three elements:

1. Counts of individual services, usually available from the patient ledger

2. Direct costs of the responsibility centers generating the intermediate products, available from the cost reports to the RCM

3. A method for dealing with costs of services that do not generate direct patient revenues

Final product costing also requires software capable of correctly grouping patients by final product and handling the conceptually simple, but numerically burdensome, calculations. The weakest link in the requirements lies in the accounting of the nonrevenue responsibility centers. Hospitals have been making cost allocations of these items for many years using a variety of acceptable approaches. The approach most advantageous under older payment methods may not be the desirable one for final product costing. The theoretical ultimate would be established transfer pricing among all responsibility centers, but almost no hospitals have made significant movement in this direction. Thus the matter of final product costing becomes one of preparing estimates or approximations using the best available data and systems, and improving upon accuracy with time. This gradual approach appears to be satisfactory; in most hospitals even a very crude approximation still serves to identify important avenues of efficiency and economy.[4]

The use of final product costs is probably less frequent than the cost reports to the RCMs. As the estimating methods suggest, no one manager has responsibility for a single final product cost. For many final products, a single medical specialty may have most of the control. Exercising that control in a manner which adequately protects the rights of individual patients and encourages the good judgment of individual physicians is a complex problem (see chapter 11). Because of these difficulties, quarterly or semiannual reports on final products are probably appropriate, supplemented with detailed information on those product groups of particular interest.

Reports on Activity Costs. The accounting files are a rich source of information for detailed cost studies below the RC level. These are sometimes called *microcosting.* Sound efforts at microcosting identify the unit costs of a specific good or service, such as a specific laboratory test or a nursing treatment. Cost studies are used for

— Comparing local production with outside purchase, often called the *make or buy decision*

— Comparing alternative methods, particularly those substituting capital for labor

— Ranking cost saving opportunities to identify promising areas in which to eliminate or reduce use

— Estimating the impact on costs of expanding or contracting a product or service

There are numerous pitfalls involved in microcosting. The most serious is the sensitivity to volume of most hospital costs. Unless fixed and variable cost details are identified, cost estimates are valid only for very narrow ranges of volume. There are interconnections between many micro goods and services; the cost of one laboratory test is actually dependent not on its own volume, but on the combined volume of several tests sharing the same fixed resources, for example, several tests prepared on the same expensive machine. (Analogously, the cost of the single nursing procedure may be dependent on the volume of several nursing procedures done on that unit.)

These difficulties seriously limit the utility of cost analysis. While it is useful in specific situations where the implications of volume can be handled, it is not helpful in more general applications. For those, it is necessary to rely on the theories of responsibility center management, specifying closed system expectations with the RCM and rewarding cost-effective behavior. Flexible budgeting, which helps the RCM deal with variations in total volume, is the more rewarding approach. It is discussed below.

Reports on Planning and Special Studies. In addition to routine reporting and specific cost analysis, the controller retains archives which can be used to explore specific questions on issues of forecasting, control, and planning. These archives are organized differently from those supporting financial disclosure. Revenue information should be recorded at a detailed product or service level.[5] Expenditures should reflect not only the functional class of resource, but also the quantity, and, to the extent possible, the revenue product or service to which they were committed. The most important use of these data is in preparing the next budget. A second use is in constructing estimates for new or revised activities. Access to detailed cost data permits careful exploration of the strategic possibilities discussed in chapter 7, that is, opportunities to reconfigure the services of the hospital by merger, divestiture, acquisition, or joint venture.

Financial Management Functions

The financial management function projects future financial needs, arranges to meet them from retained earnings, loans, donations, or sales of stock, and manages the assets and liabilities of the hospital in ways which increase its profitability. The financial management activity is relatively recent in hospitals, arising from the increased revenue base created by Medicare, Medicaid, and widespread private health insurance, and from the opportunities for obtaining credit and equity which these created. The growth in 20 years to multiple corporations, extended series of bonds issued and reissued to minimize interest costs, and deliberate investment in joint ventures for profit is as telling a story of the health care industry as the development of heart transplants. The three components of financial management—financial planning, long-term capital acquisition, and management of short-term assets and liabilities—are now essential to survival.

Financial Planning

Financial management is a forward-looking activity with a long time horizon. It begins with the generation of a financial plan which incorporates the expected income and expense for every element of the long-range plan, specifying the amount and the time of its occurrence. Although the long-range plan itself is generally specified only for five years because of the uncertainty involved, some activities such as bond repayments and major facility replacement require much longer financial planning horizons, up to 30 years. Large financial requirements must be accommodated even though they are many years distant. Discounting techniques reduce their relative impact on the near term.

Financial planning is now commonly done on computers, generating pro forma statements of income, asset and liability position, and cash flow for each of the future years. Pro forma plans show not only the amounts of cash the hospital will need, but also the sources of revenue available. For example, the hospital might plan to spend $10 million three years from now to expand outpatient services. It anticipates an increase in net income of $2 million per year from the new service. Presumably it could seek tax-exempt bonds for much of the $10 million investment, using part of its increased income to pay for the bonds. The number of questions and assumptions required even in this simple example indicates the complexity and challenge of the exercise. Obviously, forecasts of volume, costs, revenues, and effects on other services are essential, even though opening is several years away. These matters must be addressed in the proposal for the venture, as discussed in chapter 7. In addition, financial assumptions must be made about the following:

— *Price and volume interactions for the new service.* Assumptions about people's health, income, and health insurance coverage are hidden in the volume and charges forecasts.

— *Interest rate and life of bonds (dependent on a market three years hence), the hospital's overall financial position, and federal tax policy.* (Changes in the federal tax law being debated in 1986 would abolish or limit the use of tax-exempt bonds, raising the interest rate.)

— *Net revenue of the project.* Net revenue will be determined by third-party coverage and contractual arrangements. These arrangements also affect the support available for financing costs.

— *Impact of the new service on net revenue from existing services.* The shifts in activity may differ among insurance carriers, resulting in a change in net revenue different from that in gross revenue.

The first step of financial planning is generally undertaken by the CFO and his or her immediate staff, possibly with members of the finance committee of the governing board. For as many scenarios as can be practically accommodated, the computer program will produce pro forma statements. These can be evaluated by means of ratio analysis, which compares various aspects of the financial statements, such as the ratio of debt to equity, debt service to cash flow, debt service to income, and so on. These can be subjectively assessed or compared to published data to judge

— The cost and reasonableness of borrowing from various sources
— The prices required to support debt service
— The financial desirability of various proposals
— The identity and magnitude of various financial risks
— The overall prudence of the financial management

Good financial planning will consider as many alternate assumptions as possible in terms of their impact upon the long-range plan. Various assumptions might address

— The impact of the business cycle
— Proposed federal and state legislation
— Trends in health insurance coverage and benefits
— Donation, grant, and subsidized funding sources
— Alternative debt structures and timing
— Opportunities for joint ventures and equity capitalization

Fiscal plan development will also accommodate the widest possible variety of assumptions about the long-range plan itself. These might include speeding up or slowing down some programs, combining programs, and even abandoning some. Usually some modification of the long-range plan results. Pricing and operating policies for current services are also at risk; low profits raise borrowing costs and can sometimes be corrected by better cost control or higher prices. Unacceptable results at any step can force a complete reevaluation, even to abandoning the entire long-range plan.

Financial planning is used to establish the guidelines for the operating budgets. Each year's guides on price increases, revenue requirements, and cost increases should be consistent with the long-range financial plan. The plan must be revised as often as necessary; substantial departure from it threatens the financial security of the hospital and cannot be accepted as prudent management.

Despite the difficulty of the assumptions required, answers to the financial planning questions are critical to effective governance. Without them, borrowing is hasty and can be at excessive interest rates, risks go unseen until they are reality, prices are set incorrectly, projects of disastrous financial consequence can be selected, and the hospital's financial probity can be destroyed. The keys to success are similar to those of planning generally: thorough and imaginative search for opportunities and consequences, careful factual analysis and forecasting, and sufficient lead time to permit unhurried decision making. Good general accounting systems and sufficient automated support substantially reduce the required lead time. As is so often the case, success feeds upon itself; the hospital which falls behind is tempted by shortcuts and risks that erode its position further.

Financial Management of Multiple Corporate Structures

Both for-profit and not-for-profit corporations as general legal entities are permitted to form new corporations, invest in other corporations, and reverse these actions by sale or liquidation. Except for the restrictions of antitrust, there is no limit on the amount or percentage of the investment involved; it can range from negligible to wholly owned. Any combination of for-profit and not-for-profit entities is possible. The tax obligations of each corporation are considered individually as the structures develop.

This aspect of the corporate world was little used by hospitals until the late 1960s, when the first for-profit chain operations began. For-profit chains frequently structure their individual hospitals as wholly owned subsidiary corporations of a national parent. Paralleling the development of for-profit hospital chains in the 1970s, American industry in general explored conglomerates, mergers, holding companies, and other complex corporate structures. The structures were not popular in not-for-profit hospitals until the 1980s. The flexibility they offer is useful, and a wide variety of models has developed. Multiple corporate structures also provide opportunities to form joint ventures which relate corporations to individuals and to other corporations. Some experimentation with partnerships of various kinds has also occurred.

The major benefits of multiple corporate structures are, in the broadest sense, financial.

— *Risk.* The liabilities and obligations of the owned or subsidiary corporation cannot generally be transferred to the parent.

(There are certain exceptions, and the law in this area is changing.) Thus the parent risks only those assets actually invested in the subsidiary.

— *Capital opportunities*. Separate corporations offer opportunities not only to dedicate capital, but also to raise new capital, either through borrowing or equity, as discussed below. These advantages can be obtained even within the not-for-profit structure; affiliation of several hospitals operating in different marketplaces is considered by lenders and bondholders to be more diversified and therefore less risky. As a result, they will accept lower interest. Some activities are attractive to equity capital; these can be pursued only through a for-profit structure. If the parent corporation is not-for-profit, a for-profit subsidiary can be formed.

— *Taxation*. Not-for-profit corporations can be taxed on certain activities, and for-profit corporations can respond to incentives built into the tax law with nontaxable actions. It is frequently desirable to support this line of reasoning with separate corporations. These clarify the tax position and are eligible for explicit Internal Revenue Service (IRS) rulings. In addition, they can frequently be designed with a view toward minimizing the overall tax obligation.

There are other justifications for complex corporate structures. Outdated corporate charters or restrictions from long-dead donors may hinder current responses. Structures may be imposed upon the hospital corporation by another investor on terms more convenient to the investor than to the hospital. The use of multiple corporations has, to some extent, become a fad. Well-managed hospitals seek the more permanent and less ephemeral justifications, and design their parent or main corporation with sufficient flexibility to undertake any foreseeable future activity.

Although the variations are limitless, three underlying schemes can be detected either alone or in combination in specific examples:

1. *Parent subsidiary*. A corporation may establish or acquire a wholly owned subsidiary which is usually dedicated to a specific activity. The most common example may be the creation of separate corporations, usually called *foundations,* for managing endowment and frequently also for stimulating teaching and research. The foundation is usually tax-exempt; the parent may or may not be. Alternatively, the subsidiary could be for-profit for a particularly risky activity or an unusual tax advantage. It would probably be engaging in an activity categorized as "taxable unrelated income" by the IRS.

2. *Holding company.* This common model consists of one parent and a variety of subsidiaries that may differ in tax structure, purpose, location, or other parameters.

3. *Joint venture.* Two or more parent corporations invest in a subsidiary. The reasons for separate incorporation may include risk in tax, but they are also likely to include the advantages of having additional investors. The most common form of partnership activity is a joint venture partnership. Shared service organizations constitute one form of joint venture. The parents are frequently otherwise competing hospital corporations. Another common form is a joint venture with individuals in the hospital's medical staff or with a corporate or partnership structure of the staff itself. A practice called *unbundling* involves the establishment of joint ventures with hospital-based specialists (see chapter 12). The hospital is one participant; the specialists are the other. (Depending upon local advantages, they may act either as individuals or as a group, and as corporations, sole proprietors, or partners.)

Securing Long-Term Funds

The agreed-upon financial plan is used to develop capital needs and sources, including prospectuses for borrowing and equity funding and plans for soliciting capital donations. Hospitals relied largely on donated capital from both government and private sources prior to 1970. Borrowing became the overwhelming source of capitalization under cost-based reimbursement through the early 1980s. The stimulus of competition promoted a number of innovative financial solutions, including the development of corporate structures discussed above and equity funding. Equity investment for a return is impossible in a not-for-profit corporation, but it is possible for a tax-paying corporation to own a not-for-profit corporation and vice versa, opening the possibility of almost limitless combinations and variations.[6]

It appears likely that borrowing will remain the dominant form of capital finance for conservative not-for-profit hospitals. Many well-managed hospitals will choose to be in this group. Lenders require extensive documentation of assets, income, and net profit. Interest rates and even the availability of money depend upon an effective presentation. Lenders prefer and reward low risk. Thus the hospital which demonstrates good results in finance and quality is preferred in the financial marketplace. However, it can maintain that favored position in the long run only to the extent that it invests prudently to enhance its own customer base. Either excess borrowing or insufficient investment can diminish the chance of success in the long run.

Equity finance involves the formation of for-profit corporations or partnerships. It generally is appropriate for working capital and the support of developmental operating expenses, whereas debt tends to be used to finance real property and long-term assets. Although these rules are not closely followed, in general the riskier the enterprise, the more likely and appropriate capital finance. Investors generally expect returns commensurate with their risk. Venture capitalists, willing to support new and untested ideas, do so in the expectation of returns substantially in excess of anything available in lending markets. Tax laws are quite important in equity finance, both from the point of view of the corporation and that of the investor. In multicorporate situations, the institution may be both recipient of and participant in equity funding. A relatively common example has a hospital that is exempt from taxes under Section 501(C)(3) of the Internal Revenue Code forming a for-profit corporation with outside investors and then contracting with that corporation to carry out certain activities. Thus the hospital passes some of its own funds to the for-profit corporation through the contract, but it expects to earn profits from its ownership position.

Well-managed hospitals exercise extreme prudence in the use of equity finance. Evidence suggests that there are a great many dangers. Half of all newly formed for-profit corporations are bankrupt within 12 months; it is said that half of the balance fail to survive the next economic downturn. The combination of equity and debt finance introduces the notion of leverage. If debt costs are not covered by revenue, the investors' equity is used. A great many corporations of substantial size and reputation have foundered because they incurred excessive debt. Because hospital experience is almost all from the last two or three years, it has not stood the test of an industrywide recession. Thus prudence demands small, diversified investments limited to amounts which the hospital could lose without seriously impairing its mission.

Managing Short-Term Assets and Liabilities

Any operation requires *working capital*, funds that are used to cover expenses made in advance of payment for services. In addition, hospitals frequently have short-term assets available, or must borrow to meet short-term needs. The finance system manages these transactions to maximum advantage for the hospital. The process is generally called *working capital management*, or short-term asset and liability management.

Short-term financial management deals in terms of days. Income can be obtained by moving assets rapidly. Cash is never left in non-interest-bearing accounts. Other liquid assets are placed where they will obtain the highest return consistent with risk and the length of time available. (Large sums of money can be invested for small interest returns on an overnight basis.) On the other hand, short-term borrowing is minimized because it costs money. Accounts receivable and inventories are minimized because they earn no return. Accounts payable and other debts are settled exactly when due, allowing the hospital to use the funds involved as long as possible.

Most not-for-profit hospitals have acquired small endowments or permanent charitable funds. These must be invested, and the well-managed hospital invests them in a manner which is consistent with its long-range financial plan. The funds can be invested for growth or income, or they can be invested in hospital activities, such as malpractice insurance reserves or physical facilities, which return income through leases. The assistance of professional investment managers is usually advisable. The hospital must evaluate opportunities to invest in its own activities and its overall investment strategy itself; professional managers cannot make these basic decisions.

Personnel and Organization

Various skilled and unskilled personnel work in the finance system of even a small hospital. Many of these people perform tasks that are indistinguishable from those in any other corporation, while others perform tasks that require extensive familiarity with health care. The chief financial officer and his or her staff develop specifications for these jobs, sometimes subject to review by or in consultation with the outside auditor. Recruitment is generally in local or state markets. On-the-job training is often practical. Supplies are adequate, and staffing questions are rarely serious enough to attract attention from outside the finance system itself.

The position of CFO is an exception to almost all of these statements. There is a chronic shortage of CFOs, recruitment should always be national, health-specific knowledge should be highly prized, and the governing board should be directly involved in the selection. Job specifications for CFO of an independently incorporated hospital tend not to depend upon size. Similar tasks must be performed in a small hospital and a large one, to essentially the same level of professional quality. Sustaining qualified professional financial management in small hospitals is a severe problem and one that may underlie more mergers and contract management than is recognized. Contract management is available through hospitals and firms providing general management as well. Auditing firms do not accept responsibility for financial system operations—to do so would destroy their objectivity as auditors—but they do provide substantial ongoing consultation on financial matters to hospitals of all sizes.

The Chief Financial Officer

The chief financial officer is accountable for the operation of his or her system, including the financial management functions, and advises the CEO and the governing board on finance issues. She or he has more access to cash and securities than is typical in commercial corporations, where an employed treasurer assumes the functions of collections, disbursement, and asset control. The hospital treasurer is frequently a trustee who serves principally as chair of the finance committee. The lack of separation between finance and treasury theoretically increases the risk of defalcation, but convincing evidence of risk is lacking and hospitals protect themselves by security bonds and reliance on the external audit.

Training and Skills. Ideally, the CFO should have a master's degree in management or business and be a certified public accountant (CPA). Certification focuses heavily on financial accounting (the issues relating to reporting the position of the firm) and includes practical experience in auditing. It is important to note that certification places little emphasis on the two functions that distinguish hospital excellence in finance, control and financial management. Thus being a CPA is in itself a relatively weak criterion for the job, desirable but not mandatory. Formal education in management is also only desirable, principally because it makes no guarantee of ability and able managers continue to arise without its help. However, it is increasingly likely that a person seriously interested in becoming a CFO will have found an opportunity to earn both a CPA and a master's in business administration.

Experience is more important than formal education or certification. The CFO of a well-run hospital should have at least 10 years of preparatory experience, which includes exposure to the finance systems of several hospitals, familiarity with all five functions of the finance system, and demonstrated ability to assist line management in budgeting, cost reporting, and financial planning. This record can be acquired by practice with a public accounting firm on hospital accounts, and deputy experience in a large, well-run hospital. Evidence of technical skill is important and can be supported both by specimens of work and by references. Evidence of interpersonal skills, particularly the ability to work with people outside the finance department, is also important and can be supported by references. If possible, these should be solicited by telephone or direct interview with nonfinancial persons familiar with a candidate's work.

Recruitment. Recruitment should always be in national markets, and outside candidates should be considered equally with any promotion from within. Not only does internal promotion foreclose an opportunity to gain fresh perspectives, it increases the risk of defalcation because it concentrates rather than separates responsibility and knowledge. Executive search firms are available to assist in recruitment and selection. Given the importance, technical skill required, and shortage of candidates, use of such firms seems well advised. The larger public accounting firms often assist in finding CFOs and, not surprisingly, are also a major source of supply.

The External Auditor

Extensive use of external auditors was rare in hospitals until it became mandatory for participation in Medicare. Today it is almost universal, but Berman and Weeks note that the external auditor's "primary concern is not the needs of internal management, but rather the needs of external agencies and organizations . . . ." In addition, "the value and usefulness of an independent auditor lie as much in business convention as they do in operational control."[7] Their point is well taken. External auditors make a prudent survey of the accuracy of records. Although this includes review of protection of assets, it does not in any sense include either budgeting or financial management. For protection of assets as well as for cost control, the hospital's best control systems are continuous and internal rather than episodic and external. The external controls imposed by the auditor are secondary and designed essentially to assure that the primary systems are working.

Even with this caveat, the external auditor is an important element for the well-run hospital. The auditor should be accountable directly to the board's finance committee. Considerable care in selecting and instructing the auditor is justified. He or she should be free of any other financial relationship to the hospital. Technically, this means that any consultants should be hired from a different firm than the one handling the audit. While sound, this rule is frequently breached. It is unacceptable, however, to use a firm represented on the hospital's governing board: "Any direct financial interest or material indirect financial interest is prohibited as is any relationship to the client, such as...voting trustee, director, officer, or key employee."[8] While the hospital board might override the conflict of interest for banking, groceries, or the practice of medicine, it seems both unwise and unnecessary to do so for the audit. The distance and independence of the auditor are an integral part of the audit's success.

Instructions to the auditor should be formulated by the finance committee of the governing board, whose chair should receive the re-

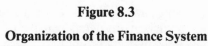

Figure 8.3

Organization of the Finance System

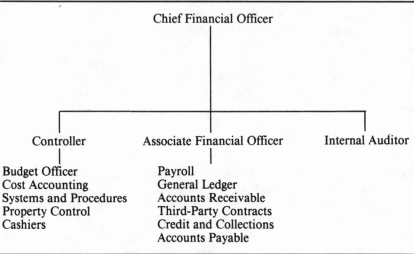

port. The instructions for audits of protection of assets should be reviewed and revised annually. It is common to use sampling techniques, with attention focused in proportion to the risk involved. This means that certain high-risk activities will be scrutinized annually, others less frequently. The revisions can bring different aspects of the asset protection system under scrutiny each year. The instructions should be based in part on advice from the CEO and CFO but should be confidential between the finance committee and the auditor. Most firms offer an oral summary and discussion of the management letter, which the board should accept.

Organization of the Finance System

Internal. The organization of the finance system, like many of its procedures, is dictated by its functions and has been thoroughly codified. Because of the use of separation of activities to protect assets, many aspects of the organization are fixed. The two critical functions, cost control and financial management, require relatively small numbers of people, with the largest numbers of personnel being in various aspects of patient accounting and collections. Figure 8.3 shows a typical organization pattern.

Financial management in such an organization would be provided by the CFO with an ad hoc team. Other variations are possible. With size, the duties under the controller and the associate finance officer would be specialized, and accountability hierarchies would develop under the specialties. Figure 8.3 reflects the assignments of information systems, admitting and registration, and materials management (see chapters 9, 13, and 15). In smaller and more traditionally organized hospitals, one or all of these activities might be assigned to the finance system.

Relation of Finance to Line. Almost every part of the organization shown in figure 8.3 is in direct daily contact with the rest of the hospital, often over sensitive matters. The key to success is maintaining a professional, productive level of exchange. Clear, convenient systems and forms make information gathering as routine as possible, permitting clinical professionals to supply what is necessary at their convenience rather than being interrupted by telephone calls. Continued attention to interdepartmental relations, through orientation and training sessions for finance personnel, also seems helpful. Two fundamentals should be universally understood: first, the accountability hierarchy of general management is responsible for setting, achieving, and departing from the expectations; second, they can carry out this responsibility best in an open atmosphere where information is widely available.

Role of Finance Committee. In the systems described in this chapter and the planning and marketing chapter, several tasks have been specifically identified for the finance committee of the board:

— Assist in selecting the CFO

— Periodically review the long-range financial plan and recommend the final version to the full board

— Approve an annual update of the long-range financial plan

— Recommend to the full board two guidelines for budget development:

  • Expected surplus from operations

  • Allowable change in total operating cost

— Review price changes and recommend pricing to the full board

— Recommend the annual budget to the full board

— Set the hurdle rate for capital investments

— Set the final priorities and recommend the capital and new programs budget to the board

— Select and instruct the external auditor

— Receive the auditor's report and the management letter

— Receive the monthly report comparing operations to expectations

While all these matters are important, the well-run hospital focuses on the future-oriented activities. Future needs well met make present needs easy.

The list makes it clear why membership on the finance committee is time-consuming and intellectually demanding. Members are important at meetings of the full board as well, and there are often overlapping appointments to the planning committee. In addition, the finance committee has routine obligations to approve the hospital's banks and financial contractors, the specific bond or stock offerings, the sale of assets and approval of contracts over predetermined levels, and the approval of officers' salaries and bonuses. Even assuming no turnover in the position of CFO, the list above can easily fill 10 or 11 fast-paced meetings each year.

Poorly run hospitals tend to get diverted into narrower, more specific decisions, approving individual purchases, remarking upon the obvious in monthly reports, focusing generally on single transactions instead of broad trends. The poorly run finance committee can devote much time to routine obligations, either because they were never integrated properly with the long-range plans and budget or because the committee is uncomfortable dealing with strategic alternatives. The routine obligations are important parts of the system of separation of activity to protect against fraud, but in the well-run hospital they take little time. It is evidence of problems if routine actions require debate or contain surprising information.

Measures of Performance

The finance activity can be modelled as a closed system, but the identification of the parameters, particularly demand and output, is confusing and arbitrary. A practical modification concentrates upon three areas in which finance makes its major contributions to the hospital's success. These are

1. Resource consumption or costs for which finance is directly accountable

2. Collection of revenue and management of liquid assets

3. The quality of information and reporting services

Resource Consumption Measures

Labor and Contract Services. The finance system has a significant number of employees, consumes much of the computing resource, and often has significant outside contracts for consultation and other services. All of these are costs which should be budgeted, as with any other unit. Accountability can be carried to responsibility centers, as shown in figure 8.3.

Working Capital Requirements. The funds needed to support operations during the period between provision of service and payment for service represent real resource consumption, although they are not emphasized by the accounting system. Hospitals encounter substantial delays in payment from third parties, often eight weeks or more. Although some contracts include advances at regular intervals to offset this lag *(interim payments)*, the hospital which minimizes short-term obligations such as payroll, inventories, and accounts payable is financially ahead. **Working capital,** defined as the amount of cash required to support operations for the period of delay in collection of revenue, is a real consumption of resources and should be budgeted as such.

The cost of working capital is the hospital's short-term borrowing rate or earning from investments, whichever is less. The amount may be offset by investing all the available cash, including any sums supplied as interim payments, but only if such payments represent a real change in the cash flow. The cost of working capital is not trivial. A medium-sized hospital spending $50 million annually with an eight-week average delay requires $10 million in working capital; this costs about $900,000 per year, the equivalent of 45 full-time employees. Accountability for minimizing the delay is through the CFO to the associate in charge of posting, billing, credit, and collection. It can be further delegated by estimating the delays attributable to each of these groups.

Other Capital Costs. Most hospitals now borrow funds for various purposes and simultaneously hold long-term investments. The earnings on investments and costs of borrowing are determined in part by the quality of financial planning and financial management. The amounts, timing, and sources of funds determine the costs for a specific project. All of these activities are under the control of the CFO, who should establish and achieve expectations for investment earnings and the cost of capital as part of her or his annual budget.

Asset Losses and Write-Downs. Inventories and certain equipment are at risk for theft, loss, and adjustments in value. It is unrealistic to expect such losses to be zero, and they represent direct and totally unproductive evaporation of assets. An expectation for such losses should be established and the RCMs responsible for the property held accountable for achieving—or, better still, *not* achieving—it. Accountability is through the plant system units responsible for protecting the physical property.

There are occasional losses of cash, and long-term assets need to be revalued from time to time because of changing conditions. One would normally expect no losses from failure to revalue assets. Responsibility for losses of assets is difficult to identify, but the finance committee should certainly consider its own role and the contribution of other managers in each important case.

Resource Conservation

Operating Revenue Adjustments. The values of revenue adjustments, principally contractual allowances for each third-party contract, bad debts, and charity, can be influenced by effective management. Careful study of third-party contract provisions, billing, and accounting procedures can reveal ways to reduce the allowances. Bad debts can be reduced by more aggressive and more efficient collection policies. Even charity allowances can be limited by careful case review and pursuit of welfare and other third-party coverage.

An expectation should be established for each allowance, and the appropriate RCM of the finance group should be held accountable.

Other Nonoperating Income. Hospitals have a variety of sources of income other than those connected with patient care. Most such income is in rents, dividends, and interest earned, but income from unrelated business is also common. There should be expectations for all major types and sources of nonoperating income, and the chief financial officer should be held accountable for these.

Net Profit from Operations. The expectation for net profit is one of the key elements of the long-range financial plan and is one of the first two short-term expectations set in the annual budget. The CFO, the COO, and the CEO share accountability for meeting it.

Net profit is extremely volatile, even under sophisticated, flexible budgeting. The net profit figure is dependent on volume, which is well outside the control of the CFO. While some sensitivity to the difficulty of achieving the net profit expectation is in order, the importance of the measure must be recognized. No other statistic so clearly reflects the long-term health of the hospital.

Quality of Financial Planning and Reporting Services

The quality of many of the functions of finance is self-evident or is measured by the output. Quality of the revenue-generating activities, for example, is measured by the adjustment; that of funds management by borrowing costs and interest income. The external audit and the management letter provide qualitative assessment of another large group of finance activities. In two of the five functions, however, the principal product of the system is information, and the quality of the work is not as apparent. These activities are no less critical to success in the long run, however, and there should be expectations for their performance.

Quality of the Financial Plan. Only subjective judgment of the quality of the long-range financial plan is practical. Worse, the people who made the plan are likely to be the ones evaluating it; nonetheless, the importance of periodic review should be obvious. By the time objective tests are available, the hospital's existence may be endangered. The following list contains questions answered affirmatively by successful hospitals:

— The plan is clear, concise, internally consistent, and consistent with the long-range plan.

— Assumptions and their implications are specified.

— Prudent and reasonable sources have been used to develop external trends, and a variety of opinion has been reviewed whenever possible.

— External events requiring modification are unforeseen by competitors as well as this hospital.

— The plan is well received by outsiders such as consultants, bond-rating agencies, and investment bankers.

— The plan develops contingencies on major, unpredictable future events.

Quality of Patient, Physician, and Third-Party Relations. The finance system has a number of contacts with members of the community and should carry these out in ways that reflect positively upon the hospital. For a great many patients carrying comprehensive health insurance, receiving the final bill can be a positive experience. Even for those who must pay out of pocket, the way in which the charge is presented can make an important difference in the patient's perception. "Guest relations" programs (see chapter 14) are certainly in order for those finance system personnel dealing directly with patients and families.

Many hospitals now sell services to physicians, bringing the finance system into direct contact with them as well. Physician satisfaction will remain a hallmark of the well-managed hospital, obviously including satisfaction with the finance system.

Finally, the finance system establishes the image of the hospital in a certain sector of the community, including banks, government agencies, self-insuring employers, and insurance carriers. The well-managed hospital anticipates a reputation of probity, candor, courtesy, and promptness. The CFO and members of his or her staff should anticipate at least informal review of these relationships and should expect to sustain them appropriately.

Quality of Budget and Performance Reporting. The finance system has a clientele for its internal budgeting and reporting activities in the general managers who must use the information. Their criticisms of it should be heeded, particularly when they deal with the accuracy and timeliness of the information. Concerns with conciseness, clarity, and level of specification are also important.

Advice from finance personnel to general managers is also a sensitive matter, and direct assessment of the opinion of general managers about such advice is wise. There is a tendency for finance personnel to enter into the expectation-setting process and the monitoring process beyond what good practice indicates. Consultation and information are likely to be helpful, but intrusion can destroy the motivation for continued improvement, because it erodes the capacity of general managers to set and achieve their own expectations.

Management Issues in Financial Management

The management issues for the well-run hospital are in the areas of financial management and cost control. Although both processes go on simultaneously, the decisions of financial management form a basis for effective cost control. They are discussed below in the evolutionary order suggested by sound planning and marketing, from the most future-oriented decisions to the most immediate ones.

The objective of financial management is to acquire sufficient capital at minimum cost—both long-term capital, which is necessary for buildings and equipment, and working capital, which is needed to support day-to-day operations. Since one important source of capital is profit from operations, even in not-for-profit hospitals, the issues of financial management include pricing of goods and services sold. They also include the management of equity and borrowing and, since 1980, issues of corporate structure. The trick to doing well with all these issues lies in financial planning. As usual, it is the farsighted institution which can take advantage of the environment rather than being totally submissive to it.

Each of these issues is worthy of a book. Good financial leadership, through the appointment of an experienced, able CFO and the use of knowledgeable consultants and board members, is obviously essential. In each issue are questions demanding the judgment of nonfinancial people, the CEO and the governing board. The discussion below will assume that the hospital has good financial leadership and will concentrate on the questions that arise in developing an integrated program which is competitive both in meeting patient needs and in price.

Developing a Realistic Financial Plan

Financial planning starts with the hospital's current financial position and some preferences for the long-range plan, short of the final, approved plan. It develops several ways in which the preferences can be financed, using combinations of cash from operations, borrowing, equity and gifts. The most promising of these alternatives are presented to general governance, and in the well-run hospital the decision is made along the following guidelines:

— Preliminary work on the long-range operational plan and the long-range financial plan is done on a high level of technical competence.

— The bias of the well-run hospital is toward liquidity and, as a result, flexibility. Well-run hospitals keep the horizon of the plans short, adopt no proposal in the absence of compelling benefit, and maintain options rather than commitments as long as possible. Commitments must be accepted as constraints, while options can be modified. Thus the later years of the long-range plan for a well-run hospital may quantify only gross revenue, services to be offered, and the anticipated size of the markets to be served. If the plan includes a building program and a borrowing program, the financial plan will include the specific commitments, and the horizon will be extended.

— The recurring question addressed is what profit, or return from operations, the hospital should seek. Whereas competition establishes prices and revenues, this establishes the maximum cost the hospital can incur. In noncompetitive situations, an acceptable cost is selected and the price is set from it. Well-run not-for-profit hospitals have tended to seek returns in the range of 5 percent of total costs. For-profit hospitals seek before-tax returns two to three times that high.

— Recurring board decisions should be made from a small number of reasonable alternatives rather than single propositions. (The strategic opportunities described in chapter 7 are inevitably unique, nonrecurring decisions.)

— In all board decisions involving planning and resource allocation, the operational plan and the financial plan are adopted simultaneously. Each such decision deals with the total organization, and any effort to isolate finance from operations would be ill-advised.

— The criteria for investment decisions must weigh risk against cost to the community. The result of increased risk is that the total cost of all of the proposals in the plan will rise, thus requiring greater benefits to make them desirable. (Usually this is expressed through an increase in the borrowing interest rate.) There are three basic causes of increased risk:

  • Prior actions of the hospital that have consumed its financial capacity

  • Individual proposals that are inherently risky

  • Too large a total set of proposals

Well-run hospitals minimize their exposure by careful attention to all three. Their bias is against risk in most situations.

— Timing is frequently important in the price of capital. Well-run hospitals allow themselves sufficient flexibility to take advantage of low interest rates and to avoid borrowing at peak rates.

— Well-run hospitals conduct annual reviews of the long-range plans in advance of the annual budget cycle. Most years these adapt and increase the specificity of generally indicated actions. Each year, the horizon is extended outward, not to commit distant future actions but to improve the understanding of near-term ones.

— Once reviewed, the long-range operational and financial plans guide development of the annual budget. Proposals must be consistent with both plans to receive serious attention in the budget discussions.

Pricing

In the past, most U.S. hospitals set prices based upon their costs and were "reimbursed," either at their stated price or at some percentage of costs. If profits were insufficient, prices could be raised. The Tax Equalization and Fiscal Responsibility Act of 1982 established the right of Medicare to set prices without regard to an individual hospital's costs. The idea proved widely popular. Within three years, most hospitals were plunged into a competitive environment where most prices were set by supply and demand. In an oversimplified model of the new condition, competition sets a realistic price, and a sufficient quantity can be delivered at that price to meet all demand. In reality, a hospital's actual cost will depend heavily on volume. A hospital seeking more profits may undercut the established price in an effort to maximize volume. Hospitals that are inefficient, overpriced, or unattractive suffer declining volume and disappear from the field.

The competitive pressure is almost entirely from group purchasers of health insurance, both government and private. It has not developed evenly across the states or even in individual communities within states. Medicare creates far greater competitive pressures in the Northeast and North Central regions than elsewhere. Pressure on state governments from Medicaid costs is widespread among the larger states, but the patterns of response have differed. Concern on the part of business and labor has differed from community to community. However, the general trend is for increased competitive pressure.

In terms of financial management, hospitals generally approach this problem by first establishing the profit required from overall operations to continue to meet the hospital's mission. This is usually expressed as a percentage or markup. However, depending on the competitive strength of the buyer, the hospital may price individual services higher or lower than the desired markup. Both options represent cross subsidies from some patients and their insurers to others, but they also represent ways of attracting necessary volumes and profits. Minimum acceptable prices are theoretically set by the variable cost of the service—if net revenue exceeds marginal cost, the offer should be accepted, assuming a better one cannot be had. Determination of the variable cost of producing each hospital service is a complex task demanding a detailed accounting system and extensive computational capability. Theoretically there is no maximum, either to profits or prices, but as a practical matter attention must be paid to the political implications of cross subsidization. The group paying the premium may take the argument into the political arena on its own terms, which may be quite disadvantageous to the hospital.

In the new environment, the well-run hospital operates in a sufficiently attractive and efficient manner to receive satisfactory volumes at prices available in the marketplace. This allows it some luxury of choice, both to decline offers at unacceptably low prices and to offer some services, such as care of the poor, which otherwise might require excessively high markups. The choice is limited and fragile, however. The role of the governing board in the new environment is to:

— Set the desired overall margin from operations as part of financial planning

— Establish pricing guidelines that require board approval for any major cross subsidization

— Support information systems and management capability which will improve the hospital's ability to compete by improving variable cost efficiency and by attracting high demand for fixed assets

— Evaluate the political and mission-related aspects of subsidies, charity, or other major departures from desired prices in a political or influence context

Use of Reserves and Debt

One of the most critical implications of the new competitive environment is for the management of reserves and debt. After working capital needs are met, earned surplus and accumulated depreciation funds constitute the major cushion the hospital has against unfortunate events in the marketplace or in operations. They are in a very real sense *reserves* against adversity. Debt reflects a commitment against future surplus and depreciation cash flows, in a sense a *negative reserve*. Reserves can be used for three basic purposes: meeting deficits, replacing capital equipment and facilities, and expansion. As a practical matter, the well-run hospital rarely has deficits. Its reserves are applied to replacement and to expansion.

The most general and far-reaching fiscal policy decision facing the governing board is the relative use of debt or reserves. The decade between 1970 and 1979 saw a dramatic change in the acceptability of debt funding, leading to a situation in which the typical U.S. hospital holds long-term debt amounting to close to 50 percent of its assets. Most of this indebtedness went to finance capital for the 15 to 18 percent annual growth hospitals experienced in that decade.

A hospital with a high reliance on indebtedness can be said to be *highly leveraged*. The implications of being highly leveraged are as follows:

— Fixed costs are increased, making the actual profit margin more sensitive to changes in volume.

— Debt-equity ratios are increased, tending to lower the hospital's credit or bond rating and raise the cost of borrowing.

— More funds are committed to expansion and replacement, supporting more new technology and more attractive facilities.

— Total operating costs increase more rapidly, because most hospital capital investments require additional operating costs.

A hospital with a low reliance on debt can be said to be *highly liquid.* The implications of high liquidity are as follows:

— Hospital operating costs are kept low; in particular, fixed cost is kept to a small fraction of the total. This allows the hospital to operate profitably at a much lower level of demand.

— Cash (or marketable securities) reserves accumulate and credit ratings improve. These allow the hospital to respond to new opportunities quickly and economically.

— Price can be reduced, leading to increased market share or greater customer satisfaction.

— Plant and equipment age and may become less attractive to doctors or patients, or both. If unchecked, this leads to declining demand.

A critical function of the finance committee and the governing board is to set the desired degree of liquidity or leverage. The decision is made via the long-range plan and financial plan, and the results are measured by the ratios of debt to equity and debt service costs to earnings. There are no general guidelines on the "right" values of these ratios, except that it is unwise to impair the hospital's bond rating without extremely good justification. The values for other communities and other hospitals can be misleading; the appropriate response must be developed out of an understanding of the local community. The following observations may be helpful:

— Many well-run hospitals have operated from conservative, or highly liquid, positions in the past. They will probably continue to do so and will be even more successful. The general bias or predisposition of the well-run hospital is toward liquidity.

— Serious threat to or actual loss of market share is the most compelling reason to sacrifice liquidity.

— Extreme positions of either liquidity or debt require justification. They are probably best justified as temporary phenomena and any hospital at such an extreme is generally well advised to be moving back toward a more usual position.

— The buyer's movement toward price competition is an expression of real concern with costs. It therefore represents strong pressure for liquidity.

— Many observers believe that the continued emphasis on lower cost will force major reorganization of the hospital and health care industry. In this reorganization, hospitals in highly leveraged positions are endangered, but hospitals in highly liquid positions will be presented with substantial opportunities for growth by acquisition.

— The best management foresees changes in the market before they occur. For example:

• The higher the health care costs of a community, the more likely it is to become concerned with reducing them. A well-managed hospital in a high-cost community, therefore, moves to liquidity in preparation for a market shift to price competition.

• Communities with very low costs may have reduced services and may risk becoming obsolete and unattractive to young professionals. Well-run hospitals in these communities make deliberate investments to counteract this danger and plan carefully for modernization when it can be done economically.

Multiple Corporate Structures

The traditional structure of community hospitals used a single corporate entity, but competition, broader scope of services, financial considerations, and new views on risk taking have encouraged the development of more complex corporate structures for hospitals. Multiple corporations isolate liabilities, offer opportunities for competitive pricing, permit investment in diverse lines of business, allow member participation and profit-sharing, and in some cases evade regulatory activity. Control can be maintained through holding companies or parent-subsidiary relationships. The well-run hospital must use the multiple corporation opportunity wisely. Blind disregard is as dangerous as foolish restructuring; each eventually impairs the assets of the enterprise.

Hypothetical Opportunities. The corporate pattern that is emerging for larger, independent hospitals is a central corporation or holding company which usually has the same for-profit or not-for-profit character as the original corporation. The hospital often becomes the dominant subsidiary of the holding company, but the holding company is free to invest in as many other corporate entities as it desires, and it may divert business to its holdings in any way consistent with market demand and rather minimal legal requirements. Thus a not-for-profit hospital might reincorporate as a not-for-profit holding company and a not-for-profit hospital, but the outpatient activities might be incorporated for profit, possibly with doctors as outside stockholders. A fourth corporation might provide diagnostic services—laboratory, X-ray, and cardiopulmonary—to both health care corporations. It, too, could be for-profit. The three working corporations could sell services to one another. Such a scenario opens several vistas:

— Doctors have been involved as investors and can be incorporated in the management of the outpatient and diagnostic activities as directors.

— Outpatient and diagnostic services can be priced without concern for the fixed costs of the hospital, presumably making them more competitive and more profitable.

— In many states with rate regulation and almost all state certificate of need laws, the outpatient and diagnostic activities would be removed from regulatory control.

— Hospital revenues would be reduced and hospital costs for inpatients increased by removing the clinic and diagnostic service support of fixed overhead, although these losses may be offset by both profits from the clinic declared as dividends to the holding company and contracts for services such as accounting and housekeeping. Pricing of these contracts may escape regulation. More important, pricing imposes a cost control discipline missing under routine overhead assignments.

Similar opportunities exist in the aggregation of several hospitals into one multihospital corporation (horizontal integration), and the expansion of the activities of the holding company into other forms of care, such as nursing homes, home care and hospices, and housing facilities for the elderly (vertical integration). The flexibility offered by these vehicles is compelling. It is likely that most well-run hospitals will avail themselves of opportunities to integrate services both horizontally and vertically.

Reporting and Disclosure Implications. Multiple corporate structure may affect the hospital's disclosure requirements and position under rate and planning regulations. For example, the hospital might set up a foundation to receive charitable donations and hospital surpluses.

Foundations are tax-exempt. They can receive grants from the hospital, as well as other donors, and can give funds to the hospital for various purposes. The funds available to the two corporations can be managed more flexibly by the governing board, while at the same time the public disclosure for the foundation need not be as extensive, and its assets and earnings are not subject to rate regulation.

A second example is the establishment of individual lines of hospital operations as separate corporations controlled by a single holding company. Long-term care, psychiatric care, and ambulatory care are often incorporated separately. In some states this maneuver avoids rate regulation, certificate of need, and licensing complexities. Hospitals which undertake unrelated businesses find separate corporations useful for isolating and reporting taxes and liabilities. These corporations offer opportunities to vary the amount of information reported; the holding company's consolidated financial statement may reveal more or less detail about various subsidiaries.

Strategies for Using Corporate Structures Wisely. The management issues raised become clear when corporate restructuring is recognized as a tool rather than an end in itself. Corporate restructuring allows more flexibility in carrying out the functions of management. It permits missions to be specialized, prices to be refined, responses to regulation sharpened, risks to be contained, and involvement in management to be increased. What it does not do is change the fundamental requirements of management. The enterprise still exists in a symbiotic relationship with its environment, still must find and complete mutually satisfactory exchanges, and still must function as a bureaucratic organization using the closed system principles of planning and control. The well-run hospital will avoid the dangers of excess that accompany any new and dramatic device. It will do that by

— Relating all corporate restructuring to the mission and long-range plan of the institution

— Justifying each corporation in terms of the mission

— Establishing new corporations in response to permanent or very long-term benefits

— Exercising caution in entering activities new to the managerial and clinical personnel

— Recognizing that corporate restructuring does not affect either the underlying benefits the community is seeking or the basic mechanisms of control of costs and quality

— Avoiding the use of corporate restructuring as a substitute for failures in planning and control

Management Issues in Cost Control

The purpose of operations budgeting, capital budgeting, and monitoring is to achieve control of cost and efficiency over the range of demand required by the external exchanges. The guidelines for doing this are included in the descriptions of the functions. A hospital pursuing these guidelines will encounter difficulties. The well-run hospital succeeds because it solves two problems better than its competitors:

1. It emphasizes expectation setting through the budgeting process as a central activity of management offering inherent professional challenges and rewards.

    a. Within the operating budget, much effort is put to finding economical but realistic and achievable labor cost expectations.

    b. Steady progress is made toward flexible budgeting, transfer pricing, and other improvements promoting intermediate product efficiency.

    c. The capital and new programs budget process is carefully designed to encourage participation, educate the participants, and result in decisions which are not only wise but also credible and acceptable to hospital members.

2. It uses its information system, organization structure, incentives, and sanctions to encourage cooperation and to discourage defensiveness.

Using the Operations and Capital Budget Processes

If a hospital makes a serious effort to implement the operations budget shown in figure 8.2, it will find that the questions attracting the most debate and emotion are those of equitable allocation of resources. These occur in both the operating and the capital budget. Most RCMs will be seeking funds for new programs and capital expenditures, as well as a level of operating costs that will allow safe, comfortable operation of their units. All members of the organization will want assurance that there is equity among units in meeting external exchange demands for economy and quality. If the annual surveillance and budget guidelines have been properly explained, they will understand that external demands must be met. They will still need to be reassured that no other work group has a more comfortable operation or an inside track on the capital funds. The tension between member needs for comfort and safety and external exchange needs for economy and quality is inevitable at all levels of the organization.

Proper handling of this tension is important. The goal is to divert it from defensiveness and self-protection to collaboration and cooperativeness. Several observations can be made about tension and its implications. One is that it becomes inevitable as soon as resources are in short supply. Its absence in hospitals during the 1970s is related directly to the easy access to funds which prevailed then. A second is that it is universal. Many people incorrectly see the tension as between the "bosses" and the "workers" or between the clinical and the governance systems, or even as a characteristic of specific individuals. Third, the tension deals with perceptions and process at least as much as it does with actual resource allocations. For much of the hospital, the question is not "What is the correct resource?" but "How do we reach an equitable, economical, acceptable solution?" Resolving that question for two major decision sets, labor costs and new programs, changes the budget from an onerous, threatening chore to a professional opportunity.

Using the Operations Budget To Encourage Productivity. Because hospitals are labor-intensive, the most substantial operating costs involve staffing. Each RCM must accept a certain level of staffing or, under flexible budgeting, a certain level of staffing per unit of output. The process by which staffing for the coming year is set will have a major effect upon tensions and, as a result, upon willingness to cooperate.

Although many hospital managers think first of outside standards for staffing, in fact, external standards may lead to suboptimal results. Human beings have a well-demonstrated ability to work safely and contentedly over a wide range of activity. The pace implicit in most work standards is such that most people can routinely achieve 120 or 130 percent without discomfort or danger.[9] For a variety of reasons beyond the worker's or RCM's control, hospitals rarely operate at such levels. The work load varies unpredictably in many hospital settings, requiring routine overstaffing to meet peak demand. Many professionals are obligated to determine the patient's needs for themselves and as a result partially set their own work load. The actual work to be done, the equipment to do it, and the methods to be used are not static; what is best next year will be slightly different from what is best now. The imprecise measurement of quality and the desire for improvement in quality also limit the precision of work standards.

In such a situation, insistence on an external standard of efficiency may be destructive. Even if the standard is achieved, there remains the very reasonable possibility that better performance is possible if a new, broader, and more energetic search is undertaken. The external standard blocks that search, both by supplying a false sense of accomplishment and by being arbitrarily imposed rather than developed from within. If the external standard is too high, it leads directly to the frustration and defensiveness which the hospital seeks to avoid.

Ideally, each RCM will be motivated to seek the best possible standard, and there will be no need to impose external solutions. Not only the RCM but the workers themselves will set expectations which will require effort to achieve, and they will anticipate and achieve satisfaction from reaching them. Few organizations of any kind have achieved the ideal consistently, but the well-run hospital comes closer than its less able competitors. The increase in cooperation which results may be more important to success than the immediate gains in RC efficiency, because a foundation is laid for further improvement.

It is a cardinal rule in the well-managed hospital that the RCM and his or her work group set the efficiency standards in an environment that rewards the continued search for improvement. To create this environment, the hospital relies on a set of rules for effective human relations. These rules are not new, although they have recently been emphasized in the quality of work life movement. They have only occasionally been systematically applied to budgeting, but they are as important in this activity as in any other.[10] They can be briefly stated as follows:

— The RCM receives training in advance covering the hospital's budget philosophy, the importance of the outcomes expectations, the reasons for being given the opportunity to propose expectations rather than being forced to accept those of others, and the value of incorporating the viewpoints of work group members.

— The RCM's supervisor offers a full explanation of the budget guidelines, assistance in setting expectations, if necessary, and encouragement to set realistically improved expectations.

— The RCM is the first person to propose the budget expectations for the coming year. He or she proposes a comprehensive set, including resources, output, efficiency, and, to the extent it can be quantified, quality.

— Each supervisory level is strongly encouraged to start the expectation-setting process by conferring with members of lower levels. Formal submission by the RCM, in the form of a signature on the initial budget request, is required.

— The information system of the hospital provides the RCM with three kinds of information about the efficiency expectation:

  • A record of output, labor consumption, and efficiency over several recent periods, permitting the RCM to search for conditions of high and low efficiency within the RC.

  • Comparison data on other hospitals, emphasizing the range of performance rather than measures of central tendency.

- Relevant external work standards.

— The forms and processes for setting expectations are simple and oriented to a complete review of resources required at various levels of operation. They are formatted for easy data entry and computer assistance, and require little or no arithmetic on the part of the RCM.

— Management engineering services are available to the RCM on request, although the RCM must accept the cost of such services as part of the total cost expectations.

— The reward system of the hospital is structured to emphasize both increased productivity and maintenance of a satisfied work force.

- Merit increases and other tangible rewards are clearly associated with setting and achieving improved expectations.

- It is understood that new programs and capital requests from units achieving commendable expectations face an easier approval process.

- Intangible rewards such as praise and public acknowledgement are used lavishly to recognize both setting and achieving expectations.

Moving to Flexible Budgeting. When systems and habits of budgeting are well established and RCMs are comfortable seeking annual improvements in performance, the hospital can benefit from flexible budgeting. A fixed budget holds the RCM accountable for constant use of resources throughout each reporting period, based on a forecast of demand established at the time the budget is negotiated. A flexible budget holds the RCM accountable for varying use of resources, depending upon the demand encountered at the time. In RCs where demand fluctuates, the fixed budget will create periods of inefficiency when demand is low and periods of overload, leading to poor quality or overwork, when demand is high. Most RCMs will instinctively avoid overload by staffing over average demand. As a result, the flexible budget will not only be more efficient on the average, it will at the same time reduce the danger of overload.

The simplest form of flexible budget assumes that a responsibility center can produce up to the limit of its capital equipment. Each unit of output below the limit will require a certain quantity of resources. The capital costs will be fixed, as in traditional budgeting. Thus for any given level of demand below the limit, the expected expenditures of the RC will be

Total Budget = Fixed Costs

+ (Number of Units) [(Unit Labor Costs) + (Unit Supplies Costs)].

If, for example, an RC produced 100 units a month on the average, its fixed budget might be

Labor costs	$1,000
Supplies costs	250
Equipment costs	200
Total costs	$1,450

Under flexible budgeting, the expectation would be

Labor costs	$10.00 per unit
Supplies costs	$ 2.50 per unit
Equipment costs	$200.00

Total expectation would depend upon production. At 100 units it would be the same as the fixed budget, $1,450, but at 80 units it would be $1,200 and at 120 units, $1,700.

Three assumptions underlie the use of flexible budgeting:

1. The workload of the RC is measurable in units which require equal quantities of at least some of the resources. (In the example above, both the first unit and the 120th require $10 of labor and $2.50 of supplies. If, for example, all units over 100 had to be prepared in an overflow space, they might take more than $10 labor each.)

2. The use of the resources required in varying quantity can be controlled by the RCM. (In the example, the RCM must be able to hire people in relatively small aggregates. At $5 per hour, the variation from 100 to 120 units means 40 hours of work, a half-time person if the reporting period is the usual two weeks. A smaller variation, say five units, requires adjusting for only 10 hours and may be difficult to do.)

3. The demand can be predicted far enough in advance to allow adjustment of the resources. (If the activity is related to unpredictable emergencies, the RCM must staff for 120 units.)

The RCM can rarely be held solely responsible for meeting these conditions. Redesigning work flows and accountability makes it possible to meet them in some RCs, but in others the assumptions can never be met. The number of places in the hospital where flexible budgeting will not work is surprisingly large; for example:

— *Difficulty in establishing a measurement unit that varies uniformly with output* poses problems for social service, educational activities, medical records, security, and planning and marketing.

— *Difficulty in adjusting resources* poses problems for all small RCs with minimum staffing requirements and many RCs requiring highly skilled professional labor, such as doctors or uniquely trained technicians.

— *Difficulty in predicting demand* poses problems for emergency services, intensive care units, coronary care units, obstetrics, newborn care, and infant care.

The well-run hospital applies flexible budgeting only where these difficulties can be overcome at reasonable cost. In practice, this means that flexible budgeting is likely to be a useful tool where there are relatively large numbers of people with interchangeable training, such as nursing, laboratory, accounting, and food service. Fewer than half the RCs are candidates for flexible budgeting, although more than half the total cost is in these RCs.

The return from flexible budgeting increases as the following conditions are met:

— The guidelines for sound human relations in budgeting and control have been applied, and a cooperative environment exists.

— The three assumptions for flexible budget applications have been met.

• Demand has been studied for ways to stabilize it as much as possible, including studies of the interrelation with other units, possibilities of promoting new stable demand, and possibilities of deferring some demand or scheduling it during off-peak periods.

• Staffing sources have been carefully studied to develop less costly ways of responding to variation in demand.

• Recurring variation has been met by improved scheduling of workers.

• Incentives for extra output to meet temporary peak demand have been given to permanent full-time personnel.

• Cross training has been provided to increase the pool of workers available for specific tasks.

• Overtime, part-time, and temporary employment that can be adjusted on short notice have been planned.

Figure 8.4a

XYZ Hospital—Flexible Staffing Budget

Instructions:
1. Top portion: To be completed by responsibility center manager, with approval by immediate superior.
2. Volume: Please show intervals of anticipated activity, in the designated output measure for your RC, reflecting the lowest level at which staffing changes due to increased volume. You may skip ranges where no change occurs.
3. Hours budgeted: Show 8 hours for a full-time shift, and normally scheduled hours for part-shift personnel. If you anticipate overtime, show the number of hours as a plus: for example, "8 + 1."

Department _____

Unit _____ Shift _____

Prepared by _____ Date _____

Approved by _____ Date _____

Personnel Hours Budgeted by Class

Volume	Title Grade									

— The RCM understands the nature of the demand variation and staff adjustment and is prepared to implement flexible budgeting expectations. The RCM must have a plan to translate demand forecast into explicit staffing patterns. Such plans are convenient for establishing the flexible budget. Figure 8.4a shows the form used by one well-managed hospital, and figure 8.4b gives an example for a conventional nursing floor. The

Figure 8.4b

XYZ Hospital—Flexible Staffing Budget (Example: Figure 8.4a)

Instructions:

1. Top portion: To be completed by responsibility center manager, with approval by immediate superior.
2. Volume: Please show intervals of anticipated activity, in the designated output measure for your RC, reflecting the lowest level at which staffing changes due to increased volume. You may skip ranges where no change occurs.
3. Hours budgeted: Show 8 hours for a full-time shift, and normally scheduled hours for part-shift personnel. If you anticipate overtime, show the number of hours as a plus: for example, "8 + 1."

Department _____ Surgical Nursing _____
Unit _____ 3 West _____ Shift ___ Day ___
Prepared by _____ ABC _____ Date _11/17/87_
Approved by _____ DEF _____ Date _11/24/87_

Personnel Hours Budgeted by Class

Volume	Title	HN	AHN	RN	LPN	Aide	Aide	Clk		
	Grade	10	08	06	04	03	02	01		
20			8	16		8		8		
22			8	16		16		8		
24		8		24		8		8		
26		8		28		8		8		
28		8		24		8		16		
30		8		28		8		16		
32		8		32		8		16		
34		8		36		8		16		
36		8		40		8		16		
38		8		44		8		16		
40		8	8	32		8	8	16		

form is simple, but the computing algorithm is complex, resulting eventually in a budget showing anticipated hours and dollars for each class of nursing personnel.

Transfer Pricing and Accounting Improvements. A number of other enhancements of the budgeting system can assist RCMs in improving their performance. Like flexible budgeting, these move from lesser to greater levels of precision, first in the accounting of costs and second in the budgeting of costs. It is often desirable to identify much more precisely where resources are actually spent. Improvement in the accounting of use of supplies is an example: if supplies are accurately costed to a small unit, such as hematology, rather than to the larger clinical laboratory, accountability is improved. General use items such as food service, housekeeping, laundry, heat, telephone, and electricity have rarely been accounted accurately to the responsibility centers. Often new reporting and information systems are required to support the more detailed accounting. Thus the effort to improve productivity must be paralleled by upgrades in the finance system, information services, and human resources management.

When the basic accounting of resources is in place, it becomes possible to view each of the responsibility centers as analogous to an independent business, buying and selling services to each other as well as selling them to the patient or customer. The prices for external sales are increasingly set by competitive market forces. There is value in attempting to set an analogous transfer price for those services not sold externally. Conceptually, the transfer price allows the buying RCM to look on the purchase as a variable cost resource to be used as effectively as possible. Simultaneously, it allows the selling RCM to recover earnings and an implicit profit. It permits comparison with similar transactions in the outside world; if the hospital's cost-based transfer price is materially different, questions of relative efficiency and quality need to be asked. The issue of transfer pricing is most relevant to the management of the human resources and plant systems (see chapters 14 and 15).

New Programs Decisions and the Capital Budget. The criterion for all capital investment is optimization of long-term exchange relationships between the hospital and its community. For the hospital to thrive, new projects, expansions, and replacement of old investments must always be selected on the basis of this criterion, which must balance both member (internal) needs and patient (external) needs. The nature of professional behavior is such that the best managers and clinicians will always have proposals which cannot be funded, so considerable tension surrounds the selection process. The process must not only identify the best proposals, but also seem equitable to organization members.

A reasonable selection process for the new programs and capital budget develops out of the long-range and financial plans, and makes deliberate use of the planning-marketing activities for programmatic improvements described in chapter 7. That process uses a planning team with both line and planning members to develop a proposal which is as objective as possible. Assuming that it has resulted in several proposals which are consistent with the long-range plan and objectively argued, how does the well-run hospital reach its final decision on implementation for the coming year? The proposals selected to be implemented will constitute the budget for new programs and capital expenditures and as such will affect the revenue, cost, and cash flow budgets.

The following steps are helpful:

1. The finance committee has direct input into proposal development by setting a hurdle rate reflecting the prevailing attitude of the hospital toward risk and liquidity. An annual adjustment in this rate is wise, to accommodate fluctuations in the interest rate and other considerations reflecting the business cycle.

2. Proposals accumulated during the year are submitted for initial review by ad hoc committees within each of the five major hospital systems. The task of these committees is to rank the proposals submitted. That is, clinical proposals are ranked in the clinical system, accounting proposals in the finance system, and so on. Within the larger systems, subcommittees may rank sets of related proposals.

3. Ranking should follow established guidelines for both process and criteria:

   a. A process which allows each committee member a secret vote on the rank is preferable, because it reduces recrimination, collusion, and status differentials.

   b. Membership on the committee should reflect contribution to the hospital's mission, but it should also offer broad opportunity to reward successful managers. High turnover of individuals is desirable, even if the representation of various groups is kept constant.

   c. Discussion and debate should be focused upon the criterion of optimizing the hospital's exchange relationships.

4. Second review by an executive-level committee with representation weighted to clinical systems should integrate the rankings of the initial committees. The board planning committee may accept the initial rankings as advisory and may refer back for reconsideration. In rare cases, it may revise the original rankings, but it should do this only with written explanation.

5. Final recommendation for acceptance should be taken from the combined ranking by the finance committee. Disagreement between the finance committee and the second review may be referred to the full board in rare cases. Theoretically, any

proposal with a positive cash flow at the hurdle rate should be accepted. However, the intangible nature of the return of many hospital projects makes this only a general guideline.

6. Acceptance by the board is normally at the time of adoption of the operating budget. Contingent acceptance is possible and often desirable. Thus a proposal may be accepted if cash flows at midyear reach a specified level, or if demand for certain services exceeds expectations.

Monitoring Performance Against Expectation

A system that emphasizes budgets and expectations reduces the importance of routine reporting. Monitoring is always required, but in the ideal case it is used only to set the next expectation and distribute rewards. Realistically, there are several areas where attention to system design will improve results. These include emphasizing exceptions in report design, seeking success rather than failure, and using tangible rewards flexibly and carefully.

Emphasizing Exceptions in Report Design. Monitoring emphasizes the rare exception so it can be studied and corrected. For each resource or revenue item budgeted there is a difference between expectation and actual performance, both for the current period and for the cumulation of periods since the start of the budget. Reporting under flexible budgeting takes full advantage of cheap computing capability. For each variable resource there are potentially three exceptions: difference in wage or price, difference in demand, and difference in the quantities of resources consumed per unit of demand.

Several thousand expectations can be generated and reported each month, with similar numbers of actual values. Some hospitals swamp their management with a comprehensive report containing all these numbers. Well-run hospitals use computer programs to reduce this flood of information automatically; that is:

— *Actual values and expectations are suppressed or placed in an appendix.* These statistics are useful only in tracking serious departures from expectations and in setting future budgets. They are available when needed for those purposes.

— *Trivial variations from expectations are suppressed; substantive ones are highlighted.* Usually, the threshold for suppression or highlighting differs with the level of reporting. For example:

• Individual resource variations may be reported to RCMs, but only totals are reported to supercontrollers.

- Current values may be reported to RCMs, cumulative values to supercontrollers.
- A lower suppression threshold than that used for supercontrollers may be used to report to RCMs.

— *Care is taken to highlight items for which one is more directly accountable.* For example, the RCM is usually accountable only for the quantities of resources consumed. Price and demand variation should also be reported, but in a subordinate position.

By following these guidelines, one can summarize performance in a few words or numbers, unless a significant departure from expectations has occurred. Information processing and report design can condense any controller's report, even the CEO's and the finance committee's, into a few lines or a page indicating the degree to which expectations were exceeded and specifying significant or recurring failures.

Seeking Success Rather than Failure. The key to easing the tensions arising from routine monitoring of the budget is to establish achievement as the rule and failure as a rare exception. The emphasis of the well-managed hospital is on improvement, not correction, of performance. The effort properly goes to setting next year's expectation, not achieving this one's. One would normally expect to see many RCs exceed their standards as the year advanced and incorporate their successes into the next year's standard. The proper role of the supercontroller is to encourage this improvement and incorporate it into the next budget; the supercontroller who spends most of his or her time tracking failures in current performance has been diverted from this job.

A second important principle is to give the manager of the failing unit at least one reporting period to correct the problem. If the supercontroller enters too quickly, the manager's role is usurped. The supercontroller finds herself or himself trapped in the management of the unit, a situation that is destructive of overall responsibilities. The strategy of delayed entry also avoids involvement with the random, nonrecurring problem.

Using Tangible Rewards Flexibly and Carefully. It appears to be best to use considerable judgment and flexibility in the reward structure. Although some hospitals have experimented with formal incentive programs based on achievement of expectations for cost and efficiency, it is not clear that these hospitals have excelled. A merit increase established retrospectively, but known to be based upon achievement of expectations, may be superior to a bonus arranged prospectively, with fixed compensation for specified achievements. The added flexibility should be used to

— Reward both achievement and expectation setting, so that, for example, failure against an ambitious goal is identified separately from achievement of an inadequate one

— Recognize the achievement of the organization as a whole

— Recognize collaboration and cooperation with other units when it results in overall achievements more valuable to the hospital than improved performance by the unit alone

— Consider the extent to which the manager successfully compensated for the impact of elements beyond his or her control

— Incorporate important elements that must be judged subjectively, such as the various dimensions of quality of care

Notes

1. See the suggested readings, especially Berman and Weeks, for discussion of the operation of the finance system, and various citations therein for standards and regulations.

2. Howard J. Berman and Lewis E. Weeks, *The Financial Management of Hospitals,* 6th ed. (Ann Arbor, MI: Health Administration Press, 1986), pp. 417–598.

3. R. J. Swieringa and R. H. Moncur, *Some Effects of Participative Budgeting on Managerial Behavior* (New York: National Association of Accountants, 1975).

4. J. D. Suver, W. F. Jessee, and W. N. Zelman, "Financial Management and DRGs," *Hospital & Health Services Administration* 31 (January-February 1986): 75–85; S. A. Finkler, "Flexible Budget Variance Analysis Extended to Patient Acuity and DRGs," *Health Care Management Review* 10, no.4 (1985): 21–34.

5. G. L. Stanley, *Hospital Safety and Disaster Policy and Procedure Manual* (Manon, IL: Hospital Physician & Consulting Service, 1977).

6. J. S. Coyne, "Measuring Hospital Performance in Multi-institutional Organizations Using Financial Ratios," *Health Care Management Review* 10, no. 4 (1985): 35–55.

7. Berman and Weeks, *Financial Management*, pp. 71–72.

8. American Institute of Certified Public Accountants, *Code of Ethics,* article 101.

9. W. M. Hancock, S. Pollack, and N. K. Kim, "A Model To Determine Staff Levels, Costs, and Productivity of Hospital Use," *Journal of Medical Systems,* forthcoming.

10. Swieringa and Moncur, *Some Effects.*

Suggested Readings

Berman, H. J., and Weeks, L. E. *The Financial Management of Hospitals,* 6th ed. Ann Arbor, MI: Health Administration Press, 1986.
Swieringa, R. J., and Moncur, R. H. *Some Effects of Participative Budgeting on Managerial Behavior.* New York: National Association of Accountants, 1975.

9

Hospital Information Services

Electronic data processing is an intellectual advance comparable to the use of steam in manufacturing: both were not only major changes in themselves, they set the stage for unforeseeable developments in the future. The effects of the steam engine went far beyond immediate increases in industrial output: they included the ability to transfer more work from human beings to machines, to locate plants close to markets rather than power sources, and a great many other changes, desirable and undesirable, contributing to the Industrial Revolution. Computers may or may not have as extensive an impact, but it is already clear that their implications reach beyond the obvious. Underestimating their potential effect is as dangerous as underestimating the difficulties that accompany installation of them.

Electronic technology can be viewed as having three broad phases: capture, analysis, and heuristics (in which the machines and the human operators, or in some cases just the machines themselves, revise operations). The first phase simply replaces human clerical activity with machines, which are faster and more accurate. Systems are not otherwise changed. No new historic files are created, and no new analysis of potential achievement is involved. Such a transition occurred in hospital business offices beginning about 1965. Complicated processes for calculating patient bills and payroll were replaced by simpler electronic systems.

The second phase creates automated information systems. In the second phase, use is made of the capability of electronic systems to store and retrieve very large amounts of information quickly via dimensions other than the one for which the systems were originally intended. (That is, patients' bills can be retrieved not just for individual, named patients, but for groups of unnamed patients, such as "all inpatients discharged in February.") This allows people to study performance and to set reliable expectations. The data first used to prepare bills and paychecks can now be analyzed for trends, variations among groups, and implications for efficiency. Hospitals began to enter the second phase about 1975. The first steps simply integrated various files into the general ledger and routine financial reports.

The technology used in the second phase defines the hospital's information system and implements the open and closed systems of hospital management. Simply put, the concepts on which this book is founded require quantitative expectations for substantial shares of hospital activity, particularly the clinical system. Through electronic analysis of large volumes of data, the information system supports the negotiation of expectations and the monitoring of achievement for the clinical system. In so doing, it permits the use of formal relationships to strengthen the collegial ones in clinical activities and greatly enhances the hospital as a bureaucratic organization.

The third phase, in which electronic systems are used to assist in patient care and in managing hospital services, has only begun. In the future, doctors will turn to the computer for the clinical histories of their patients and optimal suggested treatments, and nurses will look to the computer to give them detailed work schedules and to suggest areas in which human attention is most needed. Using its own analytic capability, the computer will not only suggest what to do next, but also get better over time. (That is, given a new patient with heart disease, the computer will suggest to the doctor which treatments have proven most effective for similar patients and to the nurse that there will be a certain number of heart disease patients requiring a specified list of treatments and activities.) It will use routinely the techniques of statistical analysis now used only for research and special studies.

By the middle of the twenty-first century, the doctor will guide an electronic system which suggests a plan of care for each patient based on analysis of both the patient's history and detailed data about specific treatment options. Forecasts of all patients' needs will be available to each patient service unit. Systems will optimize schedules, order supplies, and prompt completion of the original assignment and follow-up of any unexpected occurrence. Complete records will be available to establish expectations and monitor performance for the doctor and the nurse, as well as for every other hospital group and service; the vast data files available will permit great precision in judging the success of both future and past efforts. Everyday care will be routinely supported by electronics and scientific analysis more rigorous than that applied to the most intensive care today.

The changes set in motion will generate resistance. Just as steam power can be said to have contributed to Marxism and trade unionism, information systems will stimulate controversial responses. Two hundred years after the introduction of the computer, about 2150, there will still be some longing for "the medicine of the good old days," and real virtues will be identifiable to support it just as many people now long for and respect the individual craftsmanship of the eighteenth century.

If this vision is correct, hospitals are only now entering the second phase of the application of electronic data processing, and information services are in their infancy. Yet the combination of exchange pressures from technology and from interest in economical health care suggests that a generation of hospital managers will focus on information services. Three observations are helpful in understanding such a profound development: it will take many decades, it will be accompanied by much turmoil, and the improvements in outcome will be spasmodic, gradual, and occasionally negative. Management will have a dual role as development proceeds. First, it must guide organizations through the turmoil as efficiently and humanely as possible. Second, it should influence the result toward the needs of patients and customers in the long run, because that will ensure superior care and because it is through meeting those needs that hospitals will thrive.

To manage the change humanely and effectively, the well-managed hospital will rely upon an information services plan covering several years of new implementations and integrated with the general long-range plan and the long-range financial plan. The hospital that plans optimally will have a competitive system at all times, with a minimum of lost time in installation. The plan will specify the systems to be installed, the order in which they are to be installed, and the processes to be followed in implementation. In the context of process, the plan must address timing, criteria and methods for selecting components, methods of coordinating and integrating diverse groups and systems, ways of meeting users' needs for training and support, and incentives for acceptance, mastery, and exploitation of the new technology.

In this chapter, however, I address more immediate concerns:

— Purposes and definition of automated information systems

— Current and future functions performed by information services

— Factors guiding the development of information services

— Closed system measures for operations of information services, and ways to establish expectations and assess performance against these

— Ways of addressing three management issues in information services, namely, decentralizing equipment, assigning accountability, and using outside contractors

Purpose, Definition, and Theory of Information Systems

The purpose of information systems is to support improved control, that is, improved ability to achieve expectations. Information systems contribute to improved control in three different but related ways.

1. They improve the accuracy and speed with which transactions between major units and systems are recorded and communicated (the capture phase).
2. They provide current performance data which can be compared against expectations (the opening of the analysis phase).
3. They provide access to large data files for improvement of expectations through a more complete understanding of casual relationships (continuation of the analysis phase, which develops into the heuristic phase).

Information systems should include both capture and analysis. This book uses the following definition:

An information system is an automated process of capture, transmission and recording of information important to management; once recorded, this information is permanently accessible and can be analyzed from many aspects.

Thus, not every computer application in the hospital is an information system, but all information systems contain performance-monitoring information that is important to management. The definition also stops short of requiring the heuristic phase, although all heuristic systems will qualify. As of 1987, most hospitals have several information systems.

Information systems must be integrated if they are to provide maximum benefit to management. Much of the following discussion will deal with integrated information systems, defined as follows:

An integrated information system is a set of two or more information systems organized to provide immediate electronic access to information in each.

An example of an integrated system would be one containing both medical records and patient accounting. Very few hospitals have integrated information systems. Integration will occur over several stages of increasing sophistication in accuracy and detail. The result will permit analysis and heuristics of many of the closed system dimensions: demand, output, revenue, and costs. As of 1987, few hospitals had significant integration of systems outside the area of accounting and financial management. Integration and heuristics are the frontier of data management in the well-managed 1980s hospital.

Evolution of Hospital Information Services

The Value of Information

One distinction between well-run and poorly run hospitals is that well-run hospitals enter the evolutionary process sooner, and progress through it more smoothly. This is at least as true in information services as in any other area—perhaps more so, because the information itself is a powerful and potentially disruptive stimulus. The well-managed hospital makes more progress because it is organized to handle both the information and the debate which arises from it. Progress stems from the debate as new levels of control are identified and achieved. Improved control is supported by four complementary theories.

Four Important Theories of Control. When the electronic capability emerged, four major theories of control were available, from accounting, medicine, manufacturing, and human behavior in organizations. Each is relevant to the design of hospital information systems.

Cost accounting and managerial accounting were particularly applicable to resource control issues. Cost accounting dwelled upon the importance of precise identification of both resource and use, and it achieved its precision by improved nominal scaling, identifying more homogeneous units of activity. The theory of control used in managerial accounting assumed that expectations could be set in a budgeting process and that the variance from expectations could be traced to changes in price, volume, or performance of the line manager.[1]

Medical auditing was a similar, but less well developed, theory which assumed that expectations could be set for clinical performance. Certain diagnostic and treatment steps follow from certain present conditions. Quality can be assessed, in part, by conformity with those steps, or at least by thoughtful consideration and rejection of them. Early efforts to implement this notion were hampered by lack of reliable classification of conditions, that is, lack of satisfactory nominal scales. It soon became clear that, although the concept could be correct, computer assistance was required to track classes refined enough to be homogeneous among patients.[2] The DRGs of the 1980s were originally conceived of as homogeneous treatment groups.[3]

Statistical quality control arose in manufacturing processes. It allowed judgments to be made about the quality of a batch or a production process by sampling procedures, which reduced the cost substantially. Reliability requires strict adherence to sampling protocols, which are designed to ensure that each member of a defined set has an equal chance of being sampled. For repetitive operations or similar situations, the sample can be a very small fraction of the set and still be reliable. These techniques are used by hospitals in inspections and surveys. For example, nursing care plans or patient accounts can be sampled and inspected for completeness and accuracy; overall level of performance can then be measured, and potentially correctable areas can be defined. Similarly, surveys can be taken of samples of patients, community members, and hospital members to evaluate their overall satisfaction and areas of dissatisfaction.[4]

Human relations theories state that attention to objectives, participation, and incentives are as important as the reliability of classification and reporting in achieving control.[5] In fact, it is clear from theory and from practice that in some situations very precise control can be achieved without quantitative reporting. But objectives, participation, and incentives depend upon building groups of individuals who internalize a homogeneous set of values. This is difficult to do for large, diverse organizations. Quantitative measures and theories of performance such as managerial accounting and medical auditing can be used in controlling the organization as long as the importance of clear and relevant objectives, of negotiating expectations from these in a genuinely participative manner, of systematic feedback using reliable measures, and of appropriate tangible and intangible incentives are all clearly understood. Computers can be used to support negotiation of expectations, prompt and reliable feedback, and a record on which to base rewards. They can also be used to build larger numbers of work groups, thereby keeping each group more homogeneous.

Importance of Homogeneous Measures. All four of these theories assume that reliability will come from homogeneity, that is, that like activities and patients can be identified. In a conceptual sense, all use nominal scaling as the means to identify homogeneous groups or sets and then calculate values for more sophisticated scales, which form the basis of their management expectations. Patients, however, are notoriously diverse. Doctors and hospitals deliberately tailor activities to that diversity. Data systems therefore must deal with numerous segments of the total activity in order to achieve homogeneity. Thus, while "labor cost" is an unreliably heterogeneous measure, "intensive coronary care registered nurse–hours per patient-day" is a component that might be homogeneous among hospitals or in one hospital over time.

Similarly, "care requirements of patients with heart disease" is unpromising; "nursing care required within 48 hours of severe myocardial infarction" may be homogeneous. If it is not, the search for homogeneity will probably involve two further specifications, for age and for concurrent disease.

The magnitude of the information problem becomes apparent when one realizes that the implication of specifying homogeneous sets of information is to multiply data rather than to add them, and that a community hospital has about 10 major kinds of services for 100 major kinds of ailments. Five expectations each (say, volume, quality, cost, efficiency, and profit) amounts to 5,000 expectations ($5 \times 10 \times 100$) and an equal number of measures. The management process leads to specifying some subset of these more precisely in order to improve reliability. The number of data elements inevitably grows in response to efforts to improve. The capability of the modern information system is essential because it permits this additional specificity.

Duality of Hospital Systems. The reality of hospitals is that one group of professionals—attending doctors and nurses—focuses on patients' individual needs organized around diseases, while another group—the clinical support services—focuses on responses organized around specific tests or treatments. Both groups are supported by extensive scientific knowledge, professional protocols and certifications. Patient care calls for the effective integration of both systems. To do this, the information service and the rest of the hospital organization must first support each group. From an information services perspective, this creates dual reporting structures. Information summarizing patient care must be reportable for patients grouped by disease, nursing specialty, or physician, across all services those patients received: laboratory, X-ray, surgery, and so forth. It must also be reportable around the service given, grouping the activities of each nursing unit or clinical support service across all patients, diseases, and clinical departments.

It is common to label the first focus, around similar patients, as final product, clinical, or patient grouping; and the second as intermediate product, departmental, or responsibility center grouping. While the labeling is confusing, the concept must be recognized and understood. There is no known good way of running a hospital that does not adapt the information service to this duality of activity.

Technological Developments

Computer capability has reached the threshold of utility for hospital information services in only about 35 years. Each new generation of data-processing hardware and software has provided 100 or 1,000 times the power of its predecessor for the same cost, and at least one more such startling advancement appears likely within the decade. Univac, the first commercial computer, circa 1945, was the only one of its kind, filled a large room, and was programmed by manually connecting wires. Forty years later, the same capability was available in a box, tens of thousands were being sold each month, and programming was usually accomplished by purchasing software from commercial vendors.

Evolution of Hardware and Software. *Mainframe computers,* developed in the early 1960s, offered the capability to handle patient accounting and payroll. These machines were physically large, required closely controlled temperature and humidity, and were programmed in efficient but incomprehensibly cryptic languages. As they developed, the machines became larger, cheaper, faster, and easier to maintain. Special environmental requirements were reduced. Mainframes could store and process much larger files of data and could support several simultaneous remote users. These advances supported the development of specific programming for hospitals, shared services, and the growth of companies serving hospitals with software and data-processing facility management.

The technological gain generates two kinds of cost savings. More computing power can be purchased for each hardware dollar, but the expanded capacity encourages centralized software development and support. Centralizing software development for widespread application is both cheaper and more convenient. Software developers intent on selling the expanded and inexpensive capacity soon developed the concept of *user friendly* software, that is, methods of presenting the necessary decisions and actions in terms comfortable for nontechnical users. This development permitted direct use of the computer by doctors, nurses, and other persons not highly trained in it.

The advent of transistorized chips in about 1980 made smaller computers effective and created a new technological balance. The freestanding, or totally decentralized, application became feasible with the newer hardware, represented by refrigerator-sized *mini's* and the personal computer, or *PC*. Minis and PCs are smaller, are cheaper, need less attention, and use standardized, user friendly programs. These advantages promote flexibility and decentralization. As software becomes more sophisticated, the cost of developing it quickly moves beyond the reach of the individual hospital. Commercial companies now develop and market most of the useful software in hospitals. This process steadily expands the number of direct users and the software at their disposal.

The need for integrating information systems has kept the central hospital information service, usually a relatively large mainframe computer from becoming obsolete. Small hospitals frequently meet their central computing requirements by sharing remote facilities. Very small hospitals can use self-contained mini-computers. Large ones commonly own an on-site mainframe.

Applications. By a wide margin, most computer applications before 1983 involved accounting.[6] Computerized accounting functions in hospitals had progressed to the beginnings of heuristic capability, with sophisticated *data retrieval* and *interactive modeling* in areas such as pricing, budgeting, and income recovery from third-party contracts. All well-run hospitals had the following systems; the best had data base–oriented oriented accounting systems and were working on the problem of integrating data bases:

— Patient accounting for inpatients and outpatients

— Payroll, payroll cost reporting, and employee benefit recording

— Supply ordering, inventorying, and accounts payable

— General ledger and general financial accounting

— Cost reporting for third-party payers and revenue adjustments

— Budget preparation and direct cost reporting

Efforts to automate medical records abstracting, medical order entry, laboratory and X-ray applications, nurse scheduling, and patient scheduling had been successful in leading hospitals by the mid 1980s, but the two most successful nonaccounting applications appear to have been order capture and laboratory operations. A reasonably comprehensive clinical system involving *order entry* was demonstrated in the 1970s at El Camino Hospital, in Burlingame, California.[7] It was expensive and not entirely trouble-free. Sales of it and similar systems were slow even as late as 1987. Much greater market success occurred with the more limited system of *order communications.* The distinction between the two relates to whether the doctor or nurse enters the order directly on the computer (order entry) or writes it for later entry by a clerk (order communication). The difference is about a fourfold increase in the cost of the hardware and software to support the system. Several brands of order communications systems were marketed, and by 1985 nearly 1,000 had been sold.[8]

Several aspects of hospital clinical laboratories encouraged automation. Rapidly growing demand supported innovations. Testing itself used analog electronic equipment which provided easy translation to digital signals for control systems. Pathologists, who run clinical laboratories, are among the most quantitatively and statistically oriented medical specialists. As a result, a large number of systems was installed, or, more accurately, developed by laboratory personnel in larger hospitals.[9]

Functions

Information services are emerging in hospitals as a result of three major changes in exchange expectations:

1. Technology of medical care itself is becoming more extensive, more powerful, more dangerous, and more costly, thus requiring more precise control.
2. Technology of information systems is becoming more powerful, permitting improved control at lower cost.
3. External economic pressures, illustrated most clearly in the competitive approaches to health care finance, encourage improvement in the cost-effectiveness of hospital and medical care.

Well-managed hospitals are responding to these changes with a steady increase in automated systems. Managers of hospital information services are accountable for four functions. (In practice, most information services personnel are employed in the second function, which involves day-to-day information processing:

1. Maintaining the information services plan
2. Integrating information capture, communication, and routine concurrent processing
3. Providing archival computer support for recurring management decisions
4. Analyzing historic and comparative information for forecasting and expectation setting

Maintaining the Information Services Plan

There is every reason to think hospital information systems will continue to develop rapidly. Maximizing the benefits of these developments requires coordination with other programmatic developments, integration of automated systems, identification of the most valuable systems, plans for the recovery of costs, and careful timing. Well-managed hospitals rely on an information services plan and a procedure for developing and evaluating new applications. The plan is part of the hospital's long-range plan, and its implementation is through the capital and new programs budget.

As is the case with the programmatic portion of the long-range plan, the information services plan consists of a set of carefully selected and organized proposals. Figure 9.1 lists 10 steps in improving an information system. The basic process parallels that used in general invest-

Figure 9.1

Ten Steps to Information System Improvement

1. **Identification**—identifying desired system improvements from survey of current capabilities and exchange needs. Changes should be expected to yield improved control: better mean or smaller variance on a measure of demand, output, quality, efficiency, resource consumption, or resource conservation.
2. **Justification**—demonstrating the feasibility of the prosposal, quantifying anticipated control capabilities. It is preferable to state an expectation for change in each mean or variance and a probability of achieving it.
3. **Valuation**—determining the worth of the control improvement to the hospital, even though this is often difficult to set precisely. The sum of these values, discounted by probabilities of achievement, is the maximum total price that should be paid for the improvement.
4. **Specification**—identifying and describing available products within the price limit. Products must be evaluated on compatability, expansibility, and maintenance.
5. **Vendor Selection**—selecting the vendor offering the greatest long-term value relative to price for each improvement proposal. This process is complicated by the fact that both valuation and product specification have several dimensions, and all must be accommodated.
6. **Ranking**—ordering the list of several competing improvement opportunities on the basis of price and value.
7. **Selection**—designating the set of improvements to be implemented, incorporating the interactions among projects.
8. **Installation Planning**—developing a sequential plan for installation, with interim achievements at specified dates and, at least for substantial improvements, a PERT chart and critical path analysis.
9. **Installation Supervision**—monitoring progress against plan, revising plan as necessary.
10. **Confirmation**—comparing completed installation and control improvements to justification expectations and maximizing actual achievements. This activity involves both systems and operational considerations. It leads back eventually to Identification of another round of improvements.

ment decisions, described in chapter 8. As in the general case, it is usually wise to cycle through the steps more than once, checking with the key cost-benefit ratio that drives the ranking (step 6) first crudely and then with greater precision.[10] Each of these ten steps is discussed in more depth below.

Although the steps in figure 9.1 can be simplified, it is dangerous to omit them. Well-run hospitals seem to be able to simplify steps 1 to 6 efficiently, to make wise decisions at step 7, and to follow through to step 10, assuring that the operational improvements they desired really occur. It is likely that success feeds itself. Good long-range plans, well-designed organization structures, and effective use of existing systems give the well-run hospital insights into improvements with a minimum of effort. Weaker institutions make inferior choices or belabor the selection process. The weakest fail to follow through, thus getting no benefit from whatever efforts they eventually mount.

Identifying Opportunities for Improvement. The underlying philosophy of information services planning is simple and invariable: an improvement will be selected because it has the potential of bringing about greater operational control over the marketplace, or closed system costs, or quality. The driving force for systems improvement is always operational, whether in the hospital's ability to respond to new exchange opportunities or to improve closed system performance. Improvements should be justified by specific gains in one of these areas.

Improvements can occur only when advances in the external technology permit, but technological advance per se never drives the information services plan. Possible new systems, even on very crude or simplistic levels, should be identified for further study if they hold any reasonable potential for improvement over the existing system. New or expanded information systems are justifiable only when the resulting benefits clearly exceed the costs of implementation and maintenance. There are several general sources of benefit:

— Communication of automated data can eliminate manual capture of the same data at several places.

— Identification and posting errors, losses, and delays are reduced by use of common files, elimination of handwriting, and simultaneous updating.

— A well-constructed capture system can reduce oversights, query conflicting statements, flag expiration dates, and generally assist the forgetful human mind.

— Policy can be applied consistently over much wider domains, among individuals who have no direct contact with one another.

— The speed of electronic processing can facilitate solutions to recurring problems such as staffing and scheduling.

— Collateral records, audits, cross tabulations, and summaries can be obtained more easily, permitting more extensive analysis, improved homogeneity, and more reliable forecasting.

Developing Promising Possibilities. The second and third steps test any proposal with potential benefits for practicality in the context of the total hospital operation (justification) and in terms of economic return (valuation).

Justification should show that the proposal is technically feasible (preferably by reference to an existing successful implementation), consistent with the current services, and consistent with the existing plan. A quantitative estimate should be made of each identifiable improvement on a specific closed or open system expectation. Closed system expectations include demand, output, efficiency, quality, cost, and revenue. Open system parameters are measures of demand, market share, community support, and resource acquisition.

Step 3, valuation, is an effort to measure benefits relative to competing proposals and to the hospital's mission. The philosophy underlying benefit is one of contribution to the owners, usually reflected in the growth of the enterprise.

The first step in valuation is to describe and quantify the anticipated benefits as completely as possible. Cost reduction and revenue increase (in competitive environments) are the clearest and most common methods of valuation for information systems. A third measure, long-term impact on net profit, is the touchstone for for-profit companies. A fourth, useful for not-for-profit hospitals, is long-term increase in market share under competitive conditions. Market share is in itself an important measure of satisfaction to the owners. Bigger share translates into higher volume in the future. This, in turn, also reduces fixed cost per unit. Most proposals should be studied from all four approaches.

A practical approach translates as many benefits to dollars as possible and carries the others as intangibles to be used in step 7.

The time value of benefits should be considered. Benefits often accrue several years after start-up expenditures. Discounting techniques consistent with those used in other planning and budgeting activities translate all dollars into values as of a given time.

Particularly in the not-for-profit setting, care must be taken to assess the full impact of revenue and profit increases. In the absence of market tests under competition, these gains to the hospital may represent increased costs to the hospital's owners, who must pay for care received.

There is always the risk that an anticipated benefit will not occur. It is good practice, therefore, to assign some subjective probability of occurrence to the dollar values forecast. In the most formal approaches, Delphi and similar techniques are used to generate Bayesian probability distributions for varying risks. Formal techniques are rarely necessary. The concept of subjective probability can be used in a much simplified form, such as by estimating the risk in two or three categories, to reach a rough probability distribution. Well-run hospitals understate probabilities of achievement, and the history of systems and applications in hospitals supports their pessimism.

The recommended valuation process reduces the chance of selecting the potential improvement at four different points. Only clearly described, feasible projects are considered, revenue and profit implications are carefully considered, future benefits are discounted, and, finally, all risk probabilities are conservative. This minimizes the risk of a fruitless attempt at improvement. It appears to increase the risk of overlooking some important opportunity, however. Experience dictates the balance selected; truly important opportunities attract such attention that they are not often overlooked, and they are soon translated to dollar benefits. Any hospital with an excess of resources and no pressing opportunities under these strict assumptions is free to loosen them.

Selecting the Best Supplier. Two steps are usually necessary to identify good sources of information software. The first selects the product, the second negotiates price. Step 4, specification, is the determination of one or more acceptable sources or vendors for the system desired. Usually there are several competing vendors, and sometimes there is the possibility of in-house development. In selecting a supplier, six elements recur: effectiveness, comparative features, compatibility, expansibility, maintenance, and price. As in the case of valuation, the six must eventually be compared, despite their disparity.

1. *Effectiveness*—ability of the vendor's system to achieve the desired benefits. The evidence on this point should be as clear and complete as possible. Effective systems are those which have been extensively tested with proven results. All others are experimental, or, if they do not yet exist, developmental. The probability that the specific system will prove effective should be consciously evaluated. For systems already used by several dozen hospitals to achieve the expected benefit, the probability is high. For experimental systems, the probability is low, and for developmental ones, lower. It is likely that far fewer than half the systems, programs, or enhancements promised by developers ever reach fruition.

2. *Comparative features*—differences in features within the broad constraint of effectiveness. Ideally, all important features of the system will have been identified in the justification and valuation steps. If so, any additional features offered by the vendor are by definition unimportant. Unfortunately, the opposite problem, where a feature is part of the valuation but is not offered by all vendors, is more difficult. The hardest case, where each of several different vendors lacks a different feature, is not uncommon. The best solution to this problem is to estimate the

impact of the deficiencies on valuation and use the reduced valuation in further steps. The second best solution is to estimate the cost of correcting the deficiency and add that to the purchase price. The disadvantage of the second solution is that the integrity of the system may be disrupted by the modification, creating problems of effectiveness, compatibility, expansibility, and maintenance.

3. *Compatibility*—ability to *interface* with, or connect to, other hardware or software.

4. *Expansibility*—ability to increase capability by adding incremental units.

5. *Maintenance*—ability to keep the system in operation, which for software means principally the ability to keep it up-to-date.

Steps 3 through 5 present less of a problem than in the past. Compatibility of hardware by different manufacturers is greater than in prior years, and most equipment is now expansible as a direct result of improved compatibility. Reliability of hardware has increased, and maintenance is a less severe problem than in the past. Software, however, has become more elaborate and more powerful in ways that increase the need for maintenance.

6. *Purchase price*—initial purchase, hospital installation costs, and any future expenditure commitments, discounted to present values by the usual techniques. Price will be compared to the value developed in step 3. It is wise to establish value first (including adjustment for missing features) and price last. Many errors have resulted from the temptation to buy underpriced systems which turned out to lack important features, compatibility, expansibility, or effective maintenance.

The availability of relatively inexpensive personal computers has encouraged the use of less stringent specifications. Personal computers are frequently used for departmental information systems. The hardware can be specified so that it is uniformly compatible, reusable, and expansible. Applications software is relatively inexpensive and can be treated as disposable. The less rigorous specifications encourage experimentation and innovation. Still, certain specifications and guidelines are desirable. Well-run hospitals are using rules such as the following:

— Proposals for development of PC systems must have central authorization and must be limited in scope to the developer's area of responsibility.

— Hardware and the software *operating system* must be compatible with other hospital information systems.

— Any applications software interfacing with other systems must be compatible with them.

— Software maintenance is expected to be the responsibility of the developing department. (If the software becomes obsolete, the system will fail, but only the using departments will be affected.)

By the time step 4 is complete, the preferred vendor should be clear. That vendor will be the one with the best ratio of cost to value. At this point, all tangible values and costs will be fully accounted. Negotiation with the vendor is frequently fruitful at this point. As the field becomes more competitive, product and price differentiation will diminish. Vendor selection will rest, appropriately, on very narrow grounds.

Except for limited PC experiments, neither in-house development of new systems nor modification of purchased ones is likely to survive the cost-benefit comparison. Commercial vendors have a growing advantage in their ability to spread development costs over multiple sites. Locally written programs reduce the probability of long-term effectiveness. They are by definition developmental and are often written by people who have never written anything similar before. They present unique maintenance and expansion problems. When the original author is gone, there is usually no one to keep the code from becoming obsolete. The argument for in-house development is the need to follow unique, local customs. These customs may themselves be less than cost-effective. Well-run hospitals avoid buying systems which freeze them into further uniqueness. They recognize that "invented here" probably means worse, not better.

Competitive Selection. Steps 6 and 7 compare the proposal to other proposals, both for information services and for other systems. Only a small percentage of the opportunities considered at step 1 survive steps 6 and 7. The criterion for ranking various systems improvements (step 6) is the ratio of benefit or value determined at step 3 to cost or price determined by the vendor selection at step 5. Although any project offering an attractive ratio of value to price should theoretically be implemented, the ranking tends to support more careful review and encourages implementation of the best project, rather than simply a good one. Well-run hospitals informally rank several reasonable alternatives and include a much shorter list of projects in the annual new programs budget. This gives them broad surveillance of potential opportunities without commitment either to unpromising systems or very costly evaluations.

Step 7, selection, is based upon the ranked list of opportunities and is an investment decision which must be considered in the context of competing uses of hospital capital and other resources. Given that the projects are ranked by cost-benefit ratio, the simplest procedure would be to establish the number of proposals to be accepted. However, the actual selection process is complicated by the interaction of different projects. The ranking may be changed because a certain system improvement is related in some previously unconsidered way to other projects outside the information services arena. There may be resource limits other than cost which restrict selection of useful systems improvements. Installation of systems is disruptive to operations, and it demands highly skilled management; therefore, many hospitals limit the amount of systems work they will allow at any one time.

Installation. The final steps plan, install, and verify actual recovery of benefits for the selected systems. An information service improvement usually affects not only data-processing personnel and existing systems, but also operating personnel, and sometimes operating procedures. The larger and more widespread the impact, the more serious is the need for careful advance planning. Experienced vendors are equipped to develop installation plans quickly, but they must have assistance from knowledgeable local managers.

All systems installations should be charted according to program evaluation review techniques (PERT), with critical path determinations and explicit target dates. Although this may seem excessively formal, the PERT preparation is easier for smaller projects and proportionately as likely to reveal avoidable conflicts and problems. In large projects, the PERT plans should be the focus of widespread discussion among operations management, to make sure all important considerations have been identified in advance. Tasks should be defined in such detail that explicit checkpoints arise frequently, permitting easy monitoring of the installation.

All revision and replacements of basic capture and communications systems should be operated in parallel off-line mode to the systems they replace until acceptable results are achieved. Major expansions or new systems should be installed in test locations, with evaluations conducted for periods appropriate to the extent of the innovation.

Even if they are well planned, major innovations are rarely "on time and under budget." ("under budget" being usually more important). There are three keys to effective installation monitoring, step 9:

1. Prompt recognition of departure from schedule
2. Ability to accept delays without excessive cost

3. Ability to revise the plan continuously through the installation, creating new checkpoints

The last step of installation planning tests the internal effectiveness of the real system, either by parallel operation or by planned test against expectation. Once the system is effective, the line organization can work on achievement of benefit expectations. One advantage to explicit effectiveness review at the end of installation is that it clarifies the accountabilities; the installation team shows it has fulfilled its task, and the line must confirm the existence of the anticipated benefits.[11] It is essential that the anticipated benefits be appropriately incorporated into annual budget expectations and other operational plans and that subsequent performance be monitored to see that they are achieved.

Computer Operations

As automation spreads in hospitals, it is used for more routine and more timely communication. Patient identification, scheduling, medical orders, supplies and meal orders, personal assignments, personal telephone service, bed assignment, and financial authorizations are now computerized. Many must be available around-the-clock with only modest delays. Basic portions of the medical record and the accounting record are computerized and must be processed within a few hours. Errors and delays may be costly or may introduce serious hazards. Expensive mainframe equipment must not only be protected against damage, it should be heavily used in order to lower unit costs. The more elaborate and extensive automation becomes, the more serious the problems introduced by inaccurate data, inefficiency, or interruption of service. Thus an important function of an information service is support of timely, reliable, efficient operations.

Capture of Information. Information should ideally be captured only once for each item. All important information should be audited at entry to ensure accuracy. Once captured, the data should be transmitted where needed by networks. Traditional information capture was on paper forms, which were subject to error and loss. Modern systems use video screens with on-line audits. Networking for multiple users and archiving under modern retrieval systems require rigorous initial formatting.

For any data capture involving information likely to be shared among hospital units, information services should advise on the design and maintenance of audits, capture forms or screen specifications, networking, and retrieval capability. The information services unit has complete responsibility for the management of certain kinds of information, for example:

— *Patient registration and placement record.* Sometimes called the "administration, discharge, and transfer file," this information includes descriptions of present and immediate past patients. These are critical to clinical communication, billing, scheduling, and communication with patients and families.

— *Files of patients' unit record numbers.* Patients are usually assigned a unique, lifetime record number that must be retrieved when the patient returns for care, even after a long absence. A special file accesses not only the patient's name and number, but several confirming attributes, such as date of birth, sex, race, and mother's name.

— *Patient surveys.* Direct querying of patient and family satisfaction is an increasingly important device for marketing and outcomes quality assessment. Patients' attitudes are important elements in the quality of clinical services, particularly nursing and medicine, and also in the quality of plant services, particularly parking and food service. It is believed that positive attitudes can minimize the risk of malpractice suits. To be reliable, surveys must use carefully designed protocols, rigorous sampling routines, and extensive follow-up to reduce nonresponse.

— *Central patient scheduling systems.* Although patient scheduling begins in the individual clinical departments, there are obvious benefits to central coordination. Central scheduling systems are rare at the moment but are likely to develop rapidly.

Role of Traditional Medical Records. The largest and most accurate data system in the hospital outside accounting is in the medical records department, whose activity has often been viewed as part of clinical services. As automation becomes more complete, the role of this department is changing radically:

— Use of terminology, codes, indexes, and standards maintained by the department becomes more widespread. For example:

 • Diagnostic and treatment codes have become essential parts of the third-party charge documents under Medicare and several other contract systems.

 • Patient identification must be enlarged from name, number, and hospital location to include relevant demographic and clinical information for support services. Inpatient and outpatient records must be more closely coordinated as outpatient care encompasses more critical activities.

- Common terminology is required over a wide variety of clinical events and responses.
- The department's role in teaching terminology and codes to users and auditing results to assure uniformity becomes its most critical activity.
- While the paper medical record remains the comprehensive archive and the document that can be transported outside the hospital, its automated abstract becomes the source of information for increasingly numerous and critical decisions.
- As automated files become more accessible, the medical records department must assist in effective use of them. Many barriers to effective use relate to insufficient understanding of definitions, limitations, organization, and interpretation of terminology and codes. Classification of disease and statistical interpretation become the second most critical activity.
- As the paper record becomes a backup document, the role of medical records as manager of the hard copy library drops to third in importance among departmental functions.

The implication of these changes is that the medical records department is a central component of information services; the contribution it makes to the construction, use, and storage of the automated file is analogous to its historic contribution to the paper medical record.

Operation of Mainframe Equipment. Mainframe computers are operated by specially trained persons. Larger machines have a supervisor and a small crew. The machine itself requires periodic service, and both data and programs occasionally must be physically handled as tapes or disks. The tape or disk records contain sensitive, irreplaceable information that must be protected against both misuse and damage. Much mainframe software requires an operator's periodic attention. Small items of software maintenance are also the responsibility of the operators. When extensive order communication or other clinical activities are supported on mainframe equipment, operations are usually around-the-clock. Mainframe computers are also operated continuously to support *batch processing* of major programs such as the daily update of accounts receivable. One of the efficiency considerations is the fraction of time the machine and crew will be occupied. Larger machines perform work faster but are more expensive unless fully utilized.

Hardware and Software Maintenance. All computers, including personal computers and minis, which are *unattended* in their operations, require software that must be supported in several different ways. When it is selected, software must be reviewed for compatibility with the hospital's overall service, and usually it must be modified slightly. In time, changes must be made in local software to accommodate changes in the mainframe, expanding system needs, and changes in external conditions. Software for PCs is frequently purchased from outside vendors, who also contract for maintenance of it. The information service is accountable for the specification and supervision of these contracts.

All computers require occasional scheduled and emergency hardware maintenance. Networks also require periodic attention, both for maintenance and for adjustment to changes in user needs. Although most maintenance is now provided by contract with specially trained and equipped service agencies, the supervision of this work is an important function of the information service.

Supporting Recurrent Management Decisions

Departmental Decision Support Systems. Once data have been captured, initial expectations set, and a pattern of expectation improvement established, it is possible to identify many recurring management decisions that can be made routine and eventually computerized totally. These departmental information systems use recent data. The more advanced systems are designed to undertake elementary modelling, showing the impact of a given set of decisions on measures of departmental performance. They become important tools for planning and budgeting, as well as aids to day-to-day decision making.

Well-managed hospitals now have information systems in many areas, including clinical support services, nursing, human resources, and plant systems. They perform various tasks, but the following elements are frequently present:

— *Personnel scheduling,* work schedules for individual employees which accommodate patient care needs but are also sensitive to employee desires

— *Patient or activity scheduling,* schedules for the performance of specified work (such as housekeeping or routine maintenance) or for the optimal use of physical facilities (such as beds, operating rooms, and X-ray machinery)

— *Recording and process control,* automated tracking of orders and specimens, preparation of reports and records, and word processing

— *Inventory management,* automated reorder, distribution, and accounting for routine supplies

— *Message capability,* software to permit multiple users of departmental systems to communicate with each other and, through networking, with other systems

— *Educational and training programs,* automated prompts on the recommended method or procedure for new personnel or infrequent situations

— *Quality assessment,* Measures of process and outcomes quality obtained by automated sample selection, questionnaire design, and statistical analysis

— *Job assignment and human resources accounting,* provisions for skill profiles of employees and for day-to-day adjustment of actual work to reflect unpredictable variation in demand for personnel

Several examples of these systems are discussed in chapters 12, 13, 14 and 15. The central information service has four functions with regard to software that aid departmental decision making:

1. Provide the necessary historic files for setting internal parameters, samples, and so on

2. Provide current information through networks

3. Monitor analytic techniques and parameter settings

4. Recover permanent or long-term general performance measures

Supporting Analysis of Historic Information

Information captured in the hospital information system today is tomorrow's history. Analysis of historical performance is one of the major ways of setting future expectations. A history of several preceding periods is usually necessary. Because the hospital must be responsive to exchange needs, the expectation-setting process must include external data about exchange partners and competitors as well as its own history. Many demand, cost, and revenue expectations are driven by community factors. For example, population and hospital market share are external measures entered by the planning staff to supplement internal data. Similarly, hospitals require information on the local supply of doctors and employees for the long-range plan and annual recruitment activities. Data on activities of competitors is necessary to establish market share; competitors' information is also important to establish comparative sources of expectations. Again, data over several years are desirable. The well-managed hospital acquires much of the external data in electronic form and enters the balance to build integrated internal and external files covering several years. Carefully developed filing, retrieval, and analysis are required to use these integrated sources effectively.

Goals of Information Retrieval. The volume of information that integrated information systems generate is almost impossible to comprehend. Even with highly efficient coding, the sheer magnitude of the information presents problems of storage and retrieval. Although virtually limitless storage capacity is now available at low cost, the cheaper the storage, the more expensive the retrieval. Many hospital expectations must deal with relatively rare events, occurring at frequencies well below 1 percent. If, for example, the storage were simply a sequential ordering of events by time, many thousands of events would have to be inspected in order to develop a representative history on the one in question. Information retrieval uses established nominal classifications to make the search more efficient. Instead of searching through all events, the search will be through all the relevant categories of events. For example, in seeking an expectation on the care of pregnant women who are diabetic, the obstetrics department need search only the file of pregnant women; it might further simplify the search process by specifying two files, "normal pregnancies" and "complicated pregnancies." Search time would be significantly improved. A hospital with 10,000 patients per year could expect to have approximately 1,000 in the "normal pregnancies" file and only 100 or so in the "complicated pregnancies" file. If the classification and coding are accurate, all the diabetic mothers will be in the file of 100 "complicated pregnancies."

A structured retrieval system using a nominal scale is said to be a **hierarchical data system.** For the same volume of information, it is more expensive than a sequential data system in terms of storage requirements, but it is much cheaper in terms of retrieval requirements.

Hierarchical data systems require the user to judge in advance the likely kind and quantity of information to be used and, therefore, to design in advance an appropriate classification system. Data required to answer frequently asked questions must be easy to retrieve. The most serious design problem arises when the categories are themselves subject to change as the system is used. The retrieval hierarchy is fixed in advance. A seemingly modest change in category (for example, the inclusion of mothers with a family history of diabetes as well as those with an established diagnosis) disables the hierarchical system. If the question (in this case, "Does the patient have a family history of diabetes?") was not captured, the information system is useless. More commonly, the desired question was captured but not used in the hierarchy, so a substantially larger set of cases must be searched. Information retrieval technology is involved in the solution to that problem.

Relational Retrieval Technology. Ability to store information in electronic form advanced rapidly during the 1970s. Parallel advances in retrieval ability occurred in the 1980s. The technology of **data base management** has substantially solved the problem of retrieving previously identified categories. As more data were stored, hierarchical retrieval systems permitted increasing numbers of preset retrieval categories. The state of the art is **relational retrieval,** which allows the establishment of a category retrospectively (assuming, of course, that the necessary information was entered in the first place).

Relational data base management provides a major advance in capability of analyzing historical and comparative information. The concurrent development of *hard disk storage* for personal computers has opened the way for substantial extensions of data analysis. Relational data base management requires prospective formatting of data entry and, often, more precise and detailed codes. Thus a decision must be made to change to relational systems, and historical files must be built from that point forward. It is possible, of course, to reconstruct old files, but that is viable only in special situations. Well-managed hospitals began to move to relational technology in clinical areas under the stimulus of Medicare prospective payment. Relational technology also became available in capital equipment accounting and human resources files. By 1985, it was available for general accounting data.

Relational technology and advanced hierarchical technology with several possible search dimensions permits the low-cost, prompt retrieval of relevant data for expectation setting, planning, and other management purposes. It sets the stage for analysis, display, and understanding of past and comparative performance, and from that the development of improved expectations.

Analytic and Graphic Software. Large quantities of data reveal their secrets through analysis, which must be presented clearly to decision makers. Analysis is performed by statistical software that is capable of summarizing quantitative data, testing hypothesis about it, and analyzing possible causes of variation. Graphic packages permit the prompt generation of colorful displays, which help many people understand the meaning of statistics. Statistical and graphic packages are useful in monitoring cybernetic processes and evaluating alternative expectations.

Supporting Forecasts and Analysis of Future Scenarios. Monitoring actual performance and studying historical and comparative information generally lead to the development of alternative expectations. A central purpose of management in a well-run hospital is to find the optimal set among these numerous alternatives. The optimal set is that which best fits long-term exchange needs, but the needs themselves are ambiguous and changing, and the expectation possibilities are numerous and inter-related, making selection of the best set perhaps the most demanding test of managers' judgment. Well-managed hospitals now assist their governance group by constructing scenarios for major decision alternatives. Computerized scenarios are actually complex models that establish the relationships among various kinds of expectations, producing alternative profiles of likely results.

A common example is a model showing the impact of alternative strategies in medical staff recruitment on volume of patients, market share, and service requirements. Another example is a model showing the impact of starting one service upon demand for others. The results of these two models are frequently used to feed financial models analyzing cost, price, and profitability of proposed services.

Software for modelling several financial activities is well developed and is now available commercially, usually through time sharing. Software for examining alternative pricing decisions and designing future capital debt structures is in widespread use among well-managed institutions. Also emerging is software that addresses marketing-related issues of expansions, acquisitions, and changes in final product profiles.

Although the use of financial and statistical modelling requires much expense and effort, it is rapidly becoming standard practice for all decisions at the strategic level.

Developing a Central Information Services Organization

At present, most hospitals have a strong central information service in the finance system, one largely devoted to financial affairs. They also have a growing variety of hardware and software, performing departmental functions, that is more or less integrated with the financial system. Finally, they face steady expansion of these activities, probably for several decades into the future. This section addresses the organizational issues involved in moving the hospital toward more extensive and more effective reliance on information technology.

Sources of Hospital Data

There are four large streams of data which record the fulfillment of the hospital's major economic exchanges:

1. *Patient medical records*—the orders for work to be done and the results, as well as the record of progress. Automated information capture, in the form of order communication and of re-

sults reporting systems and electronic case abstracts, is proceeding rapidly. The order is the basic document for most charges, and the diagnosis and treatment are used in many reimbursement decisions, making the patient record a major support of revenue accounting.

2. *Revenue accounting*—counting, pricing, billing, and collecting funds for care delivered. Automation is very well developed, and integration with patient records proceeds as these are automated.

3. *Expenditures accounting*—developing costs for all the supplies and services purchased by the hospital. Two component systems, *payroll* and *materials management,* are the most important for control purposes. A third, *general ledger,* provides most other cost data. Automation is extensive. Currently, attention is focused on early and detailed capture of information and improved systems of reporting and retrieval.

4. *Departmental and miscellaneous*—many different sources of data, usually organized around the need of a single department or operations subsystem, such as nursing or planning-marketing. Often these sources are important for quality, resource acquisition, or maintenance (such as employment data in human resources). Sometimes, as in the case of internal audit data or physical inventories, their function is to improve the reliability of one of the three larger streams.

The Future of Hospital Information Services

Near-Term Directions for Expanded Capability. The exchange pressures for hospital efficiency are stimulating rapid development of information services. The intermediate product responsibility centers need flexible budgeting, patient scheduling, employee scheduling, quality criteria and protocols, and concurrent monitoring. The clinical services want increasingly sophisticated analytic machinery to develop their final product expectations. The need for human judgment, and particularly medical judgment, about the information will increase, with the result that ease of access and user-oriented presentation will be required. The data used for control in the clinical services will be used simultaneously by the governance system to decide directions for expansion and contraction of services.

To support these needs, large volumes of information about each patient, each doctor, each clinical service, and each cost center must be integrated. Data systems will capture patient records more completely, integrate file structures, broaden on-line access, and expand retrieval, analysis, and display capabilities. Many of these improvements may be achieved at constant or reduced costs, but the overall expenditure for information services is likely to grow substantially.

Considerable tailoring to the approaches of various professions and departments will be necessary, but several common types of data expansion can be foreseen:

— *Revenue control.* Automated patient registration will become universal and will be the foundation of revenue data, clinical review data, and scheduling systems. Patient revenue accounting will move to more detail on services rendered, more complete tallies of insured and patient-pay portions, and historical tallies by employer or insurance group. Detail on outpatient and long-term care will become increasingly important.

— *Budgeting and accounting control.* Hospitals will identify and report more cost centers than they do now. They will move to flexible budgeting and variance reporting. Reporting of historical and expected future costs on both a fixed and a variable basis will be an essential part of clinical review data.

— *Clinical review.* As order communication systems become more widespread, larger sections of the medical record will be automated. Abstracts of patient care will become larger and more detailed and will be integrated with cost and revenue data. Capture of basic counts of clinical activity will become routine and will be used in concurrent review. More complete information, including costs and quality measures, will be used in retrospective review and criterion setting.

— *Final product cost accounting.* Using both clinical and accounting data, actual costs of care to homogeneous, final product patient groups will be calculated and forecast in terms of alternative levels of demand. Analyses of this kind support decisions on the expansion and contraction of services and form a basis for contracting with health insurance carriers.

— *Risk management.* Order communications systems and departmental systems will automate capture of the **incident report,** basically a notice of an untoward event that raises the possibility of liability. With the integration of departmental systems into a coordinated unit, risk management data from incident reports will increasingly be compiled for both retrospective and concurrent analysis by a central unit.

These expansions of data will be supported by growing expansions of hardware and software:

— Mainframe hardware capacities will grow, permitting enlarged files for data on both cross-sectional and historical dimensions. Integrated, lifetime patient records will become a reality, as will detailed files of closed system measures for intermediate products.

— Personal computers will become smaller and cheaper. Hardware will contain current summaries of data and will permit easy access to mainframe files, as well as conveniently supporting a variety of management functions.

— Software improvements will support nearly instantaneous integration, abstracting, analysis, and display of information for clinical and managerial personnel. Recurring decisions, both clinical and managerial, will be supported by analytic software providing:

- *Statistical control.* Many control functions in a hospital must recognize the inherent uncertainty in medical practice and the variability of human conditions. The correct action depends upon knowing not only the current value of a given measure, but also its distribution and the probabilities associated with that value. This need has long been recognized in places like the clinical laboratory, where formal statistical quality control is a requirement. Needs in management areas such as inventory and staffing have become more clear.

- *Scheduling systems.* The unpredictability of hospital events has discouraged efforts to schedule, but unscheduled events require large, costly reserves of standby resources. Recent work has made it possible to reduce standby requirements substantially by frequent scheduling decisions. Both patient services (beds, operating rooms, and so on) and personnel will be scheduled in order to eliminate delays and idle capacity.

- *Forecasting, marketing, and strategic planning.* Detailed financial planning using computer analysis programs has become routine in hospitals in the past few years. Competitive pressures are likely to extend this analytic approach to other areas, such as new clinical program evaluation, personnel and facility forecasting, resource use analysis, and marketing studies.

Figure 9.2

Development of Hospital Information Systems, 1985–1995

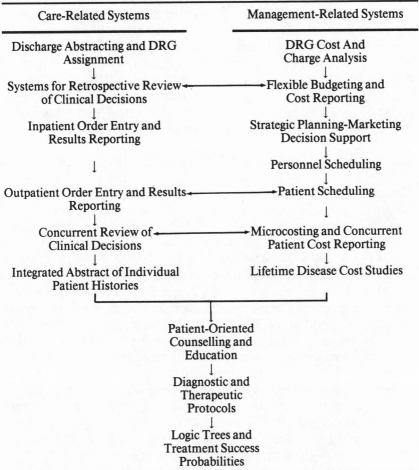

Care-Related Systems	Management-Related Systems

Discharge Abstracting and DRG Assignment ↓
DRG Cost And Charge Analysis ↓

Systems for Retrospective Review ← → Flexible Budgeting and of Clinical Decisions / Cost Reporting ↓

Inpatient Order Entry and Results Reporting
Strategic Planning-Marketing Decision Support ↓

↓
Personnel Scheduling ↓

Outpatient Order Entry and Results ← → Patient Scheduling Reporting ↓

Concurrent Review of ← → Microcosting and Concurrent Clinical Decisions / Patient Cost Reporting ↓

Integrated Abstract of Individual Patient Histories
Lifetime Disease Cost Studies

Patient-Oriented Counselling and Education ↓

Diagnostic and Therapeutic Protocols ↓

Logic Trees and Treatment Success Probabilities

Long-Term Trends. In the longer term, systems will progress as they have recently, in two major streams, clinical and managerial, but with much more emphasis on integration. The benefits sought cannot be achieved without integration. The two general streams are likely to develop in the directions shown in figure 9.2, moving from current issues of information capture, flexible budgeting, and real-time integration to increasingly elaborate systems to aid managers and practitioners at all levels. Systems which assist front-line personnel at their daily tasks will be attractive. This will be equally true whether the front line people be doctors or housekeepers. Designing sophisticated control systems using the data captured in real-time applications is not as difficult as convincing front-line workers to put data in when the data do them no good.

The need for parallel development is clear, because economies do not result from use of the care-related systems alone. Were retrospective review to indicate ways to reduce cost per case, by shortening length of stay, for example, little real savings would occur until budgets were redone to lower occupancies and eliminate personnel from the payroll. There is a similar need for close coordination between patient scheduling and outpatient order entry and between further utilization review improvements and further cost accounting refinements.

Organizational Components of Information Services

The two organizational questions involving information services are, "What are the components or subunits of a coordinated service?" and "To whom does the service report?" Even well-run hospitals differ in their approach to these questions today, and there is clearly neither consensus nor widely available evidence. Of the two questions, the latter is probably less critical. As a result, expediency, personality, or experience weighs heavily, and equally capable hospitals can reach opposite decisions. The issues and opportunities for information services accountability are discussed in the final section of this chapter.

The internal organization of information services is governed by the need for improved control. Sufficient activities and authority must be aggregated to make the information service effective in the context of the hospital's mission. Well-managed hospitals have sought centralization and common direction of input, data processing, and user services to support their steadily increasing use of information. As a result, the activities grouped under information services have been growing. The best hospitals appear to be moving to a structure like that in figure 9.3. The four functions are assigned to about three subsections, and the director is aided in the overall effort by a broadly constituted advisory committee.

Information Services Advisory Committee. A committee of key users of information services is an important adjunct to a well-run department. The committee's purposes include broad representation in the development of systems investment priorities and communication to assure effective systems design and uniform interpretation. On a different level, the committee offers opportunities to increase line participation in important decisions and to encourage acceptance of information systems. The charge to the committee includes:

Figure 9.3

Internal Organization of Information Services

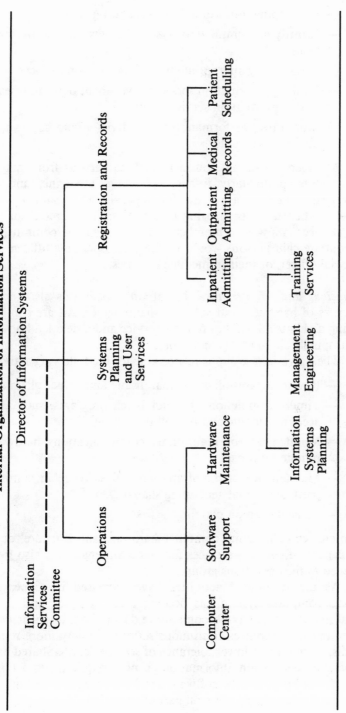

— Developing uniform definitions and typologies

— Identifying central data systems needs and proposing expansions

— Encouraging appropriate use of information services

— Ranking information services investment opportunities, as part of the information services plan

— Monitoring performance of the division and suggesting possible improvements

Membership should routinely include persons from major using departments, particularly finance, planning, medicine, and nursing. Membership can be a reward for supervisory personnel who have shown particular skills in using information. The director of information services is always a member and may chair the committee. Other appropriate chairpersons would be the chief operating officer, the chief financial officer, or their immediate deputies.

Operations and Maintenance. Mainframe operations also include the activities of hardware and software maintenance. All are similar in requiring highly technical but reliable service and a detailed knowledge of the hospital's data-processing history.

The operations group is responsible for the following activities:

— Routine operation of the mainframe and its peripherals

— Timely completion of major batch programs, such as patient accounts update and payroll processing

— Maintenance of mainframe, communications hardware, and remote terminals

— Maintenance of mainframe and all software in common use, particularly that generating shared data

— Consultation on planning issues

Maintenance of personal computer hardware and software, or at least supervision of contract services for that maintenance, is also frequently assigned to the operations group.

As the automated activities have increased in scope, the networked computer system has become more complex and the operational requirements have become more demanding. In particular, order communication requires continuous service of many more remote terminals, with a much lower tolerance of service delays. Shared data such as patient registration information is now required almost instantly through the hospital. The software and hardware for entering it, checking it, and transmitting it are all part of operations.

Operations are often contracted to firms that manage data-processing facilities. The contracting firm is expected to name a senior data-processing manager with technical skills and knowledge comparable to those of a manager the hospital would employ. The on-site manager is supported by the broader experience and specialized knowledge of the contractor's other employees. The skills of this group are often useful in information services planning and systems installation. A role remains for hospital leadership: the advisory committee would remain in place, for example.

Systems Planning and User Services. Well-managed hospitals are now stimulating the spread of computer applications. Clinical applications which improve quality and help reduce final product cost are becoming more reliable and more useful. Applications in the human resources and plant systems are growing. Computer modelling, quality control, and forecasting have become routine in the governance system. There are major benefits to be gained from a positive stance toward this technology, but most departments will need assistance, and the whole must be coordinated in order to realize the benefits. A well-managed information services unit will have people who devote significant parts of their time to applications planning and implementation, helping middle managers use the cycle described in figure 9.1.

Management engineers are frequently helpful in this activity. They are trained not only to evaluate and install computer software, but also to help managers develop work methods that get the greatest benefit from the investment. Many of the existing programs for departmental management arose from engineering studies and operations research. Information systems planning also helps management engineering. Management engineering is often perceived by line managers as an implied criticism or a threat; it is useful to be able to approach methods improvement with the promise of aids to the work offered by the computer.

Training in using information systems is a natural extension of planning and installation, and it is frequently essential to realization of benefits. Training is important both for new installations and for continued operations. Personnel turnover and systems development make ongoing training essential. Although well-designed software packages now contain training routines designed for the novice user, a local source of advice is frequently important. Interfaces between departmental and central processors are frequently a source of confusion, and these are rarely covered in training material from outside the hospital. A good information service orients users to the hospital's system, provides user guides to the interface programs and protocols, gives advice on request, and trains personnel in specific systems when the need emerges.

Registration and Records. Key financial and clinical records are organized around the individual patient. Basic information on name, date of birth, address, marital status, next of kin, sex, and race is used to assign a permanent unit number to each patient. On subsequent visits the same information is used to retrieve the number and the patient's medical history. Basic payment and diagnostic data are also important. This information must be referenced to frequently during both inpatient and outpatient episodes of care. Medical communications are identified by the patient's unit number, and medical records are accumulated using it. Most of the financial record is built from medical communications, using the unit number. It is important that these references be quick, inexpensive, and accurate, making one-time capture of the identification data and subsequent electronic transfer highly desirable.

Registration data are collected by personnel in several sites where patients are received, such as the emergency room, inpatient admitting office, and various clinics. The archives for the identifying information, the unit number, and the medical record are in the medical record department. In addition to managing the archives, the department is expert in the diagnostic and treatment codes used to describe disease and its care. (The International Classification of Diseases is a nominal scaling system which permits the grouping of similar patients for statistical and retrieval purposes. Correct application of it is fundamental to monitoring quality and, since the development of DRG payment systems, to hospital finance.) The medical records department also uses the codes to compile statistics and to retrieve records grouped by clinical condition.

As electronic use of patient registration information becomes more common, a case builds for assigning both collection and archiving —that is, registration and records—to information services. To do this, the existing medical records organization and activities in patient reception areas must be organized under information systems. It is possible to centralize each function separately.

The prominence of the medical records department prior to the development of automation attests to its importance in quality and effectiveness of patient care. The importance and precision demanded of medical records have increased rather than diminished. As noted, much of the access to and generation of medical record information is already automated. It appears inevitable that the medical records department will become an integral part of information services. As retrieval technology becomes more widespread and heuristic use of patient data files becomes more common, the need for combined technical skills in coding, retrieval, statistics, and interpretation will make this a critical component of information services.

The registration and scheduling function for inpatients and outpatients incorporates the initial contacts between patient, attending doctor, and hospital. Unlike medical records, this function is geographically dispersed. The set of financial, legal, and demographic information collected is copied electronically thereafter. The need for this information to be reliable and the close connection to medical records are arguments for assigning the activity to information services.

There are several arguments against locating patient registration in information services. The activity has profound implications for marketing and patient relations, and clinical knowledge is required to do it well. These considerations suggest a clinical locus, perhaps nursing. However, many hospitals have already moved admitting away from clinical supervision. Registration is probably most commonly part of the business office. Information services has a clear advantage as a locus, because it can handle the promotional, interpersonal, and clinical concerns as well as provide the reliability required. The solution now emerging is to allow clinical personnel to make the physical contact with the patient and to support them with a well-designed registration system that reminds them to ask all the necessary questions, edits data for accuracy, and can easily and comfortably be used by people with clinical and human relations skills.

A more compelling reason for the assignment of registration to information services is that the registration function can be extended to patient scheduling. This step, now being taken in the leading hospitals, makes management of patient demand a central part of information services. Patient registration is done as early as possible, using mail and telephone contacts to acquire information from the patient and doctor before arrival. Needed services are then scheduled using a program that at the least maintains the logs of future activity for the clinical units and at best includes a computer algorithm to optimize service and efficiency jointly (see chapters 12 and 13).

Measures of Performance

Criteria for Judging Performance

The test of an information services is in its ability to serve clinical and financial needs. Information services should have closed system expectations for demand, output, and resources established in recognition of open system needs of the hospital as a whole. The measures which quantify the expectations reflect the unique nature of information services. Performance expectations are set as they are elsewhere in the hospital, using a negotiation process centered around the annual budget.

The sources of expectation are also conceptually the same. Prior history and the experience of consultants will be used frequently. As usual, expectations should be set so that they are achieved or exceeded in the vast majority of cases. Monitoring will be important to identify future improvements, to reward the information services committee and information services personnel, and to suggest corrections in the rare cases where expectations are not achieved.

Some Feasible Measures

Figure 9.4 shows available measures for information services following the closed system framework, as applied to a large service with both remote PCs and a central mainframe. Most of these measures are derived from standard cost accounts, the operating logs detailing activities of the computer itself, and activities of the director and the information services committee. Some require special surveys and might therefore be used less frequently.

Ten Essential Measures

Ten measures on figure 9.4 are emphasized in italics. These are the most important measures for a centralized or large shop. They also are relatively easy to obtain and to translate as needed so that they are useful for smaller or decentralized operations. Even a PC dedicated to serving a small clinical unit should be at least subjectively assessed periodically on the emphasized performance measures.

1. *Service delays*—An expectation for satisfactory timeliness should be based upon the need for information rather than the capacity of the system. That is, because slow service can be very serious for the user, the definition of "slow" should be determined in part by the user. *Delay* is defined as a failure to meet the user's expectation. *Peak,* or maximum, processing delays are a more sensitive measure than averages and are therefore often preferable as an indicator of basic capacity and timeliness.

2. *User satisfaction with promptness*—Supplementing the objective measure of peak processing delays, users' satisfaction with promptness should also be obtained by a survey integrated with a survey of quality, as indicated below.

3. *Outside opinion of planning progress*—An outside consultant's opinion is important for keeping up to date on opportunities and safeguarding against isolation.

4. *Timely batch operations*—Recurring and batch mode activities should follow a predictable schedule, since the output quickly becomes an integral part of many persons' workday.

5. *Timely Improvements*—Completion of new projects on time requires an explicit timetable, as indicated in the planning steps. Once implementation expectations are established, the deadlines should be met or the causes of failure promptly understood and corrected.

6. *Batch operating hours as a percentage of expectations*—Since many tasks, or *runs,* of programs must be completed daily or more often, the total elapsed time compared to schedule or expectation is an indirect indicator of efficiency, supplementing direct resource consumption measures.

7. *User satisfaction with quality*—The opinion of the user is an inescapable focus of quality assessment for a service department. Formal surveys are particularly necessary where the operational unit is remote from the information service. See measure 2, user satisfaction with promptness, above. The two surveys should be combined.

8. *Cost of operations and systems planning*—The cost of information services operations should be kept distinct from the cost of information systems planning and development. For larger operations, budgets for supplies, labor, and capital will improve cost control. For smaller applications dedicated to single departments, estimates of supplies and capital costs are usually sufficient.

9. *Cost of improvements*—The cost of improvements, large or small, should be developed as an expectation at the time the project is approved and monitored throughout the project. Repeated failure to meet expectations is symptomatic of planning and development problems.

10. *Confirmation of expected operational gains*—Each approved proposal for improvement carries with it an expectation for the source and amount of benefits. These benefits will only be achieved if deliberate follow-up is the rule and the expectations are incorporated in annual budgets. Achieving the benefits may require the efforts of both services and the line personnel. In any case, a record of achievement should be reported and understood, with rewards for success and sanctions for unacceptable failure.

Figure 9.4

Performance Measures for Information Services

Measures in italic type are a recommended minimum set,
even for small hospital systems

Demand

Operations

Processing delays for on-line service—mean or peak times to respond to terminal requests

Unscheduled downtime—percent of scheduled availability not met

Information errors—number of transactions noted as missing or requiring correction

Programming or service request delays—days to completion of special requests

User evaluation—subjective estimate of satisfaction with operations

Planning

Profile of available services—expectation arises from planning process

Consultant's report—outsider's judgment of effectiveness of planning process and extent of services offered

User evaluation—subjective estimate of satisfaction with planning and development of new services

Outcomes

Output

Operations

Transactions per minute—direct measure of machine activity level

Scheduled program completion—completion of daily runs on time, a measure of effective operation

Planning

Achievement of planning targets—record of specific milestones of new systems implementation, a measure of effective planning

Efficiency

Operations

Entries or accounts processed per hour versus expectation derived from manufacturer's standard and analysis of software—measure of CPU efficiency, reflecting software, operations, and hardware maintenance

Hours for completion of assigned tasks versus expectation—measure of operations efficiency, usually addressed to a combined personnel-computer activity

Scheduled downtime—measure of operations efficiency

Keystrokes or documents processed per hour—measure of labor efficiency

Programmer maintenance hours per month per major software program —measure of software and programmer efficiency

Special requests filled per available hour of programmer time—efficiency of user service group

Planning

Subjective, retrospective measures only—how efficiently a planning goal was achieved, evaluated after the fact by the planning team and, the information services committee, or both

Quality

User satisfaction—surveys to evaluate planning and operations subjectively

Audits—consultants hired to audit operations, planning, and detailed components such as specific software or design criteria   *Continued*

Figure 9.4 Continued

Resources
  Resource consumption
    Operations
      Total cost as percent of total hospital operating budget—global measure
      of resource consumption adjusted for size of operation
      Total cost per year—measure of system resource consumption; expecta-
      tions and achievement studied in components:
        Labor cost—short-term cost control measure
        Supplies cost—short-term cost control measure
        Machine rental and space costs—long-term cost control measure
    Planning
      Systems improvement programmatic budgets—resource commitment to
      ongoing improvement, by topic or anticipated activity
  Resource conservation
    Operations
      There are no direct measures; performance of line operations on revenue,
      cost, and profit may be indirectly attributable to information services.
    Planning
      *Confirmation of expectations on costs revenues and profits for imple-
      mented new services*—measure of effectiveness of information services
      planning

Management Issues

This section addresses three important accountability questions for information services planning and operations:

1. How should the large mainframe relate to decentralized processors?
2. Is finance the correct locus of accountability and organizational
   control for an increasingly universal tool?
3. When is it desirable to use outside contractors for information
   services management?

Centralized versus Decentralized Processing

The critical role of information in controlling the bureaucratic organization makes it a coveted commodity. The need for verifiable data dictates a reliable, unbiased processing source and seems to rule out a
decentralized model, in which each operating system designs its own information support. Yet in practice, many hospitals are becoming less
centralized as small PCs and minicomputers are used in management.

The trend toward decentralization has come about not only because of technological advances in smaller machines, but also because central machines have no free time, require special programming, are designed for a few specialized tasks, or are staffed by people who have neither interest in nor understanding about operational questions. A freestanding machine quite often overcomes all of these weaknesses. On the other hand, it creates an independent, unmonitored set of files which may depart from others in content and format, does not communicate readily to existing machines, causes duplication of data entry, harbors errors, and encourages separatism in setting and achieving expectations.

The management options are to enforce use of the central machine, to permit decentralization, or to encourage networking. The apparent answer is networking, or what might be called *regulated decentralization*. Regulation requires use of common data sets such as the patient identification file and constrains hardware and software to permit practical interfacing. Decentralization allows the individual software to meet needs defined principally by its users rather than by information services. Advocates of centralization note correctly that the technology for effective networking is not firm; yet most hospitals have moved too far on the path to decentralization to return to centralized service, and the technology for comprehensive centralized service is also lacking. It is unlikely that centralization will return easily, because the investment in decentralized hardware and software is large and growing. Even a major advance in large machine capability will not overcome the existence of many PCs and minicomputers. At the same time, however, this means that each proposed improvement must be evaluated for location and integration and must be supported as necessary, whether on the mainframe or at a remote but networked processor.

Locus of Responsibility

Because of the historical emphasis on accounting applications, most of the data-processing activity of hospitals was the responsibility of a subordinate of the chief financial officer. The choice of organizational location was originally justifiable because the computer largely processed finance system information. The implication of the location was to raise the priorities of finance applications, further strengthening the authority of finance over information services.

Managerial use of information systems is determined in large part by the technical environment. Given a commitment to networked decentralization, it remains true that the largest processor, the most software, and the critical files are in the finance department. Well-run hospitals are examining the de facto accountability of the chief financial officer. There are several reasons for moving the information system to governance or explicitly broadening the CFO's charge:

— Clinical applications, particularly providing routine patient management and improved measurement of demand, output, and quality, are the area of greatest need. Control of information by the governance system encourages clinical participation and permits a more rapid redirection of resources toward this need. (The integration of medical and accounting records is an outstanding example.)

— Managerial control requires cooperation among several different hospitals' systems. Clinical expertise must be supported by human resources, finance, and plant services in order to address current and emerging information problems. Evenhandedness and an atmosphere of cooperation are easier to achieve when governance personnel mediate the interaction.

— The importance of data retrieval and archives outside finance is steadily increasing. Quantitative planning, marketing, and environmental analysis has increased in importance. Computer support requires new files and new software directly accessible by planning personnel. Many of the files must be collected on mainframe and networked hardware. This suggests locating the control of information capture in governance.

— Information is too valuable to be allowed out of the immediate control of general management. A bias toward the needs of finance is almost inescapable as long as accountability is to the chief financial officer.

Many well-run hospitals are reassigning accountability for information services to a member of the executive group. Some operations and software maintenance personnel may also report to finance or to clinical units, creating a matrix-like organization. When properly designed, locating information services in the executive allows it to meet its obligations to all users, based upon their ability to translate information to improved performance. The goals of the information group become hospitalwide, and the competing claims of clinical, financial, and governance systems can be more evenhandedly evaluated.

Use of Outside Contractors

Five kinds of assistance from outside contractors are available for information services:

1. *Finance*—Leases and mortgages on hardware are generally available from a variety of outside sources. Software is usually available for purchase or lease from the software vendor. Thus capital for information services is rarely a problem, even though substantial sums are involved.

2. *Consultation and planning*—Assistance in selecting hardware and software, analyzing current capabilities, and developing a plan for improvements' is available from accounting firms and other consultants.

3. *Remote processing (shared services)*—Several large companies do complete data processing on remote computers shared by several hospitals, using standard software and charging a monthly rate plus a volume fee. The hospital thus avoids ownership of the hardware and software as well as extensive planning for improvement, because the company plans changes and offers them for sale.

4. *Facilities management*—Operation of on-site data-processing services under contract is offered by a few companies specializing in hospital's needs. These companies also arrange for financing for the facilities and can be hired for consultation and planning.

5. *Software support*—Computer programs which implement hospital information goals have become increasingly complex, and outside agencies' requirements for data have become more common. These trends make it feasible for commercial companies to develop software that is usable in a great many hospitals. The companies providing the software also maintain it, incorporating changes imposed by outside agencies and technological advances. They sometimes offer customization services as well.

Most hospitals avail themselves of at least the first two levels of assistance. The decision of where to finance capital equipment is quite independent of what is being financed, but the availability of special options and alternatives for computer hardware adds to the supply of funds and thus helps lower the cost of financing generally. Sometimes companies seeking to sell information-processing equipment or services will use their financing capability to make the purchase attractive in itself, by purchasing accounts receivable or addressing broader financing questions.

In a complex, rapidly moving technical field, the use of a consultant is often prudent. Few, if any, hospitals have the expertise to forecast developments in hardware, software, and applications. Consultants can assist with the first eight steps in figure 9.1. They can be particularly helpful in the earliest steps. Both management consulting firms and public accounting firms offer consulting services, as do the firms providing direct information services. There are advantages to each type of company, but the key criterion should be a record of successfully identifying rewarding applications, whether they are in the finance, clinical, or some other system of the hospital.

Consultants who provide remote processing or facilities management are probably biased toward their own services and products, but those who do not provide services themselves may lack detailed practical experience. Much of the advice provided by accounting firms and other consultants without operational experience is more useful in planning system improvements than in installing and operating them. Development of criteria increasingly requires clinical as well as financial expertise. Not all consultants have clinical expertise.

Shared services tend to be selected by smaller hospitals. Relatively complete financial accounting applications are available at an attractively low price. Flexibility is quite limited, and there is little customizing. Improvements must be selected from among the offerings of the company.

Contract facilities management has appealed to the largest hospitals. Employees of the contracting company, rather than the hospital's own employees, manage the information services capability, or some part of it. Contract management is more expensive than remote processing, but it offers much more flexibility for the same price as inhouse operation. The contract company generally has a large inventory of available software and is willing to develop individual programs using this inventory to lower cost.

Both shared services and contract management offer maintenance of hardware and software, training for replacement personnel, and a library of software relevant to hospitals. These assets are quite valuable; skilled programmers are expensive and difficult to recruit. In addition, the companies have substantial experience in hardware planning and upgrades. Unsophisticated hospitals tend to underrate the value of experience, but for any kind of major system, the second installation is usually only half as difficult as the first. Hospitals using either contract management or remote processing thus have the advantage of experience, both in their general information service planning and in installing system improvements. It is the value of experience that allows such firms to be competitive with in-house operations.

The evolution of improvements in information services under the two outside forms is quite different. Shared services offers few choices to the hospital, protecting it against unwise investment but offering little help in selecting desirable improvements, even from its own list of products. Contract management, on the other hand, has no incentive to limit the hospital's choices and usually will profit from an excessive program for improvement. Thus, even with a facilities management contract, hospital governance has the responsibility and the opportunity to select improvements anu pace the evolution of the information system.

Some well-run hospitals hire both service and consulting firms. Although the cost is high, the test of the result is in improved operations. If the information services committee can incorporate the full set of information, balance the competing viewpoints, and devise a more effective program, the cost is justified.

Outside software support is increasingly common and no longer debatable. A large number of software companies now provides packaged software for almost every feasible application. Although many hardware and operating system configurations are served, those supported by IBM have by far the largest amount of software available. Software manufacturers have grown in size. Successful companies now offer integrated packages for a broad spectrum of applications. These packages will grow in sophistication and drop in price over the next several years. The day of the hospital's writing its own software from scratch is practically over.

Notes

1. R. Anthony and J. Reece, *Managerial Accounting,* 2d ed. (Homewood, IL: Irwin, 1975).

2. M. T. MacEachern, *Hospital Organization and Management,* 3d ed. (Chicago: Physicians Record Co., 1957), p. 243; P. A. Lembcke, "Evolution of the Medical Audit," *Journal of the American Medical Association* 199 (1967): 543–50.

3. Robert B. Fetter, et al. "Case Mix Definition by Diagnosis-Related Groups." *Medical Care* 18 (1980 suppl.): 1–53.

4. John R. Griffith, *Quantitative Techniques for Hospital Planning and Control* (Lexington, MA: Health-Lexington Books, 1972), pp. 209–44.

5. D. Katz and R. L. Kahn, *The Social Psychology of Organizations* (New York: Wiley, 1966).

6. Charles J. Austin, *Information Systems for Hospital Administration,* 2d ed. (Ann Arbor, MI: Health Administration Press, 1983), pp. 41–64.

7. Rosanna M. Coffey, *How a Medical Information System Affects Hospital Costs: The El Camino Hospital Experience* (Washington, DC: U.S. Department of Health, Education, and Welfare, DHEW publ. no. (PHS) 80-3265, 1980).

8. HBO and Company, *Annual Report* (Atlanta: HBO, 1986) and other vendor information.

9. T. D. Kinney and R. S. Melville, eds., *Mechanization, Automation, and Increased Effectiveness of the Clinical Laboratory* (Bethesda, MD: U.S. Department of Health, Education, and Welfare, 1976).

10. Compare Center for Health Management Research, Lutheran Hospital Society of Southern California, *Automated Hospitals Information Systems: How To Decide What You Want* (Chicago: Pluribus Press, 1984).

11. *Automated Hospital Information Systems: Getting the Most from the System* (Chicago: Pluribus Press, 1984).

Suggested Readings

Allen, Brandt. "Make Information Services Pay Its Way." *Harvard Business Review* 65 (January-February 1987): 57–63.

Austin, C. J. *Information Systems for Hospital Administration,* 2d ed. Ann Arbor, MI: Health Administration Press, 1983.

Austin, C. J., and Harvey, W. J. "Hospital Information Systems: A Management Perspective." *Frontiers of Health Services Management* 2 (November 1985): 3–36.

Buss, M. D. J. "How To Rank Computer Projects." *Harvard Business Review* (January-February 1983): 118–125.

Institute of Electrical and Electronics Engineers. *Proceedings, Annual Symposium on Computer Applications in Medical Care.* Silver Spring, MD: Computer Society Press, 1977 and subsequent years.

Skurka, M. *Organization of Medical Records Departments in Hospitals.* Chicago: American Hospital Association, 1985.

The Clinical System

Introduction to Part III

Providing health care is the central function and distinguishing purpose of the community hospital. The core system of the enterprise, and the one which distinguishes it from almost all other human endeavors, is, therefore, the people and activities involved in the delivery of care. The clinical system of a hospital determines how good it is in both an abstract and a pragmatic, marketing sense, because it determines attractiveness, cost, and quality of all the hospital's important products. The committed clinical resources are an important limitation on what the hospital can attempt. To do things beyond the interests and ability of the clinical personnel is dangerous, and to modify so complex and extensive a resource is time-consuming. Thus the clinical system determines not only what the hospital is, but also what it might become.

Clinical care is a central component not only of hospitals, but of all other health care organizations. It exists in doctors' offices and becomes a complex system as solo offices grow to group practices. Clinical care is central to other outpatient care, home care, and nursing home care. Hospitals are much larger than most other health care organizations, both in number of members and scope of services provided. As a result of their larger and more sophisticated clinical system, they can and do take on all other clinical roles.

The term *clinical* derives from *klinikos,* the ancient Greek word for bed, as representative of the sick person. Etymologically, at least, the emphasis is on bedside care. Today, clinical care is at the patient's side more than at the bedside. In either case, clinical care is inevitably given close to the physical presence of the patient. The clinical system, as a result, is usually a local one, rarely involving great geographic distance. Its primary focus remains a triad of patient, doctor, and nurse, but in the modern hospital many other care givers have joined the team.

Part III describes the clinical system, beginning with the organizational needs of the medical staff, moving to the issues of quality and economy of clinical care, and then addressing the roles of clinical support services and nursing services. Normally, the book defines each part of the community and describes it in terms of its purpose, functions, membership, organization, measures of performance, and issues. One function the medical staff organization shares with other clinical units —control of quality and economy of medical care—is so complex and important that it requires a chapter to itself. It is discussed with its components, issues, and measures in chapter 11.

— *The Emerging Roles of the Medical Staff.* Chapter 10 states that the medical staff will strengthen its activities in quality control and administrative decisions, tying the individual doctor more closely to her or his colleagues and tying doctors as a group more closely to the hospital.

— *Maintaining Quality and Economy in Patient Care.* Chapter 11 summarizes the complex issues involved in this function, which has emerged as the central theme of exchange demands and, as a result, the central issue for hospitals. The medical staff leads in the effort to maintain quality and economy, but the responsibility is shared by other clinical groups and the governance system.

— *Clinical Support Services.* Chapter 12 describes how these services, once called *ancillary services,* grew into the lifesaving contributions of medical technology for many patients. They now form the basis of the clinical contribution that distinguishes hospitals from smaller organizations. Not surprisingly, they are also a major element in costs.

— *Nursing Services.* Chapter 13 shows that nursing, the ancient bedside function most deserving of its Greek roots, has become an essential counterweight to the high-tech care process. Nursing is important to both inpatients and outpatients and substantially improves cost and quality of care.

10

The Emerging Roles of the Medical Staff

Doctors have been ascribed magical powers, granted extraordinary privileges and confidences, and expected to assume extra moral obligations since the dawn of human existence. The twentieth century has seen a revolution in this social contract. The magical powers have become reality through scientific advance. The privileges and confidences have been divided among many specialists, each concerned with a particular organ system or method of treatment. The anticipation of moral obligation has been replaced by the suspicion and retribution of malpractice litigation. Still, the doctor remains the leader of the clinical team, perhaps simply because any venture as complex as modern medicine must have a leader. Thus, at the core of hospital clinical activity is a group of doctors organized into a medical staff. There is typically one doctor for every hundred or so admissions. Larger hospitals have several hundred members representing a wide variety of specialties. Historically, physicians developed their economic support as agents for their patients rather than as employees of the hospital, but both forms are now common. Whether they are employed or not, doctors are members of the hospital with critical roles to play both within their own organization, the hospital medical staff, and within the larger hospital organization.

This chapter begins with a description of the privilege relationship, the unique arrangement among doctors, patients, and hospitals. It goes on to discuss the purposes, functions, and issues of the medical staff organization. Like all bureaucratic organizations, the medical staff organization's most important function is to permit its members to achieve the best possible performance. Carrying out this function in the modern clinical care environment is so complex that it is the subject of a second chapter, 11.

Definitions: Privileges and the Hospital-Doctor Relationship

The Concept of Privilege

Elements of Privilege. If it is to be successful, any relationship between professionals and their organization must recognize the profession's unique obligations and skills. For priests and dioceses, lawyers and law firms, and engineers and manufacturers, tradition has established certain characteristics of a successful alliance. Similarly, the relationship of physician and hospital must accommodate the doctor's relationship to the patient. The traditional solution develops a contract around the concept of the physician's privilege to attend (that is, treat) his or her patients within the hospital and the hospital's obligation to use its resources for the good of the community. The privilege agreement contains the following five elements:

1. *Bylaws*—The governing board and the medical staff, that is, the doctors collectively, establish certain mutually acceptable rules and regulations defining the privilege of using the hospital's capital and human resources for patient care. These rules define the concepts of privilege, the doctor's relationship to his or her patient, and the doctor's obligations for peer review. They also define how the medical staff and the hospital make decisions affecting the doctors.

2. *Privileges*—The governing board extends the privilege of using the hospital for patient care to each doctor within these rules. Those privileged are called **attending physicians.**

3. *Independent doctor-patient relationship*—Each doctor establishes her or his own relationship to each patient and is expected to pursue diligently the obligations of that relationship.

4. *Peer review*—Doctors receiving privileges are also expected to participate in peer review of the quality of care, both as a reviewer and as a subject of review. The hospital can expect that privileges will be curtailed should the clinical performance of the physician fail to meet the expectations of his or her peers.

5. *Representation*—Doctors are expected to participate in implementing and revising the bylaws. This means that the rules are

developed by and enforced by the doctor and his or her peers, so long as the governing board agrees the rules are also beneficial to the community or the owners.

The contractual consideration on the part of the hospital is access to resources, and that on the part of the doctor is willingness to participate in the implementation and revision of the bylaws. As a contract, privilege is subject to all the legal provisions normally pertaining to business contracts.[1] Each of the five elements has well-tested merits but is evolving as technology and society create new exchange pressures. The general direction of evolution is toward a closer, more extensive relationship between the doctor and the hospital.

Bylaws and their extensions allow the trustees to protect a community resource and to encourage higher quality of medicine. For the doctor, they clarify what must, what can, and what cannot be done. They also address the doctor's rights as a member of the medical staff, including rights to representation. Their strength is their flexibility— they can cover any eventuality where agreement can be reached. Their weakness is most commonly omission—silence or ambiguity regarding a matter that later becomes controversial. The form and content of bylaws reflect solutions to the problems of the past; they grow steadily as consensus is reached on previously unresolved matters. Models of content are available from the American Hospital Association, the American Medical Association, and others, with most of the consensus reflected in the criteria of the Joint Commission on Accreditation of Hospitals.

Privileges are more closely controlled in modern hospitals than formerly, reflecting society's movement toward centralizing part of the responsibility for quality. Typically, a doctor will have privileges, renewable annually, to care for certain kinds of patients consistent with his or her specialty on a level of independence consistent with his or her experience and professional maturity. The social pressure for control of privileges has been expressed most dramatically through the courts in malpractice decisions, but it is also reflected in newer financing mechanisms such as capitation health care plans (HMOs) and selective contracting with hospitals (PPOs).

Each doctor is responsible for his or her own relationship to patients. The doctor is traditionally the patient's agent and is expected first and foremost to meet the needs of each individual patient to the best of his or her ability. Therefore, the basic judgment of quality is the patient's, expressed in the right to choice of physician and to discharge the doctor at will. However, there are many areas where patients lack knowledge and are unable to assess quality. One of the functions of the hospital medical staff (that is, the doctors working collectively) is to assist the patient by assuring a basic level of technical competence for all its members. The importance of the collective function has grown steadily as patients develop relationships to hospitals, prepayment plans, and physician groups rather than to truly solo practitioners. Collective quality assurance supplements rather than replaces sound doctor-patient relationships, however.

Each doctor is expected to accept both the responsibilities and the rights of management, to not only abide by the rules, but help enforce them and keep them current in a rapidly changing world. Because each accepts this responsibility, only doctors need judge other doctors on medical matters. This concept of peer review is a central element of professional autonomy. It is highly prized by most doctors, and they invest much time and energy in carrying out their obligations.

The medical staff organization also provides for representation of the doctor's personal viewpoint and economic needs, either through its hierarchical structure or through elected representatives. Doctors may play a major role in the writing and amendment of bylaws. The right of representation is also highly prized by most doctors. Both in peer review and in representation, the autonomy of medicine is limited by society. The final approval of the bylaws, and the right to appoint or not to appoint to privileges, rests with the governing board.

Flexibility of the Concept of Privilege. Like most sophisticated, participative systems in the modern world, the system of privileges and peer review is imperfect, occasionally expensive, and inefficient from the perspective of somebody who is certain of what is right and who feels her or his colleagues either do not matter or could not possibly disagree. The very fact that it prevents trustees, executives, and doctors from regarding themselves as infallible is its chief virtue. For this reason, the most popular capitation models borrow heavily from it, and models which do not emphasize the primary relationship between individual doctors and individual patients, such as military medicine, are strikingly unpopular.

A more positive virtue is the robust flexibility of the system. Because it is a system for writing and enforcing rules within limits of mutual agreement, independent patient relationships, and peer review, rather than simply a list of rules themselves, it can be adapted to almost every conceivable circumstance. Among other examples of its flexibility, it is noteworthy that the system permits but does not require cash and other tangible payments as part of the consideration. Early in this century, doctors contributed substantial unpaid effort to hospitals. The trend has been in the opposite direction, toward compensating physicians, since World War II. Many well-run hospitals compensate the doctors who assume critical and time-consuming leadership positions.

Capitation payment systems are sometimes tied to hospital privileges, with funds flowing through the hospital to member doctors.

Other major elements of flexibility have to do with the roles of specialties. Doctors in rural hospitals traditionally have much broader clinical privileges than doctors in larger, urban hospitals with many specialists. Standards of peer review are similarly broad. In large hospitals, however, specialists are judged by and write the rules for their own specialty.

Finally, there is flexibility to cope with the evolution of both the science and the economics of medical practice. The complexity of modern medicine now demands a team effort. Physicians, as traditional leaders of the clinical team, are called upon to write scientific rules and expectations for other professions. The "competitive" approaches to economy require that these rules be extended to cover issues of appropriateness and efficiency previously left to individual judgment. Even more striking, well-run hospitals are recognizing the importance of doctors in major planning and budgeting decisions and are extending the role of the medical staff in these areas.

Trends in the Concept of Privilege

Exchange pressures upon community hospitals have supported greater complexity, sophistication, and consequence for the concept of privilege throughout this century. The trend has accelerated in the latter half. Many hospitals before World War I had open staffs, permitting any doctor to admit and treat patients. Others routinely excluded female, black, and Jewish doctors from privileges or were open only to an arbitrarily defined group.[2]

Coincident with the revolution in medical education sparked by the Flexner report[3] and financed by the Carnegie Foundation, medical practice began to be more uniformly guided by science. Hospital privileges became the principal vehicle for distributing the benefits of scientific medicine to local communities. Concern with the quality of medical care, expressed principally by the doctors themselves, led to closed staffs, where only approved doctors could practice.

The origins of the accreditation system lie in actions taken by the American College of Surgeons to improve the quality of surgical practice—and studies in the 1920s revealed substantial basis for concern over quality. *Fee-splitting* (where the surgeon paid a bounty to the referring physician), *ghost surgery* (where a well-known doctor collected a fee in keeping with his reputation, but a lesser-known one actually did the work), and *unnecessary surgery* (where examination of the tissue removed failed to reveal disease) were relatively widespread.[4] These and other evils were mostly the concern of the medical profession until the 1950s, when courts began holding doctors responsible for their errors in greater numbers and the doctrines of charitable and governmental immunity protecting hospitals from suit were overturned.

In the 1970s the courts and legislatures also turned their attention to the rights of individual physicians. Under theories of nondiscrimination and antitrust, the concept of privilege was expanded to include due process, equal opportunity, and the avoidance of restraint of trade. These actions were consistent with major improvements in civil rights and a broadened application of "free market" concepts in U.S. society generally.

In the 1980s the role of the medical staff was again broadened, this time to incorporate concepts of control of costs as well as quality. Prospective per case payment, adopted first in New Jersey and shortly after by the Congress for all Medicare recipients, required that hospitals deliver care through their medical staffs at fixed prices. For about half the hospitals in the United States, this mandated prompt changes in the quantity of services ordered for each patient, bringing the organized staff into what previously had been an individual doctor's decisions. "Competitive" private financing schemes, HMOs and PPOs, extended the concept of control of cost beyond the *case,* or hospital stay, to the care of the patient over the contract period. Implicitly, by relying on free choice of carrier in an annual reenrollment, they also reinforced the need to respond to patient's desires.

Three exchange concepts emerge from this history: the interplay of diverse ideas, such as scientific medicine, competition, and civil rights; the variety of groups able to influence the hospital-doctor relationship, such as the profession itself, courts, legislative bodies, and buyers of large insurance or prepayment contracts; and the cumulative nature of the adaptive process between organizations and society. By 1985, the five elements of the privilege relationship had stretched in well-run hospitals to include scientific quality, customer responsiveness, nondiscrimination, due process, antitrust, and cost control.

Symbiosis of the Hospital and Attending Staff

Interdependence of Doctors and Hospitals. In his or her role as the patient's agent, the physician orders or at least influences the demand for all hospital services. As a result, no community hospital can survive without a medical staff. On the other hand, the commitment is mutual. Many doctors, particularly surgeons, cannot practice medicine without privileges. Internists and family practitioners are less dependent upon hospital access, but it remains important and few would give it up. Although people often use marriage as an analogy for the hospital-doctor relationship, the biological concept of symbiosis is more apt. Doctors and hospitals can only survive through mutual dependence.

Doctors are the clinical and scientific leaders of hospitals. They have the most extensive training and the legal and public recognition to resolve many procedural questions of diagnosis and treatment. They are expected to guide the selection of the drug inventory and the materials and equipment used in surgery and other invasive activities. Hospitals rely upon doctors to report and evaluate technical advances. Doctors also assist in specifying details of treatments and procedures for nurses and professional therapists. In several cases, notably laboratory, radiology, and anesthesia, doctors actually manage the activities as **hospital-based specialists** rather than as attending physicians. These specialists supervise nonphysician employees directly, but they also influence the opinions of their attending colleagues on clinical and scientific issues.

Emergence of the Conjoint Staff. Under price competition, the medical staff's contribution to general management has become increasingly necessary. Not only should doctors have a role in selecting the formulary and the surgical instruments, they should address more fundamental questions as well. On one hand, these questions deal with the further consensus on clinical expectations, or standards of practice: what the staff believes should universally guide care for heart attacks, or pregnant women at term, or metastatic cancer. On the other, they add medical wisdom to the economic issues facing the board: what specialists' skills should be available locally, how many beds must be provided, what forms of prevention and health promotion are cost-effective.

Without much question, the trend in hospital-doctor relations has been toward intensified symbiosis. As demands for closer collaboration have increased, the medical staff organization has been strengthened, and the relationship between doctor and hospital has been more tightly defined. There are several terms for the emerging relationship. The one used here is conjoint staff, described by sociologist W. R. Scott.[5] The conjoint staff participates more actively in all the affairs of the hospital. It is more effective in its own peer review. It plays a bigger role in directing the activities of other professional groups. It is a more articulate representative of its members' needs. As such, its functions extend beyond the management of bylaws issues to the management of hospital issues. With greater representation comes greater responsibility.

The well-run hospital is developing the conjoint staff concept, by whatever name. The discussion in this chapter and subsequent ones assumes that the concept will continue to spread, driven by exchange demands for economy combined with convenient access and choice of physician.

Purposes

Purposes of the Conjoint Staff

Exchange theory suggests that the success of the conjoint medical staff is determined by fulfillment of mutually rewarding desires on the part of the owners of the hospital and the doctors. The generic purpose of the conjoint staff is to identify, fulfill, and, if possible, expand those desires. The theory also suggests that, because the medical staff is part of the larger hospital organization, it will share many purposes with other units. That is, *conjoint* emphasizes similarities, not differences, in purpose. In particular, the other clinical units of the hospital will have to share a common direction with its physicians. Unique purposes of the medical staff should occur where physician desires are unique, for example in areas relating to compensation and privileges.

Following this line of thought, one may group the purposes of medical staff organization under three headings:

1. *Purposes shared with all organizations*—These relate principally to the relationships between individual members and the organization:

    • To support a system of recruiting, selecting, and promoting persons whose capabilities most closely reflect the desires of the community

    • To provide equal opportunity for all qualified members of the organization and to assure their rights by due process

    • To maintain communications between members of the organization and decision-making bodies in a manner that promotes full understanding, responsiveness, and fairness in matters affecting the work environment

    • To aid in the resolution of conflicting desires between its members and its departments

2. *Purposes shared with other clinical organizations*—These relate principally to health care per se:

    • To promote the clinical knowledge and skill of its members

    • To establish and achieve appropriate expectations governing the cost and quality of patient care for specific services and specific patient groups

3. *Purposes unique to the medical staff organization*—These relate to the unique roles of doctors in society:

    • To advise the governing board and the executive office on appropriate expectations for quality and cost of patient care generally

- To aid in the resolution of conflicting desires between clinical professions
- To advise the governing board on long-term directions in health care and the appropriate scope of health care services

Traditional Views of Staff Purpose

A more traditional view of staff purpose emphasizes the differences rather than the similarities between the medical staff and other units of the hospital, and it tends to emphasize the rights of doctors more than their obligations. Bylaws of the traditional staff, as opposed to the conjoint model, might eliminate the recruiting purpose, diminish the cost and quality expectation purpose, and diminish the advisory purposes of the staff. Most of the activities related to these purposes would be left to individual doctors or groups outside the hospital. An extreme view, and an uncommon one, holds that the staff's purpose is to defend medical rights; this would have the staff acting more as a union than as a unit of the organization, thereby creating an adversarial relationship with everybody else in the hospital organization.

The traditional model reflects two aspects of American society which are no longer true. First, the extreme power developed by physicians relative to other exchange partners of hospitals was based in large measure upon monopoly. Shortages of physicians required concessions by others to maintain an adequate supply. Second, the exchange demands of society have substantially increased. Hospitals are no longer immune from malpractice suits. Payment mechanisms no longer support "reasonable costs," whether by the hospital's or the doctor's definition. Racial, religious, and sexual discrimination are no longer publicly acceptable. The concept of competition among providers is broadly endorsed, and competition enforces a discipline that rewards collaboration and penalizes internal strife.

Evolution from Traditional to Conjoint Views of Purpose

The notion that a collaborative rather than an adversarial response will be successful is implicit in the conjoint approach. Yet traditional divisions of responsibility are widespread, and adversarial views of medical staff purposes are very real in many American communities. Hospitals are not alone in the need for transition. Parallels can be seen in several major unionized industries in the 1980s, such as airlines, steel, and auto manufacture. These industries have encountered serious trouble and have had to revise their management approaches, as must hospitals.

Many hospitals will revise as they go. The first step for a traditional organization is to avoid destructive conflict. Even an adversarial organization can be used to communicate exchange demands and meet them effectively. Properly pursued, the exchange theory purposes themselves will improve the relationship. Carrying out the purposes unique to the medical staff and establishing good communications lead to discussion of the issues at stake. The more vigorously they are pursued, the more widespread and clear will be the issues, the viewpoints, and the solutions.

There are two crucial questions which must be addressed simultaneously. First is the role of the organized staff in health care decisions. The complexities of modern medical care are such that the doctor's professional knowledge and skill are continually required for high-quality hospital care. The economy now being demanded by the marketplace requires two additional elements: a continued search for less expensive ways to achieve the desired outcomes and coordination of the efforts of many different people. While doctors acting as individuals can meet quality needs and search for economy, a collective, organized activity can be more fruitful.

The second crucial question is the willingness of executives and governing board members to incorporate doctors into decision-making processes. Decisions begin with structure, such as doctor representation on the board, and continue through long-range plans, budget decisions, and pricing, promotion, and operational decisions. Realistic participation in these decisions is the quid pro quo for the conjoint staff, and it is more important than any tangible compensation.

Well-run hospitals and their medical staffs have recognized the need for the conjoint approach and have moved to implement it. Hospitals which aspire to be well run are using education, persuasion, and their ability to appoint physician leaders to gain consensus on the new approach.

Functions

The major categories of medical staff functions parallel the purposes, but similar and related activities are grouped together:

— Recruitment
— Representation, communication, and resolution of conflicts
— Planning and advising
— Education
— Credentialing

— Maintenance of clinical quality and cost expectations

The functions are closely related, and the order is largely one of convenience, since all must be done well. Because of its complexity, the last listed function, maintaining clinical expectations, is discussed in chapter 11.

Recruitment

Recruitment as a Joint Activity. Either doctors or hospitals can recruit on their own; however, the more they recruit jointly, the more successful they are likely to be. This is due in large measure to the complexity of competitive offers. Compensation frequently includes arrangements for office facilities, income guarantees, malpractice coverage, and introductions to referring physicians or available specialists. As membership in HMO or PPO groups becomes more common, these, too, must be in the recruiting offer. Home financing, club membership, and other social and family issues are frequently important. The hospital's buying and financing power is frequently essential to assembling the elements of tangible compensation. At the same time, doctors want to work where their colleagues are friendly, complex offers require early assurance that medical credentials are acceptable, and selecting the right candidate principally involves assessment of clinical skills. These factors require medical staff participation in the recruitment process.

Physician Needs Planning. Physician recruitment is an integral part of the hospital's long-range plan. In order to meet community expectations, the planning activity of the hospital must analyze future needs for physicians and prepare to meet them. Normally this is done by considering population growth and aging and by reviewing the age and specialty distributions of current staff members.

The question of how many doctors should be privileged in each specialty is not simple. Too few doctors cause inconvenience and possibly danger to the community. Too many doctors can reduce the income of current attending physicians. More doctors tend to increase costs. New specialties often require large capital investments and new operating costs. If the additional costs duplicate investments at other local hospitals, they may lead to competitive price disadvantages. Additional physicians also increase services, however, and if the services are attractive to patients, they increase revenue. If this revenue is obtained without exploiting either monopoly advantage or peculiarities of the insurance mechanism, it reflects a genuinely cost-effective benefit to the community. New doctors may greatly improve quality, reflecting more recent scientific advances. They may also benefit some current members of the medical staff. For example, recruiting obstetricians tends to increase market share of pediatricians relative to family practitioners. Additional doctors may support a broader array of hospital services, permitting larger and more varied practices generally.

In the well-run hospital, the planning staff generates a proposal for desired replacements and additions to the medical staff by specialty from an analysis of retirement and expansion needs. The advice of the current staff on the proposal should be incorporated through the medical departments. The medical executive committee may comment upon conflicting medical viewpoints, but the importance to the consumer suggests that the planning committee of the board is more appropriate for resolution. The physician recruitment plan must be integrated with the plan for services and facilities. The final decision on desired specialties and numbers of attending doctors rests with the governing board, as part of the long-range plan. Once these decisions have been made, the well-run hospital and its medical staff begin joint recruitment for the desired individuals.

Joint Search Committees. An aggressive joint recruitment effort is justified by the long-range expectations for quality and cost of care. Although supplies of physicians have increased rapidly in recent years and will reach surplus levels in many specialties, good doctors will always be important to the success of the hospital, and they will always be in demand. The hospital that fails to recruit will lose out to the one that does.

Recruitment has become a relatively well codified activity, carried out by a search committee representing both the executive and the medical staff. It includes the following components:

— Establishment of criteria for the position and the person sought
— Establishment of compensation and incentives
— Advertising and solicitation of candidates
— Initial selection
— Interviews and visits
— Final selection and negotiation

Right of the Hospital To Deny Privileges. Any community hospital may deny privileges to a specific applicant on either of two grounds. The clearest is failure to comply with properly established criteria governing quality of care and good character, discussed below as credentialing. The most likely outcome of credentialing decisions is not denial of staff membership, but limitation of areas of hospital practice. The second is that the doctor overtaxes the facilities available for the kinds of care he or she expects to give, or, rarely, overtaxes facilities in general. Thus a hospital is not obligated to accept a cardiac surgeon if it has no cardiologist, or if it has no cardiopulmonary laboratory, or if it feels it has enough capability for cardiac surgery already. These decisions are clearly in the domain of the governing board, but the well-run hospital implements them through the medical recruitment plan.

Representation, Communication, and Resolution of Conflicts

Infrastructure of Physician Representation. Doctors are not unique in their need for representation; bureaucratic organizations must address the needs of all those who work in them. The issues of representation are the usual ones of employment contracts, broadly, compensation, the work place, and participation in management decisions affecting the member. The goal of representation is the minimization of conflict. It is achieved by recognizing potential issues early, providing for their full discussion, rewarding innovation and compromise that reduce objections, and relying as a last resort on a respected mechanism for deciding inescapable conflicts promptly and fairly.

The formal documents of the privilege relationship provide the basis for representation and communication. The bylaws of the hospital and of the medical staff and the written contracts of staff members specify not simply the rights and obligations of each party, but also the methods by which communication is encouraged and disagreements are resolved. Well-run hospitals use such documents as a foundation for the ongoing resolution of issues that arise. They are aided in this task by a carefully fostered tradition of mutual respect, open discussion, and progress based on consensus. Success feeds upon itself; hospitals with good systems of representation have good communications, which they use to identify issues early, and then avoid them or resolve them promptly.

There are three basic approaches to representation of exchange needs, with countless variations.

1. *Management-dominated approaches*—The most important function of middle management is to represent the needs of the workers to higher levels and to see both that needs are met and that questions are answered. For the medical staff, this representation is provided by department and selection chiefs, directors of medical education, and medical executive committee members. The staff is often involved in the selection of these individuals, thereby influencing the organization.

2. *Member-dominated approaches*—Attending staff members can represent themselves by consensus, through formal action of

the medical staff. The joint conference committee is established to permit full and candid discussion between representatives of the medical staff and the governing board. In many cases, an elected office, usually called president of the medical staff, supplements management-dominated communication. This is common where chief of service and chief of staff are physicians employed by the hospital. Unions express workers' views directly. Although formal collective bargaining for medical staffs has attracted some attention, particularly in the 1970s, it seems to have limited appeal. The adversarial postures implicit in unionization are probably not consistent with other exchange needs and are less responsive than collaborative approaches.

3. *Collaborative approaches*—A third approach to representation deliberately blends both management and worker perspectives. Quality circles, suggestion systems, worker-set incentives, and other devices recognize not only the moral, but the practical necessity of hearing front line as well as front office opinions. Active participation of staff members in the working committees of the collateral organization is the way this is implemented for medicine. The work groups developing new programs are especially critical.

The approaches listed above simultaneously develop consensus on expectations, coordinate activities of the staff, and represent the staff. The difficulty is gaining active participation and prompt communication of views without burdening staff members unduly. This often can be accomplished by sensitive design and administration: doctors can be welcomed to committees, work groups, and task forces where they make a specific contribution and can be excused from meetings where nonmedical issues are addressed. Meetings can be arranged when necessary rather than periodically. Agendas can be developed with an understanding of the need to save time. Advance preparation and distribution of relevant background material make a noticeable difference, as does proper preparation of the chair.

Where communication and trust are well developed, informal devices can be used to great advantage. If all staff members are confident that they will know of decisions important to them in time to react and that they have an avenue to make their views known quickly, much time spent in formal communications can be eliminated. In well-run hospitals, nonmedical managers make a deliberate effort to maintain informal communications with the medical staff. Many successful CEOs and COOs undertake the monitoring function personally. One successful president and CEO says, "I try to stop by the doctors' lounge at least five times a week."

Board Membership for the Medical Staff. The practice of providing one or two seats on the board for the medical staff has become almost universal, as discussed in chapter 5. Exceptions are mainly limited to those institutions whose corporate charters or enabling legislation preclude such participation. In most hospitals, doctors are nominated for these seats by more or less formal means. Other doctors may also serve on the board, although they are presumably selected for their personal, rather than their professional, abilities. Rarely do doctors constitute a substantial minority; in fact, doctors can dominate the governing board only when other members fail to exercise their independent judgment. The more serious danger is quite the opposite: the board and the medical staff may assume that these few individuals, representing only a fraction of the specialties, ages, and financial arrangements of the staff as a whole, fulfill the complex representation needs of all doctors.

Other Representation. The hospital building a conjoint staff also makes sure physicians' views and needs are represented through at least the following:

— The design of the bylaws and the hierarchy of the medical staff organization avoid skewing control toward any one specialty or group within the staff, except insofar as they reward high-quality care and other performance in support of the hospital's interests.

— Doctors' advice is solicited on the revision of the mission and the long-range plan. To the extent possible, strategic planning decisions are decentralized to a level where advocates and opponents of a specific proposal can affect the outcome (see chapter 7).

— Medical staff planning solicits the opinion of existing staff and involves them in the recruitment process.

— A representative committee of physicians ranks proposals in the capital and new programs budget (see chapter 8).

— Credentialing, physician quality review, and expectation setting for physician performance are carried out by the medical staff, subject only to effective discharge of the responsibility (see chapter 11).

— Budgeting, other clinical quality review, and expectation setting involving physicians and others incorporate physicians' viewpoints appropriately. For most clinical services, this means a visible avenue for physician input on costs, quality, amenities, prices, and promotion.

— Orientation and performance appraisal for medical staff leadership emphasize the obligation to represent views and meet needs of individual doctors.

Advisory Planning and Marketing Functions

The right of the medical staff to representation is balanced by the obligation of the staff to provide competent professional advice on medical matters. The rights of the conjoint staff include fair representation of economic concerns; the obligations involve sharing scientific knowledge and relevant market information. One important distinction of the conjoint staff is the emphasis on communication to meet both the rights and obligations of the medical staff in planning and marketing matters. These include assistance with planning decisions from mission setting to new program implementation. They also include new staff roles in quality assurance, promotion, and pricing.

Staff Role in Planning. The mission and plans of the community hospital must integrate the needs of external exchange partners such as the purchasers of health care, the owners or the community at large, and the members, including the doctors. The medical staff organization should allow for doctors' comments on the value of specific technology and its economic impact on staff members. The participation of doctors in mission and planning discussions helps the medical staff understand the viewpoint of others.

The planning process described in chapter 7 envisions ongoing hospital implementation of a well-stated mission by sequences of increasingly precise proposals for new or revised activities. The sequential nature of the process is central to the quality of decision making. As ideas move to proposals and proposals move to action, there is time to obtain multiple views, resolve conflicts, and reduce risks.

Each idea or proposal must identify the extent of demand, the system necessary to provide an adequate response, and expected costs, revenues, and benefits. Finally, there must be a process for selecting those proposals with the most favorable cost-benefit ratios. Doctors have important perspectives on each of these steps. Their most important contribution is their understanding of health care services, including the economic impacts upon various practicing physicians. The conjoint model implies that doctors are important in the work groups developing factual material but that they also participate in the evaluation itself.

Methods for conducting the necessary reviews and evaluations implementing a sequential planning process are discussed in chapter 7. Doctors' involvement should be structured similarly to that of other technical contributors. Like other expensive steps in proposal evaluation, the participation of doctors can be almost casual on small projects, although it should never be overlooked. Projects to which no doctor's opinion is relevant are rare; they are probably limited to plant replacements that have no implications for patient care. (Food service and air conditioning, for example, could profit from at least cursory physician review.) The conjoint staff suggests three additional concerns:

1. All clinical projects should include medical review of their scientific merit, demand estimates, procedures and equipment contemplated, likely benefits to patients, risks to patients and staff, and project life. In cases where the specialty involved also has economic concerns, independent evaluations may be solicited. Serious disputes on these technical matters are themselves an indicator of project risk and should be presented as such.

2. All important projects should be reviewed for their impact upon the physician recruitment plan. Subjective estimates should be verified as thoroughly as possible. Two errors appear to be common:

    • The promise of much new technology is overstated. "Lifesaving" is only applicable to those few conditions where the patient cannot be moved to another facility. To be "essential for recruiting the best people," the item must be available at a visible fraction—say, 20 or 30 percent—of truly competing institutions and in the immediate plans of a majority.

    • Proposals for the common good, that is, plans and investments which make modest contributions to large groups, are sometimes overlooked because they may attract less persuasive advocates than proposals with dramatic but less universal benefits. Deliberate review of a proposal's universality is a step toward redressing this imbalance.

3. All important projects should be given independent economic review by each specialty group. There are three reasons for this:

    • Independence allows unbiased comment on boundary questions where one specialty's gain is another's loss. Clear statements of position are the first step to resolving disputes.

    • Specialties may wish to comment on certain diseases or technologies for reasons that are not clear to others. Universal review is a protection against oversight errors generally.

• A general knowledge of the interests and activities of other groups helps each specialty plan its own proposals and formulate its specific responses.

Differences of opinion between specialty groups arising from independent review should be resolved via the medical organization hierarchy, which can rank the projects in terms of their desirability for larger groups of the staff. That is, projects advocated by the surgical subspecialties should be collectively ranked by surgeons of all kinds, and that ranking should be integrated with similar ones from medicine and other specialties by the medical executive committee. The consensus ranking for all clinical proposals should be integrated into the new programs and capital budget by the planning committee or a specially designated capital budget committee with medical, executive, finance, and board membership.

Extending the logic of staff participation in new service selection and design, one should note that existing services require periodic attention as well. The leading indicator of need is frequently volume or market share which fails to meet expectations.

Medical staff help in analyzing services with unsatisfactory market share is cheap and effective. Doctor or patient concern with quality, access, amenities, or satisfaction is a cause of deteriorating demand. Soliciting doctors' opinions helps both to identify the problems and to stimulate correction of them. The medical staff begins contributing to this area by participating in the setting of clinical expectations for other professions, as described in chapter 11. Although preventive efforts are always preferable, either prevention or review after the fact may lead to more strategic judgments on additional investments in new equipment, increased operating costs, pricing, and promotion. When this occurs, opportunities are identified and the improvement process is elevated to the planning and capital budgeting cycle.

Staff Role in Promotion. Doctors have traditionally been the recipients of hospitals' promotional efforts. Under unrestricted pricing, these efforts consisted largely of providing the most extensive and the best of everything. In the new environment, however, the question is more complex: both doctors and hospitals must include price in their promotional considerations, although the tradition of emphasizing doctors will continue. The systematic incorporation of physicians' views and the resolution of conflicting interests described here as the conjoint staff can be considered promotional in themselves. They are invitations to more complete and more satisfactory membership by attending physicians. Doctors can also be important contributors to promotional efforts aimed directly at patients: they provide a vehicle for reaching the patients directly and they can suggest appropriate content for promotional material. Conjoint staffs will use the promotional capabilities of the hospital for the collective benefit of the doctors, as well as for the hospital.

Staff Role in Pricing. Most services must recover their fair share of the profit the hospital requires. Although occasional services should be subsidized, the well-run hospital treats each case as a separately justified exception. Both for-profit and not-for-profit hospitals begin their price-setting exercise with an estimate of costs and required profit; however, the relationships between cost and price are quite complicated. For most services, cost per unit of service depends upon volume. With much of the resource requirement fixed, or committed, the larger the share of market attracted, the lower the unit cost and the price. Doctors are the key to attracting market share, and their selections frequently depend upon the quality and amenities offered to them and their patients. In the competitive environment, their views are both more important and more patient-oriented. Paradoxically, one way to reduce the cost of some services is to increase the current or variable expenditures in ways that enhance market share and total volume, thereby reducing overall average cost. In most cases, however, the key to adequate demand will be good planning and competitive pricing.

Doctors are also familiar with substitutes and alternatives, including referral to other hospitals. That familiarity gives them an advantage in pricing services that is becoming more apparent in cost-competitive markets. Both cost and price decisions are undertaken in the annual budget process. Physician involvement in this process may prove to be increasingly valuable.

Staff Role in Quality Assurance. A potential conflict of interest arises from the doctor's obligation to act as agent for the patient and her or his participation in pricing and promotional decisions. The conjoint staff model suggests a different philosophy, however. It implies that the doctor must affiliate himself or herself more closely with the hospital and carry out agency responsibilities within the organization. That is, faced with a less than satisfactory service, an attending physician should work to correct the deficiency under the conjoint model. Under traditional models, he or she might more readily have admitted the patient to another hospital. With the closer, more permanent ties of conjoint staff, the moral obligation is to correct poor quality or to change affiliation.

A real conflict of interest exists if the hospital's advantage diverges from the patients' or doctors'. The most common examples involve decisions about whether to offer certain services: convenience for certain patients and income for certain doctors will be enhanced, but the community as a whole will benefit more from other services. Those who "lose" to an argument of the general good must content themselves with recognizing their gains as citizens of the larger community, including the knowledge that their future proposals are likely to be judged fairly.

Fortunately, a basic level of quality will remain essential to the hospital's interests; as a result, true conflicts of interest will be minimized. The conventional belief that higher quality costs more money is by no means certain. Some improvements in quality reduce costs, and many managers believe that the *search* for quality will itself suggest improvements in systems design that will save money. The cost of a service, new or old, is related to systems design. Doctors can suggest ways of improving design that will reduce the final cost without impairing quality. Unit cost is also a function of demand. A well-designed system, endorsed by doctors, is more likely to attract adequate demand.

Education

The organized medical staff of most hospitals has two educational functions; that of larger hospitals has three. All staffs are responsible for promoting the continuing education of their own members and for assisting in the clinical education of other members of the hospital. Larger hospitals have responsibilities for postgraduate and occasionally undergraduate medical education as well.

Continuing Education for Attending Physicians. Continuing education for doctors is now strongly encouraged as part of licensure and specialty certifications. A variety of educational programs is offered outside the hospital; however, these do not substitute for the continued study of patients in the hospital. **Grand rounds** are formal presentations on subjects of direct importance. **Ward rounds** and clinical-pathological, mortality, infection, and adverse effects conferences and committees review actual cases in the hospital.

In well-run hospitals, these activities are focused on issues of scientific dispute or potential revision of practice. Grand rounds can stimulate reconsideration of treatment methods. Other conferences can provide collective review of recurring difficulties and can focus educational content on debatable issues. Focusing staff education has a double benefit: it avoids competition with other, more elaborate programs, and it increases consensus about the most acceptable methods. This consensus is essential to using clinical expectations effectively. Using educational approaches helps assure that every doctor fully understands the expectation, develops group pressure to encourage compliance, and, by changing behavior beforehand, eliminates personal confrontations over failures.

How much to invest in staff education is a difficult judgment. Programs are often expensive to mount, but they are more expensive to attend. The opportunity cost of doctors' time is very high, and educational time must be judged in the context of other demands from family, practice, and, particularly, other medical staff functions. Education outside the hospital is often as useful, but availability differs by community. Subjectively, and according to JCAH philosophy, every doctor should have access to sufficient educational opportunity to keep herself or himself current. This requires, and JCAH specifies, at least monthly meetings of clinical departments (or, in small hospitals, the entire staff) on educational topics. Attendance is required. Beyond this minimum, it is probably wise to decentralize decisions about staff education to the lowest feasible unit of the staff and to accommodate the programs they suggest when attendance figures indicate cost-effective investments.

The pressure for improving quality and appropriateness of care is causing leading medical staffs to use their in-house educational forums in new ways. These focus much more on identifying and improving patient care protocols—that is, statements of consensus on diagnosis and treatment (see chapter 11).

Education of Other Hospital Members. By tradition, preparation, and law, the doctor is leader of the health care team. With this leadership comes an obligation to educate others, not only other clinical professionals, but also trustees, executives, and other management personnel. A particularly important part of this education deals with new clinical developments. New approaches to care frequently require retraining for personnel at several levels, and doctors should at least specify the content of that education. In addition, trustees and planners rely on the medical staff to identify new opportunities for care, and to make the implications of these clear in terms that promote effective decisions. Many of these educational requirements are met through participation on various committees and day-to-day associations. The needs are closely related to expectation setting, and well-run hospitals identify and plan for necessary education in the process of implementing expectations.

Postgraduate Medical Education. Medicine has acknowledged its obligation to train new doctors since Hippocrates. Clinical training of medical students occurs in a limited number of institutions that incorporate such training in their mission. In 1980, about 15 percent of community hospitals offered training positions for **house officers**, licensed doctors pursuing postgraduate education. The content of this education is controlled through certification by individual specialty boards and is coordinated through the AMA. House officers are paid stipends during their training because they provide important direct service, because hospitals feel they are a valuable source of recruits, and because their presence has long been thought to improve overall quality of care. An important benefit to both the community and the attending staff is that house officers are expected to cover patient needs at times when attending doctors are not present. In addition, many of the programs suitable for house officers are appropriate continuing education for attending physicians, and educating house officers is educational in itself.

The formality and cost of educating house officers have increased greatly in recent decades, and the number of doctors available is likely to decline. As a result, many hospitals will face serious questions about continuing their programs. Most who abandon medical education will have to recommit some of the expenses to continuing education, and new arrangements for providing physicians around the clock will be necessary.

Well-managed hospitals will be best equipped to retain postgraduate educational programs. They will be more successful in recruiting, and they will pursue patient care management issues in ways that improve quality and reduce cost. House officers are generally heavy users of costly services. One avenue for saving costs is the development of better expectations for care, emphasizing to the house officer and the attending physician alike legitimate opportunities for economy. Presentation of financial data along with clinical data promotes consideration of the cost-effectiveness of specific diagnoses and treatment steps. Under DRGs, HMOs, and PPOs, economies are translatable to larger profits for the hospital. These, in turn, may support a larger or more attractive educational program.

Credentialing

The Joint Commission on Accreditation of Hospitals now requires that all privileges be granted for specific, limited clinical activity, that they end annually, and that they be renewed only when there is a consistent record of acceptable quality.[6] The American Medical Association has noted that malpractice risks demand similar approaches.[7] Increasingly, doctors sharing risks for their income through HMOs and PPOs want realistic review of their colleagues' privileges. As a result, the process of privilege review, that is, **credentialing**, has become an ongoing staff activity with growing impact on the quality and economy of care.

The responsibility for privileges review is centered in a committee of the medical staff called the credentials committee. Although the executive office must support the activities of this committee with a variety of records and data, the key evaluations require clinical knowledge and must be made by physicians. The opinion of specialists must be sought when appropriate. Many larger hospitals use the credentials committee as a coordinating body, with initial review in the specialty departments. Since the decision has a direct effect on both the hospital's and the doctors' income, it must be made under due process and subject to appeal in order to protect the rights of individuals, and it must be recommended to the governing board, which is ultimately responsible for all medical staff appointments. The hospital is liable for failure to provide due process, failure to remove incompetent doctors, and failure to establish appropriate standards of practice. The individuals participating in the process are liable for arbitrary, capricious, or discriminatory behavior.[8]

This somewhat ponderous mechanism differs from the usual employment relation between an organization and its members principally in providing more adequate protection to the doctor. The CEO and the management staff, for example, serve at the pleasure of the governing board and can be discharged at any legally constituted meeting for any grounds not discriminatory or libelous. Only civil service, union contracts, and the tenure system of professors provide individuals rights similar to credentialing.

There are six major elements supporting a well-designed credentialing process, but four, and often five, of these are produced by units of the hospital other than the credentials committee:

1. Bylaws
2. Committee membership
3. Clinical standards or expectations
4. Information and data support
5. Limitation of privileges
6. Operation of the credentials committee

Bylaws. The bylaws specify both the processes through which credentialing occurs and the structure which supports those processes. That structure is usually based on the medical and surgical specialties. With the emergence of a specialty board in family practice, even the most general areas of medicine can claim a relationship to scientific investigation in a clearly defined body of knowledge. Well-run hospitals now credential their doctors not for the practice of medicine, but for certain specific procedures, even though only the largest hospitals can create meaningful organizations for the full array of specialties that offer national certification.

Most authorities view the medical staff bylaws as the principal source of due process protection for both the individual and the hospital. The bylaws establish all procedural elements, including application requirements, timing, review processes, confidentiality, committees and participants, methods of establishing expectations, sources of data, and appeals procedures. Bylaws are generally developed by the medical staff, with detailed legal review before adoption by the governing board. Regular review and updating of bylaws is important. Once bylaws are approved, the credentials committee must follow them. Failure to do so in one case but not in another is potentially discriminatory.

Committee Membership. The ideal member of the credentials committee possesses the attributes of a good judge: he or she is patient, consistent, thorough, factual, and considerate. Clearly, clinical knowledge and skill are required, but detailed knowledge is more valuable in expectation setting than in evaluating credentials. Credibility is also important. Ideally, each member of the staff should know and respect the committee. On large staffs this is impossible, but each department can know at least one member.

The usual method of selection—nomination by the departments of the staff and appointment by the medical executive committee—is satisfactory as long as the actions of the committee are prudent and consistent. The governing board's right to reject nominees for cause or to dismiss the committee and seek new nominations under clearly established conditions is a useful protection for the rights of the community and the patients. Appointment by an individual, such as the chief of staff, probably vests too much authority in a single person. Similarly, physicians with other important leadership tasks should not serve simultaneously on the credentials committee, and membership should rotate fairly frequently. Although the executive office should staff the committee, there is little evidence that having nonphysician members is beneficial.

Clinical Standards or Expectations. In medicine, as in other activities, the best way to judge capability is against objective standards or expectations established in advance. This requires measures about what actually happens; a process of education, monitoring, and control; and deliberate efforts to make performance comply with expectations. All accredited hospitals have expectations of their attending staff; well-run ones have more extensive expectations. As discussed in chapter 11, large numbers of people are involved in the process. In well-run hospitals the credentialing activity is separated from expectation setting and monitoring, both to save the committee time and to permit fuller exploration of clinical issues in a scientific rather than a judgmental environment.

Information and Data Support. The record required by the credentials committee has two major components: the credentials themselves, that is, those documents and references testifying to the education, licensure, certification, experience, and character of applicants or staff members; and information from groups monitoring clinical activities in the hospital for current staff members. The applicant is often charged with collecting the documents, although these should be scrutinized and verified if any discrepancy emerges. References should be solicited by members of the search or credentials committee. The monitoring of clinical activity is the responsibility of the departments or specialty groups of the medical staff. Because of the large number of people involved, it is increasingly common to assign the compilation of all this material to hospital employees supporting the quality review, utilization review, and risk management processes.

Limitation of Privileges. The attending physician system uses ongoing peer review to limit the hospital activities of each doctor to areas of his or her competence. National programs for specialty board certification have a similar, but not identical, objective. The boards aim to certify what a doctor is particularly well trained to do. Because scientific development, training, and certification all parallel the specialty structure, the first decision on limitation is assigned to the specialty departments or divisions in larger hospitals. They recommend that the credentials committee renew, extend, or curtail privileges. Privileges are stated in terms of ability to treat a specific kind of patient or to perform an identified diagnostic or treatment procedure. The statement may be either full, allowing the doctor the right to act completely independently, or restricted, requiring either consultation with or direct supervision by a doctor in the specialty most commonly associated with the privilege. In small hospitals without specialty organizations, privilege decisions are made directly by the credentials committee.

It is increasingly common to insist upon full certification in a specialty as a condition of membership, or, in the case of young doctors still completing their training, a specific program and timetable for earning certification. Thus the prototype for limitation of privileges is that set of activities normally included in the specialty. Well-run hospitals have several additional constraints on the specific activities for which privileges are granted:

— Agreement and compliance with final product protocols for quality and economy (see chapter 11)

— Outcomes reasonably comparable with those of other members of the specialty, at the hospital and elsewhere

— Maintenance of a minimum number of cases treated annually to ensure that the skills of both the physician and the hospital support team remain up-to-date

— Restrictions based upon the capability of the hospital and the supporting medical specialists (An individual doctor may be qualified to receive a certain privilege, but the hospital may lack the necessary equipment, facilities, and complementary staff.)

— For new or expanded privileges, evidence of successful treatment of a number of cases under supervision, either at the hospital or at an acceptable training facility

Limitation of privileges is designed to identify that set of activities which the doctor and the hospital can do well. It is possible to apply the limitations excessively, creating problems in the recruitment and retention of medical staff members. One problem arises from excessive reliance on the judgments of specialty boards. The specialties sometimes conflict with one another or reflect self-interest. Family practitioners and general internists argue that they can handle a great many uncomplicated cases without referral, while obstetricians, pediatricians, and medical subspecialists argue that their specialized skills are more likely to promote quality. There are two parts to resolving these arguments. The first is correctly identifying the needs of each patient. The identification of the complicated case and the patient at risk is as important a part of the quality of medical care as the selection of the appropriate treatment. The American Board of Family Practice has emphasized its members' ability to identify the patient truly needing referral. The second is the nature of quality. It may be wise to sacrifice some elegance in the treatment of a specific disease in order to avoid further fractionation of care among specialists. The higher the value placed on comprehensive care, the stronger the generalists' argument. Many thoughtful analysts believe that comprehensiveness is undervalued in American health care and that the balance has shifted too far toward specialization.

The second major problem arising from excessive limitation of privileges is its effect on doctors' incomes. A decision to limit all obstetrics to obstetricians and all newborn care to pediatricians may destroy the income potential of family practitioners and reduce the availability of doctors throughout the community. It also will increase the fees charged per delivery. The fee structure of American medicine tends to reward procedures more than diagnosis and specialization more than comprehensiveness and continuity. While this might be taken as a reflection of patient demand, many analysts believe that it is an artifact of the monopolies which some specialties held for many years after World

War II and which were unfortunately reflected in health insurance plans. Regardless of the origin, the result has been relatively low incomes for family practitioners, general internists, and pediatricians. The disparity has generated some sensitivity, and a hospital which limits privileges to these groups excessively may find itself in an uncompetitive position.

The criteria for limitation of privileges affect the medical recruitment plan and the long-range plan of the hospital because they are interrelated with doctors' incomes and hospital support services. As a result, resolving the level of limitation is an important function of the medical executive committee, although specific limitations are usually proposed (and disputed) by the various specialties. Limitations should also be monitored carefully by the executive office, acting on behalf of the board under general policy guidelines in the medical staff bylaws, for compliance with the hospital's mission and all aspects of its long-range plan.

Operation of the Credentials Committee. Credentialing deals solely with the question of conformity to hospital expectations: does the individual achieve the established standards as well or as often as is required for continued membership? This specification of responsibility is essential to avoid duplication with specialty case review, to keep the tasks of the credentials committee within reasonable limits, to encourage due process, and to separate potentially painful decisions from the reward-oriented process of setting and achieving clinical protocols. Credentialing activity focuses on the new doctor, whose skills are as yet untested, and on the few who are clearly having difficulty meeting minimum standards. Most doctors are challenged and rewarded by the opportunity to improve, and in the process the minimal standards for credentialing are surpassed.

The well-run credentials committee rarely takes negative actions. The better the hospital, the stronger the probability that physicians will be reappointed. Credentialing is the final safeguard of medical care quality, and significant numbers of failures are symptomatic of serious difficulties.

The credentials committee faces certain predictable problems, among them the impaired physician. Doctors, like other human beings, can be disabled by age, physical or emotional disease, personal trauma, and substance abuse. The prevalence of these difficulties among practicing physicians is hard to estimate, but it is generally conceded to be between 5 and 15 percent. Thus a medium-sized hospital could have a dozen doctors either impaired or in danger of impairment at any given time. The response of the credentials committee should be tailored to the kind of problem. Aging and uncorrectable physical disability must force reduction of privileges. Particularly well-managed hospitals attempt to provide alternative activities for those who desire them. Alcoholism, abuse of addictive drugs, and depression may be more common among physicians than among the general public. Treatment for depression and substance abuse is clearly indicated, and programs designed especially for doctors can be reached through state medical societies. Arrangements can be made to assist the impaired doctor with his or her practice during the period of recovery, thus assuring that patients receive acceptable care without unduly disrupting the doctor-patient relationship or the doctor's income. In larger hospitals there is often a committee or group set up specifically to deal with this problem. Although it usually keeps affected physicians' identities secret, its activities must be coordinated with those of the credentials committee. While every reasonable effort at rehabilitation should be made, the credentials committee is ultimately accountable for the suspension or removal of privileges.

The actions of the committee may be reviewed by the medical executive committee or referred directly to the board. As noted in chapter 5, the board is not obligated to accept the committee's actions; rather it is under strong, independent obligations to due process and to protection of the rights of patients. In well-run hospitals, disputes of credentials committee actions are rare and usually arise from individual appeals rather than board or executive committee disagreements.

The operation of the committee must also incorporate elements of due process. It is wise to assign a trained hospital employee, rather than a volunteer committee member, to carry out all procedures under the direction of the chair. Formal procedures for advance notice, agenda, attendance, and minutes are mandatory. Doctors under review should have the opportunity to see the information compiled about them and to comment upon it. Because the committee should function at a secondary level, evaluating the sum of the year's activities rather than actual patient care, the need for new direct testimony is minimized. When it is necessary, the statements should be carefully identified and recorded. The summary of the individual's activities should be compiled in writing and documented. Review of procedures by legal counsel is desirable, and counsel should attend any appeals session. The doctor is also entitled to counsel.

The serious economic and medical care consequences of the actions of the credentials committee place its members in some danger of being sued, although many states have laws protecting such committees' actions and sources of data. The well-run hospital protects committee members and others in the credentialing chain with insurance, legal counsel, and, above all, prevention of lawsuits through the maintenance of due process and sound evidence in support of the committee's decisions.

Maintenance of Clinical Quality and Cost Expectations

Obviously the function of the community hospital and its conjoint medical staff is to provide high-quality, economical care. The activities of the conjoint medical staff establish consensus on elements of care ranging from mission setting through all phases of planning, physician recruitment, credentialing, and coordination with other clinical professionals. Quality and cost expectations determine the hospital's accreditation status and its ability to compete (see chapter 11).

Membership, Organization, and Compensation of the Conjoint Staff

Membership Categories and Classes

Categories. Society grants the physician virtual autonomy in diagnosing, prescribing, preventing, and treating disease of any kind. More restricted health care professions and licenses also exist. Some of these, such as nursing and physical therapy, limit practitioners' actions with respect to diagnosis and prescription. Partially as a result of such limitations, these professionals have tended to be salaried employees of hospitals and similar organizations. Other professionals are given authority to diagnose and prescribe for specific parts of the body, and these persons are more likely to establish fee-for-service practice. Their contribution is recognized under Medicare and private health insurance, and they are entitled to hospital privileges within their licensed domain. Because their domain is limited, these professionals work under the supervision of physicians.

There are several categories of medical staff membership, reflecting the needs of the various professions. Often the non-physician categories of the staff are grouped as "affiliate staff," or some similar title. The categories include:

— *Physician,* requiring a medical or osteopathic degree and license, privileged to treat hospital patients within limits established by further training or experience. The privilege statement may require consultation or supervision in specific kinds of situations.

— *Dentist,* requiring a dental degree and license. Dentists with specialized training and certification in oral surgery are commonly privileged to do surgery in the mouth and adjacent areas of the head and neck. A physician must supervise general care and presurgical workup.

— *Podiatrist,* requiring a podiatric (formerly chiropodic) degree. The privilege is analogous to dentistry but is limited to surgery upon the hand and foot.

— *Optometrist,* requiring an optometry degree and rarely privileged, although sometimes employed by large hospitals. The license permits diagnosis and prescription for defects of the eye that can be corrected with lenses. (Ophthalmologists have an unlimited license for performing surgery on the eye and treating diseases of the eye, as well as prescribing lenses.

— *Psychologist,* requiring a degree and certification in clinical psychology. Privileges are granted for treatment of emotional and mental disease by analysis, advice, or methods other than drugs, surgery, or electroshock. Supervision by a physician usually includes a physical examination for contributing organic illness. Psychiatrists, the related physician specialists, frequently collaborate with psychologists. (Surgery and electroshock are largely discredited in treating psychological illness at present.)

— *Chiropractor,* generally not privileged in hospitals. The clinical value of chiropractic diagnosis and methods of treatment is in dispute.

— *Nurse anesthetist,* registered nurse with additional training and certification. Nurse anesthetists are frequently employed, rather than privileged, and always work under the supervision of an anesthesiologist or surgeon.

— *Nurse midwife,* registered nurse with additional training and certification in obstetrics. Relatively rare in the United States, nurse midwives are privileged to attend uncomplicated obstetrical deliveries at home or in the hospital. They are required to refer complicated cases to obstetricians and to seek consultation when in doubt.

— *Nurse practitioners,* registered nurses with additional training in elementary diagnosis and treatment, maintenance of chronic illness, and prevention. They are usually employed under a specialist's supervision for specific tasks such as well-baby care or care of stable diabetics. They also complete admission history and physical examinations and monitor recuperating and chronic patients in uncomplicated or stable condition. Nurse practitioners are sometimes employed by privileged physicians and work in the hospital under their supervision.

— *Physicians' assistants,* persons trained at the bachelor's degree level to perform activities similar to those of nurse practitioners.

With the growing surplus of physicians, the continued existence of several of the other professions is doubtful. Further, HMOs and PPOs are not obligated to contract with any of the nonphysician practitioners, and they can be expected to do so very selectively. As insurance markets shift to these forms, demand for nonphysician services will fall precipitously. Although patients will continue to purchase services directly, most services will be office-based. Hospitals are obligated to extend privileges to nonphysician professions only to the extent that they conform to the same expectations of quality and economy held for physicians. In the future, opportunities for employment will be more common than privileges for nonphysicians. Privileges, if available at all, will be justified by unique contribution. Dentistry, for example, has a long and successful history and is likely to continue as a privileged practice. Several of the nursing specialties have shown their competence and popularity with the public and are willing to practice for less income than doctors. These nurses are more likely to continue as salaried employees.

Classes. Most hospitals have the following privilege arrangements for physicians, with similar titles for the nonphysician categories:

— *Resident,* licensed doctors who are usually salaried and are not permitted to collect fees, also called house officers. Their voting privileges and participation in staff decisions are severely limited. About a sixth of U.S. hospitals have formal training programs for the resident staff. Others may employ physicians in a similar status without the training commitment.

— *Probationary,* doctors joining the medical staff and presenting appropriate credentials without observed experience; also used for impaired physicians or doctors substantially failing to comply with expectations. Persons in this class are moved to active status as soon as they have shown capability, but for a brief time their patients are followed closely by more senior staff members. Those failing to show competence must be dropped from the staff. Voting rights may be limited for probationary members. (A variety of euphemisms is used for this class of membership, principally to avoid public attention. It is even possible to construct the bylaws so that the class is not explicitly identified, if voting rights are identical to those of some other group.)

— *Active,* doctors fully privileged in their area of competence, expected to participate in the obligations of medical staff membership and to take an active part in decisions. Active staff privileges are extended one year at a time, but failure to renew must be based upon documented cause. Doctors may be active at more than one hospital, carrying the burdens of dual membership. This arrangement is common in medium-sized cities. Officers are often limited to the active group.

— *Consulting,* doctors active on some other staff, participating less frequently in care of patients at this hospital. In small hospitals this class is often for referral doctors who visit weekly or on call to assist in complicated cases. In larger hospitals it is sometimes used to permit doctors from other hospitals to admit limited numbers of patients. Consulting doctors generally have limited, negotiated obligations in decision making and no voting rights.

— *Courtesy,* temporary privileges extended to doctors substituting for staff members who are ill or on vacation or to doctors who can present valid reasons for admitting a very small number of cases and who can document their privileges at another accredited hospital. These doctors have no voting rights or decision-making obligations.

— *Emeritus,* limited privileges extended to doctors no longer in active practice. These doctors have no voting rights or decision-making obligations.

The bulk of the responsibility, authority, and patient care of the institution lies with the active attending staff, although the other classes of membership serve important purposes. The resident staff is important in larger institutions: not only does it provide much patient care through its training activity, it is a major source of recruitment. Although house officers usually have no formal decision-making rights, well-run hospitals solicit their opinions, particularly on matters directly affecting them. Showing sensitivity to the views of house officers helps young doctors think constructively about their relationship to the hospital, encourages a favorable response to a later offer to join the attending staff, and promotes recruitment of other house officers. Smaller hospitals rely more heavily upon consulting staff, and an analogous sensitivity helps extend the benefits of the relationship beyond the individual cases seen.

Formal Organization Patterns for the Conjoint Staff

The evolution of the medical staff organization in this century has been from a social or collegial group to an organization that establishes increasingly precise and extensive sets of expectations for its members and enforces compliance with them. The process was influenced heavily by science and technology. The more extensive, precise, and powerful the medical armamentarium became, the greater was the need for agreement on who was to use it and how. Clinical areas that had been ignored were first vaguely and then quantitatively addressed. The competitive environment of capitation and selective contracting requires the well-run hospital to develop with its medical staff clear expectations on the final products of care. Inevitably these will involve all the elements of the closed system model: demand, output, efficiency, quality, process, costs, revenues, and profits.

The conjoint staff is a larger, more integrated structure aimed at creating a meeting of the minds among all those involved. The consensus must include not only issues of quality, but also of planning and scope of services directly affecting each doctor's practice. The quid pro quo for more precise expectations for clinical and final products is greater participation in the economic issues reflected by the long-range plan, the physician recruitment plan, and the selection of potential new programs and capital equipment. Although both the conjoint staff and the traditional one may have formal organizations resembling that shown in figure 10.1, the units of the conjoint staff will address a broader agenda, set more precise expectations, and be more closely bound to the agenda. It is also likely that there will be more full-time and employed doctors in its operation. A number of committees and collateral organization devices are necessary under either form of organization. These are discussed in chapter 11.

Medical Staff Responsibility Centers. It may be useful to consider that, because of his or her extraordinary authority, each member of the medical staff is analogous to a first-line supervisor or responsibility center manager. Certainly, the physician has and should have extraordinary authority. However, for the hospital and the conjoint medical staff to succeed, an accountability hierarchy must exist and eventually develop and apply specific final product protocols and other expectations about quality and economy of care. To coordinate medicine, nursing, and the clinical support services effectively, the protocols must involve related disease groups. Two factors determine the level of formality: the scientific differentiation of treatment and the need for representation and coordination of differing economic viewpoints. By far the usual solution is to group doctors by clinical specialty. Although one can contemplate multispecialty teams as responsibility centers, they have not been found practical for community hospitals. The members of a given specialty constitute the smallest formally accountable group, or responsibility center. Such a unit is called a **section** (less commonly division or service), and is accountable for meeting the expectations established by and through the bylaws and for representing members' needs to the

Figure 10.1
Organization of the Medical Staff

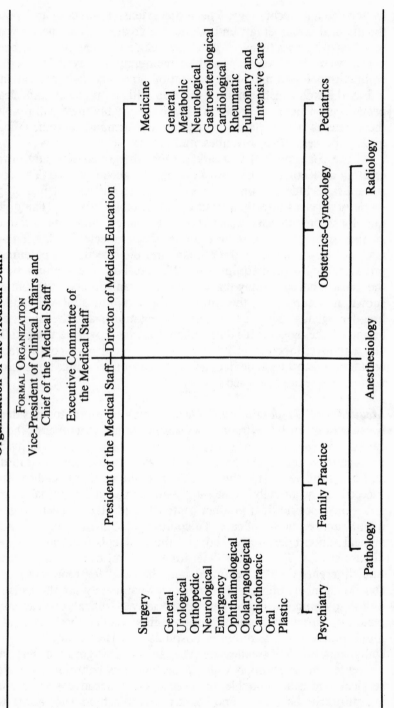

larger organization. Sections that have a common origin are grouped into **departments**, and the older clinical specialties have retained departmental status. (A confusing tradition also applies the term *department* to the much larger units of nonmedical organization, such as housekeeping or emergency.)

Unfortunately, there has been no consistent logic in determining sections and departments. New specialties have reflected similar techniques (radiology), patient needs (obstetrics), and philosophy of health and disease (family practice). Technique supported the historic split between medicine and surgery. (Another confusing duplication of terms occurred when both the entire profession and the specialties not using surgery were labelled *medicine*. The term *internal medicine* is sometimes used to make the distinction.) Surgery was divided into general (principally abdominal), orthopedic, urological, obstetrical-gynecological, neurosurgery, otolaryngological, ophthalmological, plastic, thoracic, and cardiovascular. Medicine was divided into psychiatry, dermatology, gastroenterology, endocrinology, hematology, neurology, cardiology, pulmonary disease, and rheumatology. Most of these specialties follow the major biological systems, but the parallels are inexact and differ between medicine and surgery. In some cases, holistic theories crossed these divisions and created specialties, namely pediatrics (which then split further to medical and surgical subspecialties paralleling the adult care pattern), infectious diseases, oncology, and family practice. (*General practice,* once a common descriptor, has largely been replaced by primary care specialties, principally family practice, general internal medicine, and pediatrics, but also obstetrics-gynecology and psychiatry.)

Although these competing theories suggest grounds for debate and sometimes create conflicts, there is currently little chance of modifying them at the level of the community hospital. The structure is determined in the medical faculties, implemented by the medical specialty boards, and continually reinforced by educational and continuing education activities. Whether obstetrics or family practice should deliver babies and how accountability should be split for the mother and the infant are interesting intellectual questions. Few community hospitals can afford to do more than develop clear, well-understood compromises about the answers. As a result, the medical accountability hierarchy follows the specialty certifications of medicine with special recognition of the older specialties, and the major division occurring between medicine and surgery.

Compensation of the Medical Staff

At the start of this century, the doctor was expected to pay for privileges in many ways. House officers were unpaid, except for room and board, and probationary and young attending physicians were expected to contribute significant amounts of time to clinics, that is, outpatient services for the poor. All doctors were expected to volunteer whatever time was required for the operation of the medical staff, including all the time necessary for educating house officers. In some hospitals, particularly those operated for osteopathic physicians, doctors were expected to pledge a portion of their income to support the hospital, usually its physical facilities. The only salaried doctors were in the hospital-based specialties, pathology, radiology, and anesthesiology.

These views began to change after World War II and were revised radically after the passage of Medicare and Medicaid in 1965. In well-run hospitals, only vestiges of the old system remain. House officers' salaries are roughly comparable to nurses'. Although many clinics remain, many of the patients using them pay for care. The term has lost its association with indigency and is now virtually a synonym for "health center" or "group practice." Doctors who work in clinics are compensated through fees or salaries. Hospitals began paying salaries to key officers of the medical staff in the 1960s, and the practice has spread slowly since. Medical education is usually directed by an employed doctor. The practice of contributing to hospital fund drives continues, but at a much less intense level. Arrangements with hospital-based specialists vary with the hospital, the specialty, and the individuals involved (see chapter 12).

The well-run hospital now pays a great many doctors. Even hospitals of 100 to 200 beds pay an average of two full-time-equivalent doctors; those over 400 beds average about 20 each. (The counts include any "personnel who were on the payroll, including trainees" and are subject to varying interpretation.[9]) There are several ways of compensating doctors in addition to salaries. These include income guarantees, subsidized office space or personnel, assistance with malpractice insurance and continuing education, and provision of low-cost services. The trend toward providing doctors with tangible returns in addition to privileges is likely to continue.

Reasons for Compensating Conjoint Staff Members. There are two basic reasons for a hospital to compensate a staff member. One is that the staff member provides a valuable service directly, as in the case of house officers, staff leaders, and hospital-based specialists. The other is that the doctor helps fulfill the health care mission of the institution, or, in the case of for-profit hospitals, provides a valuable source of patients. In the second case, the doctor is treading upon difficult ethical ground. It has long been held that the doctor as agent must select the best possible care for the patient and that any compensation the doctor accepts from someone other than the patient automatically sets up a conflict of interest. Fee-splitting and bribes from specialists for referrals have long been censured by ethical physicians and the JCAH. Two features of the conjoint staff absolve it of fee-splitting: it is selected on the basis of quality and economy, and it is accepted by an informed customer as part of a medical care package. That is, payment is not hidden, and the agent relation to the patient is explicitly shared.

Newer methods of payment have established an agency which holds the institution far more responsible and encourages it to select competent doctors on behalf of the patient. An analogous hospital obligation has arisen with respect to malpractice. The patient can express his or her choice by selecting the prepayment plan, the medical group, the hospital, or the doctor, in various combinations. Each of them shares the agency obligation, and they are bound together by it. Thus the second reason for compensating doctors is that the conjoint staff embodies the joint agency increasingly being demanded by the public. Hospitals and doctors which carry it out effectively will attract more economic support.

Methods of Compensating Conjoint Staff Members. Medicine as a business is as complex as any other, containing elements such as tax laws, the need for equity or retirement funds, differing access to capital markets, and returns to scale which permit larger units to perform some tasks more economically than smaller units. Because of this complexity, the opportunities for devising compensation under conjoint staff arrangements are almost endless. The following array suggests the major avenues. Combinations are usual.

1. Direct compensation:
    * *Salaries and fees.* These differ from each other only in how compensable work is defined. Salaries are more common for long-term, less defined commitments. Fees tend to be associated with tasks rather than time and are more common for direct patient care services.
    * *Income guarantees.* These usually short-term arrangements are set up to accommodate the natural growth of practice, and are often offered to newly recruited physicians.
    * *Joint ventures.* Equity units may be sold or may accrue to physician partners in for-profit ventures ranging from HMOs to non-health-related businesses. For example, staff members may be awarded shares of stock or options to buy shares in an outpatient surgical subsidiary. Ownership provides a powerful incentive to the doctor and creates different tax and time considerations than salaries do.

2. Indirect compensation:

- *Group insurance and annuity purchase.* Most insurance is less expensive when purchased through a group. Health, retirement, life, and disability plans are commonly provided to employees of the hospital. Malpractice insurance may be an important form of compensation for the conjoint staff.

- *Mortgages and leases.* Size and tax considerations favor the hospital with a generally lower capital cost, which can be used to subsidize doctors' offices. Other mortgages and leases (for home, office equipment, and automobiles) are sometimes offered to attract young physicians establishing practices.

3. Supplies purchases: Hospitals may be able to obtain supplies for doctors' offices at lower costs than the doctors can.

4. Compensation in kind:

- *Access to the patient services and equipment of the hospital.* Traditional privileges are still essential for successful practice of a great many medical specialties. Privileges are increasingly being extended to outpatient as well as inpatient care.

- *Physician coverage.* Night calls are significantly reduced by having house officers and employed doctors on duty. Emergency rooms provide backup for office care. Coverage for physicians on vacation is usually arranged on an individual basis, but the medical staff organization facilitates it.

- *Continuing education.* Regular programs are sponsored by well-run hospitals, and the expectation-setting activity of the staff should be educational in itself.

- *Direct office services.* Hospitals provide copies of patient records, billing and management services, and offices for transient use. Access to the hospital's computer and computerized records is increasingly advantageous.

Measures of Performance of the Conjoint Medical Staff

There is a difference between the effectiveness of medical care, the topic of chapter 11, and the performance effectiveness of the medical staff as an organization. Although one might say that effective care is the result of an effective organization, there are other considerations in organizational effectiveness. Like other units of the hospital, the conjoint medical staff is held to expectations regarding its effectiveness, and measures of its achievement are desirable. The areas in which measurement is available include:

— Organization structure, contributing to both quality of care and equity of treatment for staff members
— Quality, utilization, and cost
— Medical staff budgets
— Hospital-related records of individual doctors
— Measures of the current and future makeup of the medical staff relative to hospital planning and marketing

Structural Measures

Structural expectations deal with the way in which important decisions are made—who participates, what criteria are used, what procedural rules apply. They are principally stated in the staff bylaws. As such, they are fundamental supports of equity, quality, and effectiveness and are frequently referred to by the JCAH and the courts. Structural expectations are part of the foundation for good relations with the medical staff. Not only do they guarantee the rights of each individual, they encourage candid and productive discussion of issues. Adherence to these bylaws is the best legal defense the hospital has for actions it and its staff take regarding individual doctors.

Structural expectations change slowly, as new issues are identified and resolved. The well-run hospital usually has a stable structure in full or substantial compliance with the requirements of the JCAH and local licensing authorities, and with the major suggestions of its legal counsel. This structure also promotes equality of representation. Well-designed bylaws state how candidates are nominated for various offices, the specialty composition of committees, and the rights of individuals to appeal.

Erosion of the structure is a more serious danger in the well-run hospital than incorrect initial design. It occurs through failure to observe the written provisions. Structural measures are measures of compliance with structural expectations. Attendance at meetings of the staff and its committees, particularly educational sessions, must be recorded and counted for the JCAH. Other measures are often single events that are handled with the zero defect approach. They include such items as complete applications and documentation, appropriate approvals and committee routings, and notices required by the bylaws.

The key to compliance is to make individuals clearly accountable. Checklists summarizing steps for important decisions are useful and once completed, can serve as measures. Occasional audits are also useful; for example, JCAH inspectors attempt to check on actual compliance with structure as well as the existence of it. Failures can be avoided by systematic attention: new officers must be trained, bylaws and regulations must be reviewed and brought up to date, and unusual situations must be identified to assure appropriate application of the rules. Members of the executive staff assigned to various medical activities are frequently de facto custodians of structure, principally because medical staff officers have shorter tenure.

Aggregate Data on Quality, Utilization, and Cost

Many issues of quality, cost, and utilization reflect upon the skills of individual physicians. Few would dispute, however, that any given group of doctors can perform better as a whole if it has a sound organization. Thus, one indicator of an effective conjoint medical staff organization is steady improvement in such matters as outcomes measures of quality, evidence of malpractice risk, cost per case, and quantities of services used on a case-specific basis.

Budgetary Measures. Hospital expenditures for doctors and medical staff activities are substantial. Large hospitals spend almost 5 percent of their payroll for doctors other than house staff and slightly more than 5 percent for house staff. The growth of the conjoint staff will increase hospital expenditures for medical staff management. It is important to establish cost centers for the activities involved. These should parallel organizational accountability and apply to any doctor directly controlling substantial expenditures for education, monitoring, or assessment of clinical performance. Annual budgets for these activities should be established in the usual manner.

Measures for the Medical Staff Plan

Statistics on current activity are provided as noted above. Data on age (or graduation from medical school) and specialty are provided from staff membership files. A common approach to planning uses records of doctors' past activity to forecast future demands. Three problems must be addressed in such an approach:

1. The doctors currently on the staff may not be active in the future.

2. The preference of the doctors for using this hospital may change.

3. Doctors' expectations may not coincide with those of other doctors or the community.

The concept of the conjoint model assumes that these problems will be addressed through full discussion and negotiation. Implementation of the concept demands that there be expectations regarding the nature of future demand at the level of the individual doctor or at the specialty level. The starting point for discussions to set expectations should be a record of each doctor's age, specialty, and past activity with the hospital. Additional information may be obtained by questionnaire or telephone survey, but negotiation and discussion are still desirable. The hospital's long-range plan should address doctors' expectations regarding demand (with due recognition of the uncertainty and risk involved), resolve conflicts between doctors' expectations and likely community demand, and modify medical staffing by recruiting, terminating, or changing the duties of doctors. Achievement of the plan is a measure of the effectiveness of the staff organization and its leaders.

Measures of Staff Management

Many of the statistics on economic activity of the hospital also measure achievements of the conjoint medical staff. Most major measures of demand, such as admissions and outpatient visits, are measures of physician activity as well. The information system which supplies process measures of clinical activity (chapter 11) also supplies data on each doctor's economic exchange with the hospital. The data required for setting clinical expectations provide a full description of each doctor's activity as well. The same system provides data which can be used to set expectations for individual physicians and to assess their achievement of them, a useful exercise if rewards are incorporated in the conjoint organization.

Keeping the required records on individual physicians can be viewed as similar to more common human resources information systems. The record on each doctor should include salary or other cash payment, provision and utilization of nonsalary benefits, application credentials, history of privileges, major measures of activity, record of continuing education or additional training, and record of disciplinary action. Salary and nonsalary benefits are becoming increasingly important and complex as hospitals tailor individual programs to attract and keep doctors who meet their needs. Records of continuing education, additional training, and disciplinary action should be presented annually to the credentialing committee.

Individual rather than statistical use is made of this information, but the maintenance of these records is demanding. The information in them should be kept confidential, but the physician himself or herself is entitled to review it. Maintaining records is an appropriate function of the office of the chief of the medical staff. Large hospitals are finding it difficult to compile disciplinary records because several different units of the staff may have raised questions independently about the same individual.

Management Issues

The conjoint model, with its provision for greater participation and representation of doctors in decisions and emphasis on quality and economy in patient care, appears to be improving hospitals' chances of survival. The discussion that follows reviews the exchange issues underlying the struggle for survival; how some of the problem areas of the traditional staff organization have been solved by well-run hospitals; political and representational characteristics of the conjoint staff that make it attractive to practicing doctors; and economic advantages of the conjoint staff. Chapter 11 presents the central customer-related exchange issue, how the conjoint staff can assure quality and economy of patient care.

Forces for Change in Medical Staff Organization

The supports for the conjoint staff lie in the desire of the American people for free choice of physician, voluntary rather than governmental patterns of health care and hospital insurance, and convenient, exceptionally well-equipped hospitals under local control. The conjoint staff emerged in response to a perceived need for more economy with minimum sacrifice of these goals. There are alternatives to the conjoint staff, however, and whether it succeeds depends upon its appeal to patients, insurance buyers, trustees, and doctors, whose daily exchanges build or reject the model.

The traditional medical staff structure of the voluntary not-for-profit hospital has two powerful assets. First, the attending staff arrangement allows great freedom in the patient's choice of doctor and corresponding freedom in the doctor's practice. Second, it has attracted the support of social, political, and economic leaders in the community. On the other hand, it is easy to misunderstand and even easier, judging from the record, to mismanage the traditional medical staff relationship. Its failures are legion, and it is generally regarded as the most difficult aspect of hospital management. Most plausible scenarios suggest that it will not survive. One alternative is to move to the conjoint model. Another is for doctors to become employees of large, multistate hospital corporations—health care Sears Roebucks. A third would be for large bureaucratic organizations of doctors, resembling a cross between today's group practices and national public accounting firms, to either own hospitals outright or contract with the health insurance carriers who own them. The diversity of the United States strongly suggests that several models will survive, as several do now. The one or ones that thrive will be the one or ones that answer the most exchange needs.

Successful health care organizations and their medical staffs must supply four elements:

1. Convenience and choice of doctor, with the array of other clinical services and facilities necessary for comprehensive, convenient patient care
2. Cost, quality control, and efficiency sufficient to be competitive
3. Access to capital to support facilities, equipment, and a pool of professional personnel
4. Social acceptability and political influence in the local community and centers of government

Against these needs, the conjoint staff emphasizes the following assets of the older model which appear to have continuing value:

— A large group of attending doctors offers the patient a choice of physician.
— The principles of traditional medical staff organization are more fully implemented. Peer review, annual reappointments, and limitation of privileges are used to motivate quality and economy among individual doctors.
— Community participation in hospital operations, including trustees representing community leadership, is retained and encouraged.

It also expands the organization's ability in the following areas:

— The hospital corporation is exploited as a source of both human and financial capital, providing effectively for doctors' professional and economic needs.
— The ties between doctors and hospitals are strengthened by increased representation of doctors in decision making, direct financial affiliations in a variety of ventures, and a shift away from adversarial and toward collaborative thinking.

Some Nonissues in Well-Run Hospitals

To be successful in using the conjoint model, it is necessary to have been effective with the traditional one. Well-managed hospitals have clarified the responsibilities of the participants in the traditional model over the years so that the rights and obligations of the parties are well understood and responses are habitual. There are precedents for solving most problems that arise, and participants are accustomed to relying on precedence or extending it rather than seeking new methods. The methods for introducing new ideas and resolving disputes are particularly critical. They ensure that everyone's view will be heard and respected. When these habits and customs are in place, the range of ideas that can be addressed is broadened, and the speed with which consensus can be reached is increased. Hospitals which had achieved this level of sophistication by the early 1980s are likely to be successful in the future.

Formal Decision-Making Processes. Well-run hospitals use a formal process of decision making and rarely, if ever, depart from it. This process is essential to orderly representation. It reassures each member of the organization, including doctors and managers, of his or her rights and ensures that no individual will gain unfair advantage for his or her views. It helps avoid conflict by soliciting questions and opinions while modifications are still possible. It resolves conflicts by providing an accepted route for appeal. It is also a convenient device for specifying who will do what if the proposal is approved.

This should not mean that discussion is stifled by formality. Informal discussion can actually be stimulated by clear understanding of how the final decisions are made, because everyone knows how the informal discussion will be reported for formal action. In hospitals which have achieved a sound process, all the people in leadership positions know how various questions are answered, follow these methods, and expect their colleagues to follow them. Attending physicians who do not know specifics are confident that they can find out when they ask. In well-run hospitals, departures from the decision-making process are rare because they are destructive. Wise board members, executives, and medical staff leaders insist upon following tradition, and avoiding shortcuts and ad hoc decisions.

Rights and Obligations of Attending Staff Members. The well-run hospital uses its decision-making process and other elements of its formal organization to reinforce the rights of individuals and specialty groups. Each attending physician at a well-run hospital knows clearly his or her rights and obligations. Doctors have the right to be heard on issues within their area of professional competence and on issues affecting their livelihood. The fact that each doctor has the right means that none can dominate decisions unfairly. In medical staff politics, this frequently translates into treating the various specialties evenhandedly, respecting both their needs and their contributions to overall patient care rather than simply to hospital activities. Primary care specialties tend to use the hospital less than referral specialties. Their contribution to quality and economy is more obvious in capitated payment systems, however, and well-run hospitals will give their views appropriate respect.

The doctors have two obligations: to maintain standards of clinical care and to support the decision structure itself. In well-run hospitals clinical standards are extensive and specific, and they grow by the steady action of the appropriate clinical units. By contrast, the rules for supporting the decision structure are kept to a minimum. Well-run hospitals understand that most doctors will ignore excessively detailed rules but will follow a few sound guidelines. They administer these guidelines with considerable flexibility, having learned to tolerate much temperamental and individualistic behavior. Rather than discourage noncompliance (and possibly creativity) by sanctions, they encourage cooperation by reward, making conformance easy and equally effective in expressing the individual doctor's needs.

Executive Contributions to a Well-Run Medical Staff. Successful medical staff management appears to be built upon two principles. First, the executive staff provides guidance, education, and logistic support and monitors almost continuously to make sure the system is working. Second, as is the case in all closed systems, great effort is made to make the system proactive rather than reactive and to encourage rather than correct.

The executive staff of well-run hospitals routinely does the following to support its medical staff:

1. Provides orientation and assistance to committee chairs and other officers of the medical staff. It is important that these persons, like the administrative representatives, know both the general and the specific objectives of medical staff management.

2. Provides scheduling, amenities, agenda preparation, and minute-taking services to all committees and clinical departments of the staff. Often representatives of the administration are secretaries of important committees. In that capacity they can handle these logistics and help the committee keep sight of its goal. While some of these details may seem trivial, in fact agendas determine both the efficiency and the effectiveness of meetings. Evenhandedness begins with finding a convenient meeting time. Accurate minutes are essential to efficiency, to resolution of disputes, and, most importantly, to the perception that rights have been observed.

3. Uses its administrative representatives on committees to monitor the process of decision making itself, making sure that these

representatives understand the overall functions of the medical staff organization, the specific objectives of the units they are assigned, and the need for an open, equitable process.

4. Supplements its formal participation in committees and departments with an informal presence. It is important that even the chief executive of large hospitals be perceived as accessible by members of the medical staff. Many successful CEOs make informal visits to the medical lounge. Their assistants are encouraged to be similarly visible.

5. Maintains an up-to-date biography on the service of individual staff members and suggests personnel and chairs for various committees, ensuring that doctors gain skills in management as they progress to more central responsibilities.

6. Recommends to the board the acceptance of medical staff officers and committee members. The board's review of such nominations should be one of process rather than substance, because the executive office and the medical staff would normally have completed all necessary substantive review and negotiation ahead of time.

7. Reports on the effectiveness of the medical staff organization per se to both the medical executive committee and the board, suggesting areas for improvement and soliciting suggestions from staff members.

8. Suggests future topics and helps develop medical staff agendas that meet both the hospital's and the doctors' long-term needs.

Political Aspects of the Conjoint Model

The successful hospital or health care organization of the future must be attractive to practicing doctors. The goal of both the doctors and the hospital is to have excess demand for staff membership. Excess demand promotes quality, marketability, and financial stability. One way to achieve this goal is to provide financial compensation to doctors, possibly even specific incentives for compliance with joint goals. A second way is to offer greater opportunity to participate in decisions. A thoughtful doctor will soon perceive the interrelation of the two: "If a significant portion of my income is tied up in the success of this hospital, I should seek a say in how it is run." To be successful, the conjoint model must offer the doctor both greater participation in the organization and greater financial reward than competing alternatives.

Staff Participation in Decision Making. The conjoint model must develop additional rights for doctors in the decision-making process. This will involve a reformulation of the processes by which management decisions are made. New modes of participation will develop around the following areas where the governance system and the medical staff share concerns:

1. *Clinical expectation setting*—Methods of reaching a more formal consensus on a variety of matters directly related to patient care must be developed by the individual specialty departments. Mechanisms for integrating various specialty viewpoints must be developed, probably using subcommittees of the medical executive committee.

2. *Hospital operating procedures and policies*—Doctors require a highly efficient work place, well-trained personnel, and an environment as attractive to their patients as possible. Their participation in operating procedures and policies, including the formulation of policies for nursing and ancillary services, will increase under the conjoint staff model, but methods for handling this increase have not yet emerged. Committees may be unwieldy, resulting in increased roles for middle managers, who will be responsible for assimilating various viewpoints and designing a system that accommodates as many as possible. Dual reporting of clinical managers such as nurse supervisors to appropriate medical specialty divisions is likely.

3. *Long-range planning*—Doctor participation at all levels, including mission setting, will be enhanced. Proposals with clinical content will require doctors on the development team. The medical executive committee will review and comment on the overall plan and resolve interspecialty differences.

4. *Pricing and promotion*—Doctors' opinions will be solicited on specific price and promotion strategies, recognizing the differing views of the specialties.

5. *Capital and new programs budget*—Rank order of clinical proposals will be handled by an interspecialty subcommittee of the medical executive committee. Doctors on the appropriate board committees can defend clinical projects against other needs.

6. *Work-related questions and disputes*—Like other members of the hospital team, doctors require prompt and reliable responses to questions and fair, equitable, and expeditious resolution of disputes. Answering questions will be the obligation of line managers of clinical activities, including specialty

chiefs. A method for resolving disputes between doctors and other professionals must emerge. The principal disputes are among medical specialties, and they will continue to be resolved by the medical executive committee.

7. *Medical staff recruitment*—Formal solicitation of physicians' opinions on recruitment needs by specialty will be part of long-range medical staff planning. Interspecialty conflicts will be resolved by the medical executive committee or the board planning committee. New staff positions will be filled through searches undertaken by a joint medical–executive office committee.

8. *Bylaws*—Doctors will continue to write their own bylaws, subject to governing board review. Because of the increasing complexity of bylaws, advice from the executive office will increase.

9. *Credentialing*—The increased economic ramifications of credentialing will lead to a substantial increase in participation at several levels. Specialty divisions, sharing a limited, common income pool, will want more control over reappointment. The medical executive committee will resolve questions between specialties. The credentials committee will become an important secondary review body, protecting the rights of both doctors and patients.

10. *Selection of medical staff leadership*—As staff management becomes more complex, more doctors will become professionally committed to it. These leaders will compete for paid positions and will be selected jointly by the executive office and appropriate units of the medical staff. Doctors may continue to elect a president or other individuals explicitly for representation; this post will be a secondary, not primary, means of participation, designed to ensure that other mechanisms are working.

11. *Board representation*—Doctors will continue to serve directly on the governing board, but, like the presidency of the medical staff, the function will be secondary, not primary, in representing specific needs.

This list of rights is already noticeably more extensive than those of other members of the organization. It is rivaled only by the influence of certain governance groups like the executive staff or the finance committee. It also suggests that the problem will be not so much finding ways for doctors to participate as finding time to participate. Doctors will want not so much to take seats at committee tables as to assure that they are represented effectively at those tables. Thus, the role of the employed physician chief will increase, and the role of committees will be to oversee these executives.

Economic Issues of the Conjoint Model

More than most businesses, the practice of medicine operates in *niched,* or highly segmented, markets. A doctor defines the market he or she will serve by selecting a specialty, and then a location, and finally a hospital. The long-term financial success of these decisions is frequently dependent upon the decisions of the hospital. Thus the doctor as a business person has a stake in the hospital's success. The hospital is also aided by the doctor's success. It is entirely appropriate that the privilege relationship be viewed as an economic collaboration.

Purposes and Criteria of Economic Collaboration. The purposes of economic collaboration between the doctor and the hospital are twofold. From the doctor's perspective, the principal purpose is to increase her or his personal income or net worth. From the hospital's perspective, the purpose is to increase the overall effectiveness of the institution, however measured. Any successful economic collaboration must meet both objectives.

Finding mutually rewarding opportunities is complex. There has been a steady trend toward increased compensation from the hospital to various members of the medical staff. As noted above, this trend is likely to continue. However, new methods of economic collaboration are beginning to emerge. From the hospital perspective, rewarding opportunities involve cost reduction, volume enhancement, market share increase, or profit improvement. Not-for-profit hospitals are less attracted to equity enhancement and not at all to tax avoidance.

Doctors' personal income and net worth can be increased in several ways, including reduction of costs, enhancement of volume, increases in average billing per patient, and deferral of income. Which way is preferred depends in part on the circumstances of the individual doctor and in part on the tax laws. The nature of a solo or small group professional practice limits opportunities to develop equity for retirement and other needs. Young doctors have generally incurred substantial debt and need assistance with office start-up costs and other capital expenses. Older doctors may need retirement assistance and health care benefits. As these issues suggest, much ingenuity is required to design effective collaboration, even where the collaborative activity is clear.

Joint Investment Ventures. One area that has attracted considerable interest is the establishment of joint ventures between the hospital and its attending physicians in specific areas. **Joint ventures** involve mutual contribution of capital to some activity or program with the promise of future return. The best areas for joint ventures are those in which both parties contribute more than simply capital, making the joint effort more powerful than alternatives. The hospital's other contributions include market visibility, quality assurance, political influence, and the management infrastructure of information systems, recruitment capability, and specialized counsel. Doctors bring essential clinical skills, reputations, and ability to refer patients. Examples of successful collaboration include HMOs and PPOs, malpractice coverage, doctor's office buildings, and outpatient centers for surgery and other forms of care.

Joint ventures require management that is responsible to both owners. They are not managed by the hospital but are established as separate corporations or limited and other formal partnerships. As in the case of other business ventures, board membership or management committees are carefully structured to reflect contributions to long-term success. Inevitably, many directors or managers will be doctors. The individuals selected must represent the medical constituencies participating in the venture.

Joint ventures are more likely to succeed when they are carefully and independently reviewed by each party. The hospital's review should be the same as it would give any other new program or strategic opportunity. This means that the issues of long-range plan and long-range financial plan, consistency with mission and objectives, and return on investment must be weighed by the governing board. On a conjoint staff emphasizing participation, it also means review by the medical staff representatives in terms of the response of the medical staff as a whole. The review of participating doctors is less formal, but they as individuals must judge the desirability of the investment.

Experience with joint venturing is limited, so there is little evidence of long-term success or failure. Expert opinion, however, stresses attention to the contribution of the collaboration per se. It is likely that successful ventures will be those in which the partners can do significantly better because they collaborate. Ventures done as well by others or by either party alone are unpromising candidates. The best joint ventures appear to be those which provide or finance health care in directions consistent with the hospital's mission. It is likely also that the better focused the mission, the more successful the joint venture, and that successful joint ventures will stimulate closer concordance of hospital mission with the financial objectives of its medical staff. Thus the implication of joint venturing in the very long run is a closer philosophical tie between the hospital and its staff.

Other Economic Incentives for Conjoint Staff Membership. There are other financial mechanisms besides joint venturing for motivating the medical staff. Hospitals can provide staff members with salaries, perquisites, and services in kind. They increasingly do this on a selective basis, rewarding those who make the largest contributions to hospital goals. These distributions differ from joint ventures in that there is no investment or risk on the part of the doctor. Perquisites can include price reductions on goods and services such as office supplies, educational programs, life and health insurance, or accounting. Discounts are more prevalent than outright contributions of goods and nonmedical services to doctors, but providing record keeping and temporary or transient offices is not uncommon. Education and selected clinical services are frequently provided to the doctor at no charge. Arrangements for malpractice insurance coverage have recently become important.

One of the most valuable rewards is so commonplace it passes unnoticed. All hospitals with emergency rooms provide a certain amount of backup to their doctors, as well as a few referrals of new patients. All those with house staff also provide night coverage of inpatient emergencies and routine coverage that can easily reduce the number of trips a doctor makes to the hospital daily. If the hospital is a half hour away from home or office, an average of one trip per day can be worth over $2,000 per month to the typical doctor. The conjoint relationship will exploit these rewards by deliberately limiting privileges to doctors who contribute to the hospital's goals as well as their own.

Notes

1. Arthur F. Southwick, *The Law of Hospital and Health Care Administration* (Ann Arbor, MI: Health Administration Press, 1978), pp. 427–65.

2. Paul Starr, *The Social Transformation of American Medicine* (New York: Basic Books, 1982), pp. 169–79.

3. Abraham Flexner, *Medical Education in the United States and Canada: A Report to the Carnegie Foundation for the Advancement of Teaching* (New York: Carnegie Foundation, 1910).

4. P. A. Lembcke, "Evolution of the Medical Audit," *Journal of the American Medical Association* 199 (1967): 543–50.

5. W. Richard Scott, "Managing Professional Work: Three Models of Control for Health Organizations," *Health Services Research* 17 (1982): 213–40.

6. Joint Commission on Accreditation of Hospitals, "Standards for Medical Staff—Requirements for Membership and Privileges," *Accreditation Manual for Hospitals* (Chicago: JCAH, 1984), p. 89.

7. American Medical Association Task Force on Professional Liability, *Professional Liability in the 80's, Reports 1–3* (Chicago: AMA, 1984 and 1985).

8. Arthur F. Southwick, *Law of Hospital*, pp. 432–65.

9. American Hospital Association, *Hospital Statistics* (Chicago: AHA, 1982), pp. 21, 237.

Suggested Readings

Begin, J. W. "Managing with Professionals in a Changing Health Care Environment." *Medical Care Review* 42 (Spring 1985): 3–10.

Freidson, E. "The Reorganization of the Medical Profession." *Medical Care Review* 42 (Spring 1985): 11–36.

Kaluzny, A. D. "Design and Management of Disciplinary and Interdisciplinary Groups in Health Services: Review and Critique." *Medical Care Review* 42 (Spring 1985): 77–112.

Scott, W. R., and Lammers, J. C. "Trends in Occupations and Organizations in the Medical Care and Mental Health Sectors." *Medical Care Review* 42 (Spring 1985): 37–76.

Shortell, S. M. "The Medical Staff of the Future: Replanting the Garden." *Frontiers of Health Services Management* 1 (February 1985): 3–48. See also in that issue commentaries by John C. Aird and Stanley A. Skillicorn, Richard H. Egdahl, and Edward J. Conners.

Southwick, A. F. *The Law of Hospital and Health Care Administration.* Ann Arbor, MI: Health Administration Press, 1978.

11

Maintaining Quality and Economy in Patient Care

Introduction

Role of Clinical Expectations

Every time a nurse gives an injection, he or she makes several specific checks on the site, the drug, skin preparation, and equipment. Every time a surgeon starts an operation, the equipment he or she normally needs is prepared in advance. The roles of surgical team members are coordinated using a large pool of shared knowledge. Every time a patient tells a symptom to a doctor, the doctor's response is predictable for that symptom, plus other information at his or her command.

Definition of Clinical Expectations. The consensuses reflected in these everyday events constitute **clinical expectations** about the process of care. One can define the term for hospital management purposes by emphasizing its application to the activities of professionals, the recurring nature of the situation addressed, and the need for a consensus rather than an individual professional's opinion or patient's need.

> **Clinical expectations are the consensuses reached on the correct professional response to specific, recurring situations in patient care.**

Although there is not an expectation for every possible event, there are hundreds of thousands of them already in existence.

The primary function of clinical expectations is to make cooperation among different individuals and professions possible. They are necessary to allow any level of sophisticated teamwork to exist in health care. Reflecting this primary function, many clinical expectations are the work of the professions themselves, developed from necessity. Secondarily, they become a convenient statement of contracts with patients and insurers. The courts and the marketplace have reinforced the right of consumers to have their care conform to clinical expectations developed by professionals. Driven by technology and economic growth, clinical expectations become more extensive and more numerous over time.

Clinical expectations are not an unmixed blessing, because they raise the danger of regimentation. Clearly, treating every operation or heart attack identically overlooks the reality that every operation and heart attack is different, principally because it occurs to a different person. Thus, another side to the issue of quality and economy has to do with abandoning or going beyond the expectations. Doctors and most other professionals have not only rights, but also responsibilities to tailor care to the individual. These are largely defined by the expectations themselves. One may treat *this* heart attack differently, but the very difference is defined by the expectations of all heart attacks.

Analogous sets of expectations support every form of social interaction. Society anticipates that its members will comply with expectations. It relies on them to enforce laws, to support prosperity, to encourage equity, and to improve the quality of life. It uses a variety of rewards and sanctions to encourage compliance. Simple but important expectations tend to be upheld by strong sanctions. For example, violations of individuals' rights to their persons may draw imprisonment sanctions. Achievements of difficult, important expectations, such as aiding a stranger in danger, win recognition and rewards. All ethical, formal bureaucratic organizations, including hospitals, are responsive to social expectations. They also rely heavily on expectations to subdivide tasks and accountability. Like society, they anticipate compliance and reward it, and they use varying sanctions for noncompliance.

Types of Clinical Expectations. Clinical expectations as whole include care activities for practitioners working outside the hospital. The hospital's focus is upon a subset of the whole. It is a very large subset, because hospitals participate in so many kinds of care and because the expectations for complex care, like organ transplants, build upon hundreds of simpler tasks, like injections. Clinical expectations can be divided into three types:

1. **Activity or procedure expectations,** such as those for injections or physical examinations. These expectations are established by the profession most often involved, although that profession must be responsive to others and to society. Activity expectations are the most stable over time and between patients. Hospitals per se have contributing roles in setting or changing these.

2. **Intermediate product protocols,** which establish the normal set of activities for complex procedures such as surgical operations. They specify the quality and resource requirements of support services used in patient care. They have tended to be established unilaterally by the support service. They are now frequently established collaboratively between the service department and the users, who are attending physicians.

3. **Patient group protocols,** which define normal care of a common group of patients, such as uncomplicated pregnancies at term. They specify the quality and content of final products, that is, service groups delivered to patients. They usually are established by physician specialties, but they often involve the integration of several professions and specialties.

Individual patient care plans are also important; they define care and objectives for each patient, accommodating unique needs and characteristics. They specify additions and departures from the relevant group and product protocols. Medical care plans are the sole responsibility of the attending physician. Nursing care plans, described in chapter 13, must complement the medical plans. Other professions also develop care plans, but they are often of limited scope.

Ideally, a professional providing care to a patient habitually conforms to consensus expectations, making coordination possible because his or her efforts become predictable. Using the group protocol as a point of departure for individual care plans greatly reduces the communication required. Recent public actions have demonstrated the importance of all three types of expectations. The courts use clinical expectations as standards in malpractice cases. The federal government uses group norms, a crude form of expectations, to establish Medicare payment. HMOs and related economy-oriented insurance schemes require conformation to standard criteria supporting admission or surgery.

Plan for the Chapter

The well-managed hospital relies heavily on all three types of expectations. It can expect to do so increasingly in the future. Yet the ways in which it uses expectations are subtler than most people realize, and understanding these subtleties may be the key to their success. This thesis is expanded in the remainder of this chapter, as follows:

— *Philosophy.* Well-run hospitals emphasize setting expectations rather than monitoring them. They select the areas to be covered by expectations carefully, develop them patiently by consistent processes, and anticipate nearly universal compliance. They reward compliance consistently, in several ways, and only rarely must correct deviation with sanctions.

— *Expectation setting.* Those expectations selected by the hospital for formal study and development are a limited set chosen for maximal improvement in overall performance. There are strategies to determine what kinds of expectations should be selected, how many, and who should be involved. The processes of development themselves follow procedures designed to enhance acceptance and compliance.

— *Monitoring.* The most important role of the monitor is to guide the expectation-setting process by revealing directions for improvement. It serves only secondarily as an early warning for trouble. In well-run hospitals, the use of monitoring for direct individual sanctions is rare.

— *Measures.* The most sophisticated use of expectations draws flexibly and imaginatively on a large data base of patient-related activity. Care activities which cannot be quantified are poor choices for expectations.

— *Information system.* Expectation setting as a principal role places new and very different demands upon the clinical information system.

A Philosophy of Clinical Effectiveness Control

Supporting Self-Direction of Physicians

The philosophy advocated here assumes that the formalization of expectations will be increasingly important but that the well-run hospital will use this process to encourage both acceptance of the expectation and independence from it, where justified. The professional will be self-directed, but her or his direction will be consistent with collegial and organizational goals for quality and economy.[1]

Underlying this approach to clinical performance is a sophisticated version of the cybernetic model of human and organization behavior. A simple conception of feedback and control assumes correction of exceptions that do not meet the expectations. A subtler approach recognizes that prevention of exceptions by offering positive incentives and prospectively encouraging individuals to modify their behavior is better. The most sophisticated conception perceives two further truths of organization behavior. First, any real expectation in an organization is always less than ideal, so there is always an opportunity for individuals to exceed the expectation. Second, powerful incentives can motivate the search for that opportunity. Self-direction to performance which often exceeds expectations is best of all. It not only allows each worker to do his or her best, but it frees the organization from costly and painful problems of enforcement.

The well-run hospital encourages self-direction in the organization as a whole, not just in the medical staff. Supportive environments emphasize the value of each worker's contribution to the organization. They encourage questions and assure that they are answered. They provide the proper tools to do each job, and they use realistic methods. They have open channels of communication and processes of decision making, so no worker needs to feel excluded. They deliberately capture the workers' opinions in the process of management.

These virtues are often touted, but they are difficult to achieve. Some organizations do eventually achieve them, however, with a deliberate effort to maintain consistency over both time and a variety of decisions. Behind the attitudes and the specifics lies a basic technical capability: accounting and laboratory and nursing must be well run in a technical sense; governance must understand the virtue of the environment being built; and so on. Planning and marketing are particularly important: adjusting to a changing external environment without disrupting a supportive corporate environment is difficult. Maximum lead time is often the key.

Studying well-run hospitals suggests that the following characteristics are emphasized:

— There is evident an underlying commitment to patient care and humanitarian values. Each doctor understands that she or he is privileged to practice the best medicine and to represent his or her patients' needs vigorously. Each employed professional understands that the employment contract is on behalf of patients and that excellence will be rewarded.

— There is a similar commitment to the rights of all workers, including respect for each individual's contribution, open exchange of information, and prompt response to questions.

— There is widespread participation in the development of expectations.

— There is a climate encouraging organizational change which also reassures members of their security. Otherwise, anxieties develop and protectionist positions are taken. The major components of reassurance include consistent procedures and processes; well-understood avenues for comment and prompt, sensitive response; avoidance of imposed consensus; and recognition of the importance of dissent.

— The expectation-setting process generally emphasizes scientific sources and is approached as a stimulating intellectual challenge. That is, it is approached as a rewarding rather than a burdensome event.

— All expectations unambiguously identify mandatory and contraindicated categories of actions, but in so doing they specify the range of individual judgment and provide a practical procedure to follow when mandates should be overridden.

— Expectations are routinely achieved. Their achievement proves their practicality and establishes social norms encouraging achievement. Those that are frequently breached are withdrawn for further study.

— Expectations dealing with order, documentation, timeliness, and courtesy are accepted as essential. Violations are met with prompt, measured sanctions. For example, the penalty for incomplete medical records, temporary loss of privileges, is quickly and routinely applied. As a result, well-run hospitals have few incomplete records.

— In contrast, a spirit of fairness and helpfulness characterizes discussion of departures from more serious expectations. The fact that such departures are rare permits extensive investigation. Sanctions are used reluctantly but predictably in the case of repeated unjustifiable practice.

— Recruitment emphasizes the philosophy of the hospital, so it attracts doctors and employees who are congenial to its orientation.

Rewarding Clinical Self-Direction

The well-run hospital realizes that encouraging all its professionals to do their best for their patients requires more than tangible rewards or sanctions. Thus it effectively uses intangible rewards stemming from membership in a social group committed to quality. Several premises underlie the use of membership rewards; many of them relate to maintaining a balanced effort reflecting a widespread commitment:

1. One goal of clinical performance management is to make good individual patient care plans routine. Individual attending physicians select the specific diagnosis, treatment, prevention, and support for each patient.

   To achieve this goal, all possible rewards are directed toward building a capable attending staff. Rewards include reappointment, professional recognition, nomination to leadership, invitation to participate in joint financial ventures, encouragement of referrals, and occasionally community and social opportunities.

2. The patient group protocol should be a convenient starting point for the individual care plan. To the extent that this is successful, three things happen:

   a. The protocol is widely used and becomes habitual.

   b. The several professions can use it to anticipate care events.

   c. The doctor can use it as a shorthand or outline to guide his or her decisions and his or her communications to others.

   Habitual use of protocols permits the medical staff to concentrate on improvement rather than correction. Since most rewards are directed toward effective individual care, the remaining incentives must be used to encourage such habitual use. The most powerful is consensus in setting the expectation. Sanctions for noncompliance are the last resort, but these must be used promptly and judiciously when needed.

3. Nursing should rely on its care plan in the same way as the attending physician relies on the medical plan. The nursing care plan should supplement and complement the medical plan. Medicine and nursing should develop collaboratively both patient group and intermediate product protocols.

   a. Intermediate product protocols in nursing emphasize expeditious integration of the tasks of various clinical professions: (1) completing nursing tasks promptly, (2) scheduling and coordinating nonnursing events so that they can be completed promptly, and (3) immediately identifying and reporting departures from the anticipated clinical course.

   b. Nursing care plans emphasize: providing emotional support to patient and family; educating the patient in health needs, thus reducing the danger of further illness; and integrating nursing care with medical care.

4. Intermediate product protocols in the diagnostic services (laboratory, radiology, and cardiopulmonary) strive to define each test with increasing clarity. Many diagnostic tests involve judgments of probability, both in the selection of them and in their results. Reducing the uncertainty surrounding each test is a way of improving the accuracy of selection; it involves enhanced statistical analysis of results and uniformity of administration. A test which gives a more uniform result, with more clearly defined abnormal values, saves money in two ways:

   a. It can be more precisely selected, that is, ordered only when it is likely to contribute new knowledge of the patient's condition.

   b. It is less likely to cause expense by generating an erroneous result.

5. Intermediate product protocols for treatment (operating rooms, intensive care, pharmacy, and rehabilitation therapies) should be assessed as follows:

   a. The contribution of the treatment to patient care outcome should be evaluated in light of presenting symptoms and needs.

   b. The methods and resources used in each treatment should be increasingly standardized to reduce cost and stabilize quality.

6. Revisions of patient group protocols and of intermediate product protocols cause changes in the cost of products and create needs for revisions of budgets, plans, and marketing activities. The hospital can provide tangible rewards for clinical personnel as these revisions are successfully completed. Well-run hospitals are using collaborative planning, budgeting, pricing, and capital budgeting activities discussed elsewhere in this book to translate improved clinical practice into greater efficiency and economy. In doing so, they capture the economic advantages of improved expectations. A hospital which fails at these tasks of the governance and finance systems generates cynicism among its clinical personnel; achievement is a reward per se for most professionals.

Setting Expectations for Clinical Practice

Much more consensus about the best response in clinical situations exists in the literature and unwritten knowledge of the various professions than will ever be written as hospital policy. Policies are set when the three types of clinical practice expectations—activity, intermediate product protocol, and patient group protocol—are adopted for collective use. Although different members of the hospital will be involved, the processes in setting clinical expectations are similar to those of other hospital groups. They also resemble consensus-building processes of human endeavor more generally.

This discussion reviews sources and strategies for managing the expectation-setting process. It assumes that the three types of clinical expectations are set similarly and that a balanced program addressing all three is desirable. Special concerns for expectations directly affecting attending staff prerogatives are discussed after the more general issues.

Sources of Expectations

The sources of clinical expectations are the same as those of other expectations essential to hospital operation:

— *Historical.* These expectations are drawn from previous years' performance. For example, last year patients with a certain disease stayed six days. A simple expectation would be that they will stay six days next year as well.

— *Comparative.* These expectations differ from historical ones only in that they incorporate the experience of several institutions; an example would be the regional average length of stay for patients with a certain disease. The legal standards for malpractice, that is, things which most appropriately trained professionals would do in a specific circumstance, are essentially comparative expectations, as are many recommendations in clinical textbooks.

— *Scientific.* These expectations are based on random or controlled clinical trials, usually as reported in the scientific literature or in textbooks rather than as conducted at the hospital.

— *Subjective.* These expectations are based on consensus of intent, desire, or ethical considerations. Clinical expectations may rule out procedures or treatments inconsistent with the mission of the hospital or mandate those felt to be an inescapable part of that mission. Examples include expectations on abortion, "natural death," cigarette smoking, and dietary restrictions imposed by religion.

Economy is an important criterion of expectation setting. No expectation should ever cost more to set than the value of the actual change of behavior it invokes. While many seek scientific documentation for clinical practice, high-quality scientific validation is often difficult to find. As a result, well-run hospitals use all four sources of expectations, collecting the historical evidence, assembling comparative expectations, compiling the scientific literature, and noting the implications of ethical and mission-related concerns.

Tactics for Expectation Management

Some unit or group of hospital management must manage the expectation-setting process, guiding the agenda, ensuring the acceptability of both the process and its results, and monitoring the expectation statements per se. This management obligation falls on the executive unit, particularly the medical executive committee. Members of the committee who are employed by the hospital frequently bear most of the accountability for process control.

Timing and Extent of Expectation Development. Obviously, expectations are only of value if they help individual practitioners improve. Material improvement in behavior takes a substantial investment of resources and requires finite time. The tempo of expectation setting involves judging the need, the opportunity, and the resources. Need is often reflected in financial terms—loss of markets and revenue, unsatisfactory costs and profits, high premiums for malpractice insurance. Opportunity is measured by comparing actual practice to best practice, with attention to the real value of that difference. The goal of the strategy is not perfection, but remaining a leader in meeting exchange demands. On the other hand, complacency is self-defeating—it is considerably more difficult to catch up than to keep up. Well-run hospitals search for their most critical resource, whether it be leadership, organization structure, or information support. They seek to fully employ that resource but not to go beyond it. If that rate of speed is insufficient to meet market demands, they turn their attention to expanding the critical resource.

A well-run hospital concentrates its expectation-setting efforts on the areas of highest potential reward and limits them in order to avoid unnecessary frustration. Within these guidelines, the selection strategy can be broad, attempting an overall improvement by focusing on care elements central to most or all patients, or it can be specific, identifying particular risks or costs where improvement is possible.

Well-run hospitals will pursue broad and specific options at differing times. Specific strategies involve a few doctors and other professionals and a small set of patients and diseases. They are therefore easier to manage. Broad strategies involving several departments have great potential—"If everybody saves one-half an intensive care unit day per patient, the result will fund a linear accelerator"—but they have serious logistic and technical problems. The risks are analogous to the classic military problem of troop disposition: too long a line weakens the middle, while too short a line can be outflanked. *Focus,* or specificity, seems to be the usual choice for well-run conjoint staffs. It may be better to have three specific campaigns on ICU use in family practice, surgery, and internal medicine than one allegedly coordinated effort.

Management of the Expectation-Setting Process. The medical executive committee should guide the process of expectation setting by encouraging appropriate participation, setting time lines, and negotiating controversy. In general, expectations must be set by consensus among people who are materially affected. Leadership thus should go to the group or specialty with the central interest. It is wise insofar as possible to support the interest groups and curiosity of the clinical personnel.

There should be an annual review of progress and selection of new targets, preferably timed to precede the annual budget cycle, because the expectations influence intermediate product volume and cost forecasts. Committee or task force membership and agendas are selected simultaneously with the targets. The intellectual and professional reward of self-improvement is the most powerful motivator, and the second most powerful is the common need to respond to economic pressures. Good conjoint staff leadership frequently reminds its members of these rewards and is careful to reinforce them in the assignment process. Expected timetables for reports are set at the time of assignment, and foreseeable needs for consultation outside the unit are also identified.

The group charged with developing expectations should have access to all relevant professional skills. Single department or division assignment works well for surgery, where there are few territorial disputes; however, in medicine several specialties treat most common diseases. Nursing and support services can do many things on their own, but they will need to collaborate with each other and medicine on patient group protocols and other issues. An interdepartmental committee can review the information, resolve differences, and recommend the expectation to the departments or the medical executive committee.

One alternative to establishing an interdepartmental committee is allowing the modal specialty to pursue the expectation, perhaps with one mandatory consultation with others. An opposite alternative allows competing departments deliberate freedom—family practice and oncology may both pursue cancer care expectations. The conflicts which will inevitably arise can be accepted, rather than resolved, if it can be agreed that the two units are justified in using different criteria. One rational possibility is that the patients retained by family practice are not the same as those referred. Their needs might be viewed as including more holistic care, without intensive intervention. (It is interesting to think about the differences in expectations between the two departments on issues such as indications for referral to hospice care.)

The process of formalizing expectations can sometimes be speeded up by beginning with expectations proposed by authority and relying upon local review to resolve inconsistencies or difficulties. A growing number of authoritative expectations is now available in medical literature. In general, even if large sections are rewritten, starting with a possible expectation clarifies and speeds development of the finished work.

Expectation setting can be a divisive process. It is the responsibility of the medical executive committee and hospital management group to avoid unnecessary conflict by seeking areas where agreement appears obtainable and by abandoning major controversies. The amount of energy spent should be a function of the expectation's importance. The more frequently an expectation is relevant to care, and the greater the risk to the patient, the more time it is appropriate to spend on resolving differences. Many arguments are better abandoned; time changes all perspectives, and in the interim the debate can be ended by allowing alternatives, as discussed below.

Improvement of Expectation Statements. Any well-written expectation, clinical or not, should be unambiguous. This is easy if the action or outcome itself is unambiguous but difficult if the subject is vague, debated, or conditional. The problem of writing clinical expectations is that much of medicine is in the debated or conditional area. Relatively few elements of care are uniformly indicated or contraindicated. As a result, expectations can assess only a small part of the body of good medicine, and there is a danger of regimentation, standardizing what should be left conditional. There are four ways around this problem, and all are employed by the well-run hospital. They are incorporated in the expectation itself, through appropriate wording.

1. Optional or conditional activities can be clearly identified, with possible expectations left as suggestions.

2. Expectations can be applied to a sample of cases and an appropriate percentage of achievement specified. Since no doctor can always diagnose appendicitis, for example, a tolerance for a percentage of misdiagnosis is usually established. Sound laws of statistics show that, although any single case is disputable, diagnostic skill will be reflected over relatively small numbers of similar cases.

3. Expectations can incorporate what is usually but not always mandatory or contraindicated, with provisions for the attending physician to justify exceptions. While the justification required can be quite elaborate, it frequently is sufficient to

accept any evidence indicating that the doctor is aware of the expectation and is departing from it in good faith.

4. The expectation can be set separately on smaller, well-defined groups, where the indicated actions are less ambiguous. For example, patient age or comorbidity can be specified, or diseases can be more narrowly defined. A variation on this approach establishes **conditional expectations,** a branching logic to allow the conditions for certain actions to be incorporated.

The use of the fourth approach requires more data, both for setting the expectation and for monitoring it. As data capture becomes more common and data processing less expensive, this approach becomes more practical. The expectations of practice and their monitoring will become more elaborate and more refined as this occurs.

Special Considerations for Patient Group Protocols

Patient group protocols are the most extensive development in clinical expectations, and they constitute a challenge to the success of the conjoint medical staff. Patient group protocols specify the desired selection and use of intermediate products comprising the final product: that is, whether or not certain tests should be done, how the results should be used, how much time may elapse between events, how unsatisfactory results should be pursued, what the patient's condition should be at discharge or termination of treatment, and what steps should be taken to improve patient and family satisfaction. It is clear that patient group protocols rely heavily on the achievement of uniform intermediate products. Intermediate product protocols—the expectations which guide the clinical support services and nursing, discussed in chapters 12 and 13—address the question of whether the tests and treatments themselves were performed correctly.

At least in an informal and often in a formal sense, patient group protocols have existed since the great clinical-scientific advances of the late nineteenth century, when unanimity on certain responses to certain symptoms emerged. They specify certain actions as universally desirable, thereby foreclosing the doctor's judgment based on his or her examination of the individual patient. Although it may be said that science forecloses individual judgment, it may be more nearly accurate to say that science changes the domain in which judgment is appropriate.

The increasing interest in patient group protocols that has occurred since 1980 represents another shift in viewpoint about the domain of standardization. The domain of consensus is being extended rapidly, by patients and health insurance buyers rather than by professionals. It now includes economy and patient satisfaction as well as science. Patients' expectations of doctors and hospitals, reflected in malpractice decisions, have expanded steadily, with tacit public support. The Medicare payment system demands an expectation for the cost of each hospitalization by DRG, and designates the hospital as the enforcement vehicle. A less specific discipline is enforced by HMOs via capitation and the right of patients to change carriers, doctors, and hospitals annually; HMO providers often rely on specific protocols to attain the required economy and satisfaction. Often, PPOs and related insurance schemes specify key elements themselves, as is the case in preadmission certification or concurrent review of length of stay.

Scientific documentation of diagnostic and treatment alternatives is increasing rapidly. Expectations for physicians establish three categories of action: mandatory, optional or conditional, and contraindicated. Specific actions relating to prevention, diagnosis, treatment, and maintenance or rehabilitation are placed in a category. For example, a protocol for well-baby care would list as mandatory several specific immunizations for primary prevention and tests for secondary prevention. It might also mandate certain omissions, tests that had become obsolete, for example. A sophisticated protocol would list acceptable ranges for normal behavior and conditional steps to rule out disease suggested by the secondary prevention examinations. (Once disease is diagnosed, the baby is no longer "well" and care leaves the domain of the protocol.) It also would identify common concerns of parents and conditional responses to these. Certain actions would also be contraindicated. For example, to make sure the care was economical, an upper limit might be placed on the number of well-baby visits, and the frequency might be reduced as the child matured.

As is the case with individual medical decisions, the protocol might be incorrect. There is risk of both omission and commission; commission can include an unnecessary act or the wrong alternative. Even in the relatively simple well-baby example there are real dangers. Certain vaccines have proven ineffective, and certain tests have raised false or unnecessary concerns. If protocols are effectively used, these mistakes are universalized. Not only is a larger percentage of the patients put at risk, but the variety of physician actions which might reveal the error is suppressed. Thus clinical expectations in general, and final product protocols in particular, introduce an opportunity to do harm as well as good. The risk of protocols generally lies in overspecification, the suppression of individual variation which obscures the opportunity to improve.

Decision Theory and Support Service Selection. Conceptually, care is appropriate when the marginal cost of service is exactly equal to the marginal benefit, that is, when the last service ordered contributed more value through improved outcome than it cost, and the next service which might be ordered will contribute less than it costs. Real medical care proceeds in multiple and interacting logical sequences, but each considered step is a simple binary decision, to be answered either yes or no. There are thousands of such decisions, mostly answered no, in a given episode of care. Many considerations recur. That is, a laboratory test may be considered today and again tomorrow. The recurrence is often independent of the decision; whether or not the service was ordered today, it can be reconsidered tomorrow. The binary decision is reached by each doctor's internal calculus, an amalgam of her or his training and experience. Obviously, given the number of decisions and the difficulty of measuring the costs and benefits, that calculus must be fast, reliable, and robust.

There are usually costs and benefits to be evaluated for both possible answers. There are only a few easy decisions, those where one side heavily outweighs the other. For example, immunizations are almost always appropriate. For patients with severe diabetes, insulin is required. For most realistic problems, decisions are more complex, more numerous, and require faster response. When the costs include death or disability and the decisions must be made quickly, the skills of the physician are tested.

The doctor's evaluation centers on probabilities, since few things in medicine are certain. Thus a doctor treating a patient with a pain in the abdomen weighs first the probability that it is self-limiting, knowing that most afflictions in fact cure themselves in a few hours or days. Next, he or she considers alternative interventions: drugs or surgery for direct treatment versus laboratory tests, imaging, or optical scope for refinement of the diagnosis. Having selected the most promising of these, the question is, "What are the probable outcomes of proceeding and not proceeding and their relative values?" It appears that the doctor's decision-making process can be modelled as decision theory, although it is known that the actions of real doctors are considerably more complicated than the theory.[2] Taking the most drastic of the interventions, surgery, the possibilities look something like the list in figure 11.1.

The figure shows that the decision depends upon the probability that the patient has appendicitis or a disease treatable with the same surgery and upon the values placed on the costs of surgery and the costs of waiting. The question can be readdressed hourly until the patient either improves or is operated upon. For a given set of symptoms, the surgeon assumes a certain probability of appendicitis and certain values for the costs of doing and not doing surgery. He or she is indifferent when

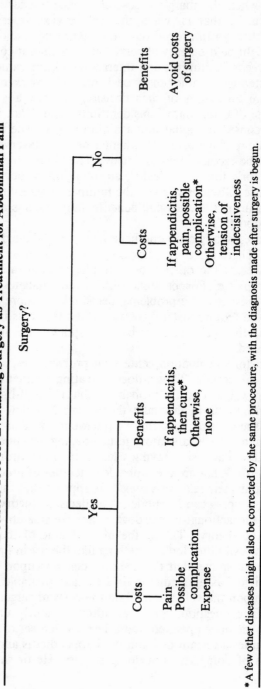

Figure 11.1

Decision Tree for Evaluating Surgery as Treatment for Abdominal Pain

Surgery?

Yes

Costs
Pain
Possible complication
Expense

Benefits
If appendicitis, then cure*
Otherwise, none

No

Costs
If appendicitis, pain, possible complication*
Otherwise, tension of indecisiveness

Benefits
Avoid costs of surgery

* A few other diseases might also be corrected by the same procedure, with the diagnosis made after surgery is begun.

(Probability of Appendicitis) (Value of Cure)
+ (Probability Not Appendicitis) (Cost of Surgery)
= (Probability of Appendicitis) (Cost of Delay)
+ (Probability Not Appendicitis) (Value of Cure).

If we let

p = Probability of Appendicitis at the Point of Indifference
$(1 - p)$ = Probability Not Appendicitis
V = Value of Cure
I = Cost of Surgery (or other intervention)
D = Cost of Delay
(D and I will always be less than 0),

then the equation is

$$(V + I)\, p + I\, (1 - p) = Dp + V(1-p)$$

or

$$p = (V - I)/(2V - D).$$

It may be helpful to assign some arbitrary dollar values to these concepts. Using negative signs for costs, let us assume that cure is worth $10,000, surgery is worth $- $5000, and delay is worth $- $1000. Then

$$p = (\$10,000 + \$5000)/(2 \times \$10,000 + 1000)$$
$$= (\$15,000)/(\$21,000)$$
$$= .72,$$

or slightly less than a 3 in 4 chance of appendicitis. Higher cost of delay, lower cost of intervention, and greater value of recovery lead to lower probability of appendicitis required to justify surgery. If delay is fatal and intervention is lifesaving, infinite value might be assigned. Then one would operate for *any* probability of disease, no matter how small, and, in fact, medical treatment for life-threatening emergencies is administered on almost that basis.

Like most models, this one simplifies reality and is not entirely correct. Few doctors consciously review probabilities in the way the model suggests, and even fewer would attempt to estimate and solve an equation or a diagram like figure 11.1. Evidence suggests, however, that even the simple form shown here predicts real behavior. For a very low cost intervention, say a $5 laboratory test, if the delay costs are high there is a strong predisposition to do the test. Even if there were no cost of delay, if the test contributes substantial value it will be done for a low probability of a positive result. This is also consistent with reality. Finally, in the actual case of appendectomy, better understanding of the costs and benefits, and, in particular, better control of the costs of delaying surgery, has led to a steady decline in the number of appendectomies performed and in the number which are done but reveal no appendicitis.

Use of Decision Theory To Improve the Ordering Decision. Decision theory suggests three routes to improving the contribution of medicine to health, that is, to improving the appropriateness of care.

1. Increasing the value of intervention:
   a. Finding a new intervention
   b. Increasing the variety of cases for which an intervention is appropriate
   c. Improving the discriminatory power of diagnostic tests, that is, the ability to detect whether or not the patient has a certain disease or condition
   d. Improving the results of therapy
2. Reducing the cost of intervention:
   a. Reducing the danger of harm to the patient
   b. Reducing the resources consumed by the intervention
   c. Increasing the variety of cases for which an intervention is appropriate (Because many interventions require substantial fixed costs, increases in the volume of an intervention can reduce costs.)
   d. Reducing the pain or discomfort associated with an intervention
3. Reducing the cost of delay:
   a. Speeding or improving the transmission of orders for intervention
   b. Reducing delays between orders and intervention
   c. Reducing conflict between interventions
   d. Reducing preparation failures
   e. Minimizing intervention failures and repetitions

The support service itself improves the appropriateness of care when it adds a new intervention or increases the effectiveness of an existing one; reduces the dangers, expenses, or discomfort associated with either intervention or delay; or reduces the cost associated with delay. The attending physician improves appropriateness when he or she makes fewer selections with negative value, reaches the correct alternative faster, or includes more interventions with a positive value. The patient group protocols support better care when they make these actions easier. It is worth noting that they do not improve care by detecting inappropriate decisions except insofar as they prevent future errors.

Logic for Selecting Patient Group Protocols. Hospitals must obviously be highly selective in their protocol development. Whole medical texts are devoted to the protocol elements of a single disease or disease group. Hospital protocols must be limited to important diseases and conditions and to those items most likely to be sources of variation in behavior. Many subjects are easily ruled out. Items which invariably occur or never occur need no formalization. Items which have little or no cost and no discernible effect on the outcome are too trivial to formalize. Items on which no consensus can be reached represent unresolved questions that for the present cannot be formalized. The hospital must focus upon those items where substantial value is at stake and substantial variation can be reduced. *Value* in this context is the ratio of benefit to cost. Thus an item is appropriate for incorporation into hospital patient group protocols if it reduces variation in a manner that affects the outcome (or benefit) for the resource use (or cost).

Unfortunately benefits and costs are not measured in ways which make it easy to apply these concepts. Well-managed hospitals tend to focus first on variation in benefit, particularly unexpected death, disability, complication, patient dissatisfaction, or risk of malpractice. These concerns are given primacy over costs; protocols are selected which minimize the patient's and the hospital's exposure. These methods may or may not be more costly than the original norm. In any case, the study of quality issues frequently reveals cost-saving opportunities as a byproduct.

In controlling costs, the well-managed hospital attempts to build consensus about care of high-cost patient groups and high-cost elements within those groups. Likely targets are identified in a four-step procedure:

1. Patient groups are ranked by total (not average) annual costs consumed.

2. High-cost groups are studied to identify those with high variability in members' costs.

3. Within each selected group, the total annual cost is subdivided by element of care, and costs are ranked by element.

4. High-cost elements are studied to identify those with high variability among patients. The range, and particularly the minimum, of current performance is a useful measure of variability. The maximum usually involves only a very small number of cases, and the norm, or modal, performance has no merit if the minimum is still safe and effective.

Value can also be extended to the specification of individual items. Value is related principally to two factors, patient satisfaction and the maintenance of optimal health. Patient satisfaction builds long-term revenue and helps ensure success for the doctor and the hospital. The maintenance of optimal health results in lower lifetime expenditures for illness. Obviously both goals are desirable for patients covered under capitation insurance. Both are also highly ethical; they incorporate the noblest virtues of the healing professions. Identifying opportunities for improvement by developing expectations is more difficult. The following four areas may suggest avenues:

1. *Data on adverse effects, untoward outcomes, incidents, complaints and malpractice*—The data are compiled from a variety of sources and are studied for common patterns of disease, physician, specialty, or hospital department by risk management groups.

2. *Patient and family satisfaction survey*—So long as representative samples are involved, this information can also indicate fruitful avenues. (When self-selected or haphazard responses occur, variation in response may appear as variation in satisfaction, making investigation less profitable.)

3. *Readmission data or total annual costs of claims per patient*—Optimal management of chronic degenerative diseases, for example, may be that which minimizes the number of hospitalizations for the population for the year or for a specified period preceding death. Hospital files are not generally automated to recover this information and may be incomplete. Insurance claims files are a better source; however, even specific cases of readmission, relapse, or recurrence can suggest opportunities.

4. *Clinical literature and the subjective opinion of respected clinicians*—Certain styles of medical practice are clearly more cost-effective than others, and they should certainly prevail in the absence of dissent or contradictory evidence.

Monitoring and Achieving Expectations

Traditional versus Conjoint Views

If the conjoint medical staff pursues the model of building consensus around clinical expectations incorporated in intermediate and patient group protocols, it will depart substantially from traditional models. The most notable change may occur in the monitoring process. Traditional models of medical staff organization devote considerable time to monitoring for compliance on a limited set of stable expectations. Conjoint staffs will learn to build consensus on an expanding set of clinical protocols. They will reward far more often than they punish. Their monitoring will emphasize three roles:

1. Indicating areas where development of further expectations is likely to be fruitful
2. Identifying instances where performance has exceeded expectation, to be considered for reward
3. Flagging and documenting instances of repeated exception, where disciplinary sanctions must be used

These expanded roles will require a stronger clinical information system, characterized by flexibility, extensiveness of data, coordination of data, and analytic capability. The use of the information system in identifying and establishing expanded expectations has been addressed earlier in this chapter, and the requirements are discussed in chapter 9.

Improvement of Individual Performance under the Conjoint Model

Power of Self-Review. The goal of the expectations is to change behavior, and the best time to change behavior is *before* an action or decision has been taken. The true goal of expectation setting is universal acceptance and compliance. When this occurs, the individual professionals monitor themselves, as they do for most professional actions. This is the most important form of monitoring, because it is cheap, nearly universal, and subject to more rapid correction than any other. Formal and group monitoring efforts are never more than complements to this central self-monitoring activity.

In the well-run hospital, monitoring and expectation setting are intertwined. Relying heavily on education, encouragement, and support to prevent departure from expectations means that only a few individual violations occur and that only a small, low-profile activity needs to be devoted to correcting them before they become widely known and erode the social pressures for conformance. In addition, monitoring detects exceptionally good performance, and the conjoint staff organizes the formal rewards to recognize it.

Use of Rewards and Sanctions. The traditional staff had rewards, but they were informally applied, largely intangible, and in some cases even invisible. Good doctors on traditional staffs had personal satisfaction, the admiration of their colleagues, and occasionally a higher rate of referral and thus the economic ability to support higher fees. Although fee variation may be lowered under the conjoint model, collegial admiration can be made more public, and tangible rewards can be increased through opportunities to participate in joint ventures, incentive payments, salaries, and opportunities to reduce the costs of practice. The conjoint staff will compensate its leaders appropriately and will select them from among good doctors. It will establish office arrangements and support for economical, high-quality practice, and it will give priority to those who support its concept of good medicine. Through HMOs and PPOs, it will provide direct incentive payments to successful practitioners.

The clinical expectation takes the carrot and stick approach—the strongest possible tangible and intangible rewards for cooperation and predictable sanctions for noncompliance. The sanctions are virtually automatic in procedural matters such as incomplete charts. The information system must check procedural compliance routinely and flag violations promptly. Little human judgment is involved, although issues such as illness and data system errors must be considered.

Substantive matters are handled quite differently. It is assumed that every professional wants to do his or her best for the patient. Repeated departure from standard suggests a potentially complex situation requiring investigation and sophisticated judgment. The monitoring system identifies the problem, supports the investigation, and designates the person or group accountable for resolution. For both procedural and substantive areas, two or more levels of judgment and accountability are desirable. One, the primary monitor, is normally expected to follow through with appropriate action. The second acts only on request or in the event of failure of the first, or in the case of repeated violations by the same individual involving several different primary monitors.

Guidelines for Monitoring. The conjoint model will be much more a model of line hierarchical accountability than the traditional model. Reliance on a long list of collateral organization structures, mostly committees, will be replaced by reliance on the individual attending physician, responsibility center managers in the other clinical areas, and the medical specialty groups as accountability centers.

Several guidelines support efficient monitoring:

— The monitoring process begins with expectation setting, in the sense that any formal expectation must include a way in which it can be monitored. (This requirement is a major factor in reducing the staff's monitoring work load.)

— The information system supports the monitoring process. Monitoring can be universal, continuous sampling, intermittent sampling, or ad hoc sampling, depending upon the cost of acquiring data and the value of the potential improvement. It also can be manual or partially or fully automated. Whatever the case, the information system must deliver complete, prompt reports on both achievement and nonachievement.

— Information is reported first to the individual doctor or other professional, who is allowed time to respond before any further action is taken. Similarly, the primary monitor is allowed time to respond before the secondary monitor intervenes.

— Clinical chiefs and hospital line managers participate personally at key parts of the monitoring activity, but all other work is done by staff employees or, increasingly, computers.

— Errors, or failure to achieve expectations, are used in three ways:

  • To devise educational programs for the staff generally
  • To guide systems revisions, including new work methods and equipment and revisions of expectations
  • To pursue a program for correction with individual practitioners

— Individual corrections programs are designed to correct defects rather than to punish.

— Rewards and recognition are provided for exceptional achievement and often for the effort of monitoring itself.

Overview of the Traditional Model

Conceptual Foundations. Traditional medical staffs monitor their own performance by relying upon individuals, expecting a very high level of compliance. Substantive violation is reviewed by a complex set of committees (described below) which are usually responsible for setting expectations also. The medical staff officers and leaders usually establish this collateral organization of committees. Only occasionally do department chiefs, service chiefs, and medical staff vice-presidents act as responsibility center managers in the traditional sense. They have an obligation to intervene in the patient care activities of individual doctors in emergencies,[3] but they avoid routine use of their authority. In contrast, nonmedical professionals use their senior members frequently to provide direct advice, as, for example, the CFO and the external auditor do on accounting, or nursing managers do on nursing.

Doctors' avoidance of individual supervisors is a matter of style rather than a fundamental revision of closed system theory. This style is consistent with respected and effective theories of human behavior in organizations. Doctors' preference for group-oriented monitoring styles occurs even in the most structured staffs, such as closed-panel HMOs.[4] It appears to have at least two underlying causes. One is that the social concepts of colleague and supervisor are inimical. Doctors are simply uncomfortable pursuing corrective action with their colleagues. The other is that medical practice can be impaired by excessive standardization and second-guessing. The danger of interfering unproductively in the complex doctor-patient relationship calls for caution.

The organization theories supporting this style of behavior hold that help sought by the individual is more valuable than that imposed by the organization.[5] The best traditional medical staffs encourage superior clinicians to respond on an informal basis. In what are sometimes called "corridor consultations," respected "clinical opinion leaders"[6] provide informal advice on patient management which may be more influential than the comments of a formally designated leader.

Despite the persuasiveness of these arguments, it appears that more effective individual response must be achieved in order to meet external exchange demands. Public concern with the quality of care is expressed both through malpractice litigation and through the desire for public display of quality statistics. Concern over costs and willingness to provide incentives for reducing costs are now well demonstrated. It appears likely that patients will demand quality and amenities as well. Hospitals and physician groups which cannot meet this demand at a competitive price will face economic difficulty.

An example of the weakness of traditional staffs is presented by the troublesome problem of impaired physicians. Even on the best staffs, doctors get old, sick, and distracted by personal and financial difficulties. Physicians are more susceptible to mental illness and substance abuse than the population at large. Each of these hazards reduces their clinical effectiveness. The prevalence of these problems is not known precisely, but available evidence suggests that from 5 to 15 percent of doctors have noticeable impairment. This means that most hospitals will have several such problems at any given time.

Well-run hospitals support rather than punish the impaired doctor. They provide direct clinical assistance and supervision, and they insist that the doctor's underlying problems be treated. Only after these measures fail do they withdraw staff membership. In order to respond in this constructive way, the staff must be able to identify these problems promptly. The traditional model, with its emphasis on committees, divided or obscure accountability, and corrective rather than constructive responses, has great difficulty doing so.

A conjoint model emphasizing specialty group accountability is more promising. It should be the function of line clinical managers (in medicine, department and section chiefs) to spot and protect the impaired physician and his or her patients. Chiefs can intervene where necessary more quickly, more sensitively, and more effectively than a committee. Appeals might be heard by a standing or ad hoc appeals committee.

If committees are used to handle problems of impairment, they should be designed for that purpose alone and should operate nearly anonymously. Using traditional committees or conjoint committees which are also involved in expectation setting is burdensome on members' time, unduly adversarial, inflexible in the kinds of sanctions and responses that can be used, and distracting from the more important activities of those committees.

Clinical Committees. The result of reliance on the collateral organization is that a large hospital can have several dozen committees charged with setting expectations and monitoring collective performance on specific elements of quality and economy. The committees are often organized around medical staff departments but involvement of other professions has increased in recent years. Well-managed hospitals are encouraging that trend, but the corrective functions undertaken by these committees discourage candor in the presence of other professions.

The following are traditional committees:

— *Tissue committee.* This committee is responsible for the identification of cases in which the pathologist's diagnosis, based solely on examination of tissue removed, fails to support the diagnosis leading to surgery, suggesting that the surgery could have been avoided. The committee establishes criteria for evaluating each such case and for judging the acceptability of each surgeon's overall diagnostic record. (This committee was prominent in the early activities of the American College of Surgeons, in the 1930s. Although still a contributor to surgical quality control, its significance has waned with the development of a much wider variety of procedures and more precise criteria for preoperative diagnosis.)

— *Surgical committee.* The surgical committee has replaced the tissue committee in importance. It reviews a variety of measures, such as preoperative diagnostic test requirements and routines for postoperative care, relating to the quality of surgical care generally. Its reviews are frequently for educational purposes or criteria development and are oriented toward specific diagnoses or procedures. Membership should include representatives of the major support services for surgical care—anesthesia, laboratory, operating room, postoperative nursing, rehabilitation therapies—as well as others indicated by the hospital's organization. Large hospitals must use subcommittees. The *operating room committee* is often a subcommittee.

— *Medical committee.* Analogous to the surgical committee, the medical committee reviews nonsurgical cases for educational topics, development of criteria, and procedures. Development of criteria has lagged because of the complexity of medical care. Membership should include nursing, laboratory, diagnostic imaging, radiation therapy, rehabilitation therapies, cardiopulmonary diagnosis, and pharmacy. Subcommittees usually follow the major subspecialties; cardiology and oncology include much of the inpatient activity.

— *Other departmental committees.* Analogous committees for family practice, obstetrics, pediatrics, psychiatry, and subspecialties are used in larger hospitals. One advantage of departmentalization is that it groups common diseases and treatments. The use of departmentalized committees for monitoring not only spreads the work load, but increases the scientific consensus which can be obtained. As a result, it tends to improve both the efficiency and the effectiveness of the committees themselves. There must be enough activity and sufficiently interested physicians in each area to provide an effective forum.

— *Mortality committee.* This traditional interdepartmental committee reviews all deaths occurring in the hospital in order to identify preventable contributing factors, occasionally including behavior of individual physicians. Review is more effective if it can be developed within each specialty. Obstetrics now assumes that death will never occur and holds extensive review in the rare event that it does; pediatrics can make similar assumptions except for newborns. Postsurgical and posttrauma deaths should be reviewed by surgery and anesthesia. Medical deaths include many very old patients for whom no prevention is appropriate; in such cases, the mortality committee may play only a secondary role.

— *Utilization review committee.* Designed as a primary controller of utilization, this committee has generally encountered much difficulty. The line organization is preferable for monitoring individual exceptions, and the clinical departments for establishing patient group protocols.

The emerging role of the utilization review committee may be to establish the strategy and plan for clinical expectation setting generally, as a subcommittee of the medical executive committee. It should monitor a variety of issues related to effectiveness or economy of care, principally length of stay and very expensive therapy or diagnosis, such as ICUs, tomographic imaging (CAT scan), and some drugs. The committee may still help the medical specialty or department involved to set appropriate expectations for the indications, procedures, and reporting of results involved in these expensive items.

— *Infections committee.* This committee establishes criteria and monitoring systems for nosocomial (hospital-acquired) infections and pursues methods of controlling or eliminating them. Infection control frequently involves nursing, other clinical professions, and the plant system. It uses epidemiological methods to monitor infections, which are reported to it by both nursing and medicine using a unique reporting system. The epidemiological methods used are also applicable to risk management. The infections committee may become a subcommittee of risk management in the future.

— *Emergency care committee.* Expectations covering quality and cost for all professions working in the emergency room, as well as arrangements with outside agencies such as police, fire, and ambulance services, are the responsibility of the emergency care committee.

— *Disaster preparedness committee.* This committee is responsible for the hospital's plan for meeting civil and presumably also military disasters, occasions upon which a very large influx of seriously ill or injured patients must be accommodated. Disaster preparedness involves every system of the hospital. Monitoring is accomplished by walk-throughs and simulations, which must be held at least annually and evaluated by the committee.

— *Pharmaceuticals committee.* The **formulary,** or list of drugs the hospital will inventory, and rules governing prescription and administration of these drugs are determined by the pharmaceuticals committee. Intravenous fluids and **controlled substances** (narcotics) are usually included. Nursing, pharmacy, and medical staff are all involved in these activities. Although this committee would not directly set patient group protocols on drug usage, its actions clearly must be coordinated with them.

The committee has tended to address the forms, brands, and prices of drugs required. It is also moving to important questions of drug interactions, substitutions, and clinical contraindications, and to supporting the pharmacy department in a consulting role. Given the complexity of modern drug therapy, there is substantial opportunity in this area.

— *Medical records committee.* This committee is responsible for the content and organization of medical records, including timely completion of them. Nursing, the medical records department, information systems, and finance are frequently involved, as are doctors. The committee is moving to an information systems design role, guiding the measures of performance and the information system providing them.

— *Risk management committee.* Risk management functions can be performed by employed staff reporting to the chief of staff or to the medical executive committee. An advisory committee can be established because of the importance of the activity to the medical staff. The committee's functions consist of:

- Epidemiological analyses of incidents (that is, events in which a patient, visitor, or employee may have been injured) reported by nursing, medicine, or any supervisory personnel

- Study and revision of procedures to reduce hazards identified by epidemiological analysis, observation, or reported experience of other hospitals

- Compilation of actions of various committees evaluating performance of individual physicians in order to report to the credentials committee prior to annual review of privileges

— *Others.* Hospitals establish a number of other standing and ad hoc committees where the advice of several professions is important to maintaining quality and economy of care. Dietetics committees address special diets, construction and equipment committees plan facilities, forms committees design forms, and so on.

Toward a New Structure. The number of these committees suggests that doctors may have a reasonable case when they complain that they are "committeed to death." The variety of them, and particularly the lack of a common taxonomy, suggests that redundancy, conflict, and omission are clear dangers. There is reason to think the system is too poorly structured to survive, but a clear alternative is difficult to design. The problem appears inherent in the complexity of the hospital itself: patients with varying needs make selective use of a disparate collection of services. The well-managed hospital is learning to use patient group protocols to identify the needs of similar patients and intermediate product protocols to ensure uniform service.

Separately, these two steps leave too many problems unaddressed. The essential integration of them comes through the medical department committees with both physician and nonphysician membership. Without question, such coordination is an important source of efficiency and economy. For example:

— Each profession encounters specific problems with patients requiring guidance. Individually, these are the responsibility of the attending physician, but common responses are needed for groups of patients (for example, ischemic heart disease patients receiving physical therapy).

— There are issues in work methods or equipment which go beyond the skills of the profession involved.

— There are interactions among various modalities (diet, drugs, X ray, laboratory tests and so on) that must be identified and managed.

— Many care activities are sequential, thus the timing and ordering of clinical events affect overall length of stay.

— Patient compliance with treatment routines depends upon instruction, assistance with logistic problems, and assistance with emotional problems. Several different professions are involved in this process. Their concerns should appear coordinated to the patient in order to reinforce the message. (In chronic disease such as hypertension and diabetes, compliance is a major factor in reducing complications and hospitalizations.)

— Care of the dying involves substantial stress for professionals as well as the patient and his or her family. Management of this stress is becoming a collective effort, often incorporating the clergy as well as the employed team and the attending physician. (The issue may be important in economic as well as humanistic terms: about one-quarter of all Medicare expenditures occur in the final year of life.)

Analysis of the kinds of problems that must be addressed indicates that medical department–oriented committees with multiple professional membership will emerge as the central expectation-setting and monitoring bodies. Such committees may follow major hospital departments as well, and integration may be accomplished by appointing members jointly. Risk management, utilization review, infections and the more topical committees will either atrophy or assume a secondary role in support of the medical executive.

There are two potential failings of this proposition, even in well-run hospitals:

1. *The committees are profession-centered rather than patient-centered.* As a result, they are at risk of missing many coordination questions which arise around the unique impact of illness on each patient.

2. *The periphery seems to get more attention than the center.* Nursing has physical control of the patient, responsibility for delivery of many other modalities, most of the patient teaching and emotional support responsibility, and the most extensive family contact. The typical head nurse, however, deals with a half-dozen clinical departments with no clear committee or individual resource. Social work is similarly orphaned in most hospitals.

Solutions to the latter problem seem to have emerged where only one or two medical specialties have patients on a particular nursing unit; maternity, neonatology, and psychiatry commonly meet those conditions. Unfortunately, the expense of dedicating nursing units is exorbitant except for the largest hospitals. Most hospitals can segregate their patients only approximately, and then into larger groups such as medicine and surgery. At that, the scheduling system, which maintains the predictable censuses so important in controlling the cost of nursing care, tends to do so by scattering nonsurgical patients onto surgical floors.

One management scheme for improving the quality and effectiveness of nursing care and its coordination with other professions may be to designate specific nursing liaison responsibility to salaried medical chiefs. Physician managers have recently emerged in intensive care and emergency. Alternatively, nursing might have several management committees, representing the major medical specialties, to coordinate it with medicine.

Solutions to the profession-centered focus must come from committee design and the information system. At least one member of each clinical committee should be encouraged to play an ombudsman role. Relevant information on patient satisfaction, from surveys, complaints, and informal reports, should be routinely summarized for each clinical committee.

Measures and Information Systems for Clinical Performance

The subtlety and variety of human beings and their illnesses generate a potentially overwhelming amount of information. Codifying and quantifying data have been and continue to be a central intellectual task, representing with a few keystrokes the patient, the disease, the diagnosis and evaluation, the treatment, and the result. The demanding task of classifying diseases is representative: the current classification is the ninth international revision,[7] and there is active debate about the best means of grouping the several thousand conditions and afflictions which it identifies.[8] Management-oriented doctors like Codman,[9] Mac-Eachern,[10] Lembcke,[11] and Slee[12] have struggled with the problems of measuring patient care. Their concepts, formalized and extended by Donabedian,[13] have been widely challenged, but until recently data-processing capability has lagged behind them. Information-processing technology has reached a useful level. The gap narrows as medicine itself becomes more precise, classification methods are improved, and data-processing capability increases. Clinical performance measurement will be revised continuously over the next two decades.

The challenge in designing clinical information systems is to improve the value of care by assisting the clinical professions to select and provide the optimal intervention for each patient. The system that could do this would have four parts:

1. *Prevention*—prompting of prospective users to prevent oversight or error. Examples of this include computer screens and paper forms which suggest the information or criteria applicable to a given intervention.

2. *Monitoring*—identification of compliance with established expectations, with the capability of describing and analyzing noncompliance.

3. *Expectation design and improvement*—presentation of retrospective comparisons and trends that support revision of existing expectations or the formulation of new ones.

4. *Education*—methods of reporting which summarize arguments for existing or proposed expectations.

Manual systems for these purposes have existed for decades in hospitals. Automation introduces a substantial improvement in the speed, precision, and comprehensiveness with which these activities can be pursued.

At present, it is possible to automate readily most of the quantifiable data in the medical record. Laboratory results, drug orders, X-ray orders and some results, patient acuity, physiological capability, kinds of surgery and other invasive treatments, and, most important, diagnosis, have been scaled and can be computerized economically if accounts receivable records require coded descriptions of illness and treatment.

The current limitations are in the accuracy and completeness of the classification and coding systems, in the spread of hardware and software necessary to capture and analyze data, and in the development of expectations from available information.

Community hospitals need to utilize existing measures more effectively in expectations development. Many hospitals have hardware, software, and stored information which they have not yet assimilated and translated into useful expectations. Developing human organizations and information systems for expectation setting is a more rewarding starting point than investment in hardware, software, or classification improvement.

The following discussion reviews cost measures, quality measures, and systems design for improving clinical expectations.

Cost Measurement

Measures should be available for both costs and quality and for all three types of clinical expectation: activities, intermediate product protocols, and patient group protocols. Resource or cost measures are generally acquired from the accounting system; the accounts receivable system, the cost accounting system, and the budgeting system are used.

Sources for Counts of Care Activities. The critical element in the cost of final products is the quantities of various activities and intermediate products. The cost of patient care can be viewed as the sums of activities (blood gas examinations or doses of antibiotics), grouped to intermediate products (laboratory or pharmacy) and finally to similar cases (all patients with coronary artery disease). One may begin by assuming that any activity which is eliminated without identifiably increasing the risk of unfavorable outcomes is cost-effective. Counts of each activity are necessary. These come from the patient billing, or accounts receivable, system. Systems now being marketed can specify and store detail well beyond the foreseeable needs of most hospitals. The starting point for improvement, therefore, is a detailed billing record which can link the activity counts to the diagnosis or treatment group. More advanced work will require increasingly precise cost estimates.

Sources for Unit Costs. Unit cost estimates, and forecasts of unit costs under proposed conditions, are constructed from the financial accounting system of the hospital. This system records resources used by type (*natural accounts,* such as labor, services, and supplies) and responsibility center (*functional accounts,* such as emergency room, hematology laboratory, and housekeeping). To estimate the cost of a single activity, such as a test for high-density lipids (HDLs) in the blood, the classification system must be very precise. Further, the labor and equipment times devoted to HDLs must be recorded exactly. Most important, the real questions involve not today's, but tomorrow's cost of HDLs and so must come from the budget, not the history of costs: "What will be the savings if we reduce HDLs by 30 percent?" Forecasting requires not only patient billing systems and financial accounting systems, but also strong budgeting systems.

Hardware and software capability now exist in cost-accounting and flexible budgeting systems to support the several hundred responsibility centers required. In well-run hospitals, the accounting system can give reasonable cost estimates for intermediate product and major activity groups, such as blood tests, with some ability to forecast costs of changes in volume. Specific activities, such as testing for HDLs in the blood, usually require ad hoc cost studies. These are relatively easy to perform in limited numbers.

Well-run hospitals can now provide most cost data necessary for clinical expectations, but special studies or estimates will be required for activities or situations that depart dramatically from normal operations.

Quality and Benefit Measurement

Quality and benefit measures are still not quantified to the degree that accounting costs are. Process and outcomes measures are more valuable than structural ones. Process measures usually contribute to activity, intermediate product, and final product measurement, while outcomes are used mainly in final product or patient group expectations.

Sources of Quality Measures. The normal sources of quality and benefit measures are as follows:

1. *Routine departmental records and data,* such as laboratory quality control statistics, radiology machine logs, patient schedules, and charge vouchers. These are increasingly automated, but specific plans are needed to ensure retention of detail for historical analysis.

2. *Routine medical records,* which contain patient descriptions, orders, reports, medical notes, nursing notes, outcomes, and dispositions. Notes and most reports are not yet automated.

3. *Sampling surveys,* such as nursing quality audits and patient satisfaction surveys. These are ongoing or periodic and are distinguished from routine data by the fact that they cover less than the full universe of events.

4. *Incidents and noncompliance reports,* such as reports of accidents, equipment failures, and oversights. These are nonrepresentative counts or descriptions. One should not infer that all similar cases are reported.

5. *Special surveys,* which are conducted on a one-time basis.

The preferred source, both for cost and accuracy, is always routine records. However, many items used in measuring quality are too complex for routine assessment. Measurement costs mount when nonroutine sources are used, and the rule that the value of real changes in behavior should exceed the cost of the expectation monitoring system still applies.

Outcomes Measures. Outcomes measures of the quality of the final product usually assess aspects of the patient's condition on discharge. The clinical performance measurement system should record outcomes and produce them at any level of aggregation, from the individual patient to the entire patient population of the hospital. The measures available include:

1. *Counts of negative results,* for example, deaths, hospital-acquired infections, complications, and adverse effects.

2. *Tissue verification of clinical diagnosis,* that is, examination by pathologists of the tissue removed in surgery (to verify preoperative diagnosis) or in the postmortem examination (to verify all diagnoses).

3. *Patient and family satisfaction,* determined through questionnaires covering all aspects of hospitalization, but identifying contributions of individual professions or services as clearly as possible.

4. *Placement at discharge,* whether home, ambulatory care, home care, other hospital, nursing home, or other.

5. *Postdischarge course,* which would note any readmission, complication, or deterioration.

6. *Subjective assessment of condition,* for example, cured, improved, stable with reduced function, terminal.

7. *Objective assessment of condition,* using various scales of physiological function, such as scales of laboratory values for critical physiological function or scales of ability to perform functions of daily living.

Outcomes measures, while useful, present serious difficulties:

— For outpatient care, there is no clear point at which to assess "outcome," because care is and should be continuous.

— Most hospital patients, probably better than 9 out of 10, survive hospitalization without measurable negative results. Even in the few cases where negative results occur, the clinical performance implications differ drastically, for example, between cases where death is inescapable and cases where total recovery should always occur.

— Laboratory verification of diagnosis after surgery has become steadily less discriminating. "Disease" is frequently a matter of degree, and the contribution of surgery hinges on several factors beyond the degree of disease present in the specific tissue. (For example, hysterectomies, cholecystectomies, arthroscopies, and joint replacements are justified as much on contribution to the patient's functioning as on the degree of disease present.)

— Subjective measurement of outcomes is difficult and expensive to do reliably. Objective measurement, at the current capability, is relevant to only a small fraction of patients.

— Patient satisfaction, while relatively easy to assess and quite valid in terms of such marketing factors as compliance and reenrollment, reflects little about the technical quality of care.

— Finally, all outcomes measures share the problem of dependence on factors well beyond the doctor's control. The patient's general physical and emotional condition, affected by genetics and style of life, often makes the difference between successful and unsuccessful treatment.

The implication of these limitations is that most evaluations of care must rely upon process. The few available outcomes measures will be used most effectively to evaluate the process expectations and only rarely to evaluate the care itself.

Process Measures. Most process measures are counts or percentages of attributes. The process measurement has two components: an expectation reflecting consensus about care (for example, "Patients undergoing surgery with general anesthetic must have a history and physical examination for cardiopulmonary disease recorded") and counts of exposure and compliance (for example, 115 patients received general anesthetic; 110 of them had appropriate records). (Less commonly, the process measure is continuous; for example, hematocrit for group samples of normal women should have means of 42 percent and standard deviations of 2.5 percent.)

Process measures should be well documented, easily measured, scientifically noncontroversial, and flexible enough to cover most cases. The typical doctor treating the typical patient anticipates nearly universal compliance. Expectations can be improved through study of the relatively rare noncompliance or recognition of comparative, scientific, or subjective opportunities. A major use of the information system is to provide evidence of how specific processes contribute to the outcome. Although scientific research usually supports the change of critical expectations, many internal proposals for revision require data on number of cases, costs, patterns of various care givers, and disease-specific outcomes.

Reporting and Use of Clinical Expectations

Contribution of Automation to Information System Support. The functions of the information system supporting clinical expectations can be understood as capture, storage, retrieval, and analysis. These functions can be performed by automated or manual systems. The contribution of automation is as follows:

— *Capture.* Encoding and electronic recording of information permit convenient communication and retrieval. The costs of capture are generally justified by immediate improvements in speed and accuracy of communication. Storage, retrieval, and analysis for clinical assessment are frequently byproducts of information capture for accounting needs. Automated capture of clinical activity makes two vital contributions: it provides readily accessible files for study of new expectations, and it permits monitoring to prevent rather than correct departures.

— *Storage.* Retention of data in electronic form reduces the need to discard data and facilitates retrieval of previously unmanageable quantities of data. Storage problems are being addressed both by improved file design and storage procedures and by data base management systems designed to handle unforeseen problems of recovery.

— *Retrieval.* Retrieval systems must be able to locate, isolate, and recover data from the hospital's own historic files and from comparative or supplementary sources. Data from different files must be related or merged in order to address the question at hand. A key development in information systems recently was the ability to retrieve data without advance planning, made possible by data base management systems.

— *Analysis.* The ability to reduce data to useful comparative or descriptive summaries, test hypotheses, forecast, and present results in readable text, mathematical, or graphic form is essential for analysis. These capabilities are used for activities other than clinical performance and are widely available in statistical and spread sheet software. Graphics capability is also important and is easily obtained. These analytic tools assist in the development and evaluation of new expectations.

The general goal is to automate as much measurement of clinical performance as is cost-effective at any given time. Cost-effectiveness is enhanced by meeting multiple information needs simultaneously. (These issues are discussed more extensively in chapter 9.)

Monitoring and Detection of Statistical Error. There are two monitoring uses of clinical performance measures, prospective and retrospective. Prospective uses, where the existence of the expectation is flagged in advance to allow the clinician to comply or override on specified terms, are the more powerful. Opportunities for prospective applications have become far more numerous as a result of automation. They may hold the greatest promise for improving quality and economy by eliminating oversights and errors which give rise to later corrective action or which even introduce complications in the patient's care. If each patient should have a history and physical examination for cardiovascular disease prior to receiving general anesthesia, the easiest way to get it is to incorporate the request into the ordering sequence. A *prompt* will appear whenever the doctor orders surgery. If a flexible set of overrides is also designed, virtually all patients will be in compliance.

Even with high rates of compliance, retrospective monitoring and investigation of departures are necessary. They assure that compliance is achieved and help identify ways in which current expectations can be improved. The systems for retrospective monitoring should accomplish these goals at the lowest possible cost. Statistical approaches permit routine low-cost, retrospective review of departures (either overrides or suspected failures).

Retrospectively, any individual patient or care activity can be evaluated by classifying care as above or below a norm, or within or outside a range, yielding attributes measures of performance, as discussed in chapter 3. Groups of patients can be evaluated by noting the percentage that falls within the range. One advantage to an attributes approach is that, as expectations become more numerous, the percentage scores can be expanded easily, either in aggregates or in categories reflecting the expansion. Opportunities for improvement can be found quickly by scanning the aggregates or categories and selecting for study those where the statistical evidence suggests a significant variation. (As an analogy, batting average is an attributes measure. It can easily be expressed for the team, for outfielders, and for individuals. It can also be categorized by home and away games, left- and right-handed pitchers, with and without runners on base. Finally, given enough times at bat, it can be calculated for combinations—outfielder A, away games, against right-handed pitchers, with runners on base.)

Statistical evaluation of process attributes scores is readily available. The statistical problem is to design a system that will detect infrequently occurring true failures without detecting an unsatisfactory number of false positives. Because the system emphasizes compliance and not correction, it is wise to investigate only those failures where there are likely to be benefits from the intervention by the medical staff organization. Each case investigated should be a learning experience, providing a reward which encourages improvement. False positives, where no correctable factor can be identified, waste time and may create hidden costs in the form of adverse psychological reactions from clinical personnel.

The probability of significance, that is, the probability of a real change in process, can be estimated from the theoretical distribution, an easy task for modern computers. Low rates of false positives are achieved by setting the error detection threshold at a 99 percent probability of true process change for a single reporting period, or at 90 percent probability for two successive periods. Attributes events can be expected to follow the binomial distribution and can be modelled as Poisson distributions or normal distributions.

Many aspects of clinical performance can also be treated as continuous measures, providing more sensitive analyses of group performance. Such treatment is also straightforward with modern computer software, but because of the volumes of information involved it is probably appropriate mainly at lower organizational levels and for special studies. It is used extensively for quality control within the clinical laboratory, for example.

Expectation Setting. Initial expectations will usually be adapted from published sources and professional consultants. They will be limited to the most costly or dangerous elements of care or to the most numerous patients. Over time, expectations will become both more specific, applying to more narrowly defined patient groups, and more extensive, applying to a greater fraction of the final product. For example, the anesthesiology department, considering the cardiopulmonary examination expectation above, may review several characteristics for increased specificity, such as age, sex, race, admitting diagnosis, and kind of general anesthesia. Statistics on current local practice will be needed. A sample of records may be analyzed for each of these characteristics and, if necessary, promising combinations. Once the department has decided on the improvement, say by adding "over 45 years of age" to the expectation, counts must identify age in order to report compliance, adding this dimension to the reporting system.

Expectation setting must always deal with uncertainty: it is never clear in advance what will result from a study of ways to improve a specific expectation. Uncertainty turns to risk in the case of the information system, where large investments can be made to support gains in quality and economy that are never realized. The well-run hospital takes strategically consistent risks in this regard. Except for those few hospitals whose mission includes pioneering, the hospital should adopt information technology that has been thoroughly tested and successfully applied in other hospitals.

Summary of Information and Measurement Needs

In summary, the measurement and information system supporting the development of process expectations in the well-run hospital has the following characteristics:

— An automated discharge abstract records demographic, diagnostic, surgical, and outcomes data on each patient, identifies the accountable doctors and nursing units, and identifies the more detailed medical record.

— Counts of services by type or group are available from the patient billing record, and the billing record can be merged with the abstract to permit identification of any given subgroup.

— Estimates of costs at current volumes can be attached to individual intermediate products and groups of smaller ones.

— Estimates of cost changes associated with expected changes in volume of intermediate products can be prepared from budget sources.

Efforts are being made to develop more extensive and precise groupings, more accurate estimates of costs, applications to outpatient settings, and more current data for prospective monitoring. The effort to support clinical performance expectations is a multidimensional one, and balance among the dimensions is important. The information system should be available to support the clinical organization, but investment can be deferred until the organization has developed. The automation of data collection can be balanced against the extent of the expectations, and the precision of cost estimates and cost change estimates can be improved as the expectations develop. It is important to remember that only the clinical performance assessment system must be effective to improve quality, but both clinical and intermediate product cost control systems must be in place to effect gains in cost-effectiveness.

Notes

1. David Mechanic, "Physicians and Patients in Transition," *The Hastings Center Report* 15 (December 1985): 9–12; L. F. McMahon, et al., "Hospital Matrix Management and DRG-Based Prospective Payment," *Hospital & Health Services Administration* 31 (January-February 1986): 62–74.

2. M. C. Weinstein and H. V. Fineberg, *Clinical Decision Analysis* (New York: Saunders, 1980.)

3. Arthur F. Southwick, *The Law of Hospital and Health Care Administration* (Ann Arbor, MI: Health Administration Press, 1978), pp. 409–22.

4. Eliot Freidson, *Doctoring Together* (Chicago: University of Chicago Press, 1980).

5. C. Argyris, *Personality and Organization: The Conflict Between the System and the Individual* (New York: Harper, 1957).

6. John Eisenberg, *Doctors' Decisions and the Cost of Medical Care* (Ann Arbor, MI: Health Administration Press, 1986), pp. 48–49.

7. *The International Classification of Diseases,* 9th Rev. *Clinical Modification,* Vols. 1–3 (Ann Arbor, MI: Commission on Professional and Hospital Activities, 1978).

8. *Health Care Financing Review,* 1984 Supp.

9. E. A. Codman, *A Study in Hospital Efficiency: The First Five Years* (Boston: Thomas Todd, 1916).

10. M. T. MacEachern, *Hospital Organization and Management* (Chicago: Physician's Record Co., 1938).

11. P. A. Lembcke, "Evolution of the Medical Audit," *Journal of the American Medical Association* 199 (1967): 543–50.

12. V. N. Slee, "CPHA Experience in Measuring Quality," paper presented to the American Public Health Association Program Area Committee on Medical Care Administration, 94th annual meeting, San Francisco, November 1966.

13. Avedis Donabedian, *The Definition of Quality and Approaches to Its Assessment* (Ann Arbor, MI: Health Administration Press, 1980).

Suggested Readings

Eisenberg, J. *Doctors' Decisions and the Cost of Medical Care.* Ann Arbor, MI: Health Administration Press Perspectives, 1986.

Freidson, E. *Doctoring Together.* Chicago: University of Chicago Press, 1980.

Weinstein, M. C., and Feinberg, H. V. *Clinical Decision Analysis.* New York: Saunders, 1980.

12

Clinical Support Services

Today's well-run community hospital conceives of itself as a community resource for patient care with great flexibility but with the obligation to configure itself economically and efficiently. It begins this configuration by adopting a mission and a long-range plan. Consistent with its mission, it pursues a mutually supportive relationship with a carefully selected group of doctors under the arrangements of the conjoint staff. Increasingly, both hospital and staff depend upon competitive financial arrangements such as Medicare's prospective payment system, various kinds of HMOs, and preferred provider contracts emphasizing quality and appropriateness of care. As the central resource of this network, the hospital must develop services for diagnosis and treatment which are complementary to private doctors' offices, attractive to the community, and consistent with the underlying goal of health care. These services, which together with the attending staff and the nursing staff define the clinical capability of the hospital, are called the clinical support services. Their origins in anesthesia and surgery a century ago opened the era of the modern hospital. They have grown steadily in capability, complexity, and size since.

Each clinical support service is supervised by a professional, often a specialist physician. Each has extensive technology and unique procedures. Support services also have a number of common characteristics. In this book I discuss management of support services in light of those common characteristics, leaving the emphasis on their differences to texts covering each service. This chapter discusses how the well-run hospital succeeds in the quest for reliability and appropriateness of clinical support services, and is organized around the following topics:

— Definition and purpose
— Clinical functions
— Management functions
— Personnel and organization
— Measures and information systems
— Management issues

Definition and Purpose

Typically, a clinical support service activity, such as a laboratory test, a drug, or an operation, is ordered by an attending physician as part of a program of diagnosis and treatment. The physician requests the service rather than supplying it in his or her office because it requires a staff and facilities that cannot economically be provided by a small office. There are very large numbers of such activities.

In addition, hospitals are providing some support services directly to community groups. Particularly for HMOs, it is useful to encourage disease prevention and health maintenance among the population served. Health education such as prenatal classes, primary prevention such as immunization programs, disease screening such as urinalysis and blood pressure testing, and behavioral assistance in such areas as smoking cessation and bereavement have all become commonplace in well-run hospitals. These programs are not specifically related to individual patient treatment and therefore do not require the direct order of an attending physician. Medical staff guidance and support are clearly desirable, however, and the services are part of the clinical offerings.

> **A clinical support service is (1) a unit organized around one or more medical specialties or clinical professions providing individual patient care on order of an attending physician or (2) a general community service, such as health education, immunization, and screening, under the general guidance of the medical staff.**

Under this definition, nursing is a support service. It is so large and complex, however, that it merits discussion on its own, in chapter 13. Many observations about support services apply to nursing as well.

The purpose of clinical support services is to extend the health care–giving capability of the total system, including that of private attending physicians. This purpose is intuitively clear, but it contains a hidden complexity. Many of the less elaborate support services can be provided either in the hospital or in doctors' offices. Doctors derive both income and professional satisfaction from providing these services, and it is often more convenient for the patient to receive them in the doctor's office. At the same time, the services provided by the hospital become quite costly if they are not widely used. The optimal system requires enough attending doctors to satisfy community desires as well as enough support services. Thus the purpose implies that the profile of services offered at the hospital must be consistent with the physician recruitment plan, allowing doctors to perform in their offices those services which they can safely and economically provide. One of the tasks of the conjoint staff is to define and implement this profile.

All community hospitals have clinical laboratories, radiology services, pharmacies, electrocardiography services, and operating rooms. The scope of support services available is related to the size of the institution; all large hospitals have several subdivisions of these basic services and a number of additional services. Labels, groupings, and designations are not uniform, and counts are not precise. A useful classification of the nonnursing services categorizes them broadly into diagnostic, therapeutic, and general community activities. Although some services include both diagnosis and treatment, one usually predominates. Figure 12.1 shows the services a community hospital of over 400 beds is likely to have; it may have a scattering of others as well.

A serious illness may require upward of a hundred separate activities from clinical support services. Each of these must make a distinctive contribution to the overall pattern of care. It is obvious from the list in figure 12.1 that the characteristics of these activities are very different. The selection of clinical support services is the task of the attending physician, at least implicitly in the final product protocols and the logic discussed in chapter 11. The selection is recorded as an order; the business of the support services is the fulfillment of those orders. The vast differences in modality and contribution are accommodated by using uniquely trained individuals for each support service. Yet at one level of abstraction above these differences, similarities emerge. The responsibility center managers of social service and megavoltage therapy, for example, share several common functions. In the well-run hospital, they pursue the fulfillment of these functions in very similar ways. It is convenient to group these generic functions of clinical support services into *clinical* and *managerial,* the former relating somewhat more closely to the activity at hand and the latter to logistics. The distinction should not be overdrawn. The clinical service manager is responsible for both, and both are essential.

— Clinical functions:
  • Quality assurance, broadly defined to include patient satisfaction and physician satisfaction in addition to the provision of reliable and relevant clinical interventions

Figure 12.1

Common Clinical Support Services in a Large Community Hospital

Diagnostic Services
Clinical laboratory
  Chemistry
  Hematology
  Histopathology
  Bacteriology and virology
  Autopsy and morgue
Diagnostic imaging
  Radiography
  Tomography
  Radioisotope studies
  Nuclear resonance imaging
  Ultrasound
Cardiopulmonary laboratory
  Electrocardiology
  Pulmonary function
  Heart catheterization
Other
  Electroencephalography
  Electromyography
  Audiology

General Community Activities
Immunization and screening
  programs
Cardiopulmonary resuscitation
  training
Family planning, prenatal, parenting,
  and child care classes
Smoking cessation program
Alcohol education
Weight control and physical fitness
  program

Therapeutic Services
Pharmacy
  Dispensing
  Intravenous and mixture service
Operating suite
  Anesthesia
  Surgery
  Recovery
Labor and delivery suite
Emergency service
Blood bank
Rehabilitation services
  Physical therapy
  Respiratory therapy
  Speech pathology
  Occupational therapy
Radiation therapy
  Megavoltage radiation therapy
  Radioisotope therapy
Social services
Home support
  Organized home care
  Hospice
  Lifeline (transportation and
    home meals)
Clinical psychology

- Coordination and timing, integrating each individual service into an efficient program of care
- Assisting attending physicians in offering appropriate care by informing them of the cost-benefit calculus underlying various diagnostic and treatment interventions
— Managerial functions:
  - Demand management and scheduling of patients
  - Staff maintenance, recruitment, selection, and scheduling

- Budgeting of costs and revenues
- Planning to ensure the proper scope of services

The clinical and managerial functions of support services are increasingly interdependent. Quality and costs, marketing and pricing are interrelated. Careful long-range planning and accurate forecasts of demand for services has become essential to success in competitive environments. Intermediate product protocols define all aspects of services, including methods, costs, prices, and quality. The term is probably more formal than actual practice in the 1980s, but well-run hospitals certainly have recognized the interdependence of various aspects of support service management and are moving rapidly toward the style implied in the descriptions that follow. That style is one which concentrates a battery of forward-looking decisions on the annual budget exercise, expanding it well beyond simple concerns with cost. Largely as an outcome of those annual discussions, specific issues of quality, cost, service, and marketing are identified for intensive study. The results of those studies lead to changes formalized in the budgets for subsequent years.

Clinical Functions of Support Services

The clinical functions of support services are those necessary to maintain quality, by its broadest definition. One can construct four relevant groups of this complex and multidimensional subject:[1] technical quality, integration or coordination, satisfaction, and appropriateness. Technical quality, a concept essentially analogous to product consistency and service reliability, is the proper starting point for management concern. Coordination is useless in the absence of technical quality, and satisfaction is improbable. Appropriateness, clearly a part of the broader philosophical definition of quality, is attainable only after an acceptable level has been reached in the other three dimensions.

Technical Quality: Effective and Reliable
Completion of Orders

Broadly speaking, technical quality is the filling if a doctor's order in a manner satisfactory to the doctor. In most, but not all, cases, the service should also be effective, that is, it should make the contribution to care which the doctor anticipated. Achieving technical quality is a matter of doing the correct thing, doing it consistently over a wide variety of situations, and in most cases achieving the anticipated outcome. Technical quality is clearly a primary concern of the managing professional. Fulfillment of the management functions tends to support technical quality by providing appropriate staffing, training methods, facilities, and supplies. Beyond these matters, technical quality depends upon routine measurement and monitoring.

Technical quality is measured by:

— *Interim measures of performance,* such as radiation monitors, temperature records, and reagent tests

— *Process inspections,* preferably following explicit protocols and carried out by trained, unbiased observers

— *Record reviews,* including patient medical records and departmental records

— *Counts of repeat tests and unsatisfactory results*

— *Results inspection, or reported values,* such as test averages in the laboratory or inspection of filled prescriptions

— *Accuracy of values on blind,* or control, specimens

These measures can be developed from either samples or universes, as appropriate, and subjected to statistical analysis, as described briefly in chapter 3.

A well-run support service identifies a variety of measures of technical quality and uses the least expensive ones on a daily or hourly basis to assure consistent performance, even though the validity of these measures is imperfect. It bolsters this short-term effort with periodic studies introducing greater scope and validity. The frequency and extent of these depends upon the cost of unsatisfactory performance as well as the cost of the studies. By definition, an important support service tends to have high costs of unsatisfactory performance. As a result, a large part of the management effort is devoted to maintaining and improving technical quality. Measurement is an adjunct to this goal, however; process design, personnel training, and proper equipment are the vehicles that establish quality.

For most applications, technical quality is optimized rather than maximized. That is, perfect performance is appropriate only when a life is at stake. Otherwise, the goal should be to attain as high a quality as is consistent with the resources invested. For example, unsatisfactory X-ray film exposures can result from improper dose estimation, improper machine calibration, variation in the power supply, or movement by the patient. Although one wishes to get as many satisfactory films on the first try as possible, retake has a finite price. One would not invest more in stabilizing the power supply than it contributes by reducing retakes. Similarly, one would not make the examination unnecessarily unpleasant by frightening patients into absolute immobility. An anticipated failure rate is built into the monitor; satisfactory performance will be something greater than 0.0 percent retakes.

Coordination and Promptness

Each of the clinical support services contributes uniquely to patient care, but the combined impact is always greater than the sum of their individual contributions. Interactions abound: certain tests interfere with others, drugs interact, treatments impair organ systems not damaged by the disease itself. Timing is often critical and rarely irrelevant. Success demands coordination and integration; high quality within the individual services is only the starting point. The patient's attending physician is responsible for the proper selection and timing of events, but the well-run hospital carefully supports his or her efforts. Coordination of support services is a major theme of hospital management, extending from long-range planning, organization design, and information systems design at the governance level to coordination of day-to-day or hour-to-hour activities on the nursing unit. Patient group protocols, nursing care plans, and scheduling systems are keys to success. Implementation of them requires both conjoint staff approaches and effective communication with nursing.

Much of medical care is given in sequence—diagnosis precedes treatment, anesthesia precedes surgery, treatment precedes rehabilitation, et cetera. The elapsed time between complaint and cure is frequently a function of the sequencing and timing of events. The more intense care becomes, the more critical sequencing and timing are. For example, an extensive list of support service orders, including specific nursing care, must be completed prior to surgery. Delays add to the length of stay, and omissions impair quality. Intensive care service is a second example. Hourly diagnostic services are often required, and delays can be as life-threatening as inaccurate reports.

Other timing issues are cyclic. Many activities, such as attending doctors' rounds, occur daily at regular times. Results of routine diagnostic tests are most useful if they are reported in time for rounds, usually about 24 hours after they were ordered. There is no extra benefit to 12-hour reporting cycles, and reports after 25 hours are no better than reports after 48. (In hospitals with house staff, 6- or 8-hour cycles might have important benefits.) Well-run support services determine when and in what order services are needed, measure actual response time, and make an effort to minimize delays that affect the attending doctor and the patient. Demand management systems are emerging as the key to timeliness and sequencing. Automated ordering, results reporting, and patient scheduling are important in demand management, which is discussed in detail below.

Coordination is the most difficult of the four dimensions of quality to achieve. Measurement is difficult. The judgment of the attending physician and nurse may be the best monitor of performance. Under automated systems or on a survey basis, selected events can be monitored. Two steps seem to encourage coordination. One is to use automated equipment to access and integrate as much information as possible. Good laboratories report both cross-sectional and time series profiles of values for individual patients. They also use the age, sex, and full working diagnosis on each patient to interpret findings. Access to drug orders, almost within reach of current electronic capability, will also be useful to them. The second step is to encourage face-to-face communication. When support service personnel have direct access to the attending physician and the nurse, coordination seems to improve. Capable support service managers encourage such contact. Pathologists and radiologists take pains to discuss patients and services with attending physicians, because such discussions are the nucleus of coordination. They also support investigations of appropriateness.

Satisfaction: Amenities for Patients and Doctors

The attending physician plays an important role as a monitor of support service quality; his or her comments are valuable, and formal surveys should be undertaken periodically on issues of technical quality, timeliness, and coordination. The nurse is also in a central position to evaluate support services on at least some aspects of these dimensions. In addition, doctors' and patients' desires for amenities should normally be satisfied.

Customer satisfaction is essential for repeat business and favorable recommendations, and repeat business from the attending physician is the source of success for support services. Attending physicians, in turn, must satisfy their customers, the patients, both with their personal services and those they obtain as agent. In medical care, there is an additional concern. Patients who are satisfied with their treatment participate more actively in it and are more likely to respond favorably to it. Patients who are dissatisfied tend not to follow instructions.

Technical quality is probably the central factor in attending physician satisfaction, although amenities such as personal style, parking, interior design, and hours play a role for doctors as well as patients. For patients, the way they perceive themselves to be treated by nursing and support service personnel is critical to satisfaction. Perceptions can be improved by proper training and incentives. Guest relations programs for employees are valuable (see chapter 14).

It matters very little whether patients' and doctors' desires for amenities seem rational to the support service. Because of his knowledge of manufacturing technology, Henry Ford was sure that painting cars colors other than black was too expensive. By failing to offer colors and several similar choices, he lost the dominant market share to General Motors. The customer may not always be right, but he or she is always the customer. If patients want their husbands in the delivery room or out, if they want the walls tiled or papered or mirrored, if they want their babies delivered at home, the obstetrical service and the delivery room will attempt to respond. Similarly, if attending physicians want parking, or steak for breakfast, or a color television in the lounge, the well-run hospital will at least consider providing them.

Three factors limit the response of the hospital. The most powerful is price. Most people want many things they cannot afford, and the hospital's obligation is to estimate true demand at a realistic price. The second is the extent of consensus. Price tends to be a function of consensus. Mass market amenities generally cost less than custom ones, which appeal to smaller groups. Most hospitals must choose amenities on the basis of their appeal to the mass market, whereas their response to doctors' requests is extensively and deliberately customized. To also customize amenities would drive the total price too high.

The third restraint on the provision of amenities is ethical. Prudence and safety take precedence over amenities. High-risk mothers cannot be permitted home delivery. Cigarette smoking is being actively discouraged by well-run hospitals. They do not sell cigarettes, and they limit smoking areas severely.

Support Service Contributions to Appropriateness

The clinical service manager is the expert on the contribution of each service to total patient care. The proper patient group protocol and the individual patient's plan depend upon a clear understanding of where each service is effective and on the ability of the service unit to deliver the service reliably. Because of his or her expertise, the clinical service manager makes a dual contribution, assuring reliability and assisting in optimal recovery.

Clinical support services can contribute to appropriateness of care in five general areas.

1. *Quality*—Appropriateness begins with high technical quality and includes other aspects as well. All the aspects of quality outlined above are important to appropriateness, but three aspects relate directly:

    a. *Precision*—In both diagnostic and therapeutic services, a precisely standardized, reliable product encourages appropriate demand. In therapeutic services, this tends to mean uniformity across patients and time, a predictable set of actions. In diagnostic services, it means both predictability and refined statistical analysis to identify more decisively the abnormal value.

b. *Promptness*—Once a patient's care has begun, the timing of support services often has a great impact on final cost. Appropriate care provides the next indicated service without delay.

c. *Coordination*—Certain support services interact: drugs change laboratory values, tests require different physiological states, therapies are more effective when coordinated. Improper sequencing of services can cause inappropriate care. Well-run services devote considerable effort to integrating their activities with other support services and nursing.

2. *Cost*—Scope of service affects efficiency and quality; efficiency affects cost; and cost affects price. Good planning, budgeting, and cost control contribute to appropriateness. Competitive pricing tends to attract the volumes necessary to achieve appropriate quality and to make the service more accessible to the doctor and the patient.

3. *Satisfaction*—Appropriateness includes encouraging what is necessary as well as discouraging what is excessive, and satisfaction is a contributor to appropriateness. Doctor, and particularly patient, dissatisfaction may lead to avoidance of necessary services.

4. *Communication*—A dialogue on general issues of care as well as patient-specific ones promotes appropriateness. The well-run service participates actively in clinical discussions, "advertises" its services and their appropriate use, and provides reliable summaries of trends and new developments.

5. *Scope of services*—The kinds of services available locally affect the need for referral to more distant sites. Few hospitals can afford to offer all services. The key to appropriateness is the right balance of offerings within and between support services. For whatever group of patients the hospital staff treats locally, appropriate care provides complete service.

Management Functions of Support Services

The clinical support services have general management functions which can be identified by the closed system parameters of resources, demand, efficiency, revenues, and profits. Reflecting the unique needs of support services, they include scheduling or demand management, planning and capital budgeting for equipment and facilities, and budgeting for costs, revenues, and profits. These fundamentals provide an infrastructure for improving quality and appropriateness of care. The well-run clinical support service routinely meets expectations in these areas within narrow tolerances.

Patient Scheduling and Demand Management

The popular stereotype of the hospital emphasizes its emergency care, ready at a moment's notice to respond to crises which arise without warning. This is in fact an important role of the hospital. Three major kinds of demand—pregnancy at term, heart attacks, and trauma from accidents—cannot be anticipated and require immediate response. Several less common emergencies have the same immediacy. The term *stochastic* applies to events that occur at random, that is, totally independent of one another, and that, as a result, are predictable only in the aggregate and with relatively large variation. Efficiency is lower in stochastic and life-threatening situations because resources must be on standby for an unpredictable surge of demand. Delivery suites, for example, rarely average more than 75 percent of capacity.

Despite the popular stereotype, most demands made upon the hospital are not stochastic and nondeferrable. Some are quite predictable, such as well-baby and prenatal examinations and preventive care generally. Others can comfortably be deferred for several hours or days. If they are scheduled in advance, much greater efficiency can be obtained. Scheduled care is less prone to error than stochastic care, and it can be managed to the greater convenience of attending doctor and patient. Finally, scheduling permits prospective review of appropriateness.

Demand management is a process of scheduling, appropriateness review, and cost reduction with the following goals:

— Appropriate demand is encouraged by making the service convenient, competitively priced, and satisfactory to doctors and patients.

— Inappropriate demand is discouraged by participation in patient group protocol development, by retrospective monitoring and education, and by prospective monitoring.

— Demand is categorized by priority and is then met with appropriate timeliness. Deferrable demand is scheduled for a mutually convenient time.

— The reduction of variation in work load which results from scheduling is converted to lower operating costs.

Demand management requires an understanding of three major areas: the nature of patient demand, the availability of scheduling resources, and the contribution of stabilized demand to high-quality, cost-effective, easily marketed services.

Analyzing and Predicting Patient Demand. Need for support services differs not only by service, but also by patient. A scale of priorities can be developed ranging from "immediate need" to "indefinitely deferrable." In practice, simple scales with three ordinal categories are used. These categories are often called "emergency," "urgent," and "schedulable." The scheduling objective for each category is as follows:

1. *Emergency*—to be treated without delay, despite the loss of efficiency that results. Standby capacity will be built into the resource supply to the extent warranted by the emergency.

   The term *emergency* can be applied to any situation for which first priority service is desirable; it need not be life-threatening. The amount of standby protection will be adjusted downward for less serious priorities. As it is reduced, efficiency will rise. If the emergency category is life-threatening, it is common to accommodate over 99 percent of the anticipated emergency demand at substantial inefficiency.

2. *Urgent*—to be treated as soon as possible without serious impairment of either efficiency or the convenience of others. The category is appropriate where modest, controlled delay does not impair satisfaction or quality. Often, urgent becomes emergency if demand has not been met soon enough.

3. *Schedulable*—to be treated at a mutually agreed future time. Once agreement is reached, care is delivered as scheduled in virtually every case. It is thus quite predictable for patient, doctor, and service.

   It is often possible to create a subcategory which is scheduled, but which will accept an earlier date on short notice. This subcategory actually improves efficiency in some situations, and it is attractive to some patients and doctors.

The support services differ in their priority profiles. Physical therapy, for example, has no emergencies and few urgent demands. The largest support service, the clinical laboratory, faces demand in a different sense because it works on specimens rather than patients and often provides several tests upon each specimen. Its emergencies are called *stat* requests (from the Latin *statim,* immediately). It is difficult to define an urgent category. Schedulable is often defined in hours, but it permits substantial efficiencies from batching similar tests.

Uniformity and reliability of classification are the most important criteria in designing demand categories. For very expensive services, emergency might be defined by rigorously enforced criteria. In less costly situations, one might accept any doctor's statement that the request was an emergency. Without prior discussion, doctors' views would be highly variable, reducing scheduling efficiency. Uniformity can be enhanced by definitions, examples, education, audits, and, if necessary, sanctions.

In addition to the priority categories, it is important to note that demand can vary by time of day, day of week, and season of year and that different services have different demand forecasts. The trend in some is rapidly upward, in others slowly upward, and in others stable or declining. Sound marketing requires an analysis of these trends and variations and a deliberate decision on the hospital's response. The forecasts for cycles and trends accepted as hospital expectations are then built into the scheduling system and, in turn, into the resources made available.

Demand Scheduling Systems. A demand scheduling system identifies future demand, classifies it as emergency, urgent, or schedulable, and establishes the time at which it will be met. There are three levels of scheduling sophistication. An *unscheduled* system effectively treats all demand as emergency. It then either meets demand immediately and accepts the inefficiency which results, or it inconveniences doctors and patients by making the patients wait and calling them at unpredictable times. *Elementary scheduling* systems establish an allowance for combined urgent and emergency demand and schedule deferrable demand into the remaining capacity at mutually acceptable dates. *Sophisticated scheduling* systems call in patients from the urgent list to fill in gaps in emergency demand.

Elementary systems work well in situations where a large fraction of the demand is schedulable. For example, suppose 25 services per shift were demanded on the average. Unscheduled, this demand might vary from 15 to 35 on a given day. If the unit is large enough to provide 35 services, efficiency will be 25/35, or 70 percent. If 20 of the services can be scheduled at near 100 percent efficiency, capacity for about 10 units must be reserved for variation in the remaining emergency and urgent demand. Efficiency will improve to 25/30, or 87 percent.

Sophisticated scheduling requires demand in all three categories, an information-processing system that provides the operator with timely reports, and the ability to get a response from urgent demand quickly. For example, the office scheduling hospital admissions, seeing that fewer emergencies occurred during the night than expected, can summon urgent patients for admission. By doing this, a sophisticated admission scheduling system permits efficiencies of up to 95 percent of bed capacity, while still meeting both emergencies and prior scheduled commitments.[2]

The more sophisticated the scheduling system, the more it costs to operate. Data and processing requirements expand, personnel must be specially trained, and the costs of errors mount. However, well-designed systems are capable of 20 to 30 percent improvements in efficiency of use of fixed resources. They also reduce variation, so labor needs are more stable and more easily predicted. This allows more predictable work schedules for employees. Finally, they allow both doctors and patients to plan their activities. Except in cases where danger or discomfort is high, a timely, reliable date is preferable to an unpredictable delay, especially if the patient or the doctor shares in the cost of the inefficiency that results from instant service.

Scheduling is useful in all support services except those serving almost exclusively emergency demand. Its sophistication should depend on the character of the demand, and its benefits depend upon efficiency. Benefits, therefore, are not achieved through scheduling alone, but also through control of the resources actually used. This requires effective planning and budgeting, although good patient scheduling can simplify budgeting requirements by eliminating complex, flexible budget programs. Good patient scheduling also aids personnel scheduling.

Scheduling tends to support appropriate use of clinical support services in several different ways. Stable work flow reduces errors that result in repeat services. Predictable reporting reduces unnecessary emergencies or stat requests. The data required to operate sophisticated scheduling systems are recovered from the same sources as data for patient group protocols and performance monitoring.

Sophisticated automated scheduling systems are available for major support services and for admission and occupancy management. These programs keep records, print notices, and provide real-time prompts to scheduling personnel. They automatically monitor cancellations, overloads, work levels, and efficiency. Most of them can also be operated in a simulation mode to analyze the costs and benefits of alternative strategies. Simulation outputs are useful in both short- and long-term planning to evaluate potential improvements in demand categorization, resource availability, and scheduling rules.

Pricing, Advertising, and Promotion. Many of the activities under the clinical functions of support services, such as maintenance of quality, provision of amenities, and encouragement of appropriate use, can also be viewed as promotional or advertising efforts to encourage doctors to select the hospital's services over competing alternatives. Many of the resources required for clinical support services are fixed. As a result, higher volumes of appropriate work are an important way of improving efficiency and cost. Given that for most services underlying demand is fixed by the incidence of certain diseases, increased volume can come only from increasing the hospital's market share or increasing the community served.

The principal competition for many clinical support services is doctors' offices. Under the conjoint staff concept, hospitals will negotiate the profile of their clinical support services with their physicians in an effort to create an attractive joint offering for patients. The hospital emphasizes the rarer and more expensive services. The larger the community served and the more inroads made against competitors, the broader the scope of services the hospital can provide. Clinical support services are thus constantly seeking to increase demand.

Direct advertising to patients is of questionable value, because the support services are ordered by physicians, but advertising that enhances the image of the institution as a whole by emphasizing its amenities and the competitive pricing of its clinical support services is likely to be useful. Direct sales to HMOs and preferred provider purchasers will become increasingly important. Joint advertising with capitation and managed care third parties appears inevitable. Insurance carriers and hospital-doctor providers both gain from the promotion of their capabilities.

Pricing is also relevant in a competitive environment. Most hospitals offer a variety of discounts in addition to their publicly posted price. Prior to the advent of competition, line managers of clinical service departments were rarely involved in pricing decisions. As described in chapter 11, well-managed hospitals include line managers in pricing discussions and will anticipate an increasingly sophisticated response.

Integrated Demand Management. The well-run hospital strives to integrate demand management and resource allocation in the following ways:

— It stimulates demand by providing high-quality attractive amenities and service, and competitive pricing. Deliberate efforts are made to increase volumes of appropriate demand by enlarging the service community or increasing market share.

— Under the conjoint staff model, support services are assigned to the hospital or offices of its attending staff in mutually satisfying ways.

— Appropriateness of demand for at least the more expensive clinical services is carefully reviewed. Under some models of capitation and case management, prospective approvals are required for nonemergency demand.

— Carefully developed forecasts establish the likely level and character of appropriate demand, the resources required to service it, and the cost and efficiency of those resources.

— The long-range planning function evaluates the contribution of each service to the hospital's mission in light of competing opportunities for investment, striving for the optimum balance of services. Allocations of fixed resources, such as space and equipment, are established by this process.

— The character and level of demand are analyzed in terms of scheduling capabilities. In general, most scheduling algorithms permit trade-offs among the following desiderata:

• Delays in response to emergency demand

• Delays in response to urgent demand

• Cancellations of previously scheduled patients or failures to deliver service at the specified time

• Time horizons to the next available time for schedulable patients

• Variability of demand by day or shift

— The values associated with these trade-offs are established by ad hoc planning teams, which balance the needs of patients, attending doctors, employees, and efficiency in finding a solution.

Facilities and Equipment Planning

The manager of each clinical support service is responsible for review of potential expansions and reductions of activity. Given the great importance of fixed costs and efficiency in pricing considerations, the planning function is crucial. Most revisions in the scope of service require changes in capital equipment. In well-managed hospitals, these are developed in conjunction with the annual budget review and must compete with other opportunities for investing hospital funds. Managers of clinical support services are frequent sponsors of programmatic capital proposals, as described in chapter 7. The following discussion assumes that the planning process resembles the one described in chapter 7. It discusses ways in which good managers identify, describe, justify, and defend their proposals.

Identifying Opportunities. It is the function of the support service manager to identify all possible service opportunities and to develop proposals for those worthy of detailed consideration. This responsibility includes monitoring technological developments to identify innovations and obsolescence. It also includes monitoring volumes of activity to respond to growth and uneconomically low demand. Finally, it includes identification of ways in which the hospital–attending staff partnership can be enhanced by relocation of services.

At the most basic level, there are two resource allocation decisions for each support service and each of its separable components: *whether* a service will be offered; and *how much* service will be offered. In health care, the whether should depend first on quality. Many services cannot be done well unless they are done frequently. The level of demand should exceed what is necessary to support a trained, practiced team. After a quality threshold has been met, how much is a function of cost, price, and market attractiveness. Cost is frequently a function of fixed equipment capacity. Within equipment limits, higher volume translates into lower costs.

The two questions of whether and how much apply in three recurring forms:

1. Should a new service be added?
2. Should an existing service be discontinued by the hospital in favor of doctors' offices or other sources?
3. Should the resource commitment for an existing or proposed service be expanded or cut back?

The forces for revision stem from changes in both the outside and inside environments. Outside forces include:

— Shifts in demand
  • Changes in population size
  • Aging of the population
  • Changes in income, price elasticity, and amenities expected
— Technological development
  • New services
  • Enhancements
  • Replacements
  • Obsolete services

Inside forces include:

— Changes in patient care protocols

— Changes in attending physician satisfaction

The variety of sources of change encourages frequent, formal review. Support service managers in well-run hospitals address all three questions at least annually. Where a reasonable chance of a need for change exists, they develop a proposal, beginning simply and informally and elaborating as the first reviews indicate.

Under the payment systems before competition, expansion was pursued more aggressively than cutbacks of support services. Studies of the use of clinical support services suggest that many are currently overused by 20 percent or more. Under competitive market conditions, hospitals will benefit from capturing savings, reducing costs, and offering more attractive prices. To capture economies as well as respond to innovation, two steps are important:

1. Rewards, including compensation, must be established for line managers of support services who achieve important economies.

2. The medical staff must encourage support service efficiency, and the managers must participate actively in discussion with them.

Traditional payment methods for support services reward expansion and penalize reduction. This is particularly true of services with medical managers, as discussed below. In a less dramatic way, the salaries of nonmedical managers also depend upon the size of their operation. New incentive pay arrangements for support service managers must be developed to reward efficiency, cooperativeness, and quality of service, including patient and doctor satisfaction. They also must recognize contributions to the overall cost-effectiveness of the hospital.

Less tangible incentives must also be present. Paramount among these is full partnership in the decision-making group. The well-run hospital must carry out its planning discussions in a style that recognizes and encourages the active contribution of support service managers. Most of this recognition must come from medical peers.

Developing Proposals. The proposal stage is actually several iterative steps of increasing rigor and complexity. The process for proposal development and evaluation is described in chapter 7. The final steps judge the investment proposal competitively against other opportunities for the hospital. Decisions are implemented through the annual capital budget and the annual operating budget. In well-run hospitals, assistance is available from the planning-marketing group whenever necessary.

Since the proposal will be evaluated in cost-benefit terms, it is important that it be constructed in those terms. A well-designed proposal addresses all the elements of the closed system model, but it usually emphasizes forecasts of demand, costs, and benefits. The technical issues of these forecasts are discussed in chapter 7. Proper estimation of the benefits is usually the critical consideration in clinical service proposals. The support service manager should be attentive to three benefit sources, direct patient care, improved revenues, and benefits achieved through other services.

Evaluating Patient Care Benefits. Conceptually, the major benefit of an expanded service, or cost of a service foregone, is its contribution to patients' health and well-being. In reality, most service proposals involve convenience rather than new capability. Benefits must be compared to the treatment alternative with the next lowest cost. A service which supplements another one that is not overcrowded and is located ten minutes away has a value equal to ten minutes' travel, even if the service is lifesaving.

Any true addition to health care can be quantified if disease prevalence rates, population reached, and probabilities of success are known. Often the population reached is forecast as some share of a geographic market. Then the quantity of benefit is:

$$(p_1 SP)p_2 B,$$

where

p_1 = Prevalence of Disease

S = Market Share

P = Population Served

p_2 = Probability of Success

B = Benefit to Individual Patient.

In this model, $(p_1 SP)$ is the basic forecast for demand. Only the probability of success and the benefit require new information. The probability of benefit is usually suggested in the scientific literature. Thus one might use the model to estimate that an additional 200 open-heart surgeries can be done per year (that is, $p_1 SP = 200$), noting that in comparable situations there has been a demand for that much surgery and that the operation has been successful 75 percent of the time. Thus the benefit is $150B$ per year. There are clearly weaknesses in such an argument, but the debate is better informed with the estimate than without it.

Attaching a precise value to a specific benefit is often impossible, but at least subjective comparisons can be made between competing alternatives. (The benefit in the example above is allegedly longer life with dramatic improvements in health. Evidence of this is controversial, however; it appears that not everyone who has the operation experiences increases in longevity or activity.) Many persons would value prevention over lifesaving benefits and lifesaving benefits over restorative or palliative ones. Specific proposals can theoretically be scaled by a variety of techniques, including forced choice surveys and Delphi analysis. Years of healthy life restored can also be used to scale benefits, but most new hospital services improve the quality of life rather than extend life itself. Income loss avoided helps evaluate benefits, but it is problematic for retired persons and not universal. Elimination of pain and suffering is hard to evaluate; as a result, it may be undervalued in a subjective weighting.

Cost Reduction as a Benefit. Any proposal that reduces cost enough to earn an acceptable return on its capital investment should be adopted. Thus cost reduction is an important benefit of reduction and replacement proposals. Care must be taken to estimate all costs accurately, including hidden ones, and to be sure the claims for savings can truly be met. Reductions in work force that cannot be translated into reductions in real payroll are a frequent source of error. The manager should anticipate that her or his proposal will be incorporated as an operating budget reduction when it is implemented. (Other issues of cost and revenue estimation are discussed in chapter 7.)

Revenues as Benefit Measures. The best test of the market value of anything is its price on the open market. Even rare and obscure items are evaluated successfully this way. The open market condition is very difficult to meet in health care, however. Most clinical support services are purchased on the patient's behalf by a physician, paid for by insurance, provided under threatening circumstances, and not infrequently delivered by a geographic monopoly. These are scarcely the conditions for informed consumption. Prices set in competitive bids to HMOs or PPOs certainly come closer: the buyer is informed, presumably judicious, and has a choice. Well-run hospitals include such prices, and the revenues they generate, as important measures of value. Because fair competitive tests are so rare, hospitals must often consider other benefit measures as well.

The possibility of revenues achieved under monopolistic conditions and through cost reimbursement schemes should be treated with great caution. The price in such situations is frequently set in ways that automatically justify the proposal.

Increased Market Share as a Benefit. Proposals can be justified by their ability to attract attending physicians and patients using the total offering of the hospital. Thus it is frequently argued that obstetrics is necessary to recruit family practitioners, or that an emergency room adds admissions which are important enough to overcome losses on the service itself. The premise is reasonable but very difficult to prove. Requirements for attracting physicians diminish as the supply of doctors grows; the recruitment argument should be viewed skeptically. Patient recruitment is not automatic; the emergency room will add admissions only if it is successful.

Surveys of existing services provide evidence of total demand by patients in a certain category and may reveal the potential for increasing market share. Determining the value added by increased volume requires elaborate financial modelling. Arguments for the value of attracting demand are most powerful when they are presented as evidence of market focus: a service which is complementary to others serving a certain group of patients identified in the hospital mission should certainly be valued higher than one serving a diffuse or off-focus group.

Defending the Proposal. The support service manager and the planning-marketing representative are proper advocates of the proposal in the evaluation process. As advocates, they should be prepared to answer questions and make modifications as the proposal progresses. They also must be prepared to accept rejection. By the same token, it is management's obligation to see that their role as advocate is accepted by others; their current efforts should not prejudice their future ones.

The procedures supporting annual review of capital and new program opportunities are described in detail in chapter 7. Well-run hospitals emphasize these elements:

— The support service manager is clearly responsible for identifying opportunities.

— Planning-marketing assistance is readily available to develop proposals.

— The hospital's mission statement
  • Is used routinely as the guide to rank new opportunities
  • Makes the preferred direction of growth clear to the support service manager
  • Is modified incrementally as time passes

— All proposals are judged competitively with one another, in a common review process.

— There is medical review and ranking of medical projects, and support services are fairly represented on the review panel.

Consistency of both process and judgment is the hallmark of the well-run hospital. The arguments for departing from these rules almost always claim expediency. A wealthy donor, an unexpected breakdown, a unique technological breakthrough—these are the rationalizations for exceptions to the planning process. However, there are soon enough "exceptions" to engulf the process. At that point, political influence and persuasive rhetoric become the criteria guiding investments.

Consistent review processes provide a pattern that extends and clarifies the mission itself. Several themes recur when proposals are being evaluated. One theme weighs economy against inconvenience and satisfaction: What level of service delays and amenities is best? Another considers the speed of innovation: How long should the community wait for new support service technology? These are questions of management style and are discussed in chapter 7.

One major benefit of consistency is that it helps the manager to shape his or her service to complement other services. This contributes, in turn, to efficiency and to market appeal. The support service manager can tailor opportunities to match the hospital's style. The feedback which permits him or her to do this comes in two ways, through evaluation of his or her proposals and through participation in the evaluation of others' proposals.

Budgeting and Cost Control

The traditional goal of the operating cost budget is to establish the lowest cost consistent with quality. This remains an important part of the intermediate product protocol, but the interdependency of budgeting with scope of service, demand management, quality, pricing, and market satisfaction are now clearly recognized. The narrow issue of cost control appropriately comes after consideration of quality, appropriateness, demand management, and planning. This section identifies the decisions, information requirements, and roles of the management team for budget preparation in the well-run hospital. Some of the technical issues arising from continued sound budgeting practices are discussed below.

Establishing Cost Budget Expectations. Preparing a cost budget for a support service is a matter of establishing seven kinds of expectations:

1. Scope of services
2. Quality and appropriateness goals

3. Demand forecasts
4. Scheduling policies
5. Staffing policies
6. Labor productivity standards
7. Supply usage standards

Even for a small department, there are a great many different specific numbers to be set. Many of these are available as a result of the planning process; for most of them, last year's achievements provide a valuable starting point.

Roles of Management Groups. Well-run hospitals have clearly defined management roles in setting budget expectations. The *budget manager:*

— Assembles historical data on achievement of last year's budget
— Prepares hospitalwide forecasts of major measures
— Sets up guidelines for changes in total expenditures, prices, and employee compensation approved by the finance committee of the board (see chapter 8)

The *support service manager* and his or her subordinate supervisors:

— Identify changes in the scope of services and the operating budget arising from the planning and capital budgeting process
— Review progress in quality and appropriateness, setting improved expectations for the coming year
— Review the hospitalwide forecasts, extending them to the specific levels required in the department and suggesting modifications based upon their knowledge of the local situation
— Propose expectations for staffing, labor productivity. and supplies consistent with forecasts and assumptions about scope, quality, and scheduling
— Identify opportunities for long-term improvements in market, quality, and cost that should be developed during the coming year

The *executive manager* and other line superiors of the support service:

— Review demand forecasts and coordinate revisions suggested by individual services
— Assist the managers with their tasks and encourage them to aim for steady but realistic improvement

— Assure that the hospitalwide expectations for total expenditures and price increases are met

— Coordinate interdepartmental issues that arise from the budgeting process

— Identify interdepartmental opportunities for development during the coming year

— Evaluate the progress of support service managers in order to assist in the distribution of incentives

A large and subtle corporate culture underlies these three roles, but when they are achieved the hospital is well run. Issues of productivity, quality, and mission are effectively solved, in the sense that the hospital will meet the exchange demands necessary to stay in a competitive position. If one further step is taken—if support service supervisors take the expectation-setting activity to the attending staff committees concerned with final product protocols—a mechanism is established for addressing each aspect of production (quality, appropriateness, planning, scheduling, labor, and supplies cost) in an independent yet coordinated way. Four conditions are necessary for this state:

1. The ideal role to be played by each group—executive, finance, support service—is understood by all, even though it is not perfectly achieved.

2. Information systems provide data for historical, comparative, and scientific alternatives to important operating expectations and identify trends in exchange demands.

3. The norm is that current budget expectations are achieved and that next year's will be even better in meeting hospital exchange goals.

4. It is understood that those who exceed expectations will be rewarded in substantial and visible ways.

Guidelines and Information Requirements. Several elements of demand management, financial management, information systems, and planning feed directly into budgeting and cost control decisions. Ideally, a hospital starts its budgeting activity as follows:

— Historical information on demand, labor productivity, and supplies productivity is obtained. (Brand-new services should have their initial budget as part of the new programs proposal under which they were established.)

— Fixed costs for facilities and equipment are established by the planning and capital budgeting activities and need no further attention. (It is sometimes desirable to carry the capital budgeting decisions into the operating year. In effect, the service then has two budgets, one applicable if the proposal is approved, the other if it is not.)

— Hospitalwide forecasts suggest the total demand for inpatients and outpatients by major clinical services. The statistical association of service demand with these forecasts has been calculated.

— Patient group protocols define appropriate demand for costly services.

— Recent analyses of historical data establish the trends in demand for large inpatient groups.

— Demand categories, scheduling rules, and acceptable limits of delay are established in the patient scheduling system. Simulations show the remaining emergency and cyclic variation.

— Personnel scheduling practices establish the availability of workers to meet demand.

— Labor costs by job classification and individual employee are available. A guideline for wage and salary increases has been established.

— A target for change in total expenses for the hospital is established by the finance committee.

It takes many years of effort to develop the complete foundation for budgeting, but the more information of this sort is available at the start of the budget cycle, the simpler it will become to develop the budget itself. It is usually developed first on the basis of unchanged volume, then adjusted for volume change, and finally adjusted as indicated in the proposals for new programs or capital investments. In a competitive environment, the goal is to do better each year, improving quality or productivity to make the service more attractive to doctors and patients.

Achieving High Labor Productivity. High labor productivity is the result of effective planning, not only to define a popular and efficient scope of services, but also to provide proper equipment and organization. It requires a sound patient scheduling system, as discussed above. When these elements are in place, productivity is achieved by reducing variation in demand, improving staffing flexibility, and reducing labor standards per unit of output.

Reducing variation in demand is a matter of pursuing the components of the scheduling system:

— Standardizing and restricting the use of the emergency category
— Promoting use of the urgent category
— Using the scheduled category to flatten cyclic variation
— Improving the sophistication of the scheduling protocol itself

Staffing flexibility is enhanced by effective use of:

— Overtime and part-time personnel
— Float pools
— Cross training of workers
— Job enlargement
— Well-designed work groups
— Compensation by the hour or unit rather than salary

Labor standards are improved by:

— Revising the work method
— Substituting more cost-effective equipment
— Purchasing outside services where indicated
— Providing more responsive supervision
— Improving worker training
— Recognizing and encouraging increased effort
— Awarding bonuses and tangible prizes for increased effort

Although hospitals have not been forced to improve productivity until recently, the competitive environment is likely to force several related kinds of responses in clinical support services:

— Demand forecasts, patient group protocols for expensive support services, and labor productivity standards will become more common.
— Scheduling systems will become more extensive and more sophisticated.
— Flexible budgets will be used to control labor costs.
— Employment arrangements will be adjusted toward more flexibility, emphasizing part-time and overtime employment.
— Smaller units will disappear or shrink, in favor of purchased services from larger operations at lower unit costs.
— Larger units will drop highly specialized and low volume activities, leading to more focused missions.
— The very largest units, usually in referral and teaching centers, will be the only sources of a full range of services.

Establishing Prices

The "proper" price in a capitalist society is that determined by a competitive market. In practice, pricing has been distorted by such exchange factors as the inadequacy of insurance funding prior to Medicare and Medicaid, variations in benefit design, and monopolistic conditions for the supply of many services. As a result, specific support service prices have drifted far above and below their "proper" market values.

Pricing of individual support services has only recently become an important concern at the departmental level. Under cost reimbursement and monopolistic conditions, prices were generally set by the finance section. Under competition, it is important for the department to know the prices and understand their competitive implications. The best way to make this clear is to have them participate in pricing decisions. When this occurs, the departmental manager can be held accountable for a profit or loss expectation.

Prices must accommodate both cost and market requirements. There are two major approaches to pricing specific support services:

1. *Relative value scales*—Specific services are ranked by their relative difficulty or required skills. The weighted index which results is multiplied by either a market-determined base price per unit or an accounting estimate of cost per average unit.

2. *Microcosting*—Cost accounting schemes are used to estimate unit costs for very small services, such as each of two dozen simultaneously performed blood chemistry analyses.[3]

Several of the health care professions providing support services have established price schedules using relative value techniques. In this approach, the resources used in each kind of laboratory test are evaluated by more or less sophisticated techniques, and an index is constructed relative to some simple and universal service which is given a weight of 1.0. The relative value scale can be priced by selecting a dollar value for the unit test. If, say, hematocrits have an index of 1.0 and are priced at $3.00, then triglycerides, with a weight of 4.5, will be priced at $13.50. Provider scales are essentially offering or bid prices, set without testing market acceptance. They are therefore not competitive and cannot be accepted by third-party payers. They may still be used to estimate individual profit levels within the department. They are less accurate and less expensive than microcosting.

Two assumptions are inherent in both methods of costing as a basis for pricing. One relates to the absorption of fixed costs: if volume declines, costs for the same service will mount. The other establishes the overhead and profit burden to be shared by each service: the likely result is a substantial difference between cost and price. Some services will have costs well above any price the customer will accept.

Pricing in the competitive environment depends more upon market forces than upon costs. There are normally three groups of prices, depending on the source of payment:

1. *Undiscounted price,* frequently for services sold to self-pay and indemnity insurance patients. Much outpatient activity occurs on this level.

2. *Negotiated discounts,* for services sold to insurers, including so-called cost-based pricing. This method has little benefit for either the hospital or the third party and may simply be a transitional phase.

3. *Total hospitalization or an annual capitation fee,* for services sold as part of larger packages, including the Medicare prospective payment system for inpatients. The "price" to the department is a transfer price, or imputed share of the total payment. This share may be based on the department's share of undiscounted charges.

Each of these cases has a different set of implications if competition is severe. In the first case, it is important that the published price be competitive. Because costs are dependent on volume, a hospital which does not price competitively will lose volume, causing higher costs and rapid loss of profits. In the second case, it is essential that the department understand the need for the discount and its impact upon operations. This method of pricing forces attention to intermediate protocols and internal productivity. The third case forces attention to demand and patient group protocols as well as to intermediate protocols.

Successful pricing strategies begin with a recognition of the reality of competition and the three kinds of sales. The published price must be set on the basis of the marketplace and costs lowered below it to a satisfactory markup. If the market price of a certain laboratory test, drug, or X ray is $5.00, the hospital must match this price to the extent that third-party contracts permit. If overhead and profit cannot be earned at the competitive price, the hospital must cut its costs, increase its volume, promote a quality or service distinction, raise the price of other services under less competitive pressure, or forego profit. (Increasing volume is appropriate only if variable costs are exceeded by the competitive price.) If the hospital can produce a higher volume for a price of $4.00, the opportunity for increasing market share by reducing the price must be considered.

Few hospitals have paid serious attention to the pricing implications of competitive environments. Even well-run institutions have tended to price on the basis of accounting analyses, idiosyncratic history, or relative value scales. They will move toward more market-driven pricing. In doing so, they make pricing part of marketing strategy rather than accounting. Two steps appear appropriate at present:

1. Pricing will become the domain of support service managers as well as financial personnel. A key element in strategic discussions will be the relative impact of volume on price. Because all overhead and many direct costs are fixed, servicewide pricing strategies to attract volume will be more attractive than microcosting.

2. Managers of support services will be accountable for departmental profits. Estimates using transfer prices and market prices will become more important in the reporting and reward system. Support service managers will respond to price incentives to lower cost expectations. Because of the history of support service pricing, significant reductions in many prices will occur in the next few years.

Personnel and Organization

Professional Personnel

With rare exceptions, the well-run hospital seeks as manager of each support service an experienced leader in the health care profession associated with it, and staffs the service with a blend of professional and nonprofessional personnel. The roots of many services are in nursing. Some services—operating rooms, delivery rooms, and special care units, for example—still use nurses as their professionals. Baccalaureate or advanced nursing degrees are usually required for managers, and prior experience in the service is essential. Pharmacists, physical therapists, occupational therapists, and medical social workers, who traditionally have not held M.D.'s, manage another group of support services.

A growing number of support services is led by physicians with specialty credentials. Clinical laboratories, radiology and imaging, radiation therapy, anesthesiology, and cardiopulmonary laboratories now virtually require physician leadership. Medical leadership is common in emergency rooms and coronary care units. It is growing slowly in the rehabilitation services. Physicians certified in psychiatry take a special interest in supervising these services as a group.

Many physician-led services have developed nonphysician professions as well. In addition to nursing, there are registered medical technologists, radiographers, respiratory therapists, and nurse anesthetists.

Finally, under both medical and nonmedical leadership, there is a variety of nonprofessional clinical jobs, such as case aides, physical therapy aides, phlebotomists, pharmacists' assistants, and so forth.

Many of the professions have set up economic protection through licensure or certification requirements. In the services that are not licensed or certified, prevailing standards of practice require the provision of appropriately trained professionals. The definition of "appropriate" is increasingly a matter of national rather than local consensus. As a rule, a person trained appropriately for a support activity would be a physician, a professional trained in the service or a nurse experienced in it, or someone with less training who worked directly under a physician's supervision.

Larger hospitals operate training programs for many of these professionals, including physicians. Underlying economic conditions suggest that many of these training programs will be consolidated or closed. Because of the impact of competition, supplies of most professionals will be adequate for some years to come, perhaps into the next century. Declining numbers of young people through the 1980s and changes in the work aspirations of women suggest that many professions will have difficulty recruiting members. As a result of declines in both need and demand, hospital investments in education may become burdensome. One major advantage of training programs, the satisfaction they bring to supervising professionals, may be replaced with more direct recognition and financial incentives.

The system of public certification or licensure places a burden upon hospitals because of their visibility. Doctors' offices now have the privilege of using nonprofessionals to carry out many of the elementary support service tasks under the doctor's direct supervision. Thus a simple surgical procedure can be done in a doctor's office by a doctor and her or his "nurse," who need not even be licensed or registered. In a hospital, the same procedure might require the efforts of a surgeon, an anesthesiologist, a pharmacist, a recovery room nurse, and an operating room nurse. The hospital's advantage in safety and efficiency is eroded by higher costs of professional labor.

To make hospitals more cost-effective, efforts have been made to amend licensure and certification requirements. The strength of the lobbies for individual licensure being brought to bear suggests that these efforts will not be successful. The hospital may adjust many of its staffing requirements under physician supervision, however; thus they are likely to consider more doctors and fewer specialized professionals.

Compensation of Support Service Managers

The major support services led by physicians have had a century of growth and can be said to be the keystone of modern acute care: with this success has come financial success for their physician leaders. Only surgeons in certain specialties command as high a median income as pathologists, radiologists, and anesthesiologists. It was not always so, however. Substantial tension marks the history of relations between hospital-based physicians, the hospitals which pay them, and attending physicians. Although these tensions revolved around mutual acceptance and esteem, money also played a critical role, both for its symbolic and its economic significance. Method and amount of compensation of hospital-based specialists are recurring topics in the management of support services. Although it gets less attention, the subject of compensation for nonmedical professionals leading these services is also important in the well-run hospital.

General Criteria for Compensation. Compensation for managers in a bureaucratic organization should meet three general guidelines, and hospital-based specialists and support service managers generally are no exception.

1. Compensation should equal long-range economic opportunities for similar positions elsewhere. That is, the test of compensation is the market. Compensation consistently below market rates will create difficulty in recruiting and retaining professionals. Compensation consistently above market rates will impair the competitive position of the hospital.

2. Within the limits market differentials permit, compensation should reflect organizational needs. Those making the greatest contribution to the organization should receive the greatest compensation.

   This criterion implies the need for uniformity in administration of compensation and flexibility in adapting to changing organizational needs. It suggests that, while collective bargaining and other negotiating devices are satisfactory mechanisms, care should be taken to minimize monopolistic advantage or personal influence. It also suggests the need for review of monopolistic positions, reducing or eliminating them and the services they represent if feasible.

3. Compensation should encourage professional growth and fulfillment consistent with organizational needs. Incentives to improve performance in directions consistent with hospital exchange needs are part of a good compensation program.

The incentives offered in a specific compensation program are sometimes complex. Fee-for-service compensation for hospital-based specialists, for example, directly rewards volume of service and promotes efforts to satisfy attending physicians. It promotes efficiency only if the attending physicians reward it by selecting the efficient producer. Salaries offer no particular incentives for either efficiency or customer satisfaction.

Compensation for Physician Managers. Although most hospital-doctor compensation contracts involve support service physicians, it is important to note that the contract mechanism is spreading to previously uncompensated attending staff. Over a quarter of all physicians in 1981, excluding residents, had hospital contracts that included compensation. Hospital compensation for support specialists differs only in frequency; three-quarters of the pathologists and over half the radiologists had such arrangements.[4] Under hospital-owned HMOs and PPOs, all participating physicians have such arrangements, at least for a portion of their income.

The fundamental distinction in compensation contracts is between employment and independent contractor status. A third major category, the joint venture, has arisen recently. This contract provides for the sharing of equity and risk rather than simply costs, fees, or operating revenues. Each of the three major forms is quite flexible, with a number of common variants.

1. *Employment*—Employment usually implies regular payment of salary or wages, participation in benefits, and hospital employee status for subordinates. Employees are subject to payroll tax deduction and encounter certain restrictions on income tax deductions. Hospitals are often liable for the malpractice of their employees and insure them as part of the hospital's coverage. Employee status is not established simply by the wording of the contract; it depends on the locus of specific responsibilities. Employees cannot bill third parties for services covered under employment. Hospitals include all costs in their reimbursement. It is possible for a specialist to be both an employee and a contractor, for different responsibilities. Doctors can be established as a separate class or classes of employees, permitting almost unlimited variation in designing the employment contract.

    a. *Status*—Doctors may be full- or part-time. The employment contract may permit or restrict other employment or private practice.

b. *Compensation*—Employment compensation can be by either wage or salary. Bonuses such as overtime are possible under each.

c. *Benefits*—Doctors as employees can be included in group retirement, health, accident, and life insurance. Almost any other benefit or perquisite can be specified, sometimes with important tax consequences.

d. *Incentives*—Compensation can be increased through year-end bonuses for achieving specific or general goals.

e. *Limitations*—Compensation in the form of equity tends to be more difficult under employment contracts. This can be a tax disadvantage for the doctor. In addition, compensation may not cause dispersion of not-for-profit assets (technically, *inurement)* to individual doctors.

2. *Independent contractor*—The contractor arrangement allows the doctor to operate as a business for tax purposes, changing the rules for deductible expenses. Variants are theoretically even more flexible than under employment. They include arrangements which involve hospital payment to the physician, physician payment to the hospital, and those where there is no monetary transaction between the two.

a. *Fee for service*—The specialist and the hospital separately arrange for payment directly with the patient or the third-party carrier. Such arrangements are not uncommon where the analogy to surgery is strong, such as cardiopulmonary services and radiation therapy. HMOs and PPOs may contract separately with the hospital and the physician, leaving the arrangement between the two free of compensation. The hospital may compensate for supervisory and teaching services by employment or other contract.

b. *Franchise and lease*—The specialist pays a fee to the hospital, either as rent for the facilities and equipment used or as a franchise for privileges. Franchise and lease arrangements are relatively rare at present. There are barriers to covering the department's operating costs under the physicians' part of Medicare which place the parties at a competitive disadvantage.

c. *Shared revenue*—The coordination and supervision of hospital employees and the obligation to serve all attending physicians are responsibilities accepted by the specialist and compensated by the hospital. Two versions developed, both of which assumed a joint billing for services and division of the proceeds: *percent of gross,* which divides the revenue before deducting the costs of operating the service department, and *percent of net,* which divides revenue after deducting departmental expenses.

3. *Joint ventures*—These new forms parallel the development of the conjoint staff and the competitive approach generally. They are designed to share the incentives for meeting exchange needs between the support service manager and the hospital. They are complex and untested at the present time, although they show interesting potential.

The usual structure is a for-profit corporation, with equity held by both parties. The profits of the venture come from the sale of services, giving the corporation the same pricing questions as any other. Presumably, efficient management and effective pricing will lead to expanded profits. These can be reinvested, allowing equity to grow, or distributed as dividends, as determined by the corporate board.

A variant establishes the joint venture as a full or limited partnership, changing many of the tax consequences of income distribution.

Revenue implications for the hospital are profound. In many cases, hospital charges were set to recover relatively heavy overhead burdens. Unless the services represented by the overhead are also sold to the new corporation, a significant loss of revenue could occur.

Design of a sound contractual relationship is demanding, but it yields to repeated applications of sound management technique.

Compensation of Nonphysician Managers. The compensation of nonmedical managers is no different conceptually from that of physician managers, except that the nonmedical professions normally do not include fee-for-service practitioners. Employment is by far the usual arrangement. Well-run hospitals consider bonuses and incentives for contribution to the overall good. Most of the nonmedical support services are more easily marketed with other elements of patient care. This reinforces the tendency away from independent contracts and joint ventures.

Although many of the nonmedical specialty groups have indicated interest in fee-for-service compensation, the combination of their weaker bargaining power and increasing public concern over the cost of health care has prevented significant growth of any payment method other than salary. Viewed from the perspective of corporate enterprise generally, the use of a nonsalary mechanism is desirable when salaries fail to produce the desired behavior, usually when powerful, specific incentives can be devised. Thus one might contemplate piece rates or productivity bonuses in repetitive, management-defined tasks like pharmacy order fulfillment or laboratory tests. The useful incentives can be achieved through employment contracts rather than fee-for-service arrangements. Fees are becoming less relevant, even within the practice of medicine, as a result of the growth of capitation insurance.

Organization of Clinical Support Services

Clinical support services vary widely in size and activity. The largest is usually the clinical laboratory, which can have over 100 members. The smallest services have only one or two professionals. Large services are usually organized on the basis of their techniques, tools, or modalities. There is an increasing tendency toward cross training and single-team structure among those services that face declining volumes. Certainly, any internal specialization which impedes the movement of personnel adds to fixed costs. Well-run hospitals are moving in the opposite direction.

The external organization presents a serious problem of grouping disparate elements into a coherent whole. A reasonable accountability hierarchy would place a group manager over several comparable services. Unfortunately, the list in figure 12.1 represents more than 40 separate cost centers, and common themes to support rational grouping are difficult to find. Figure 12.2 reflects a structure with 8 group managers. It has three steps between the levels of responsibility center manager and chief operating officer and associates responsibility centers that, for the most part, address related problems and serve the same physician and patient clientele. The assignment of responsibility centers to group managers is only occasionally controversial:

— *Pathology,* clinical laboratory (chemistry, hematology, histopathology, bacteriology, virology), autopsy and morgue, blood bank

— *Radiology and imaging,* radiography, tomography, ultrasound, radioisotope studies, nuclear resonance imaging, megavoltage radiation therapy, radioisotope therapy

— *Pharmacy,* dispensing and intravenous mixtures

— *Cardiopulmonary and electrodiagnostic,* electrocardiology, pulmonary function, heart catheterization, electroencephalography, electromyography, respiratory therapy

Figure 12.2

Possible Organization of Clinical Support Services

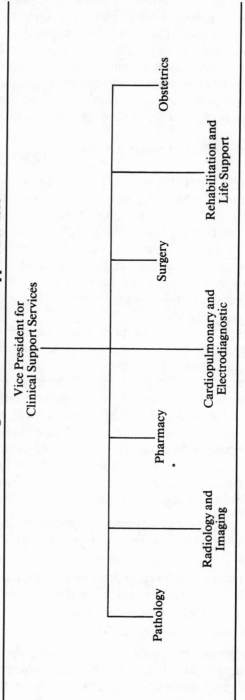

— *Surgery,* operating suite, anesthesia, recovery, emergency service

— *Rehabilitation and life support,* physical therapy, occupational therapy, speech pathology, clinical psychology, home support, immunization and screening, substance abuse, wellness programs

— *Obstetrics,* labor and delivery

— *Health promotion and illness prevention,* community education, mass screening, and support group activities

Measures and Information Systems

A wide variety of measures arises within each service and from the accounting, medical records, and planning-marketing departments. This section suggests measures that emphasize those external exchanges which affect survival most directly. These measures should be supplemented with closed system measures for demand, quality, productivity, cost, and revenue.

Measures of Market Acceptability

It can be said that a support service's contribution to the hospital's survival and growth depends mainly upon the following things:

— Satisfying patients

— Satisfying attending physicians

— Matching competitors' offerings

— Maintaining competitive price

— Minimizing incidents and hazards

A well-designed information system for a clinical support service will monitor actual achievement.

Satisfying Patients. Customer response to a service can be obtained through reliable surveys and should be reported at least annually. The cheapest method is a general, hospitalwide survey, with specific questions addressing at least the largest support services. Convenience, timeliness, and attitudes of personnel appear to be the most important concerns. Questions should be constructed from previously published sources, and modified only as necessary for the specific situation.[5] Expectations for these measures should be drawn from historical sources, because comparative data are rarely available and the responses are highly sensitive to the sampling situation and the survey design.

Satisfying Attending Physicians. A formal survey of attending physicians' views on support services is desirable annually, at least in hospitals with large staffs. The issues are usually reliability and timeliness of response, acceptability to patients, and quality of professional advice and guidance. Well-designed surveys pursue negative responses to identify correctable matters. Comparison with results from prior years is useful, and survey questions can address the hospital's standing relative to its competition. ("Rank the five clinical laboratories listed below according to your preference.") Supplementary information from the medical staff organization is useful, but it is often biased toward the viewpoint of the doctor who is already a high user, as opposed to the viewpoints of doctors who might become high users. Anecdotal and idiosyncratic evidence on physician satisfaction should not be ignored. Those services which provide adequate professional advice and guidance tend to hear of problems and opportunities through that process. The formal mechanisms in such cases simply protect against failure of the informal contact.

Matching Competitors' Offerings. The mix and scope of support services are frequently important in promoting use of the hospital as a whole. Thus it is useful to survey as formally as possible the services offered by other hospitals serving the same market. Hospital-based surveys are probably reliable sources of such information. It may be possible to integrate them with price surveys.

Maintaining Competitive Price. Because prices in a competitive environment are not controlled by a single supplier, success requires comparative data. Further, prices must be set in response to market conditions. Unless customers recognize a valuable difference in service, market share will go to the lowest bidder. The manager of a clinical support service must recognize the external price and the margin required by the hospital as a whole. He or she must then operate the service within the remaining resources.

For hospitals, pricing problems are complicated by the fact that services are sold at three different levels: the service or unit; the case or discharge; and the person-year or capitation. A package, or mix, of an intermediate product like laboratory services constitutes a case, and a package of cases constitutes a capitation rate. Despite this complexity, the hospital must earn a satisfactory margin on each level, and the margin expectation is specified for each support service. The data system must provide information on all three terms—price, margin, and cost—at all three levels—unit, case, and capita. Moving from the unit level to the case level requires estimates of the number of services used for each case group. Moving to the capitation level requires case level estimates plus estimates of the incidence per year of each case group. At higher levels, measurement system precision involves all three elements.

Source information includes:

1. *Unit cost, prices, and margins*—Internal data come from the accounting and budgeting systems. Comparative data on prices are easily obtained for all other vendors, both hospital and non-hospital.

2. *Cost or charges per discharge*—Medicare and often Medicaid pay a fixed price per discharge. Cost per case is essential to determining the contribution of these payers to profit. Publicly available Medicare cost reports permit study of the relative contribution of the service to the total for similar hospitals. Shared data services can provide case-specific comparisons.

3. *Cost per capita*—Contribution of the service to annual capitation premiums for major HMO and PPO customers can be calculated through HMO or insurance information systems. These systems are required because the patient's total annual use may include several instances or outpatient care and more than one admission. The value should be adjusted for age or made specific to the population group most at risk for the service. It is rare to have comparative data, but trends can be observed. Cost per capita is theoretically the best information for patient group protocols, because it permits consideration of readmission rates and other elements of total health care. Few hospitals have the measure now. Availability can be expected to increase in the coming years.

Minimizing Incidents and Hazards. Support services account for significant fractions of the hospital's malpractice, workers' compensation, and general liability. Data on hazards and unexpected events can be compiled monthly, but annual review is more reliable to identify trends and possible improvements. Comparative data are not reliable unless definitions and accounting procedures have been carefully standardized. For most hospitals today, historic records are the only useful guides. Case-by-case review may suggest avenues for improvement more often than statistical analysis.

Internal Measures of Performance. While external measures are essential to guide the clinical support service manager in meeting overall hospital goals, much of the detailed and day-to-day management relies on more specific measures of internal processes. The relationships between the outcomes measures and internal, or process, measures are usually complex and often only partially understood. It is important that the support service manager understand these relationships. The manager sets expectations based on last year's performance and the needs suggested by the outcomes expectations. The areas of process measures follow the closed system model:

— Demand
— Quality
— Cost and efficiency or productivity
— Profit

Measures of the Demand Process. Process measures of demand should be maintained in two areas: (1) the level of recorded requests and (2) measures of unmet demand, disruption of service, and delay.

1. *Level of demand*—These arise from automated scheduling or order entry sources and are reported in counts. They should be reported monthly or weekly, by major demand groups and pay sources. Statistical tests of significance of variation should be included. Statistical histories for specific physicians, nursing floors, and patient characteristics should be accessible when needed.

2. *Rates of failure*—These include cancellations by source (patient, doctor, or department), delays, stat requests, and services repeated because of failure or poor results. Automated clinical service systems collect all these measures. Statistically valid comparisons against history or expectations are needed in the larger units. These may require additional software and analysis.

Measures of Technical Quality. Process measures of technical quality are generally compliance statistics, that is, attributes counts of acceptance against a priori criteria. Often a criterion is established by the profession and is a subjective consensus, for example, "Is the exposure correct on this radiograph?" Occasionally absolute tests are available, as with laboratory blind tests. The measures often cover a diverse array of considerations. If several dozen are evaluated for a single patient, worker, or setting, a score can be constructed and treated as a continuous or variables measure.

Well-run support services are implementing the following steps to obtain relatively frequent assessments of process quality:

1. The more important aspects of the service are identified, and the criteria constituting good care are developed as a consensus of professional judgment. Although these criteria are usually

published in the literature of the profession, collective review and local consensus are important.

2. A survey instrument reviewing the agreed-upon matters is devised, and surveyors are trained to administer it in an unbiased manner.

3. A sampling strategy is formulated. The strategy identifies how frequently results are needed and at what levels of detail. It specifies a random selection of patients designed to meet the reporting needs at minimum cost. (Consultation with a qualified statistician is usually required.)

4. The strategy is implemented, frequently through automated ordering of scheduling systems, which also provides for recording, analyzing, and reporting results.

5. Process quality scores are tracked on the shortest horizon consistent with the sample and are aggregated to reveal information about specific personnel, activity, or patient groups over longer periods.

Measures of Cost and Productivity. The measures for cost and productivity are collected by the accounting system, but the support service manager participates in determining how detailed the data should be. Issues involving the support service include application of accounting definitions and selection of productivity standards (see also chapter 8).

— *Account center definition.* Each supervisor within a support service department should have his or her own cost and revenue centers. The combination constitutes a responsibility center. Functional account detail for the responsibility center will show labor costs, supplies costs, and so on and revenue by source of payment. Appropriate parts of the budget are similarly segregated, and the supervisor gains the ability to set and meet expectations in which she or he has participated, a critical component of closed system theory. (Information for more detailed functions or smaller work groups will require special studies.)

— *Labor and machine productivity standards.* Productivity standards offer opportunities for improvement after scheduling and forecasting gains have been achieved. Comparative standards are useful in revealing the range of competition and the known limits, but the best expectations always recognize local history.

— *Allowances for variation in demand.* Even under the best of scheduling systems, allowances for unpredictable variation in demand are frequently necessary. Setting these allowances and

.establishing the cost of them require advice from the support service manager.

— *Flexible budget variance measures.* Flexible budget systems report variances for the demand forecast and labor productivity terms. Most flexible budgets also report any variance in the purchase price of labor, such as might arise from using too high a skill level or excessive overtime. Thus the manager must minimize three variances, price, demand, and quantity of labor. Under fixed budget approaches, variations are reported only in dollars or for labor in dollars and hours.

— *Overhead.* Overhead expectations were traditionally reported as fixed costs, but this provides no incentive for economy to either the overhead department or the service department. Well-run hospitals are moving to "sell" as much overhead service as possible to the support services on a transfer price basis. The transfer price is analogous to the price the hospital would charge if it sold the service to outsiders. Use of the overhead service then becomes a flexible budget item for the support service. The overhead department becomes accountable for demand forecasts, transfer price, and "profit."

Measures of Profit. Measures of profit are determined according to established accounting rules. Once the overhead question is addressed and the support service manager is consulted about the price schedule, a profit expectation can be jointly set. Any departure from it should be traceable to some component: demand, productivity, scheduling, unit costs, overhead, or prices must also depart from expectations. If, and only if, price is competitively set, profit provides a global measure of support service management skill in terms comparable to other support services and the hospital as a whole.

Information Systems

Good information systems arise from the needs of the organization, and the needs of the support services are now clear. Fortunately, so is the technology to deliver them. The list of major components of the information system is relatively long, but several components interact, either with each other or with other services. This permits economical software and file systems.

Emerging Capabilities. Within a few years, every manager of a major clinical service will have automated support in the following areas:

— *Patient scheduling.* This function will be integrated with other information systems for both inpatients and outpatients so that a patient with several needs can have them met in an orderly and prompt manner. Within the unit, the scheduling system will use urgent and on-call patients to stabilize demand. It will capture from electronic order entry systems and master patient files the full description of the service requested and the characteristics of the patient. It will record historical data on demand by category and several patient classes, and it will show variability and departure from forecast by shift. A forecasting algorithm will report near-term personnel needs to aid in scheduling. The system will also report failures, cancellations, and delays.

— *Personnel and machine scheduling.* Software recording the personnel available to the department, with data on skills, cost, employment history, and scheduling preferences, will accept short-term demand forecasts and calculate a reasonable schedule of personnel to meet them. The schedule will be presented to the supervisor for review and correction and will then be printed in convenient form for each worker. The software will be capable of listing overtime to date for each employee, allowing equitable distribution when overtime is necessary.

— *Order processing.* Descriptive data on patients obtained from the scheduling software will be attached to each order for service. When the service is performed, these data will be used in three ways:

- To post the patient's account
- To adjust the results report for patient characteristics
- To build historical files for development of patient group protocols and intermediate product protocols

— *Results reporting.* Information on normal and nonnormal conditions will be entered by professionals, who may also enter notations in English. Results can be electronically reported to the attending physician. In the diagnostic services, prior tests can be summarized, permitting analysis of trends. Historic results files will also be accessible, leading to improvement of intermediate product protocols.

— *Patient medical accounting.* Summaries of support service activity for episodes of illness will be incorporated in a master clinical abstract file. This file, augmented automatically with billing information, will form the historical resource for patient group protocols.

— *Clinical performance assessment.* An algorithm will identify sample patients for outcomes measures of quality, generate the survey instrument, and accept responses to it efficiently. It will also prepare summary reports and analysis of trends, calculate statistical significance, and provide early warning of departures from important quality measures.

Design. The information system meeting these needs will be a network using large mainframe files and processors for high-volume activity, principally related to master records and schedules, billing, personnel, and clinical performance. Personal computers will meet local need in most departments, although clinical laboratory may require larger equipment. Patient and personnel scheduling, order processing, results reporting, and clinical performance assessment will be locally available. Interface between these machines will be instantaneous, so the support service operator will use the PC without knowing the source of the processing.

Management Issues

Well-run hospitals are recognizing that four conditions are essential to the progress of the clinical support services:

1. Maintaining between the support service specialist and manager and the attending staff relationships that encourage continued development of cost-effective patient group protocols.
2. Developing contract and compensation arrangements that encourage clinical support service managers to contribute to improvement of patient group and intermediate product protocols.
3. Integrating clinical and managerial functions more effectively through improved intermediate product protocols.
4. Capturing the economic gains from improved protocols using flexible budgeting techniques.

Building Cooperation with Other Hospital Systems

The competitive environment requires much closer cooperation among support services, the attending staff departments and sections, and the governance system. These relationships have frequently been troublesome. Well-run hospitals attempt to strengthen them by addressing both the general elements of a fruitful professional relationship and, for the physician specialist, a well-designed and well-administered contract.

(There are close parallels for the nonphysician manager and other supervisory employees.)

Fruitful Professional Relationships. Good relationships rest on candor, respect, and trust, and they are collaborative rather than adversarial. They are supported by the following general goals:

— Full recognition is always accorded both the managerial and the professional rank of the specialist. This means that no distinction is made between the political rights or status of specialists in, say, surgery versus anesthesia. It also means that physician managers of major support services, recognized in both the supervisory structure and the medical staff structure, attain considerable power. This power is counterbalanced by the marketplace and the influence of the attending staff.

— All relevant decision-making procedures are standardized and communicated widely throughout the organization, including the medical staff. The issues on the agenda, the bodies making the decisions, and the ways in which to gain a hearing for one's arguments must be clear to everyone.

— Participation in decision making is routinely adjusted to the question, so no individuals or groups need fear being omitted from a decision critical to their activity.

— Methods of appeal and resolution of conflict are clear and adhered to strictly.

Communication with Clinical Departments. Good relations between support services and clinical departments begin with good service, meeting the attending doctors' exchange needs for quality, efficiency, and price. In addition, they include a program of communications in three major areas:

1. The development of patient group protocols (or, where these are not formal, education on the contribution of the service to specific conditions), including information on:

   a. Reliability, validity, and sensitivity of diagnostic aids

   b. Effectiveness, cost, and difficulties associated with therapeutic aids

   c. Interactions between two or more services

2. The needs of the attending specialty, specifically:

   a. Clinical problem areas noted either by the support service manager or by the attending physicians

    b. Recent changes in technology

    c. Achievements of the service department in terms of doctor and patient satisfaction or technical quality

    d. System improvements and how to use them

3. Consultation with attending staff on difficult or unusual cases, emphasizing:

    a. Convenience

    b. Thorough and competent responses

    c. Support of the attending physician

Improving Contracts for Hospital-Based Specialists

Medical support specialists have had the monopolistic advantage of shortages since World War II, with the result that contracts have followed their desires and their incomes have risen far more rapidly than those of other specialists. As the market becomes more competitive because of increased physician supply, hospitals will be able to exert more influence over both income and contract terms.

Compensation. One of the easiest elements to dispense with is the actual amount of the specialist's income. The hospital should expect to pay, and the specialist should expect to receive, fair market wages. The approximate base income of the specialist can be determined from annual surveys by the American Medical Association, supplemented with local surveys as necessary. Arguments that the hospital should pay more or less than market should be viewed skeptically. Most such arguments reflect some other issue, which is better faced directly than subverted into salary negotiations.

    The cost implications of other elements of the contract are far more serious. Critical elements include goals which encourage greater contribution to both intermediate and final product protocols and professional growth. The method of payment may be the key to those objectives.

Goals of the Contract. In general, employment should enhance the flexibility rather than the rigidity of the relationship, relate the reward of the specialist to hospitalwide achievement, and enhance security for the individual. These goals should be reinforced in the contract. It is wise to have the contract summarize the areas in which quantitative expectations will be developed, describe how these will be established, and recognize their limitations in terms of overall patient care goals. Well-run hospitals discuss in negotiations the obligation of support service managers to participate in final product protocols, management of demand, and cooperative efforts with other services to increase overall hospital efficiency. It is as important to include these matters in the goals of the contract as it is to include them in the design of the compensation.

An ideal employment relationship encourages a wholesome life-style that integrates professional and personal concerns. Such a relationship supports many years of fruitful work by stimulating variety, learning, acceptance, and recognition. These elements make a job psychologically rewarding. Professional fulfillment is probably enhanced by study opportunities and sabbaticals, appropriate limits to work requirements, regular vacations and relief, the perception of fairness and flexibility in negotiating and administering the contract, and the maintenance of peer recognition for the specialist, both as a physician and as a manager. The last is supported more by actions than by the contract itself.

Selecting the Method of Payment. The many approaches for compensating the physician specialist are described earlier in this chapter.

It is worth recognizing that employment is the tried and true method of payment for managers generally. Almost universally in the commercial world, department and division level managers are first paid a salary, although substantial modifications and enhancements may be added. Few enterprises would contemplate having as manager of a major revenue center someone who was *not* an employee of the company. The responsiveness required in a competitive marketplace suggests the need for simplicity, continuity, and a unified reward structure. Employment contracts achieve this, particularly since they involve the employment of all subordinates of the physician specialist.

On the other hand, the employment contract presents several difficulties:

— *Weak performance incentives.* There are three major areas in which a salary contract may lack sufficiently direct performance incentives:

    • *Quality and satisfaction.* Fee-for-service payments provide greater incentive for attention to "customer" needs. In the case of support services, the customer is both the patient and the attending physician, and their needs include high technical quality, prompt service, and amenities.

    • *Patient group protocol,* or final product productivity. Employment offers no *direct* incentive to reduce use of support services, although it is superior to most arrangements with independent contractors, which contain financial incentives to increase use.

- *Intermediate product productivity.* Unless modified by bonuses, salary contains no incentive for productivity or competitive pricing. The specialist, like any other manager, may respond well to financial incentives.

— *Adverse effect on earning potential.* The specialist's salary is usually paid solely by the hospital, and he or she cannot bill insurance carriers for services. The hospital's payment may be limited to an amount which is independent of the support service contract. The total billed to the insurance company may be greater under fee contracts with separate billing. The selection of fee contract options to gain revenue is commonly called **unbundling.**

— *Higher income taxes.* Salary seems to lag behind other forms of compensation in protecting income from taxation. Many of the specific exemption opportunities of fee-for-service practice are relatively small and transient. The laws, and more significantly the regulations which interpret them, change frequently on minor details of business expense deductions, capital investment, and the like.

— *Invidious status comparisons to other doctors.* The fee-for-service model suggests both an agency relationship to patients and a professional self-reliance which are attractive elements of practice for many physicians. The direct patient contact enjoyed by primary care physicians can never be reproduced for referral specialists, let alone hospital-based physicians. The contrasts are heightened by salaried compensation. Invidious comparisons to "real" doctors can arise from too sharp a contrast between employed and private practice physicians. However foolish such issues may appear to outsiders, they have been an important part of much dissatisfaction of hospital-based specialists.

Fee-for-service and percent-of-gross schemes probably do not enhance either intermediate or final product productivity. The specialist is compensated for additional output, even if it is obtained at ridiculous cost to the hospital. Percent-of-net payment methods force consideration of internal efficiency. Under all three, sharp declines in specialist incomes may result from changes in patient group protocols. These may be disruptive, particularly if they are unexpected or perceived as punitive.

Joint ventures are not fully understood. They appear to have three advantages. Two of these, unbundling and tax avoidance, must be considered as transient. As such, they might be beneficial, but they probably are not compelling reasons for experimentation. The third advantage is that the joint venture, at least theoretically, marries the participants to common goals. Both intermediate and final product productivity can be rewarded, and issues involving amenities assume their proper importance. Service-by-service joint ventures might still lack incentives for collective efforts. Disagreements might be expected on such issues as new hospital investments, for example. If a hospital invests in imaging instead of laboratory diagnosis, a redistribution of the physicians' incomes results under all schemes except employment. Invidious comparisons with other members of the medical staff might take on a new cast under joint ventures, particularly if these were limited to only a few specialties. The opportunity for joint ventures, including both support service and attending physicians, is arising from HMO and PPO activities, but it represents a major unexplored shift away from the traditions of fee-for-service medicine.

Payment method is now clearly a negotiable item. The best method appears to depend on the hospital's identifying which liabilities can be controlled and which opportunities exploited locally.

Improving Intermediate Product Protocols

Well-run hospitals are working toward the integration of all aspects of support service operation. They believe that long-term cost-effectiveness will be improved by an integrated approach, which here is called the intermediate product protocols. These include quality, appropriateness, scheduling, planning, budgeting, and pricing.

A major requirement of support service managers will be sound judgment in dealing with incomplete and changing measures of performance. Quantified expectations can introduce distortion away from unmeasured elements. Yet a properly used quantitative system permits both easier achievement of expectations and focus on unquantified elements. Leadership toward the positive rather than the negative outcome will require broad clinical understanding, human relations skills, and good judgment. The well-run hospital today is developing the automated system requirements, learning to set the expectations by collaborative rather than adversarial negotiation, and developing the management judgment of the support services.

Worker participation will be critical to a successful outcome. Responding to quantitative incentives without overlooking the compassion and charity which must underlie patient care will be difficult. Workers must try harder to respond to variation in demand. Maintaining cross-trained skills also requires extra effort. Equity demands that these efforts be rewarded, and theory suggests that tangible rewards will increase the success of the hospital. The mechanisms for establishing those rewards have not yet been established.

Quality, Amenities, and Satisfaction. Quality measurements should exist, and explicit expectations should be written for as many areas of technical quality, satisfaction, and amenities as possible, even though measurement will be difficult and some can be monitored only at long intervals. (The writing prompts discussion, reduces ambiguity, and speeds communication, particularly when the written expectation is widely available.) An increasing number of quality measures exists and is routinely compared against expectations.

— *Response times and repeat rates.* Ordering systems record these automatically and treat them as quality control statistics for high-volume services such as laboratory, pharmacy, and imaging.

— *Technical quality.* The measure of technical quality is being improved by increasing specification of the patient's situation. In many cases, patient age, comorbidity, and concurrent treatment affect the test or therapy. Automated ordering supports transmission of these data to the support service specialist. For quantifiable tests, frequency distribution of values of results are being captured in increasingly specific patient sets. Using these improves the reliability of the resulting diagnostic decision, reducing false positives while at the same time increasing sensitivity to true disease. Measures of the dispersion of test results, such as the range, the standard deviation, or the coefficient of variance, are effective quality control tools.

— *Surveys of patient and attending physician satisfaction.* Formal surveys, particularly of patients, are increasingly common and are being improved to yield statistically reliable results. Although cost is shared across the hospital, it remains relatively high, and the frequency of such surveys is kept low. Random responses, usually complaints, are tracked as indicators between surveys. Informal communication with individual attending physicians is supplemented by communication with the medical staff organization units. Scheduling systems, reporting systems, and employee education are used to improve results.

— *Amenities.* Well-run hospitals are paying more attention to amenities that patients and doctors find attractive. Hours of service, delays and reporting delays, attitudes of personnel, parking, and comfort are being improved to increase the attractiveness of service.

Management of Demand. The well-run hospital is moving to improve management of demand at every level: categorizing patients appropriately, eliminating expensive, unnecessary emergencies, reducing demand for overused support services, and implementing patient scheduling systems that produce highly reliable forecasts of the actual work to be done each day. Although these activities overlap, they can be described under three headings:

1. *Patient group protocols*—The well-run support service has data on demand by diagnosis-related group and is able to present averages, trends, major sources of variation, and published consensuses about appropriate use of the service for common diseases. These data are accessible to the attending services most involved with the diagnosis. While patient group protocols may not exist formally in many hospitals yet, the attending service and the support service members know the ranges of common experience better than they did, and well-run hospitals are considering formal protocols. Demand for support services is falling as a result of these preliminary efforts to limit it to cost-effective applications.

2. *Forecasting*—The well-run hospital provides a central forecast of demand for inpatient and outpatient services as well as forecasts by major pay source. The support service expands these forecasts in as much detail as the size of the operation will support. The refined forecasts support patient scheduling, personnel scheduling, and equipment scheduling.

3. *Patient scheduling*—The well-run support service now schedules patients whenever possible, and sets as specific a time as possible. Technology for automated scheduling that is centralized for all services is progressing but is not yet common. When available, it will eliminate conflicts over timing and sequencing between support services.

Improving the Budget and Cost-Effectiveness

All of the issues of the integrated intermediate product protocols eventually affect the cost of operation, and both costs and markets should be considered in establishing prices. Thus the operating budget is developed as the final step of the protocols. At a certain level of efficiency, it becomes practical to expand the budget to a flexible format accommodating scheduled variation in demand.

Benefits and Difficulties of Flexible Budgeting. Both fixed and flexible budgets use productivity standards or expectations of output units per hour of worker time. The important distinction between the two is that flexible budgeting expects the supervisor to adjust staffing to short-term variation in demand. Fixed budgeting, common in hospitals until the 1980s, establishes fixed dollar and real resource levels for the entire year or adjusted for seasonal variations. Labor resources are frequently identified as *full-time equivalents* (FTEs) and *positions,* which can be filled on a full- or part-time basis as designated. The system is unable to achieve maximum efficiency when demand is changing.

The starting point for flexible budgeting is the identification of fixed and variable costs. The distinction based on the manager's ability to adjust expenditures, is a function of the skills and imagination of the manager and the organization as a whole. Any cost should be identified as variable and subject to flexible budgeting when the dollar savings achievable as a result exceed the cost of doing so. Costs of supplies are generally easy to control and should be flexibily budgeted in most cost centers The difficulties of flexible budgeting diminish after patient and personnel scheduling systems are installed, because they provide important information as by-products. At present, well-run hospitals are developing flexible budgeting for labor costs in clinical laboratories, pharmacies, X-ray departments, operating suites, some nursing units, outpatient clinics, and larger physical therapy and rehabilitation therapy units.

Flexible budgeting for labor costs is useful whenever the variation in demand that remains after scheduling can be accommodated by varying the work force. Three conditions must be met in order to justify the added expense and difficulty:

1. Demand can be reliably described in terms of a productivity standard.

2. Demand can be reliably forecast.

3. Personnel staffing can be varied in response to changes in demand.

These restrictions make flexible budgeting unnecessary or impractical in a surprisingly large number of situations. Nursing, social work, and some other services adjust the quantity of services given to patients on the basis of their professional judgment of need. Productivity standards are only useful when the impact of such adjustments can be described in advance. Random variation in demand cannot be forecast, meaning that staffing for it must be fixed. It is inevitable in obstetrics and coronary care, and difficult to manage in emergency service. Finally, for very small services, very specialized services, and night or evening shifts, there is often no opportunity to increase efficiency, because only one or two persons must be scheduled.

Fixed budgeting is cheaper and easier for the supervisor to manage. It is therefore appropriate unless specific advantages can be found for flexible budgeting. The principal disadvantage of fixed budgeting is that staffing is set at a level that permits service to peak loads. If these are very high—say a third more than average—there will be many shifts on which demand is less than staff capacity. However, people are surprisingly flexible. A normal work group can accommodate a 20 percent variation in average shift demand without serious danger either to themselves or to patients. Thus a great many support services can operate very well on fixed budgets.

Well-run hospitals enter into flexible budgeting when the benefits of fixed budgeting have been exhausted. They build toward flexible budgeting by addressing productivity standards, forecasting, and worker scheduling in a coordinated sequence, seeking the largest possible improvement in productivity at any given time.

Requirements for Labor Productivity Standards. Both fixed and flexible budgeting assume a reliable unit standard for labor productivity, that is, that a properly trained, experienced, and equipped worker can produce a certain average number of units of output per hour. For flexible budgeting, reliability must occur at the level of staffing assignment, usually the shift. For fixed budgeting, reliability can occur over a much longer interval, such as a pay period.

A staffing standard is always more reliable over large numbers of services. A standard will fit over several weeks, although it varies too much to be useful for a single day. One implication of the need for reliability is that flexible budgeting is more rewarding when services are of short duration (so that many are performed each day), while scheduling is more rewarding when services take a long time to perform. This condition is more likely to be met when many individual services are performed in a shift. Long surgical procedures are unlikely to fit shift-level variable staffing, whereas short laboratory tests are.

Forecasting Demand. Both fixed and flexible budgets depend upon forecasts of demand. A well-run clinical support service has historical data for demand categories by shift, day of the week, and week of the year. These data are used to forecast labor requirements for each shift. Scheduling systems make short-term forecasting easier by reducing variation in staffing requirements. They also generate a continuing file of demand data to improve forecasting.

In well-run hospitals, the finance system uses regression to forecast trends and relationships between support service demand and aggregate hospital demand, expressed in discharges, patient days, and outpatient activity. These statistical forecasts are always reviewed subjectively by the support service managers before being incorporated into the annual budget. Managers who are familiar with their service are quite accurate forecasters over horizons of several months or a year, but their insights are less useful for longer periods.

Flexible budget reports isolate the variation caused by the difference between forecast and actual demand from that caused by deviation from the labor productivity standard. Obviously, the supervisor is not accountable for the forecasting error in the same sense as for the variation from the productivity standard. However, in the long run, the forecast error should also be reduced by better data and better scheduling. Thus the supervisor's responsibilities extend to both elements of the budget variance, and rewards should reflect combined achievement.

Precision in forecasting demand is useful only to the point of controlling the work force. As forecast errors are larger at smaller volumes, greater specificity becomes counterproductive at some level of detail. A practical level of specificity uses patient aggregates, such as clinical services, or major diagnostic categories as demand groups. These assume that three measures can be forecast.

1. D, the total demand for all groups
2. p_i, the proportion of the total in group i
3. U_i, the expected units of service per discharge in group i

Then the group demand will be $D \times p_i \times U_i$, and the total service demand will be $\sum (D \times p_i \times U_i)$. This permits development of values for D and p_i over the hospital as a whole. It also permits easy adaptation to patient group protocol revisions by changing U_i.

Varying Staffing for Support Services. As forecasting and demand management improve in well-managed hospitals, the need for flexible staffing in support services will become clearer. Many of the services are driven by admissions, and under admission scheduling systems these will differ sharply by day of the week. Shorter stays demand faster turnaround on diagnostic tests, which in turn may require larger evening shift operations. Technological improvements and more precise patient group protocols will cause some services to increase and others to decline. Efficiency will require prompt adjustment of the work force as these changes occur.

There are six ways to adjust a work force to changes in demand:

1. Gain greater output per hour from increased individual effort.
2. Change the number of part-time or temporary employees.

3. Adjust the effective number of full-time employees by using voluntary or involuntary furloughs or increasing overtime.

4. Transfer personnel from assignments with declining volume to those with increasing volume.

5. Use contract, or agency, personnel.

6. Terminate workers or undertake new hiring.

Although the cost of a specific approach depends upon the situation, the higher numbered responses are generally more expensive for short-term applications. The costs may appear in training, turnover, quality, or other indirect considerations. The use of agency personnel should be a last resort because of the costs, which frequently include loss of quality as well as premium hourly labor costs.

The strategy of the well-managed clinical support service should be to:

— Develop long-term forecasts of employment needs and limit permanent employment to the lowest reasonable forecast. These steps will avoid forced terminations and improve morale among permanent workers.

— Develop a cadre of trained part-time or temporary workers. These workers may require a premium over the hourly rate for standby, training time, or similar services, but they will be less costly than agency personnel and more familiar with the hospital's needs and standards of quality.

— Provide systems support and incentives for increased output, particularly when it is necessary to meet short-term fluctuations in demand.

— Use overtime to accommodate short-term increases in demand.

— Cross train employees in several operations so that jobs can be reassigned without loss of quality.

These strategies will require substantial support from the human resources system, as discussed in chapter 14. For the larger services, they will also require both personnel and patient scheduling systems to manage the complex logistics.

Notes

1. Avedis Donabedian, *The Definition of Quality and Approaches to Its Assessment* (Ann Arbor, MI: Health Administration Press, 1980).

2. Walton M. Hancock and Paul F. Walter, *The "ASCS" Inpatient Admission Scheduling and Control System* (Ann Arbor, MI: Health Administration Press, 1983).

3. Howard J. Berman and Lewis E. Weeks, *The Financial Management of Hospitals,* 6th ed., (Ann Arbor, MI: Health Administration Press, 1986).

4. C. Bidese and D. Danais, *Physician Characteristics and Distribution in the U.S.— 1981* (Chicago: Division of Survey and Data Resources, American Medical Association, 1982).

5. John E. Ware, *An Experimental Approach to Validating Patient Quality of Care Assessments* (Santa Monica, CA: Rand Corporation, 1983).

Suggested Readings

Bouchard, Eric A. *Radiology Management: An Introduction.* Denver, CO: Multi-Media Publishers, 1983.

England, Brent, ed. *Medical Rehabiliation Services in Health Care Institutions.* Chicago: American Hospital Publishers, 1986.

Jenkins, Astor L., ed., van de Leuv, John H., assoc. ed. *Emergency Department Organization and Management,* 2d ed. St. Louis: Mosby, 1978. Published under the editorial guidance of the Hospital Committee of the American College of Emergency Physicians.

Karni, Karen R., Viskochil, Karen R., and Amos, Patricia A., eds. *Clinical Laboratory Management: A Guide for Clinical Laboratory Scientists.* Boston: Little, Brown, 1982.

American Society of Hospital Pharmacists. *Model Quality Assurance Program for Hospital Pharmacies,* rev. ed. Washington, DC: ASHP, 1980.

13

Nursing Services

Introduction

Definition of Nursing Services

Most people, when asked to evaluate their inpatient hospital care, speak first not of the doctor, but of the nurse. Furthermore, if they think well of their nursing care, they tend to rate the whole experience, even the bill, more favorably. While the patient's emphasis is in some ways naive, it is not entirely misplaced. Next to medicine, nursing often makes the most important contribution to speedy recovery. It is almost always critical to inpatient care, usually relevant to outpatient care, and central to long-term institutional care. Organizationally, it is by far the largest service of the modern hospital. In the health care field, nurses are as ubiquitous as doctors. There is virtually no place that they have not made a contribution.

Speculating on the future of hospitals, one notes that nursing is already one of three main clinical subsystems, along with the attending staff and the other clinical support services. The competitive environment suggests a bigger, more influential role for nursing. This chapter addresses this emerging potential of nursing. It assumes that nursing care is defined by patient needs and professional skills rather than in- or outpatient location. It also assumes that the well-run hospital will be interested in many or all locations for care. Finally, it assumes that well-educated nurses will pursue the broad purpose of homeostasis with a professional zeal that brooks no invidious comparison, on gender or any other ground.

Defining what nursing service is has proved troublesome to both nurses and nonnurses. In part this may be due to the extraordinary breadth of nursing's contribution. Nursing can be defined by its willingness to undertake almost anything necessary to help the patient return to or sustain independence. This role was defined by Florence Nightingale as stretching from emotional support to control of hazards in the environment. The patient need not be sick; nursing services include prevention. The patient need not survive; nursing service is important for the dying.

Nursing can also be defined by its objective of assisting the patient to homeostasis, a state of equilibrium with one's environment. This concept was also articulated by Florence Nightingale, who said in 1859 that nursing is those activities which "put the patient in the best condition for nature to act upon him."[1] This concept prevails in most of the more modern definitions, which add the goal of independence.[2]

> **Nursing is the provision of physical, emotional, and cognitive services that support or improve the patient's equilibrium with his or her environment and that helps the patient gain independence as rapidly as possible.**

The definition is limited only by the patient's needs and the services provided by others. As the support services grew to technical and professional maturity over this century, nursing relinquished responsibility for many of them. More remains than has been given away.

Purpose of Nursing

The route to homeostasis includes a nursing assessment or diagnosis, the development of an individualized plan or expectation, and the implementation of the plan by specific nursing tasks or tasks requested of other services. Prevention has always been important, including immunization, environmental control, screening, and prompt follow-up to minimize the impact of disease. It is obviously better to prevent loss of equilibrium than to try to regain it. Even for the sick patient, preventing the spread of disability is superior to correcting losses.

The nursing process of diagnosis and response resembles the medical one conceptually, but the details of a nursing care plan seek to complement rather than duplicate a medical protocol. Medicine's focus on technology has stimulated nursing's emphasis on access, mental and emotional considerations, education, motivation, acceptability, and satisfaction. As medicine has become high-tech, nursing has become high-touch.

The purposes of nursing are as follows:

— To promote health, including emotional and social well-being
— To prevent disease and disability
— To provide environmental, physical, cognitive, and emotional support in illness
— To minimize the consequences of disease
— To encourage rehabilitation

Scope of Nursing Services

Nursing service can be classified into two categories, personal nursing services, or what nurses do for patients as individuals, and general nursing services, consisting of educational, public health, and other group-oriented activities. The first is far larger and historically the center of hospital nursing activities, but the second is important in its own right and is receiving increased attention from hospitals seeking to provide resources for community health.

Personal Nursing Service. Personal nursing service encompasses most of the professional activity of nurses and employs about two-thirds of this nation's 1.3 million working nurses.[3] It can be conceived of as having three dimensions, and these direct specialization of activity: site, duration, and clinical specialty (see figure 13.1).

Referring only to these three dimensions, there are 4 × 2 × 7 or 56, potential assignments. While the largest group is probably intermediate acute medicine, it is shrinking. Intensive care nursing and various home and outpatient activities are growing. A specific hospital would be unlikely to have all 56 jobs, but the definition of hospitals permits them to have any of the jobs. Large hospitals probably have about 30 different nursing work assignments. The individuals filling these posts tend to refer to themselves as specialists. In fact, they use specialized skills and draw upon unique as well as general nursing experience, so hospitals would seek related experience when recruiting or promoting them.

General Nursing Services. Well-run community hospitals have moved decisively toward collective, rather than individual, patient services, not only as a contribution to their public health goals, but also as a way of reducing total cost of care. Smoking, alcohol, and hypertension appear to account for 10 to 20 percent of total health care costs, and these may be reducible through education. Emotional stress within the family, which may lead to spouse and child abuse, can also be reduced by edu-

Figure 13.1

Categories of Personal Nursing Service

Site
  Bedside
    Intensive
    Intermediate
    Limited
    Home
  Outpatient
    Office
    Clinic
    Emergency service
  Noninstitutional
    Neighborhood or community
    Work place or school
  Other
    Surgery
    Delivery
Duration
  Short-term, or acute
  Long-term, or chronic
Clinical Specialty
  Medicine
  Surgery
  Obstetrics
  Pediatrics
  Psychiatry
  Substance abuse
  Rehabilitation

Figure 13.2

Categories of General Nursing Service

Health Education
  Parenting and child health
    Prenatal and parenting
    Infant nutrition and development
    Child and adolescent development
  Life-style and adult health
    Sexual expression and contraception
    Exercise and fitness
    Weight control
    Implications of aging
  Chemical dependency and substance abuse
Prevention
  Primary prevention
  Screening
  Social and home services for the aging

cation and counselling. Nurses, because they are accepted by the public as knowledgeable, yet less formidable than doctors, are well placed to contribute.

General nursing services emphasize group activities for disease prevention, as opposed to care of individual patients. The scope of general nursing services is shown in figure 13.2.

Extended Nursing Roles. The nurse providing personal or general service in inpatient and outpatient settings fills a familiar role complementary to the attending physician's. Three more independent professional nursing roles have emerged. One group of extended roles involves more clinical responsibility. **Clinical nurse practitioners** receive extra training for medical diagnosis or treatment. In areas where doctors are in short supply, nurse practitioners conduct patient examinations, counsel patients, and supervise routine chronic care. **Nurse midwives** handle uncomplicated obstetrics. Both have demonstrated competence equal or superior to that of physicians within these domains. **Nurse anesthetists** are trained to work under general medical supervision.

The second extended role is that of **case manager.** This concept has arisen from the success of HMOs. HMOs depend upon adept selection of less costly diagnostic or treatment alternatives whenever possible. The case manager is a coordinator and overseer who seeks to assist other health care professionals in finding the least costly solution at any particular juncture. Nurses, particularly those with postbaccalaureate education and considerable clinical experience, are well positioned to become case managers. It is likely that case management will be increasingly popular in the coming decade. It may emerge as the best way to deal with health care of the aged, or it may lead to ideas as yet unimagined for this complex and expensive problem.

The third extended role is in hospital and health care organization management. Nurses constitute a significant group of middle management in every hospital. Some are nurse clinicians, specialists in the problems of certain patient groups. Others are general line managers, supervising large staffs and accountable for a broad range of expectations. It is wise to remember that a large nursing floor will involve 50 or more employees and will relate routinely with most clinical support services as well as finance, human resources, and plant services. The nursing department constitutes half the work force in most hospitals and generates at least half the revenue. It is routinely in direct contact with most of the rest of the hospital. In the effort to improve quality and productivity, the nursing management role will expand.

Plan of the Chapter

This chapter attempts to show how nursing contributes to the hospital's mission as one of the three major elements of the clinical system. It describes nursing as it must be understood by others in the hospital, especially members of the medical staff, governance, and clinical support services. But because these perceptions must be congruent with nursing's own, this chapter also reflects the perspective nursing managers must have in order to build the well-managed hospital. The chapter builds managerial functions around clinical ones, and organization and information systems around the combined clinical managerial need. The following major topics are covered:

1. Clinical functions of nursing
2. Managerial functions of nursing
3. Personnel and organization
4. Measurement and information
5. Management issues

Clinical Functions of Nursing

A well-managed hospital has, by definition, high-quality economical nursing care. The breadth of the commitment to homeostasis requires similar breadth of clinical nursing functions. Control of quality and economy begins with development and implementation of the nursing care plan. Implementation leads directly to other important clinical functions: communication with other clinical groups, assistance to families of patients, general prevention and health education, and, finally, case management.

The Nursing Care Plan

The nursing care plan documents the needs of each patient and establishes the expectations for nursing procedures and outcomes. Properly written, the inpatient care plan incorporates the discharge plan, although the discharge plan is sometimes segregated as a device for coordinating the many professions who must complete their work before the patient can leave. (Even when the discharge planning function is isolated, it is usually assigned to nursing.) The care plan is developed early in the disease episode and is revised as needed. It is more formal in inpatient and long-term outpatient care and is often left unwritten in brief, uncomplicated outpatient encounters. A good care plan strives to do the following:

— Incorporate all care that is cost-effective

— Exclude any care or service which is less than cost-effective

— Anticipate individual variations and prevent complications

— Organize the major events in the hospitalization or disease episode to minimize overall duration

— Identify potential barriers to prompt discharge and plan to investigate and remove them

Nursing Diagnosis. Each nursing care plan begins with a thorough nursing diagnosis, that is, the identification of actual or potential departures from homeostasis. The nurse evaluates the patient using a paradigm that reflects the scope of personal nursing services (figure 13.3) and taking into consideration the patient's total set of diseases and disabilities, general physical and emotional condition, and family and social history. Sources of information include observation of the patient, physical examination, patient and family interviews, and the physician's history, physical examination, provisional diagnosis, and diagnostic test and treatment orders. Family views are important, and a description of the patient's home environment is frequently required.

The Plan as Diagnosis Plus Response. The nursing care plan goes beyond the diagnosis to address the correctable departures from homeostasis which have been identified and to prescribe corrections for them. The plan has obvious parallels to the medical patient care protocol. It tends to be less specifically related to the disease at hand and more broadly directed to the full needs of the patient. The nursing plan emphasizes physical, emotional, and environmental aspects of treatment as well as disease. Since nursing must deal with side effects and potential complications, the nurse must be familiar with the medical protocol. If the emotional impact of the disease on patient and family will be severe, the diagnosis should recognize this as an element of comprehensive care and a potential barrier to prompt discharge. If the spouse is ill or the apartment has narrow doors, return home may be more difficult.

The nursing plan must be dynamic, tailored as often as necessary to changes in the patient's condition. It is often written down more fully, because several nurses will be involved in implementing it. Even more than the doctor's protocol, the nursing plan can be significantly aided by computer files. Models for specific diseases, analogous to the patient group protocols discussed in chapter 11, can be available on computer as a pattern. The nurse can develop a plan more quickly and with less risk of oversight by modifying a disease model to individual needs.

Figure 13.3

Scope of Personal Nursing Care

**General Physical Care, with Attention
to Afflicted Organ Systems**
  Respiration
  Circulation
  Digestion and elimination
  Feeding and nutrition
  Skin care
  Bones, joints, and muscles
  Sensation
  Sex and reproduction
Care-Related Teaching
  Reassurance and motivation
  Self-care
  Rehabilitation
Emotional Support
  Supporting illness-related
    emotional problems
    Transient reactions to
      illness and trauma
    Grieving: death, disability,
      and disfigurement
  Supporting general mental health
    Detection of mental illness
      and substance abuse
    Psychiatric nursing
    Mental hygiene
Drug Administration
  Explicit orders
  Judgmental (PRN) orders
**Other Treatments Ordered by
Attending Physician**

Nursing's Contribution to Economical Care. The nurse's professional skill and judgment contribute substantially to economical care. If the diagnosis is well made and the responses are prompt, much difficulty can be forestalled. The doctor and the nurse ideally collaborate in maintaining or restoring equilibrium, but much of the general observation of the patient is by the nurse. Although the doctor may order any service, a significant amount of care can be given or withheld at the nurse's discretion.

As an illustration, an otherwise well 40-year-old woman is admitted with gallbladder disease for cholecystectomy. If all goes well, she will have surgery on day 2, walk that evening, be off pain medication by day 4, and home on day 7 without further problems. During her week in the hospital, nursing care will avoid the following hazards: circulatory complications from inactivity, respiratory complications from anesthesia, infections at the wound site, imbalances in body chemistry, insecurity and anxiety related to postoperative condition, postdischarge complications from poor dietary habits, and drug dependency. Should any of these occur, an expanded course of treatment will be required. The new treatment will introduce new hazards, starting the cycle over. Stay and cost will escalate, and patient satisfaction will deteriorate. Should the patient be older, her systems will be more fragile, and the range of tolerance to nursing error diminishes. If she has an intercurrent disease or complication, nursing needs mount exponentially. Two new groups of hazards must be avoided, one relating to the other disease, the second to interactions between the two. Diabetes, for example, creates one list, cholecystitis and cholecystectomy a second; having both creates a third, because surgery profoundly endangers the homeostasis of diabetes.

Coordinating with the Medical Protocol. There is substantial merit to joint development of the nursing and medical protocols. Both should incorporate a specific plan and time for discharge. Many elements of the medical protocol require coordinated nursing actions. Nursing may lend valuable new perspectives to debatable components of the medical protocol and may suggest cost-effective modifications.

These considerations suggest that joint development of nursing and patient group protocols will be the pattern in well-run hospitals. It is not now, in part because both professions are still struggling with content and use of their individual protocols. Computerization is not yet widely available; while it is not necessary, it will be a great aid to doctors and nurses developing and using protocols. The care of the woman with gallstones, described above, is already better in well-run hospitals because the doctors and nurses share a deep common knowledge of diagnosis and treatment. As they formalize that knowledge they will improve their mutual understanding, and with it the quality and efficiency of care.

Nursing Services for the Patient

The activities supporting and implementing the patient care plan include:

— Personal nursing care

— Communication with doctors and support services

— Assistance to the patient's family

— Control of the ward environment
— Preventive education
— Case management

Personal Nursing Care. While the specifics of nursing are the business of the profession itself, the scope of nursing should be clear to everyone in hospital management. Figure 13.3 shows the extraordinary scope of nursing care to patients as individuals.

Patient-Related Observation and Reporting. Nursing is the only truly continuous inpatient service. Given that nurses are also frequently in intimate contact with the patient, they are ideally placed to observe and communicate the patient's condition, needs, and response to previous actions. The nurse is responsible for:

— Reporting clinical observations to the attending physician and house officers
— Recording drug administration and nursing treatments
— Receiving, coordinating, and transmitting orders for clinical support services
— Preparing the patient or specimen for support services
— Knowing the patient's location and receiving him or her back from support services
— Receiving and transmitting results of reports from support services
— Preparing and forwarding incident reports for any untoward events
— Maintaining the paper or electronic file that constitutes the medical record
— Receiving and storing the patient's possessions
— Assisting visitors to the floor

It is not surprising that prior to the introduction of computers, nearly half the nursing staff's time was devoted to written and oral communication. Computers are totally automating several of these functions and materially simplifying others. As a general rule, the faster these communications and the fewer errors, the lower the cost of service can be. The recovery of costs depends in many cases on reducing actual nursing labor.

Family Assistance. Nursing shares with medicine responsibility for communicating with the family or other significant persons in the patient's life. Nursing success in this communication is a critical element of overall patient satisfaction. Generally, the assistance falls into two categories, cognitive and emotional.

The family needs a variety of specific facts, ranging from the name of the responsible nurse to care needs after discharge. Well-run nursing units, including outpatient units, anticipate most of these factual needs and provide educational materials, both verbal and written. The broad outline of the care plan is given to the family, including the anticipated dates of key events such as surgery and discharge. This serves a dual function, relieving anxiety and permitting the family to prepare. Nursing shares with the plant system responsibility for treating visitors hospitably. It must generate incident reports on visitors and floor staff if anything goes wrong.

Illness and hospitalization are anxiety-producing events, and high-quality care strives to minimize the anxiety of both patient and family. The more stressful the event, the more nursing attention to family response is likely to be needed. Terminal illness provides a unique and extreme case, and well-run hospitals are moving systematically to minimize the emotional trauma, guilt, and anxiety associated with the death of relatives. When death is almost certain, this effort frequently centers on the hospice, a blend of home, outpatient, and hospital care designed to make death as emotionally bearable as possible. In less predictable situations, nursing support for the family is as important as nursing support for the patient, for it is the surviving family whose health can be improved.

The key to provision of emotional support to the family is thoughtfully developed protocols which anticipate common problems and provide the staff with solutions. Well-run hospitals are developing protocols for terminal illness and other high-stress events and are incorporating them into in-service education. Such programs include:

— Identifying significant personal relationships
  • Evaluating the family structure
  • Recognizing important nonfamilial relationships
— Identifying family stress
  • Stress-producing medical events
  • Symptoms of stress in family members
— Role of cognitive information in relieving stress
— Specific cognitive requirements for common events
— Professional affect and behavior allaying stress

— Techniques for assisting individuals in stressful situations
— Hospital policies on stress-producing situations, for example:
  • Postsurgical notification
  • Terminal care
  • Emergency resuscitation
  • Orders not to resuscitate
  • Assistance available to family members
— Assistance available to staff
— Dealing with professional guilt and grief

Environmental Control. Although Florence Nightingale and her followers scrubbed the floors themselves, maintaining a safe and effective environment is now the responsibility of the plant system. Nursing, however, is properly held accountable for reporting any failure of that system and for insisting that it be corrected. The inpatient or outpatient head nurse is responsible to patients, visitors, and staff for general safety, effectiveness, and expected amenities in the floor environment.

In addition to general environmental control, nursing is responsible for clinical aspects of the environment. Certain sites—for example, surgery, premature nursery, and coronary care—have become highly complex. Electronic, mechanical, and chemical environments are created for intensive patient care. They are frequently the responsibility of specially trained and experienced nurse managers. Analogies can be made to quite a different situation, the structured environments of psychiatric care. It is wise to remember that the hospital environment can be a therapy in itself. Hospitalization is occasionally ordered simply to obtain that environment or to escape one that is unsafe or dysfunctional. The head nurse is responsible for maintaining the clinical environment, whatever it might be.

Control of microbial, radiation, and chemical hazards on nursing units is a nursing responsibility. Special techniques for avoiding contamination are part of the clinical procedures of nursing. They often involve other professions and usually require coordinated development. Nursing must enforce these procedures.

Certain addictive drugs, called *controlled substances* or, less formally, *narcotics,* are regulated by the federal government. Nursing shares with medicine and pharmacy the reporting and control obligations. Well-run hospitals, recognizing that doctors and nurses have a high risk of addiction, provide preventive and rehabilitative programs.

Prevention and Health Education. Nursing has extensive and important educational responsibilities relating to the consequences of specific diseases and events. It teaches diabetics how to adjust and administer their insulin; heart attack survivors how to regain full activity; hypertensives the importance of their medication; new mothers how to care for and enjoy their babies, how to maintain their own health, and how to avoid unwanted pregnancies; and many other useful programs. If these tasks are well done, future disease is reduced. Under HMO types of insurance, hospitals receive direct financial benefits from their successes in this area. Under any insurance, patient, professional, and community satisfaction is improved. Thus expectations for patient education are an essential part of care plans for inpatients and outpatients.

Well-run hospitals go beyond the disease-specific teaching in the care plan. They educate the patient about the risk defined by existing disease, sex, age, occupation, and other demographic characteristics. Pursuing the examples above, nursing education might be extended as follows:

— For the diabetic, interaction of diabetes and oral contraceptives, smoking, and use of alcohol

— For the person who has had a heart attack, stress reduction, exercise, and smoking and weight control programs

— For the new mother, child rearing, immunizations, family relations, avoidance of child abuse, resources available to the family

A third level of nursing education is emerging and is likely to continue to grow. Hospitals are increasingly active in general education and counselling to the well population. Programs on smoking cessation, exercise, alcohol abuse, aging, sexuality, and weight control are attractive to the public and may be cost-effective in HMO populations. (Among other virtues, they suggest that self-care is virtuous, cheap, and, if carefully done, effective.) Support groups for stressful events other than disease (divorce, childbirth, job) have become popular following the disease-oriented model (postcolostomy, Alcoholics Anonymous, hemophilia). Individual counselling on these topics is apparently similarly effective. Nurses can equip themselves professionally to provide educational programs and counselling and to organize and assist support groups.

Case Management. Case management is the comprehensive oversight of an individual patient's care from the perspective of long-term cost-effectiveness. It is now rare in hospitals but may emerge in the near future. The role is especially attractive as a way of providing comprehensive but economical long-term care to the aged. The term first arose in experimental HMOs for the aged called social health maintenance organizations (SHMOs). Effective care of the aged must dedicate itself to lengthening and improving biological and emotional life while minimizing lifetime health care expenditures. Although evidence is far from complete, it appears that the best solution is one that guides the patient continuously from late middle age. The case manager maintains a long-term relationship with the patient, one that emphasizes prevention and fitness to the greatest possible extent, treats the deteriorating organ systems thoroughly but economically, provides increasing support as several organ systems begin to fail simultaneously, and arranges the last months of life in response to the patient's own wishes.

Three current functions of nursing are part of case management. They are less comprehensive and unfortunately less constructive, ways of improving the quality and cost-effectiveness of care. One is utilization review, where nursing verifies the appropriateness of admissions and checks inpatients' progress against expected discharge dates. The negative features of utilization review are serious, and it is unlikely to make a large, permanent improvement in either quality or utilization. A more positive and more comprehensive activity with a similar goal is **discharge planning.** Discharge planning, a natural part of the nursing care plan, identifies the expected discharge date at or before admission and coordinates the various services necessary to achieve the target. It is conceptually close to case management but is limited to the hospital episode and lacks the long-term continuing relationship with the patient.

The third case management function currently performed by nurses is monitoring dangerous or questionable practices by other clinical personnel. Nursing, because of its round-the-clock coverage and central communications role, is responsible for reporting employees or doctors acting in unreasonable or impaired ways and for stopping dangerous activities. They report such problems through their own hierarchy and then to the appropriate executive personnel.

Managerial Functions of Nursing

Patient care in a hospital consists of both physical activity and the written record. The physical activity requires movement of patients, specimens, personnel, and supplies. The record requires precise identification of the patient, orders by the attending physician and the nurse, responses which are frequently several steps long, and reports. The management issues of logistics (the movement of personnel and supplies) and communications (the maintenance of information) are fundamental to high-quality and appropriate care.

Nursing has managerial responsibility for numerous logistic and communication activities, including patient-related logistics and communications, quality assessment, need or acuity assessment, staffing, and plant and supplies logistics. The activities involved have been and will be greatly aided by the computer.

Patient Logistics and Communication

Nursing involvement in patient-related logistics and communications can be grouped into three major functions, initial admission, communication after admission, and patient scheduling and transportation. Although classed here as management functions because they support so much nonnursing activity, logistics and communication are a direct extension of clinical nursing requiring professional knowledge and skill.

Patient Admission. Patient admission establishes the commitment among hospital, doctor, and patient. For both inpatients and outpatients, it originates the medical and financial records and begins patient-related communication. Identification information is obtained, searches are made for record number assignment and existing financial obligation, financial arrangements are established, and a series of notices of admission and orders for care is transmitted to the several interested units of the plant, financial, and clinical systems.

Much admissions activity is automated in patient registration systems. Advance scheduling is becoming more common for both inpatient and outpatient care; the predictability is convenient for the patient and aids efficiency and quality for the hospital and the attending doctor. The systems of scheduling used are similar to those described in chapter 12.

The nurse's involvement in the acceptance and admissions process has always been prominent in the emergency room, where nursing evaluation and triage remain important. For urgent and elective patients, the following clinical factors must be addressed; their growth has drawn nursing back into admitting, a function that had been delegated to clerical and financial personnel for several decades:

— Important medical orders are now written when the patient is scheduled, before the actual admission. These normally would be interpreted and transmitted by nursing and probably should be for the newly arriving patient. Preparation for preadmission tests often requires patient education, which is normally provided by nursing.

— Patient satisfaction is enhanced by reassurance and explanation early in the care process. This is one of nursing's most significant contributions to patient care.

— Case management, including both discharge planning and prospective review of clinical orders, should begin prior to the patient's physical arrival, if possible. Nursing has increasing responsibility for these activities.

— Scheduling of patient care involves a number of choices requiring clinical knowledge. In addition, the location of patients in the hospital affects nurse staffing, quality, and efficiency.

Patient-Related Communication. During the patient's episode of inpatient or outpatient care, it is necessary to maintain a comprehensive, current medical record for the many services participating in diagnosis and treatment. Generally the information must include symptoms and complaints, concurrent disease or complication, working diagnosis, medical orders and nursing plan, and the results of diagnostic investigations and treatment to date.

During the patient's active treatment, nursing is responsible both for the maintenance of the medical record as a document and for the communication of appropriate content to other clinical services. (Permanent storage and certain summarizing functions are assigned to the medical records department.) The record is confidential, and nursing bears much of the responsibility for protecting its confidentiality. The attending and house physicians and the individual support services are responsible for their own entries into the record. Nursing enters its own *nursing notes* and handles the physical transmission of most of the rest. It transmits orders to services and receives responses back. The order and response communications are often oral or on temporary papers preceding the final documents.

The significance of nursing's responsibility is often overlooked. In fact, prior to computer assistance, communication of all kinds required about half of the time of inpatient nurses, with patient-related communications consuming the lion's share. Although the process seems simple—order, transmit, respond, file—there are many additional steps. Information from the record frequently must be added to the order. Multiple copies are required for both quality control and billing. Many orders require several steps. "To surgery," for example, will involve the floor or admitting nurse in several communications, the operating suite nurse in several more, and the anesthesia department in yet more. Even a simple drug order, "by mouth, four times a day," can trigger a dozen or more communications. The magnitude of the problem is revealed by the numbers. If each patient has 10 orders a day and each order requires 10 transactions, a 50-patient floor will process 5,000 transactions. Most will be handled by the day shift, at a rate of about one every seven seconds!

The clinical communications process is the center of current computer developments in hospitals. Because rapid, error-free transmission of data is the hallmark of computers, the automated medical record has been a dream for two decades. Progress has been surprisingly slow, reflecting, more than any other factor, unwarranted optimism on the part of systems designers, who underestimated the complexity of the task. However, electronic processing is now routine for medical orders in well-run hospitals, once nursing personnel have entered the order into the computer. Direct entry by physicians has had less success but will evolve with technical improvements in computers.

Responses and reports are also moving to automated systems. English language text, necessary for such things as the medical progress report and the nursing note, presents the greatest difficulties for automation. The development of systems for clinical support services will increase the number of automated responses. Laboratory responses are already routinely automated, and imaging and surgery will move steadily in that direction.

Patient Scheduling. Computerized orders can be scheduled by the computer to improve the efficiency of support service and nursing operation and to minimize the time required of the patient. At present, most of the scheduling required to coordinate support service and nursing activity is still done by telephone by *ward clerks,* clerical personnel responsible to the head nurse. The ward clerk generally conducts most of the record maintenance and scheduling activity with other support services. The scheduling must accommodate limitations in the patient's physical condition and competing demands. Most of the services require direct contact with the patient, and many of the services have requirements affecting others, such as being performed before meals or before certain other services.

The support service departments are rapidly developing their own computerized scheduling systems. Coordination of these into a master schedule for each patient is technically possible and can be expected to emerge piecemeal over the next several years. As it does, nursing's responsibility can shift to active monitoring of the automated process and to more effective preparation for each patient. Substantial reductions in clerical personnel on nursing units appear feasible as the automation of communications and scheduling activities occurs. Quality will be enhanced as oversights and conflicts are eliminated. A reduction in duplicated and spoiled tests and orders can be expected. Prompt fulfillment of scheduled orders also reduces stat requests. Case management can also be improved. The existence of a well-ordered advance schedule, even though it may be only a few hours before the events are to take place, permits prospective review of compliance with the patient group protocol.

Patient Transportation. Nursing is also responsible for the safe transportation of inpatients. Although many outpatients can follow guidance from plant services to reach the various clinical support services, inpatients are frequently impaired by their illness and must be moved by hospital personnel. The task is time-consuming but important to patient satisfaction. Employees who do it are usually unskilled and may be supplied by a unit of plant services (see chapter 15). They should be trained both in guest relations and in handling the medical emergencies which may arise while the patient is in transit.

Measurement of Acuity and Patient Need

The demand for nursing care on an inpatient floor or ward is a function of two elements, the **census,** or number of patients, and their **acuity,** or how sick they are. The ability of the nursing staff on the floor to adjust to this variation is limited; although nurses can work harder, the work must be done in a constrained period of time. It is important to provide a staff adequate to meet quality goals. Staffing needs are generally measured in hours required per patient, and sicker patients have higher requirements.

Measurement of Patient Need. Well-run hospitals now assess patient acuity daily on acute care units. Despite 25 years of work, there remains substantial difference of opinion as to how acuity should be measured. The most common approach to assessing acuity has been by binary or simple ordinal scales indicating departure from normal function in several physiological and psychological factors known to influence nursing time. Items include therapeutic and diagnostic needs as well as those involving eating, dressing, and elimination; the emotional state; and the amount of observation ordered by the doctor. A high score requires increased nursing care. A typical acuity scale is shown in figure 13.4. When such scales are used, values for each patient are reported by the head nurse. Computerized systems calculate acuity, assign staffing requirements to individual patients, and add up the nursing personnel required on each floor.

It is important to note that problems of variability of staff and reliability of measurement are greatly reduced by aggregating individual values by floor. Although individual patients vary three- or fourfold, aggregates of 30 or more patients vary much less—theoretically only 20

Figure 13.4

Patient Acuity Assessment Questionnaire

NPAC™

MED/SURG PATIENT CLASSIFICATION TOOL

MEDICUS SYSTEMS

PATIENT NAME		ROOM/BED	

UNIT	c0ɔ c1ɔ c2ɔ c3ɔ c4ɔ c5ɔ c6ɔ c7ɔ c8ɔ c9ɔ
	c0ɔ c1ɔ c2ɔ c3ɔ c4ɔ c5ɔ c6ɔ c7ɔ c8ɔ c9ɔ

Admission or Transfer In	1	c ɔ	Tube Care	26	c ɔ
Discharge or Transfer Out	2	c ɔ	Oxygen Therapy	27	c ɔ
Less Than 2 Years	3	c ɔ	Respirator	28	c ɔ
Age 2-6 Years	4	c ɔ	Trach/ET Tube	29	c ɔ
Unconscious	5	c ɔ	Vital Signs Q1½ - 2 Hr.	30	c ɔ
Confused/Disoriented	6	c ɔ	Vital Signs Q1 Hr. or More Often	31	c ɔ
Sensory Deficits	7	c ɔ	Monitoring - Non-Invasive	32	c ɔ
Partial Immobility	8	c ɔ	Invasive Monitoring	33	c ɔ
Complete Immobility	9	c ɔ	Prep. for Test/Procedure	34	c ɔ
UP AD LIB	10	c ɔ	Special Teaching Needs	35	c ɔ
Up with Assistance	11	c ɔ	Special Emotional Needs	36	c ɔ
Bed Rest	12	c ɔ	Multi-System Instability	37	c ɔ
Bath with Assistance	13	c ɔ		38	c ɔ
Bath Total	14	c ɔ		39	c ɔ
Assistance with Oral/Tube Feed	15	c ɔ		40	c ɔ
Total Oral/Tube Feed	16	c ɔ		41	c ɔ
I & O Simple	17	c ɔ		42	c ɔ
I & O Complex	18	c ɔ		43	c ɔ
IV's & Site Care	19	c ɔ		44	c ɔ
Specimen Collection - Simple	20	c ɔ		45	c ɔ
Specimen Collection - Complex	21	c ɔ		46	c ɔ
Isolation	22	c ɔ		47	c ɔ
Incontinent/Diaphoretic	23	c ɔ		48	c ɔ
Simple Wound and/or Skin Care	24	c ɔ		49	c ɔ
Extensive Wound and/or Skin Care	25	c ɔ	Other:	50	c ɔ

DRG NUMBER	c0ɔ c1ɔ c2ɔ c3ɔ c4ɔ c5ɔ c6ɔ c7ɔ c8ɔ c9ɔ
	c0ɔ c1ɔ c2ɔ c3ɔ c4ɔ c5ɔ c6ɔ c7ɔ c8ɔ c9ɔ
	c0ɔ c1ɔ c2ɔ c3ɔ c4ɔ c5ɔ c6ɔ c7ɔ c8ɔ c9ɔ

PHYSICIAN CODE	c0ɔ c1ɔ c2ɔ c3ɔ c4ɔ c5ɔ c6ɔ c7ɔ c8ɔ c9ɔ
	c0ɔ c1ɔ c2ɔ c3ɔ c4ɔ c5ɔ c6ɔ c7ɔ c8ɔ c9ɔ
	c0ɔ c1ɔ c2ɔ c3ɔ c4ɔ c5ɔ c6ɔ c7ɔ c8ɔ c9ɔ
	c0ɔ c1ɔ c2ɔ c3ɔ c4ɔ c5ɔ c6ɔ c7ɔ c8ɔ c9ɔ
	c0ɔ c1ɔ c2ɔ c3ɔ c4ɔ c5ɔ c6ɔ c7ɔ c8ɔ c9ɔ

PAYOR CODE	c0ɔ c1ɔ c2ɔ c3ɔ c4ɔ c5ɔ c6ɔ c7ɔ c8ɔ c9ɔ

percent as much. While one patient, just under the limit for assignment to an intensive care unit, might require 2 hours of attention in a single shift and another only half an hour, it is unlikely that 30 patients of either extreme would occur. The range of the average for 30 patients would likely be only plus or minus 15 minutes. (This is still enough to require changes of staff. At maximum, $3.25 \times 30 = 97.5$ hours would be needed, or 12.0 persons. At minimum, only $2.75 \times 30 = 82.5$ hours, or 10.3 persons would be needed.) A similar process smooths errors in patient acuity classifications, so long as they are not systematically biased in one direction or the other.

Although various alternatives to the scale in figure 13.4 have been reported, no important improvement in quality or efficiency has been shown. An important limitation is the subjective nature of the head nurse's evaluation. Although it is relatively inexpensive, requiring only a few minutes of time per patient, it is unreliable because it depends on human memory, which is fallible and can be distorted by bias. Scores usually creep upward in an unmonitored system, inflating the nursing staff requirement. Identification and correction of creep is possible, but at added system cost. Audits can control creep. Well-designed computer systems routinely test the means and variances of acuity scores for statistical trend.

More objective, automatic, and less costly methods of automating patient records are the likely improvement. One approach under development identifies nursing tasks from the automated nursing care plan and medical orders. Staff requirements are calculated directly from counts of nursing activity and medical orders. Acuity can be calculated indirectly from the ratio of required staff to average staff. A second approach being developed recognizes that acuity for patients with a common diagnosis follows predictable patterns after admission. For example, acuity of patients is high immediately after surgery, and after admission for medical emergencies. Data on nursing needs by patient group and day after admission can be used to estimate staffing and acuity. Substantial historical data would be required to establish either proposal, but either would eliminate subjective judgment.

Uses of Acuity Measurement. Acuity measurement is used to stabilize the ratio between required staff and available staff on each nursing floor. Given an acuity measure, there are two basic approaches to that goal, and well-run hospitals are pursuing both. The first is *staff adjustment,* that is, the number of personnel on a given floor or unit is adjusted to patient need. (The adjustment occurs at several different times, as discussed in the section on nursing personnel logistics, below.)

— Staffing decisions establish the average number and mix of personnel required.

— Scheduling algorithms use historic data to maintain the average need on a daily and weekly basis while accommodating nurses' work habits.

— Assignment algorithms suggest the necessary changes to a nurse staffing manager on a shift basis. Assignment flexibility is usually obtained by:

  • Developing *float pools* of nurses trained to work at several different locations

  • Using call-in and agency personnel when needed

  • Transferring nurses between floors

  • Assigning overtime

The second is *census adjustment,* that is, the combination of an admission scheduling system and a nursing acuity assessment and staffing system offers several important possibilities:

— At the planning level, stabilizing the census substantially lowers variation in floor acuity and staff need. Although a given census of patients varies in acuity, the floor census is the larger factor in the variation in staff need.

— At the budgeting level, floors can be designated for specific ranges in acuity, and some floors can be closed in slack periods. The use of intensive care units for very high acuity patients reduces variation on routine care floors, although ICUs themselves are subject to widely fluctuating need for staff.

— At the assignment level, in hospitals large enough to have several floors appropriate for a given admission, incoming admissions can be placed on floors with a high ratio of actual staff to required staff.

There are several implications for personnel and patient demand management (these are discussed below), but in general the fewer changes at the assignment level, the more efficient the system and the higher the quality is likely to be.

Monitoring Quality of Patient Care

Nursing monitors quality of its own clinical services and participates in quality and utilization review undertaken by the medical staff and others.

Nursing Quality Monitoring. Process and some outcomes measures of nursing care quality are now assessed regularly in well-run hospitals. Current methods use specially trained nurse observers and samples of patients. Quality assessment addresses mainly process issues. Figure 13.5 is an example. The approach can be broadened to capture outcomes measures, to expand appropriateness monitoring, and to include services other than nursing. Computer systems in nursing departments generate the proper samples, print out questions tailored to the patient's age, sex, and diagnosis, and provide for prompt reentry and tally of results. These surveys permit review of the following elements of performance:

— Nursing care plan
  • Comprehensiveness
  • Appropriateness
  • Timely completion and implementation
— Patient condition and physical care
  • Completion of nursing treatment
  • Patient condition
  • Patient environment
— Record keeping
  • Nursing notes
  • Support service reports
— Patient support
  • Emotional status
  • Education
  • Satisfaction

Using the performance monitoring results as a guide, nursing management can improve its quality of care by education and systems revisions, including:

— Selecting topics for in-service education
— Revising nursing procedures, or intermediate product protocols (Automation of procedural manuals promises more frequent compliance and easier revision.)
— Revising patient scheduling to reduce day-to-day variation in nursing demand
— Improving personnel scheduling and assignment to reduce day-to-day variation in available staff

Figure 13.5

Selected Nursing Quality Control Questions

MEDICUS GENERAL HOSPITAL
SCORE REPORT BY SERVICE

SERVICE: SURGICAL

		NEURO 08/85 09/85	C-ICU 10/85 11/85	4 NOR 08/85 09/85	9 EAS 08/85 09/85	10 WE 10/85 11/85	SERV-ICE MEAN
1.1	Condition is assessed on admit	60	75	83	88	100	81
1.2	Data relevant to hospital care	80	100	80	77	96	87
1.3	Current condition is assessed	95	81	83	75	67	80
1.4	Written care plans formulated	75	72	69	83	92	78
1.5	Coordination with medical plan	93	68	75	74	75	77
1.0	**NURSING CARE PLAN FORMULATED**	**79**	**81**	**76**	**80**	**91**	**81**
2.1	Protected from accident/injury	96	93	92	100	100	96
2.2	Comfort/rest need is attended	100	90	97	83	83	91
2.3	Physical hygiene is attended	100	89	83	88	100	92
2.4	Oxygen supply need is attended	100	96	75	76	92	88
2.5	Need for activity is attended	75	100	100	89	90	91
2.6	Nutrition and fluids attended	84	100	88	89	67	86
2.7	Needs for elimination attended	67	84	93	67	96	81
2.8	Need for skin care is attended	92	92	67	50	100	80
2.9	Protect patient from infection	92	75	75	100	100	88
2.0	**PHYSICAL NEEDS ARE ATTENDED**	**93**	**90**	**88**	**88**	**93**	**90**
3.1	Oriented to hospital on admit	88	86	100	94	65	87
3.2	Extended courtesy by the staff	93	67	98	86	76	84
3.3	Privacy and rights are honored	80	75	92	74	80	80
3.4	Psycho-emot attend thru commun	100	100	74	90	93	91
3.5	Taught health/ill prevention	85	80	75	88	67	79
3.6	Family is included in the care	71	80	77	53	88	74
3.7	Psycho-emot attend thru milieu	NA	NA	NA	NA	NA	
3.0	**NON-PHYSICAL NEEDS ATTENDED**	**89**	**86**	**85**	**81**	**87**	**86**
4.1	Records document care provided	72	70	63	64	93	72
4.2	Patient response is evaluated	100	100	84	80	89	91
4.0	**ACHIEVEMENT OF CARE EVALUATED**	**84**	**81**	**71**	**71**	**91**	**80**
5.1	Isolation procedures followed	100	82	83	86	100	90
5.2	Unit prepared for emergencies	85	96	97	92	94	93
5.3	Medi-legal procedures followed	NA	NA	NA	NA	NA	
5.4	Safety procedures are followed	50	0	33	100	50	47
5.0	**UNIT PROCEDURES ARE FOLLOWED**	**88**	**79**	**84**	**90**	**92**	**87**
6.1	Nurse report follows standards	90	83	75	71	92	80
6.2	Nursing management is provided	77	80	79	67	81	77
6.3	Clerical services are provided	75	56	61	69	75	67
6.4	Environmental service provided	84	74	77	87	76	80
6.5	Professional services provided	69	83	74	75	64	73
6.0	**DELIVERY OF CARE FACILITATED**	**79**	**75**	**74**	**75**	**77**	**76**

NA - Indicates subobjective not applicable

Expanding to Related Areas of Quality and Utilization Review. Many hospitals also use nurses for concurrent utilization review, a form of case management that monitors adherence to the patient group protocol on expensive components of care, especially the length of stay and discharge plan. While the samples for concurrent utilization review and nursing quality are usually different because review focuses on cases that are prone to overstay, the same computer support, trained reviewers, and results processing systems can be used.

Additional structural, procedural, and outcomes components described below can be added to the existing framework without difficulty. One important outcomes measure, survey of patient attitudes, will require more extensive training of observers. Once observers are trained in interview technique, it is a simple matter to expand the surveys to broader issues of satisfaction with the attending physician, house staff, clinical support personnel, and plant service personnel and to record completion for other clinical services. If this is done, the hospital will have a current monitor of several important elements of quality.

Well-run hospitals are likely to develop quality and utilization assessment teams who are trained to visit samples of patients, review records, and report answers to survey questions assessing the elements of nursing quality listed above, parallel questions on satisfaction with other services, and compliance with patient group protocols for appropriateness. In the process, they may verify reported acuity. While these teams could be in the governance system, much of their role is nursing.

Nursing Personnel Logistics

Nursing personnel decisions are the result of a four-step process moving toward progressively shorter time horizons.

1. *Staffing* decisions establish the number of professional, technical, and clerical nursing employees required for each nursing floor or unit. The results of staffing decisions establish scheduling and daily assignment requirements and set the nursing expense budget.

2. *Scheduling* decisions develop plans for daily availability of personnel and establish the work schedules of individuals.

3. *Assignment* decisions adjust shift-by-shift variation in personnel requirements of each floor.

4. *Budgeting* decisions translate expectations regarding staffing, scheduling, and assignment into personnel costs.

Staffing. Staff availability determines the capability of nursing units and is a major factor in the quality of care. Nursing procedures and responsibilities, in turn, determine proper number and kind of staff. Changes in procedures and responsibilities must be assessed in terms of costs and benefits. If staffing is increased or shifted toward professional levels, one should expect a corresponding improvement in the measures of outcomes—length of stay or number of patients seen per day, patient satisfaction or doctor satisfaction—to justify the added investment. Presumably, one would first see an increase in the number of procedures performed or the quality of procedures.

Decisions about the nurses needed for outpatient care are easier to comprehend and can serve as a model for the vastly more complicated inpatient staffing decisions. For example, a small clinic is staffed Monday through Friday for five identical day shifts with two classes of personnel, licensed practical nurse (LPN) and clerk, a level historically sufficient to provide satisfactory service. This decision sets the budget and establishes the scheduling which must occur. If the staffing is upgraded to one registered nurse (RN) and a clerk, one would expect greater nursing responsibilities and more procedures, such as an increase in patient education. Further, one would expect the clinic to attract more patients, or to care for them with less hospitalization, or to be more satisfactory to patients and doctors, or in some way to show a measurable improvement for the increased cost.

Inpatient nurse staffing decisions are made for each floor and shift. They establish the number and mix of personnel required for the range of acuity and census that floor is expected to encounter. Since each floor commonly has four skill levels (RN, LPN, aide, and clerk) plus a head nurse, and during a typical year will vary in demand for nurses over a range of 100 percent or more, and is operated for three shifts which are usually very different in character, the decisions are not simple. The process of making them determines the organization within the work group and its capability for undertaking professional responsibilities.

A popular trend has been toward an "all professional" staff (without LPNs or aides) and "primary care" (full, continuing responsibility for individual patients). Primary care strives to improve outcomes, shorten stay, and reduce readmission by bringing better judgment to bear on the assessment and planning process. Although promising, primary care is not practical for all units. Long-term care, for example, is provided largely by practical nurses, and primary care has radically different meanings on the night shift, in the emergency room, and in the recovery room. Various team arrangements are alternatives to primary care models. In these, the professional nurse is often team leader for a group of less highly trained personnel. Team approaches are aimed at reducing costs by substituting less skilled personnel under the supervision of professional nurses.[4]

Using either team or primary models, staffing decisions should be developed by nursing management based on careful forecasts of census and acuity combined with specific outcomes and process expectations. Conceptually, a well-designed staffing plan establishes expectations on what tasks nursing will perform, how frequently these will occur, what indications support them, and what outcomes in quality, efficiency, and economy are anticipated. For example, the following kinds of measures are directly influenced by the staffing decision:

— Process achievements
  • Content of nursing care plan
  • Frequency of recurring nursing tasks
  • Frequency of physician order tasks
  • Indications for patient-related tasks
  • Patient education
  • Allowance for in-service education
  • Other measures of quality
— Outcomes achievements
  • Length of stay
  • Readmission rates
  • Patient satisfaction
  • Physician satisfaction
— Economy achievements
  • Nursing cost per patient-day
  • Nursing cost per patient admitted

Even the best hospitals are just reaching this level of understanding of nursing's contribution to patient care; however, the well-run hospital now has acuity and quality assessment, well-developed nursing procedures, experience in the use of formal nursing care plans, and reasonable computer support for patient scheduling, patient communication, and personnel scheduling. With this equipment, it is in a position to specify improvements in these measures which might result from increases in staffing or, alternatively, to demonstrate that reduced staffing has led to no deterioration.

Personnel Scheduling. The work schedules for specific employees must be established to match the staffing plan. There is generally less need for staff on weekends, and even with the best patient scheduling there are times when patient need requires changes in staffing. Although most nurses work the traditional 40-hour week, 12-hour shifts are sometimes used instead of 8-hour shifts. Many personnel are part-time, working less than the full number of shifts per week. Absenteeism, holidays and non-patient care assignments must be accommodated in the schedule.

Nurses must fit these needs into the rest of their lives. Predictable schedules or several weeks' advance notice of changes are desired, but nurses also want to request special days off. Scheduling systems which help them do this are an important recruitment and retention device.

Computer-aided scheduling systems now meet most of these needs. A well-designed program has the following characteristics, listed in approximate order of importance:

— Staffing matches the forecast requirement; overstaffing and understaffing are minimized.

— Personnel are scheduled consistent with their designated specialization, professional competence, and agreed-upon work commitment that is, full- or part-time).

— A pool of flexible personnel is maintained to meet unexpected variation caused by changes in acuity and absenteeism. (Pool members are often specially trained and compensated.)

— Schedules for individuals are maintained two or more weeks in advance.

— Schedules minimize unnecessary transfers between units and shifts.

— Weekends, late shifts, and other less desirable assignments are equitably distributed. ("Equitably" is usually not "equally"; one nurse's preferences are not the same as another's.)

— Personal requests for specific days off are accommodated equally, so long as they are submitted in advance, can be met within cost and quality constraints, and do not exploit other workers.

There is a strategic aspect to scheduling management that complements a good computer scheduling system. Quality will depend on having adequate numbers of properly trained personnel at each work location. Obviously this begins with sound human resources management: attractive work environment, effective recruitment and selection, retention of capable personnel, and continuing in-service education. Well-run hospitals are supplementing these general human resources management strategies with special responses that capitalize upon computer-aided scheduling capability, including:

— Recruiting qualified workers who are seeking less desirable shifts and days

— Emphasizing permanent part-time personnel to match recurring needs

— Maintaining call-in lists of personnel for areas with highly variable staffing needs, such as intensive care

— Developing a float pool of both full- and part-time personnel trained to serve in several areas with high variation in staffing need

— Establishing overtime and shift length policies which recognize differing work habits and personal needs

Assignment. Computer-assisted assignment systems make the final adjustment of staffing for each day or shift. Assignment consists of assessing the staffing requirement for each unit, including patient acuity on the inpatient units, comparing that to the actual staff available, and using pool, call-in, or transfer personnel to minimize the differences. Because of absenteeism and unpredictable variation in patient need, some units will have excess staff and others shortages. The more effective the staffing, personnel scheduling, and patient scheduling, the narrower the range of differences and the less adjustment by reassignment. Commercial software offers assignment, acuity, and quality assessment; simulation for budgeting; and basic personnel records in a single package.[5]

The use of float pools, call-ins, and transfers is necessary, but it should be minimized. Float pools are difficult to sustain and generally increase costs. Call-ins from outside pools of temporary employees or agency personnel brought in on contract are even more expensive. At best, the training of agency personnel is outside the hospital's control, and the individuals are less efficient because they are not familiar with their work environment. Transfer of personnel from one location to another within the hospital presents similar difficulties. Most nurses do not like to be transferred, and the problems of cross training and unfamiliar work stations remain. Quality deteriorates as a result.

Budgeting. The expense budget for nursing is heavily committed to personnel, and the personnel budget is derived directly from policies implemented in staffing, scheduling, and assignment. Each floor or unit is an accounting responsibility center, with the head nurse as primary monitor. Fixed personnel budgets establish expectations for monthly consumption of nursing hours and costs. Flexible budgets use the staffing requirement expectations for each shift and assume that short-term variation in demand will be met by changes in schedule and assignment. Under flexible budgets, some costs vary with census and acuity, although others usually remain fixed.

Well-run hospitals now use flexible personnel budgeting for all nursing units where patient demand varies in a predictable fashion. (Obstetrics and coronary care are two units in which demand varies but cannot be predicted. Long-term care units often have insignificant variation.) Flexible budgeting for supplies is now routine for all units. In some situations, it may be necessary to maintain units which can be opened or closed in response to patient demand.

Budgets specify exactly the staff anticipated for each combination of census and acuity. The same computer aids which develop the work assignments generate the forecasts of census and acuity necessary for budgeting. Most computers have simulation features, which allow evaluation of alternative strategies. The labor expense budget is determined almost automatically once the staffing pattern and the forecasts of demand are selected.

Pricing and revenue budgets for nursing are attracting more interest. It has been traditional to include nursing charges within a general room, board, and daily care charge and to ignore the contribution of nursing to hospital revenue. There are several reasons for specifying nursing prices and having nursing participate directly in pricing decisions like other clinical support services. Nursing management can evaluate:

— Nursing prices compared to market competition

— The customer's interest in quality and satisfaction and the customer's willingness to pay for improvement

— Trade-offs among alternatives to improve patient satisfaction

— Nursing's contribution to reduced length of stay

— Relative value of educational activities

— Substitutions between nursing and other clinical support services (for example, postoperative respiratory care, use of analgesics)

— Substitutions between nursing and medicine, such as the role of the nurse clinician

The concept which recurs throughout these advantages is that examining nursing's contribution to profit allows more thorough evaluation of the effect innovations will have on the market. While it is true that most of these evaluations can be carried out using special studies within existing accounting systems, the use of a nursing price will make comparison easier and quicker.

Other Logistic Functions of the Patient Unit

The nursing staff on inpatient and outpatient units is largely responsible for several other logistic functions. For patients, the delivery of drugs, medical supplies, and food usually involves nursing. Nurses also frequently obtain specimens for the laboratory. Nursing must assure the safety and comfort of guests, doctors, and other employees using the floor.

Nursing transmits drug orders to pharmacy and receives the drugs back to administer. Error-free administration is difficult to achieve. Timing, patient condition, and coordination with other support services are frequently significant. Drugs for pain relief are frequently prescribed *PRN,* when necessary, at the nurse's discretion. Drugs have negative side effects, and the quantity required is a function of the quality of nursing care, particularly in patient education, motivation, and reassurance. Parenteral fluids present a particularly critical challenge, both to cost and outcome quality. The consequences of error can be life-threatening.

Medical supplies are also administered by nurses. Economical use is desirable, but supplies used should be accurately charged. Nursing is accountable for both the costs of medical supplies used and the revenues they generate in well-run hospitals.

Food is important symbolically and emotionally as well as nutritionally. The patient's ability to maintain maximal nutritional status is often important in health education and disease prevention. Nutritional education is done by nurses more often than dieticians.

All of these logistic functions call for close cooperation between nursing and other departments or systems. Given the volume of activity and the complexity of patient care, it is not surprising that breakdowns occur. The result is tension between nursing and other units. Well-run hospitals take the following steps to minimize both breakdowns and the tensions surrounding them:

— Support service and plant systems are strengthened to minimize breakdown. Quality of service for many of these activities is measured by their ability to satisfy nursing and patient needs.

— Specific expectations on tasks, timing, and quality of performance for other departments' activities are used to clarify ambiguous or debatable accountability. Disagreements are resolved promptly and once settled, are translated into specific expectations, with nursing collaborating on them.

— Incentives for personnel in other departments encourage both completion of established expectations and satisfaction of nursing requests as they arise.

— Incentives for nursing recognize the two-way nature of many of these relationships and reward genuine cooperation. (Nursing has many opportunities to protect equipment from damage and maintain safety and cleanliness.)

— Recurring failures of logistic expectations are promptly reported by nursing to higher levels of accountability. All management personnel respond promptly, recognizing that denying or ignoring such reports is a negative incentive to lower levels of management, both in nursing and in the failed system.

— Disputes are also referred upward quickly and are resolved by a reasonably unbiased process which recognizes the legitimacy of complaint. The process should be understood by all and accessible to all.

Planning

Nursing, like all other units of the hospital, is responsible for identifying new developments in its field, developing proposals for additions and deletions to the hospital's services, and defending these proposals against alternatives. The process for nursing proposals resembles that for other support services, as described in chapters 7 and 12.

Nursing is also likely to be involved in many evaluations of strategic opportunities, as described in chapter 7. The nursing functions are important in almost all health care activities and are central to several. Much vertical integration of hospitals into outpatient, mental, chemical dependency, and home care is more effective with nursing skills. Nursing is central to long-term inpatient care for rehabilitation or maintenance.

Many hospitals face changing demands which necessitate opening new nursing services and closing old ones. The following criteria guide these decisions in well-run hospitals:

— Consistency with mission
— Contribution to market share or attractive product design
— Level of need or demand
— Quality requirements
— Cost
— Risk
— Benefits
  • Patient benefits
  • Contribution to other activities

• Financing and contribution to profit

Appropriately, the list for nursing is not unlike that for the hospital as a whole. Like other services, nursing is obliged to review the scope of its services constantly and to seek revisions when they are potentially rewarding. Incentives for nursing managers should recognize this obligation. The techniques for review are similar to those described in chapters 7 and 12.

Personnel and Organization

Nursing as a profession and as a unit of hospital organization is almost as diverse as medicine. The profession contains within it careers reaching from the hospital to the home to general and public health services that do not involve individual patient care. Nurses' activities stretch from high-tech to high-touch. In addition, there are significant numbers of managerial jobs. The patterns of training and the hospital nursing organization reflect this diversity.

Educational Levels of Nursing Personnel

Formal educational opportunities in nursing, as in most other professions in the United States, have increased since World War II. Uniquely among the professions, nursing has retained all of its original levels, rather than simply adding years to the training requirement. There are now three professional and four nonprofessional educational levels (see figure 13.6).

Several attempts to rationalize this structure have led to a career ladder which accommodates repeated return to formal education, via LPN, associate, bachelor's, master's, and doctoral degrees. The growth of junior colleges has made this career ladder more accessible, permitting well-run hospitals to abandon diploma programs in favor of participation in associate and baccalaureate programs. Certification has not kept pace with these developments. Registration, the traditional recognition of professional nursing qualification, is available with as little as two years' study after high school. Well-run hospitals are specifying additional training beyond the RN for many assignments such as intensive care, team leaders, supervision, and primary care for acute medical and surgical floors. Beyond registration, practical experience as a substitute for formal requirements can, of course, be judged on an individual basis.

Figure 13.6
Educational Levels of Nursing Personnel

Professional Levels
Baccalaureate nursing degree—four years beyond high school in an accredited college or university are required. This is the basic skill level for head nurse and increasingly for acute inpatient staff nurse.
Certificated postbaccalaureate education
Nurse anesthetist—one year after the baccalaureate degree is required.
Nurse practitioner—at least one year after the baccalaureate is required.
Nurse midwife—less than one year after the baccalaureate is required.
Postbaccalaureate degrees
Clinical degrees—these parallel the major specialties of medicine. The master's degree requires one or two years, the doctorate four or more years after the baccalaureate.
Management degree—the master's degree requires two years after the baccalaureate.

Nonprofessional Levels
Subbaccalaureate registered nurse (RN) preparation
Diploma in nursing—This is a hospital-based program of three years beyond high school, qualifying for the RN but not the baccalaureate degree.
Associate in nursing—This is a college-based program of two years qualifying students for an RN and associate degree. The degree is accepted as partial fulfillment of the baccalaureate.
Non-RN skill levels
Licensed practical nurse (also called licensed vocational nurse)—This requires a one-year junior college program. The LPN is the most common requirement for long-term care and is even used on supervisory levels in nursing homes.
Nursing aide—only hospital in-service training is required.

Trends in Nurse Supply and Recruitment

Although significant reductions in nursing personnel may result from shorter hospital stays, lower census, and the use of computers, demand for RNs and professionally trained nurses appears to be increasing, while the number of entering students is falling. Reports of shortages were widespread in major cities in 1986 and 1987, as they have been periodically for several decades. Despite this recurring public concern about nursing shortages, there has never been hard evidence to support the existence of a widespread general shortage. In such a situation, normal markets respond by a rapid increase in wages. Since such a response has never been demonstrated for nurses relative to other health care professions, economists conclude that alleged shortages were temporary or local phenomena.[6]

Although the shortages may have been an illusion, there is a serious problem of recruitment and retention, particularly for the staff nurse who provides most acute inpatient care. A hospital needs slightly less than one full-time staff nurse per patient. A hospital with a patient census of 300 employs about 250 full-time-equivalent staff nurses. Since many of these posts will be filled by part-time personnel, over 300 individual nurses will be employed. The staff nurse job is both physically and emotionally demanding. It tends to be filled by young people who are highly mobile. Compensation is relatively low. Market prices for teachers and pharmacists are higher, although educational requirements are similar and neither of those jobs combines the hours, physical demands, and critical responsibilities of a staff nurse.

It is not surprising that staff nurse turnover is high, frequently in excess of 50 percent per year. Well-run hospitals make a deliberate effort to reduce turnover and increase work satisfaction. Retention is generally cheaper than recruitment. More important, the satisfaction of current staff nurses is quickly sensed by potential recruits, and a reputation as a good place to work is a powerful asset. Most important, there is evidence that nurse satisfaction is related to outcomes measures of patient care quality.[7] Well-run hospitals strive for a recruitment and retention advantage over their competition by repeated attention to the following concepts:

— Clarity of roles, procedures, and expectations is a major factor in reducing job stress.

— Prompt, reasonable response to job-related questions and issues is important in maintaining motivation.

— Development and implementation of a comprehensive, effective nursing care plan is the single most important factor in raising the staff nurse's contribution to patient care.

— In-service education, floor leadership, and quality monitoring provide a staff nurse with skills and guidance to develop and implement a sound care plan.

— Real contribution to patient care increases self-respect and job satisfaction. It also increases the respect of other clinical professions for the nurse's professional skills and judgment which further increases job satisfaction.

— Intangible rewards, chiefly praise and public recognition, reinforce self-respect and collegial recognition of professional achievement.

— Hours, scheduling, and work policies designed more for the staff nurse's personal convenience offer a relatively simple, easily promoted attraction.

— Tangible rewards can be used to encourage improved job performance. A nurse who is rewarded for measurable improvement in patient care, rather than for seniority, can more easily be motivated to remain in patient care practice.

The underlying philosophy of this list is that good nursing is its own reward and that the job of nursing management is to provide opportunities to do good nursing. The functions described in the preceding sections, and the systems which implement them efficiently and effectively, are the tools for the job.

Nursing Organization

Nursing tends to follow a consistent accountability hierarchy in its many sites and specialties. An individual staff nurse, or a team led by a staff nurse, constitutes an informal work unit below the responsibility center. The responsibility center manager for several geographically adjacent work units comprising a floor or ward is a head nurse. Supercontrollers go by various names, usually nursing supervisor. Supervisors either are clinical specialists or can use specialists in a staff role. This structure fits most inpatient floors and outpatient units and can be modified to fit home care. It also fits the nurse-managed support units such as operating rooms, delivery rooms, and recovery rooms. Specific policies, procedures, and skills differentiate the various services. Clearly, the procedures for operating rooms are very different from those for outpatient psychiatry. The staff nurse for chronic care is usually an LPN; for acute units, an RN or a nurse with a bachelor's degree; and for intensive care, a nurse with a bachelor's or master's degree. The skill required for outpatient care depends upon the role and can be LPN, RN, bachelor's degree, or nurse practitioner.

There are several questions about the supervisory levels of the accountability hierarchy that remain unresolved, even in well-run hospitals:

— *How to handle the size and diversity of the nursing floor.* The head nurse as primary monitor or responsibility center manager is responsible for a number of people and dollar volume that would be assigned to two levels of supervision elsewhere in the hospital. (A floor with an average census of 50 acute patients requires a nursing staff of up to 40 full-time-equivalents and represents nursing costs of $1 million and room, board, and care revenues of $3 million per year.) Round-the-clock operation exacerbates this problem.

— *How to provide effective supercontrol and meet the support needs of the nursing organization.* These needs include recruitment, in-service education, staffing, incentives, and development of procedures.

— *How to use the master's level clinical specialists.* These nurses are the best source of advice on care plan design and implementation. They can consult on cases within their expertise regardless of the patient's physical location. This advice is very useful for patients with multiple disease processes.

— *How to promote effective communication between nursing and the other clinical activities, particularly the attending and house staffs.* Close collaboration between the doctor and the nurse improves both quality and effectiveness of care. Mechanical, attitudinal, and status problems combine to make it difficult to sustain.

There is clearly much to be done, but one can be optimistic about the immediate future. The competitive environment will reward hospitals and individuals who solve nursing organization problems more effectively. The surplus of both doctors and nurses and the general aura of change and experimentation permit questions like these to be actively considered. The management tools—chiefly automated systems —to measure performance objectively and therefore to evaluate changes, are available.

Measurement and Information

The growth of automated support for patient scheduling, order entry, duty assessment, nurse scheduling, quality assessment, and detailed costs and charges accounting for individual patients has provided a platform for major advances in quality and cost-effectiveness for nursing. The gains which well-managed hospitals have made so far have largely been within the capability of individual items on this list. At least one major round of improvements is foreseeable from appropriate integration of this information. Leading hospitals are now moving toward integration emphasizing outcomes of care on a per case or per episode basis.

The discussion which follows summarizes the measures by category: demand, cost, revenue, output efficiency, and quality in order to concentrate on the opportunities available through integration. Similarly, the major data-processing systems are described in terms of their applications rather than their components.

Measures

Nursing now has a rich opportunity to measure its resource investments, its activities, and its contributions to the steady improvement of hospital performance. The typical responsibility center, such as the inpatient ward or outpatient clinic. is the unit which can set and achieve expectations on all the closed system dimensions. Budgeting sessions for nursing can now easily address the following set of measures at the process level:

— Expectations for costs and charges by functional account (that is, labor, supplies, and facilities)—are set for both the total dollars per accounting period and, under flexible budgeting, the unit costs and charges. Well-managed nursing units, supported by the full array of computer aids, now find the achievement of cost expectations routine. Summary levels of performance are monitored, and modern payroll, materials management, accounts receivable, and general ledger systems permit the exploration of any level of detail necessary.

— Demand measures include both the average and the variation in occupancy, delays for scheduled and urgent service, and counts of cancellations or disruptions in the scheduling process. Expectations are set through and achieved by patient scheduling systems.

— Nursing functions are identified, coordinated, and recorded by a combination of patient care plans and order entry systems. These not only permit much closer control of the nursing care process, but also generate outcomes measures of performance, such as rates of completion and delays.

— Nurse scheduling, assignment, and patient acuity systems now allow staffing to be adjusted to the variations in patient need which remain after patient scheduling systems have been applied. Well-designed systems provide measures of patient need, structural quality, and cost in terms of physical rather than dollar resource units.

— Assessment of process quality is routinely achieved through inspection of both patients and nursing records. Reliability has been improved by using specific questions to guide the inspection and by developing numerous questions to cover the range of patient needs. Cost and time requirements have been reduced by automation of question selection, sampling procedures, tallying, and analysis. Expectations can now be set for percent of satisfactory scores, not only in general, but also in specific levels of care, care plans, and reporting.

As systems such as these are installed, obvious avenues of improvement appear and are explored. These are frequently at the process level, but they also occur at the level of a single system and a relatively limited set of measures. The process of identifying and addressing these opportunities appears to take several years in most hospitals. The best hospitals are only now reaching the conclusion of this phase. A second, more rewarding, and more challenging phase now appears possible in these hospitals, where the three components of medicine, nursing, and clinical support services collaborate toward a goal of cost-effective care. Nursing will make its contribution by refining process expectations based upon general outcomes of patient care. That is, once the well-organized nursing unit has demonstrated its ability to achieve reasonable expectations on the process measures identified above, its next task will be to identify from outcomes data the kinds of expectations which yield the best overall results.

Outcomes Measures of Patient Care. Direct outcomes measures of nursing have been difficult to establish. The breadth of purpose and the constant interaction among nursing, medicine, and other aspects of the patient's environment combine to make assessment of nursing's contribution difficult. However, there are six outcomes areas in which nursing is important both in monitoring and in influencing favorable results. Well-managed hospitals are now measuring the following and reporting results to nursing responsibility centers. At present, expectations are still vague and approximate. As the relationship between the outcomes measures more closely related to open systems concerns and the process measures collecting nursing's day-to-day decisions are more clearly identified, the expectations will become rigorous.

1. *Patient and family satisfaction*—Nursing shares with other services the need to satisfy patient and family perceptions, and nursing's performance affects the scores of others. Well-run hospitals now routinely survey patient and family satisfaction. Expectations should be set on these scores at the time of the annual budget. Praise and compliments should be reported directly to their source, and scores should be highly visible on nursing units. Public identification and praise of good individual performance is useful. Programs in guest relations can improve results, but many issues involve professional nursing concerns and must be addressed through nursing procedures and in-service education.

2. *Attending physician satisfaction*—Nursing shares with other units of the hospital the need to meet the requirements of attending physicians. Formal surveys of the attending and house

staffs should specifically include evaluations of nursing care. Informal contacts are more common and in well-run hospitals more useful. The nursing accountability hierarchy parallels that of the major specialties of medicine, and each supervisor in it should make frequent informal contacts with his or her medical counterparts. In well-run hospitals, evaluations of nursing supervisors include review of relations with physicians.

3. *Case-specific resource measures*—When patients are grouped by diagnosis and related characteristics, it is possible to develop measures of resources used, costs, and revenues. Grouping inpatient discharges by DRG is currently popular, but the concept can be applied to other groupings and, with some serious practical difficulties, to outpatient care. Useful measures for DRG groups include:

   a. Length of stay

   b. Nursing cost per case

   c. Support service cost per case, particularly for isolated services directly influenced by nursing care

   d. Revenue per case
   These measures can be reported according to floor, either individually or in a weighted index.

4. *Readmission rate*—Nursing frequently influences the length and extent of the patient's recovery through predischarge education and motivation. Nurses who successfully train patients to take medications carefully, maintain weight, diet, exercise, and avoid smoking and alcohol abuse will see fewer readmissions over large numbers of patients than those who are less successful. The rate is difficult to measure and only partially reliable at present. Rates of readmission to other hospitals and sources of care are lacking. Focusing on specific diagnoses such as diabetes, arthritis, and congestive failure is wise.

5. *Incident reports*—Incident reports are written communications of any untoward happening of potential danger to patients, visitors, or members. They are processed by the risk management unit and provide the first evidence of hazards or liability. Although other departments submit incident reports as well, the majority comes from nursing. Prompt and complete reporting is a recurring problem because the report is frequently perceived as an admission of guilt or failure. Reporting is enhanced by clear and readily available forms (computerization is likely in the near future), nonjudgmental processing, and the constructive use of analysis to show how hazards can be reduced.

6. *Infection reports*—Hospital-acquired infections are a serious environmental concern in hospitals and are usually monitored by an infections committee which includes nurses. Although both nursing and medicine are obliged to report infections, nursing can do so more easily. Nursing is responsible for infection control techniques and should prevent nosocomial infections by continued education and reminders about infection control procedures.

Structural Measures of Nursing Care. Well-run hospitals now routinely accumulate several structural measures of nursing care. Hours per patient-day or outpatient visit, adjusted for acuity, is the most common and most important. The percentage of hours by professional personnel is also common. Personnel records should show the training, experience, and in-service education of each employee. Repair and maintenance records show the attention paid to facilities and equipment; nursing shares in the accountability for physical plant because it is expected to report breakdowns. The JCAH lists a number of other structural standards designed to encourage good nursing practice.[8]

Information Systems

Because of the amount, breadth, and complexity of information it requires, nursing relies heavily on computer service. The set of systems nursing will require in the future interlocks with those required elsewhere in the hospital. Automated interfacing will be required, linking both mainframe and PC equipment. A summary list may be helpful here (specific systems are discussed in several different chapters).

— *Patient care support systems.* All of these systems are likely to remain on mainframe or central hardware.

• *Admission and acceptance* (also called patient registration, or admission, discharge, and transfer) records basic registration information, assigns identification number, identifies hospital location of patient, communicates arrival and initial orders, and initiates both patient ledger and patient order file.

• *Admission scheduling* records classification of demand (usually emergency, urgent, or scheduled) and scheduled future date, if any. It establishes current and future availability of admission opportunities and prompts call-in from the urgent list.

- *Support service scheduling* records schedule for future support services, resolves conflicts in preparation and transportation needs, and shows availability of service.

- *Order entry and results reporting* records physician's and nurse's orders and care plans, transmits orders to support services, receives reports back from support services, and prompts recurring nursing tasks. More advanced systems will permit tailoring of individual care plans from a patient group protocol and will record nursing progress notes.

— *Managerial support systems.* These include both general accounting systems which operate on mainframe hardware and nursing department systems operating on expanded PC capability. They will shortly include systems for data base analysis including retrieval analysis and graphic display of data. Although few hospitals make effective use of this technology today, it is becoming cheaper. It, too, relies on expanded PC capability. Easy communication between PCs and the mainframe is clearly an important consideration.

  - *General accounting and budgeting* supports flexible budgeting and cost and revenue reporting, including payroll.

  - *Patient data analysis* permits the identification and grouping of individual patient records for care, charges, and quality according to any of several dimensions (responsibility center, physician, patient age, and so on). It also supports common statistical analysis and graphic representation.

  - *Nursing personnel records* include special training and assignment capabilities, work preferences, evaluations, and other data on individual employees.

  - *Nursing procedure descriptions* are instantly accessible, automatically updated nursing procedures for use by staff. They replace the paper procedural manual and may require mainframe support.

  - *Staffing and scheduling* accepts work preferences and special requests and uses demand forecasts to develop advance schedules for floor personnel.

  - *Acuity assessment and assignment* accepts tallies of patient acuity by floor and shift, and actual staff availability. It uses staffing standards to calculate required staff and records time series data on acuity scores and actual versus required staff. These provide statistical quality controls to detect significant change in recorded acuity.

- *Process quality assessment* identifies samples of patients and questions according to preset rules. It prints survey questionnaires, accepts responses, and tallies quality scores following preset rules. It can also display time series of scores graphically, providing statistical quality control of nursing care.

The well-run hospital now supports most of the information requirements on this list. Expansions and enhancements are being developed rapidly in quality assessment systems, DRG grouping, order entry, nursing procedure files, acuity assessment, and scheduling.

Management Issues

If it is true that the better the nursing, the sooner the patient will recover, the competitive environment presents a challenge to nursing management. Nursing, as one of the three major clinical groups, can make a substantial contribution to both quality and economy of care by prevention, supportive care, and case management for outpatients and by reduced use of other clinical support services, education and reassurance for patient and family, shorter stay, and discharge planning for inpatients. Costs can be reduced in all of these areas with no reduction, or perhaps even an increase, in quality. Nursing will continue to be heavily involved with the aging. Clearly, a large part of the savings will come from improved management of chronic disease. Much effort will be involved with death and the last months of life.

The picture which emerges is one of high-touch in its broadest sense: cognitive, emotional, environmental, and social support for patient and family, taking into account quality of life as well as length and emphasizing the patient's categorical right to make his or her own decisions. Achievement of this goal could spark a renaissance of nursing, a rebirth of professional satisfaction from a newly challenging and rewarding personal care role. Nursing has important obligations which must be met before new tasks can be added, however. Both clinical and managerial functions must be improved, and the effort must address quality and efficiency simultaneously.

Nursing care is improved if the patient recovers sooner, has more positive perceptions of the service he or she received, and encounters less subsequent difficulty. It is done efficiently if these goals are achieved at relatively low cost, and efficiency is improved if the same level of quality is maintained at lower cost. All of these considerations involve the doctor and the patient as well as the nurse. Thus the causes of improvement or of perceived shortfall are multiple and obscure. This should not be seen as a deterrent, however. Specific opportunities can be identified and translated into achievable short-term goals without full understanding of the network of causes.

A Clinical and Managerial Agenda

Nursing can maximize its contribution to patient care by taking the following steps:

— Establish measurement systems to provide routine guidance in patient care for each floor or unit (discussed earlier in this chapter). Particular attention should be paid to such clinical measures as

- Procedural quality measures, emphasizing the establishment and implementation of a patient care plan
- Patient satisfaction measures, assessing the acceptability of care both for nursing and for the hospital as a whole
- Outcomes measures, reflecting both clinical and economic consequences, such as length of stay, cost per case, and readmission

and to such managerial measures as

- Occupancy and acuity measures, to quantify patient demand
- Staffing, scheduling, and assignment measures, to identify personnel availability
- Accounting measures of nursing unit costs and revenues
- Communications measures of timely order completion

— Determine acceptable long-term goals for these measures. Goals will depend upon exchange needs, or community demand, as well as technical capability. Areas of greater deficiency will become priority concerns for annual improvement.

— Negotiate practical improvements in expectations for priority concerns with head nurses in annual budget activities. The budget is expanded to all closed system considerations in this process.

— Study nursing activities and systems to identify ways in which further improvements can be made toward acceptable levels of performance. Opportunities include:

- Revising nursing procedures, equipment, and staffing
- Improving personnel training and in-service education
- Improving nursing care plans
- Improving patient care information systems

- Eliminating variability in physical care and treatment procedures
- Increasing reassurance and encouragement to patients
- Providing more extensive patient education

— Study other clinical service costs to find less costly ways of meeting acceptable performance levels. Better nursing can reduce laboratory work, drug usage, social service, respiratory therapy, and rehabilitation therapy requirements.

Implementing the Agenda

The agenda above is one for measuring, collaborative goal setting, and searching for more cost-effective care at the level of the head nurse or staff nurse. Some hospitals are already far enough along on this agenda to reveal some of the concerns that must be addressed.

— The economy, quality, and efficiency of nursing are interrelated. The expected levels of performance on all of these dimensions should be established at the time of the budget negotiation.

— Improvements must be translated into cash savings through changes in the operating budget. Since about 95 percent of the nursing budget is for labor, this usually means changes in staffing. Most nursing labor budgets should be established on a flexible basis.

— Nursing computer systems should provide measures and expectations of staffing efficiency on a shift-by-shift basis, thus improving control of costs and quality.

— Admission scheduling systems should stabilize floor census and acuity by calling in urgent or schedulable patients. Outpatient scheduling systems should perform a similar role for ambulatory units.

— Patient scheduling systems should coordinate clinical support services, relieving nursing of all but monitoring activities.

— Order entry systems on nursing floors should be gradually expanded to incorporate model nursing care plans, routines for tailoring these to individual patients, automated entry of nursing notes, rapid access to procedural manuals, routine sampling and questionnaires for quality control, and direct, objective assessment of acuity.

— The nursing work force should be restructured to provide a cadre of full-time personnel and a pool of more flexible workers. Peak needs should be met by prearranged call-in contracts with properly experienced part-time personnel, and overtime or special need bonuses should be developed to encourage regularly scheduled staff to respond to short-term peaks. If current personnel work harder or longer, the need for additional employees can be reduced.

— Nursing organization should be strengthened internally, with attention to more explicit roles for supervisors and clearer, shorter chains of accountability. Nursing middle managers should be judged on the achievement, satisfaction, and turnover of their subordinate personnel.

— Accountability for staffing and labor costs should be assigned to the head nurse, who as responsibility center manager is also accountable for employee satisfaction with schedules and assignments, the number of staff transfers, and the maintenance of a high level of training and experience on each floor. A supervisory-level staff manager may be useful to support the head nurses.

— Head nurses should be evaluated on outcomes and process measures of patient care and the satisfaction of patients, attending doctors, and staff nurses. Satisfaction of professional nurses should be assessed as it is for doctors, by solicitation of comments and by formal surveys.

— Head nurses and supervisors should receive substantial rewards for consistently and realistically improving performance on outcomes measures. Nursing unit values on quality and utilization measures should be frequently reported and highly visible. Public recognition should reward exceptional improvement.

— Incentives for good performance by staff nurses must be substantially strengthened. Samples of process quality should be accumulated to permit objective assessment of the individual staff nurse's effort. Achievement should receive both tangible and intangible rewards. Routine salary and wage increases should be abolished or substantially diminished in favor of retrospective merit increases. Nonrecurring bonuses should be used to avoid excess fixed costs while offering larger rewards for successful innovation.

— The hospital's clinical organization should encourage collaboration between nurses and the attending staff. Nursing membership and active participation in clinically oriented committees should be routine. Many desirable changes are revisions to the patient group or final product protocol, for example, revision of the criteria for admission to intensive care. Others involve changing nursing's own intermediate product protocols, but these must always be understood by the attending doctors in order to avoid confusion and gain cooperation.

— Given the complexity and importance of the issues, major changes should be tried in experimental settings before being widely introduced. It is useful to distribute the experiments; in fact, the opportunity to experiment is a reward, and a positive attitude toward change can be built by assigning the opportunity as such.

The well-run hospital is already further along on this agenda than its less successful counterpart. General characteristics of farsighted planning, well-designed governance processes, objective dialogue on clinical matters, conflict resolution, and positive rewards provide support for a nursing program. Sound information systems, budgeting systems, and clinical review activities provide the foundation for objective review and revision.

Notes

1. Florence Nightingale, quoted in V. Henderson, *The Nature of Nursing* (New York: MacMillan, 1966), p. 1.
2. V. Henderson and G. Nite, *Principles and Practice of Nursing,* 6th ed. (New York: MacMillan, 1978) pp. 1–25.
3. U. S. Department of Health and Human Services, Health Resource Administration, *The Registered Nurse Population, an Overview,* Report 82-5, rev. (Hyattsville, MD: HRA, 1982), p. 13.
4. Fred C. Munson et al., *Nursing Assignment Patterns, User's Manual* (Ann Arbor, MI: AUPHA Press, 1980).
5. NPAQ, a product of Medicus Systems Corporation, Evanston Ill.
6. Institute of Medicine, *Nursing and Nursing Education: Public Policies and Private Actions* (Washington, D.C.: National Academy Press, 1983), pp. 51–88.
7. C. S. Weisman and C. A. Nathanson, "Professional Satisfaction and Client Outcomes," *Medical Care* 23 (October 1985): 1179–92; R. W. Revans, *Standards for Morale: Cause and Effect in Hospitals* (London: Oxford University Press for Nuffield Provincial Hospitals Trust, 1964).
8. Joint Commission on Accreditation of Hospitals. *Accreditation Manual for Hospitals.* (Chicago: JCAH, published annually).

Suggested Readings

Alexander, E. L. *Nursing Administration in the Hospital,* 2d ed. St. Louis: C. V. Mosby, 1978.

Finkler, S. A. "Flexible Budget Variance Analysis Extended to Patient Acuity and DRGs." *Health Care Management Review* 10 (Fall 1985): 21–34.

Hancock, W. M., and Fuhs, P. "The Relationship Between Nurse Staffing Policies and Nursing Budgets." *Health Care Management Review* 9 (Fall 1984): 21–26.

Henderson, V., and Nite, G. *Principles and Practice of Nursing,* 6th ed. New York: MacMillan, 1978.

Institute of Medicine. *Nursing and Nursing Education: Public Policies and Private Actions.* Washington, DC: National Academy Press, 1983.

Munson, F. C., et al. *Nursing Assignment Patterns, User's Manual.* Ann Arbor, MI: AUPHA Press, 1980.

National Commission on Nursing. *Summary Report and Recommendations* and *Nursing in Transition, Models of Successful Organizational Change.* Chicago: Hospital Research and Educational Trust, 1983.

Wakefield, D. S., and Mathis, S. "Formulating a Managerial Strategy for Part-Time Nurses." *Journal of Nursing Administration* 15 (January 1985): 35–39.

PART
IV

The Human Resources
and Plant Systems

Introduction to Part IV

Any complex organization includes many activities which are supplementary to its central task or purpose. The clinical system is the center of the hospital. Governance, finance, human resources, and plant support the clinical system in ways that are acceptable to the external exchange community. The two systems discussed in Part IV are devoted solely to providing the physical resources for care. Human resources supports the large work force, including doctors and volunteers, which hospitals require. Plant maintains the complex array of supplies, equipment, and facilities.

Yet to describe human resources and plant systems as playing a supporting role is to understate their true contribution. The patient care activities of the hospital can be brought to an immediate halt by an interruption in the availability of these resources. For example, a power outage or the absence of critical personnel will stop some activities of the hospital instantly and all of them quickly. Less dramatic, but more important, the performance by human resources and plant systems must parallel the quality and efficiency of other systems. It is impossible to sustain a high-quality clinical system unless it is supported by similar quality in human resources and plant. Exceptional people are attracted to, and average people perform better in, hospitals where human resources and plant systems work well. Thus efforts to build a leading institution often begin by strengthening these two systems.

Like the rest of the hospital, human resources and plant systems are shaped by exchange forces. Not only the economic and social issues surrounding patient care, but also general forces affecting community-wide employment opportunities and real estate development are involved. Specific expectations for human resources and plant services must be derived through the governance process, reflecting the hospital's mission, long-range plan, and annual budget. The two systems provide input to these central decisions, because the availability of resources and the exchange constraints on acquiring them, such as the attitudes and expectations of employees, are part of the exchange equilibrium.

— *Human Resources System.* Chapter 14 discusses the system which provides all the general support for the hospital's work force. A mutually satisfactory exchange relationship is its goal. In hospitals this includes all the elements of the employment contract that are common to several groups of workers; the boundary of human resources is usually the point where a profession or position is differentiated from others. Planning, recruitment, training, compensation, benefits management, and collective bargaining are its most obvious functions.

— *Plant Services.* Chapter 15 examines the organization which manages the complete physical environment of the hospital and provides several basic services, including food service and security, to patients, visitors, and members of the hospital. Planning is critical to long-term success, but the plant system has vital roles in maintaining safety and supporting minute-by-minute operation.

Human resources and plant services affect everyone who is involved with the hospital. From the visual impression given to passers-by to the motivation of the operating room team, specific actions of these systems contribute significantly to a favorable result. Furthermore, the hospital environment is a demanding one, often requiring great precision and narrow tolerances of human resources and plant systems. A hospital has more precise expectations for menus than most hotels, for example. It stocks a far more critical array of sizes and types of medical supplies, such as blood and surgical implants, than retail stores do of clothes, for example. It operates facilities and equipment under stricter requirements for control of temperature, contaminants, and reliability than many manufacturing processes.

14

Human Resources System

In 1983, at the beginning of the era of competition and cost control, hospitals had more than 3 full-time-equivalent employees per bed, reflecting a steady increase throughout the preceding two decades.[1] The number of professions and job categories had also increased. In addition to employees, the human resources of a hospital included doctors, services contracted through arrangements other than employment, and volunteers.

A typical medium-sized community hospital employs persons in over three dozen licensed or certified job classifications, including building trades and stationary engineers as well as clinical professions. Many of the positions are held by part-time personnel. The number of individuals employed is about 30 percent larger than the FTE count. The employed work force supports a physician group representing about two dozen specialties and numbering from 0.5 to 1.0 doctors per bed, depending principally on the number of hospitals where the doctors seek privileges. Both employees and doctors are assisted by volunteers ranging from trustees to candy stripers.

Finally, hospitals also use contract labor services, via long-term management contracts, for whole departments and shorter contracts for specific temporary assistance. Long-term contracts are common for housekeeping, food service, and data processing. Among the shorter are consultation contracts with accounting firms and planning firms, as well as shift by shift requests for nurses, clerks, and other hourly workers. The number of people involved appears to be between five and six persons per bed. Put another way, a typical 300-bed community hospital requires over 1,500 persons to complete the equivalent of 1,000 full-time jobs in about 100 different categories.

This group, referred to in earlier chapters as the "members" of a hospital, constitutes the hospital's most important asset, its human resource. Regardless of the specific relationship, each member joins the hospital in an exchange transaction. The member is seeking some combination of income, rewarding activity, society, and recognition. The hospital is seeking services that support other exchanges. Some aspects of the exchange relationship with members deserve emphasis:

— The members are absolutely essential to continued operation. Members' motivation and satisfaction directly affect both quality and efficiency. Unusually high motivation can provide a margin of excellence, while a few highly dissatisfied members can temporarily or occasionally disrupt operations.

— Membership, like the seeking of care, is a free choice for most people. Even those whose skills can be employed only in hospitals usually have some choice of which hospital they will work at and how much work they will seek. Success in attracting and keeping members tends to be self-sustaining; the hospital with a satisfied, well-qualified member group attracts more capable and enthusiastic people. The well-run hospital markets itself to its members almost as much as it markets itself to its customers.

— The members represent only about 2 percent of the hospital's service community, but because of their close affiliation with the hospital and their frequent contact with patients, they are unusually influential:

  • As a promotional force, members, both those who come into direct contact with patients and those whose unseen services determine patients' safety and satisfaction, are powerful. What they say and do for patients and visitors will have more influence on competitive standing than any media campaign the hospital might contemplate.

  • As an economic force, members are also significant. Hospitals are always important employers in a community, with a payroll of about $65,000 per bed, plus doctors' incomes and contract payments. In many communities, hospital employees are the largest single group of employees. Furthermore, about half a hospital's payroll represents income from outside the community, largely Social Security payments for Medicare. Finally, most of the employment opportunities in hospitals are in unskilled jobs. The hospital's economic impact as an employer is thus weighted to lower-middle-class females, a group presenting serious employment problems for many communities.

• As a political force, members can command increased respect for the hospital among elected officials of government and labor unions by demonstrating their support of it. While members are only about one-tenth as numerous as patients, their strength can be multiplied when the issue is important enough to motivate their families, as is often the case when substantial numbers of jobs are at stake.

Purpose of the Human Resources System

The purpose of the human resources system is to plan, acquire, and maintain the skills, quality, and motivation of membership consistent with fulfillment of the hospital's mission.

Since a properly worded mission defines community, service, and cost, this purpose accommodates both the profile of skill levels and the needs for economy defined by the governing board (see chapter 5). Motivation and quality reflect the exchange nature of membership contracts; the human resources system supplies much of the hospital's tangible transactions with its members.

The purpose of the human resources system is fulfilled by the usual process of iterative planning, beginning with the mission and a long-range human resources plan of about five years and continuing through annual revisions and specific budget expectations to month-by-month and day-by-day schedules of departmental activity. The human resource system must accomplish four functions:

1. Work force planning
2. Work force maintenance
3. Compensation
4. Collective bargaining

These functions, except collective bargaining, must be fulfilled for all member groups if the hospital is to be well run. (Collective bargaining applies only to formally organized workers.) This purpose is implemented largely, but not entirely, by the human resources department, a major organizational unit usually directed by a vice-president. The department often has full control of human resource system functions for all nonprofessional employees and extensive influence over all professional employees except physicians. Doctors and volunteers are least likely to be directly affected by the human resources department, but well-run hospitals are increasingly placing key functions of these groups under the department. Even when direct management of the relationships with these groups is assigned elsewhere, it is necessary to coordinate many of the policies. In the well-run hospital, the human resources department advises on all human resource issues. The discussion which follows emphasizes the function rather than the accountability of the department. In the final section of the chapter there is a brief discussion of the desirability of assigning accountability for specific groups elsewhere.

Functions of Human Resource Management

Work Force Planning

Work force planning allows the hospital adequate time to respond to changes in the exchange environment which require adjustment in the work force. The work force plan is a subsection of the long-range plan. It technically includes, and is always coordinated with, the medical staff plan (see chapter 10). It develops forecasts of the number of persons required in each skill level by year for the length of time covered by the long-range plan. It also projects available human resources including additions and attrition, even to specifying the planned retirement of key individuals.

Development of Plan. The initial proposal for the work force plan should be developed under the direction of the vice-president of human resources, using forecasts of activity from the long-range plan and incorporating changes in service indicated by the medical staff plan. The draft plan should include:

— The anticipated size of the member and employee groups, by major category of skill and department

— The schedule of adjustments through recruitment, retraining, attrition, and termination

— Wage and benefit cost forecasts from national projections tailored to local conditions

— Planned changes in employment or compensation policy, such as the development of incentive payments or the increased use of temporary or part-time employees

— Preliminary estimates of the cost of operating the human resources department and fulfilling the plan

The draft is reviewed by the major medical staff specialties and employer departments, and their concerns are resolved. The revised plan is shared with the plant system, because the number and location of employees determine the requirements for many plant services. The revised plan supports the long-range financial plan and is incorporated in the final package recommended to the governing board by the planning committee.

Using the Work Force Plan. The work force plan must be reviewed annually as part of the environmental assessment, along with other parts of the long-range plan. The amended plan and the annual budget guidelines direct the development of even more detailed plans for the coming year. The human resources department works closely with the employing departments to specify individual compensation changes, and work force adjustment. The financial implications of these actions are incorporated into the departmental budgets, which set precise expectations for the number of employees, the number of hours worked, the wage and salary costs, and the benefit costs.

Well-run hospitals also use the work force plan to guide human resources policies. Among these are the timing of recruitment campaigns; guidelines for the use of temporary labor, such as overtime, part-time, and contract labor; and incentive, compensation, and employee benefit design. The plan may be useful in making decisions about new programs and capital, as when the existence of a surplus work force becomes a resource for expanded services. Even such strategic decisions as mergers or vertical integration can be affected by human resource shortages and surpluses. All of these applications of the plan call for close collaboration with other executives and clinical departments. Collaboration is also desirable on short-term work force management issues, particularly training, motivation, lost time, and turnover. Improvements in these areas reduce the cost of the human resources department and can be translated into direct gains in productivity and quality by line managers.

The penalty for inadequate work force planning is loss of the time and flexibility needed to adjust to environmental changes. Many management difficulties are simpler if adequate time is available to deal with them. Inadequate warning causes hasty and disruptive action. Layoffs may be required. Recruitment is hurried and poor selections may be made. Retraining may be incomplete. Each of these actions takes its toll on workers' morale and often directly affects quality and efficiency. Although the effect of each individual case may be modest, it is long lasting and cumulative. The hospital which makes repeated hasty and expedient decisions erodes its ability to compete.

Maintenance of the Work Force

Building and maintaining the best possible work force requires continuing attention to exchange relationships between the hospital and its members. The hospital cannot remain passive. The best people must be recruited, and they are more likely to remain with an organization which actively meets their personal needs. Investments in recruitment, retention, employee services, and programs for training supervisors in human relations become a part of the intangible benefits as perceived by the employee or member. The additional cost of well-designed programs in these areas is relatively small, but the return is very high.

Recruitment and Selection. Retention of proven members is generally preferable to recruitment, because the risk of dissatisfaction is lower on both sides. However, expansions, changes in services, and employee life cycles result in continuing recruitment needs at all skill levels. Equal opportunity and affirmative action laws, sound medical staff bylaws, and union contracts all require consistency in recruitment practices. A uniform hospital protocol for recruitment establishes policies for the following activities:

1. *Position control*—One position is accountable for control of paychecks authorized, approval of recruitment requests, and keeping the work force at expectations established in the annual budget (see below).
2. *Job description*—Each position must be described in enough detail to identify training, licensure, and experience requirements and to determine compensation.
3. *Classification and compensation*—Wage, salary, incentive, and benefit levels must be assigned to each recruited position. These must be kept consistent with other internal positions, collective bargaining contracts, and the external market.
4. *Job requirements*—The specific skills and knowledge sought must be specified with enough precision to permit equitable evaluation of applicants.
5. *Applicant pool priorities and advertising*—Well-run hospitals have policies covering priority consideration of current and former employees and employees' relatives for job openings. Policies also cover the design, placement, and frequency of media advertising, including use of the hospital's own newsletters and publications.
6. *Initial screening*—It is common to have prescribed application forms and established polices for initial screening of applicants.

Screening normally includes review and verification of data on the application. It may or may not include interviews. A great many applicants for most jobs do not come close to meeting the job description and personal requirements. Particularly for high-volume recruitment, screening takes place in the human resources department so that it will be uniform and inexpensive. It is important that all applicants be treated fairly and courteously. They or their friends and relatives may fit later recruitment needs.

7. *Final selection*—Applicants who pass the initial screening are subjected to more intensive review, usually involving the immediate supervisor of the position and other line personnel. The final selection must be equitable and consistent with the job description and personal requirements. The human resources department usually monitors compliance with these criteria.

8. *Orientation*—New employees need a variety of assistance, ranging from maps showing their work place to counselling on selecting benefit options. They should be given a mentor who can help them fit into their work group. They should learn appropriate information about the hospital's mission, services, and policies to encourage their contribution and to make them spokesmen for the institution in their social group.

9. *Probationary review*—Employees begin work with a probationary period, which concludes with a review of performance and usually an offer to join the organization on a long-term basis. Often, increased benefits and other incentives are included in the long-term offer.

Modifications of the basic protocol are usually made for professional personnel and for temporary employees. Modifications for temporary employees and volunteers greatly simplify the process in order to reduce cost and delay, while those for professional personnel recognize that recruitment is usually from national or regional labor markets and that future colleagues should undertake most of the recruitment.

For the medical staff and higher supervisory levels, search committees are frequently formed to establish the job description and requirements, encourage qualified applicants, carry out screening and selection, and assist in convincing desirable candidates to accept employment. The human resources department acts as staff for the search committee while assuring that the intent of hospital policies has been met. Well-run hospitals now use human resources personnel to conduct initial reference checks and to verify licensure status and educational achievement for doctors and other professional personnel. This provides both consistency and a clearer legal record.

Hospitals are subject to various regulatory and civil restrictions affecting recruitment. Federal regulations regarding equal opportunity require that there be no discrimination on the basis of sex, age, race, creed, national origin, or handicaps that do not incapacitate the individual for the specific job. Those covering affirmative action require special recruitment efforts and priority for equally qualified women, blacks, and persons of Asian and Latin ancestry. (Religious hospitals may give priority to members of their faith under certain circumstances.) In addition to these constraints, hospitals must follow due process, that is, fair, reasonable, and uniform rules, in judging the qualifications of attending physicians. Medical staff appointments are also subject to tests under antitrust laws (see chapter 10). Hospitals are required to be able to document compliance with these rules and may be subject to civil suits by dissatisfied applicants. Monitoring and documenting compliance with these obligations is a function of the human resources department.

Retention and Reduction. Policies for promotion, retirement, and voluntary and involuntary termination must be similar in fairness and consistency to those for recruitment. For motivational purposes, they should be designed to make work life as attractive as possible, and they should permit selective retention of the best workers. This means that all collective actions should be announced and planned as far in the future as possible, that opportunities be widely publicized, that criteria for promotion or dismissal be clear and equitable, and that loyal and able employees be rewarded by priority in promotion and protection against termination. It also means that all policies are administered uniformly and that there is always a clear route of appeal against actions the employee views as arbitrary.

Well-run hospitals make an effort to interview persons who are leaving. Their candid comments can be useful to eliminate or correct negative factors in the work environment. They often serve to improve the departing worker's view of the organization as well.

Employee Services. Many hospitals provide services to their employees through their human resources department on the theory that such services improve loyalty and morale and, therefore, efficiency and quality. Evidence to support the theory is limited, but the services are often required if competing employers provide them. Specific offerings are often tailored to the employees' response. Popular programs are allowed to grow, while others are curtailed. Charges are sometimes imposed to defray the costs, but some subsidization is usual. Those commonly found include:

— Health education and promotion and access to personal counselling for substance abuse problems (Routine personal health services, other than emergency services arising on the job, have largely been replaced by comprehensive health insurance benefits .)

— Infant and child care, often important to young women

— Meals, routinely provided through food service without human resources involvement

— Social events, often recognizing major holidays or corporate events but also used to recognize employee contributions

— Recreational sports, particularly where the hospital happens to have facilities or where community programs accept hospital teams

— Credit unions and payroll deduction for various purposes

One theme of these activities is to build an attitude of caring and mutual support among hospital workers, on the theory that a generally caring environment will encourage a caring response to patient and visitor needs.

Occupational Health and Safety. The hospital is a moderately dangerous environment for workers. It contains unique or rare hazards, such as repeated exposure to low levels of radioactivity or small quantities of anesthesia gases and increased risk of infection. In practice, however, accident rates are low. Illness and injury arising from hospital work are kept to low levels by constant attention to safety. The hospital's dedication to personal and public health encourages this vigilance. For those who might be complacent or forgetful, two laws reinforce its importance. Workers' compensation is governed by state law. Premiums are based on settlements but also on process evidence of attention to safety. The federal Occupational Safety and Health Act establishes standards for safety in the work place and supports inspections. Fines are levied for noncompliance.

Much of the direct control of hazards is the responsibility of the clinical and plant departments. Infection control, for example, is an important collaborative effort of housekeeping, facility maintenance, nursing, and medicine to protect the patient. Employee protection in well-run hospitals stems from procedures developed for patient safety. The human resources department is usually assigned the following functions:

— Monitoring federal and state regulations and professional literature on occupational safety for areas in which the hospital may have hazards

— Identifying the department or group accountable for safety and compliance on each specific risk

— Keeping records and performing risk analysis of general or widespread exposures

— Maintaining records demonstrating compliance and responding to visits and inquiries from official agencies

— Providing or assisting training in and promotion of safe procedures

— Negotiating contracts for workers' compensation insurance, reviewing appropriate language where the insurance is negotiated as part of broader coverage, or managing settlements where the hospital self-insures

Educational Services. Human resources departments provide significant educational opportunities for employees and supervisors. In-service education is offered on topics where uniformity of understanding is desired. On issues to be handled uniformly among relatively large groups, human resources personnel provide the entire program. Routine offerings are usually less than two hours long, with multiple sessions when more time is needed. Classes are limited in size, and offerings are repeated to provide greater access. Topics include:

— *Orientation,* including a review of the hospital's mission, history, major assets, and marketing claims, as well as policies and benefits of employment

— *Work policy changes,* reviews covering the objectives and implications in major changes in compensation, benefits, or work rules

— *Major new programs,* permanent or temporary actions of the hospital that affect habits and life-styles of current workers. (New buildings, relocations, and construction dislocation are often topics.)

— *Retirement planning,* offered to older workers to understand their retirement benefits and also to adjust to retirement life-styles

— *Outplacement,* to assist persons being involuntarily terminated through reductions in work force

— *Benefits management,* selection of options and procedures for using benefits, including efforts to minimize misuse

Clinical departments often use their own supervisors or consultants for professional topics, but human resources in larger hospitals provides facilities, promotion, and logistic assistance. In larger hospitals, human resources can collaborate with governance and finance units on hospitalwide concerns such as the annual budget.

Supervisory training and counselling is a particularly important human resources function. In the well-run hospital promising workers are identified well before they are promoted and are trained in methods of supervision and effective motivation. Multiple presentations using a variety of approaches and media are used to establish and reinforce basic notions: the use of rewards rather than sanctions, the importance of fairness and candor, the role of the supervisor in responding to workers' questions, and the importance of clear instructions and appropriate work environments. Much of the folklore of American industry runs counter to the realities of sound first-line supervision. Thus even promising personnel need repeated reinforcement of the proper role and style. Cases, role playing, recordings, films, and individual counselling are helpful in maintaining supervisors' performance.

Guest relations has become a prominent educational offering for human resources departments. These programs use role playing, games, and group discussion techniques to reinforce attitudes of caring and responsiveness to patients and visitors. Well-run hospitals use the guest relations educational programs as part of a comprehensive effort; workers will respond more effectively to customer needs when their own needs are met by responsive supervision, adequate facilities and equipment, and hospital policies which encourage flexibility toward customer needs.

Grievance Administration. Well-run hospitals provide an authority independent of the normal accountability for employees who feel, for whatever reason, that their complaint or question has not been fully answered. Under collective bargaining, the union contract includes a formal grievance process which is often adversarial in nature, assuming a dispute to be resolved between worker and management. Under more common arrangements, a grievance procedure is still necessary. It should state workers' rights and obligations as clearly as possible, but it should emphasize cooperation, clarification, and mutual adjustment rather than the existence of two conflicting positions. The secret to grievance administration lies in forestalling formal complaints by eliminating causes, settling disputes reasonably and quickly, and collaborating with workers on solutions which go beyond the limits of conflict to make actual improvements in the work environment.

Good grievance administration begins with sound employment policies, effective education for workers and supervisors, and systems which emphasize rewards over sanctions. Effective supervisory training emphasizes the importance of responding promptly to workers' questions and problems. Good supervisors have substantially fewer grievances than poor ones.

When disagreements arise, they should stimulate the following informal reactions; these should be supplemented by the formal review process typically found in union contracts, leading to resolution by an outside arbitrator:

— Documentation of issue, location, and positions of the two parties to provide guides to preventive or corrective action

— Credible, unbiased, informal review to identify constructive solutions

— Informal negotiations which encourage flexibility and innovation in seeking a mutually satisfactory solution

— Counselling for the supervisor involved aimed at improvement of future human relations

— Settlement without formal review, either by mutual agreement or by concession on the part of the organization

Grievances which go to formal review should almost always be decided in the hospital's favor, because a high percentage in the worker's favor encourages more grievances. Even if the concession appears relatively expensive, the hospital is better off avoiding review and making an appropriate investment in the prevention of future difficulties.

Compensation

Employee compensation includes direct wages and salaries, cash differentials and premiums, bonuses, retirement pensions, and a substantial number of specific benefits supported by payroll deduction or supplement. Federal law requires withholding of social security and income taxes from the employee and contributions by the employer. Other employment benefits are automatically purchased on behalf of the employee via the payroll mechanism. Compensation constitutes more than half the expenditures of any community hospital. From the hospital's perspective, such a large sum of money must be protected against both fraud and waste. From the employee's perspective, accuracy regarding amount, timing, and benefit coverage should be perfect.

The growing complexity of compensation has been supported by highly sophisticated computer software, with each advance in computer capability soon translated into expanded flexibility of the compensation package. The latest developments in payroll programs have been increased use of bonuses and incentive compensation, as well as "cafeteria" benefits, which allow more employee choice. Well-run hospitals now use payroll programs that process both pay and benefit data for three purposes—payment, monitoring and reporting, and budgeting. This software permits active management of compensation issues in the human resources department through position control, wage and salary administration, benefit administration, and pension administration.

Position Control. The hospital must protect itself against accidental or fraudulent violation of employment procedures and standards and must assure that only duly employed persons or retirees receive compensation. This is done through a central review of the number of positions created and the persons hired to fill them, called **position control.** Creation of a position generally requires multiple approvals, ending near the level of the chief operating officer. Positions created are monitored by the human resources department to assure compliance with recruitment, promotion, and compensation procedures and to assure that each individual employed is assigned to a unique position. Position control authorization is required before employees can be paid.

It is important to understand the limitation of this activity; it controls the number of people employed rather than the total hours worked. The number of hours worked outside position control accountability is significant in most hospitals. Position control protects only against paying the wrong person, hiring in violation of established policies, and issuing double checks. It does not protect against overspending the labor budget or against errors in hours, rates, or benefit coverage.

Wage and Salary Administration. Most hospitals operate at least two payrolls and a pension disbursement system. One payroll covers personnel hired on an hourly basis, requiring reporting of actual compensable hours for each pay period, usually two weeks. The other covers salaried, usually supervisory, personnel paid a fixed amount per period, often monthly. Contract workers, such as clinical support service physicians, are often compensated through nonpayroll systems. (Benefits, withholding, and payroll deduction are usually omitted from contract compensation, although certain reporting requirements still obtain.)

Wage and salary administration includes the following activities:

— *Verification of compensable hours and compensation due.* This is applicable only to hourly personnel. The accountable department is responsible for the accuracy of hours reported. The task of the human resources department is to verify line authorization, the base rate, and the application of policies establishing differentials.

— *Compensation scales.* The well-run hospital strives to be competitive in each position where comparison can be made to other employers and to treat other positions equitably. To achieve this goal, each position is assigned a compensation grade. These grades establish consistency among similar activities within the hospital. The human resources department conducts or purchases periodic salary and wage surveys to establish competitive prices for representative grades. At supervisory and professional levels, these surveys cover national and regional markets. For most hourly grades the local market is surveyed.

— *Seniority and cost-of-living adjustments.* Since World War II hospitals have recognized changes in cost of living and the experience and loyalty reflected by job seniority. Calculating the amount or value of these factors and translating that into compensation at the appropriate time is the task of the human resources department. Well-run hospitals are rapidly diminishing the importance of both of these compensation factors. Incentive payments in the form of bonuses and merit increases are replacing the more automatic seniority and cost-of-living raises.

— *Incentive and merit adjustments.* A number of experiments in merit-oriented compensation in the decades prior to 1980 failed to yield convincing results. One major problem was the counterincentive of unrestrained reimbursement; hospitals and departments which did not economize were too often rewarded as well as or better than those which did. Another problem was the lack of reliable and valid measures of output, efficiency, and quality. The competitive market environment has eliminated the first problem, and improving information systems are steadily reducing the second. As a result, incentive and merit compensation will receive much more attention from well-run hospitals in the next few years. The issues involved are discussed below.

Benefits Administration. Many of the social programs of Western nations are related directly or indirectly to work, through programs of payroll taxes, deductions, and entitlements. These programs are fixed in place by a combination of direct legal obligation and tax-related incentives. Nonwage benefits are generally exempt from income tax, providing an automatic gain of at least 12 percent in the benefits that can be purchased for a given amount of after-tax money. Further gains stem from insurance characteristics. Life, health, accident, and disability insurance are substantially less costly when purchased on a group basis.

As a result, hospitals and other employers in the United States support extensive programs of benefits, which add up to 40 percent beyond salaries and wages to the costs of employment. (The term "fringe benefits" was common until the total cost of these programs made it obsolete.) The exact participation of each employee differs, with major differences depending on full- or part-time status, grade, and seniority. In general, there are five major classes of employee benefits and employer obligations beyond wage compensation:

1. *Payroll taxes and deductions*—The employer is legally obligated to contribute premium taxes to Social Security for pension and Medicare benefits, as well as to collect a portion of the employee's pay for Social Security and withholding on various income taxes. (A few hospitals have special pension programs which substitute for Social Security.) Most employers also collect payroll deductions for insurance programs, union dues, various privileges like parking, and contributions to charities such as the United Fund. While the deductions represent only a small handling cost to the employer, they are an important convenience to the employee.

2. *Vacations, holidays, and sick leave*—Employers pay full-time and permanent employees for legal holidays, additional holidays, vacations, sick leave, and certain other time not devoted to work. Educational leaves, jury duty, and National Guard duty are common. As a result, only about 85 percent of the 2,080 hours per year nominally constituting full-time employment is actually worked by hourly workers. The nonworked time becomes a direct cost to the hospital when the employee must be replaced by part-time workers or by premium pay. It also is an important factor in the cost of full-time versus part-time employees. Part-time positions often do not share in these benefits at all, or share only on a drastically reduced basis. On a per-hour-worked basis, they can be 15 percent less costly as a result.

3. *Voluntary insurance programs*—Health insurance is an almost universal entitlement of full-time employment. Life insurance and travel and accident insurance are also common. The employer obtains a group rate which is much lower than that offered to individuals, but most well-run hospitals pay a large portion of the remaining premium as an employment benefit. Employer-paid premiums are partially protected from income tax. These payments add about 10 percent to the cost of full-time employees. They are rarely offered to employees working fewer than 20 hours per week and may be graduated to those working between half and full time.

4. *Mandatory insurance*—Employers are obligated to provide workers' compensation for injuries received at work, including both full health care and compensation for lost wages. They are also obligated to provide unemployment insurance, covering a portion of wages for several months following involuntary termination.

5. *Other perquisites*—A wide variety of other benefits of employment can be offered, particularly for higher professional and supervisory grades. These generally are shaped by a combination of tax and job performance considerations. Educational programs, professional society dues, and journal subscriptions are commonly included. Sabbaticals, that is, extended time off for independent study, are becoming more common. Cars, homes, club memberships, and expense accounts are used to assist executives to participate fully in the social life of their community. The theory is that such participation increases the executives' ability to understand community desires and identify influential citizens. Added retirement benefits, actually income deferred for tax purposes, and termination settlements are used to defray the risks of leadership positions.

In managing employment benefits, the human resources department strives to maximize the ratio of gains to expenditure. Four courses of action to achieve this are characteristic of well-run departments; three of them relate to program design and one to program administration:

1. *Program design for competitive impact*—The value of a given benefit is in the eye of the employee, and demographics affect perceived value more than personal tastes do. A married mother might prefer child care to health insurance because her husband's employer already provides health insurance. A single person whose children are grown might prefer retirement benefits to life insurance. Young employees often (perhaps unwisely) prefer cash to deferred or insured benefits. Employee surveys help predict the most attractive design of the benefit package. Flexibility is becoming more desirable as workers' needs become more diverse. Recent trends have emphasized cafeteria benefits, where each employee can select preset combinations.

2. *Program design for cost-effectiveness*—Several benefits have an insurance characteristic such that actual cost is determined by exposure to claims. Health insurance, accident insurance, and sick benefits are particularly susceptible to cost reduction by benefit design. Health insurance, by far the largest of these

costs, is minimized by the use of prospective admission review, copayments, preferred provider arrangements, and capitation. Many hospitals as employers are encouraging participation in their own capitation or preferred provider contracts by increasing the costs borne by employees who choose other plans. Accident insurance premiums are reduced by limiting benefits to larger, more catastrophic events. Duplicate coverage, where the employee and the spouse who is employed elsewhere are both covered by insurance, can be eliminated to reduce cost. Costs of sick benefits can be reduced by eliminating coverage for short illnesses, and by requiring certification from a physician early in the episode of coverage.

3. *Program design for tax implications*—Income tax advantages are a major factor in program design. Many of them, such as the exemption of health insurance premiums, are deliberate legislative policy, while others appear almost accidental. Details are subject to constant adjustment through both legislation and administrative interpretations. As a result, it is profitable to review the benefit program periodically for changing tax implications, both in terms of current offerings and in terms of the desirability of additions or substitutions.

4. *Program administration*—Almost all of the benefits can be administered in ways which minimize their costs. It is necessary to provide actual benefits equitably to all employees; careless review of use may lead to widespread expansion of interpretation and benefit cost. Strict interpretation can be received well by employees if it is prompt, courteous, and accompanied by documentation in the benefit literature initially given employees. Health insurance is probably the most susceptible to poor administration. Careful claims review, enforcement of co-pay provisions, and coordination of spouse's coverage are known to be cost-effective.

Prevention of insured perils can be fruitful. Absenteeism and on-the-job injuries are reduced by effective supervision. Accidents and health insurance usage are reduced by effective health promotion, particularly in cases of substance abuse. Counselling is also believed to reduce health insurance use. Workers' compensation is reduced by improved safety on the job site. Unemployment liability is reduced by better planning and use of attrition for work force reduction. It is noteworthy that these activities are all affected by human resources management, through employee services, supervisory training, work force planning, and occupational safety programs.

Pensions and Retirement Administration. Pensions and retirement benefits pose different management problems from other benefits because they are used only after the employee retires. Nonpension benefits are principally health insurance supplementing Medicare. Recent developments have led hospitals to offer bonuses for early retirement as a way of adjusting the work force.

Pension design and retirement program management involve questions of benefit design and administration that are directly analogous to those of other insured benefits. Because the benefit is often not used for many years and represents a multidecade commitment when use begins, pensions are funded by cash reserves. As a result, pension issues also include the definition of suitable funding investments, that is, to what extent they should be divided between fixed-dollar returns and those responsive to inflation, and the management of the funds, including investment of them in the hospital's own bonds or stock. Finally, pension-related issues include the motivational impact of the design on the tendency of employees to retire.

The pension itself, but not other retirement benefits, is regulated under the Employee Retirement Insurance Security Act (ERISA). Regulations for ERISA specify the employer's obligation to offer pensions, to contribute to them if offered, to vest those contributions, and to fund pension liabilities through trust arrangements. These regulations leave several elements of a sound pension and retirement policy to the hospital:

— The amount of pension supplementing Social Security

— The amount, kind, and design of Medicare supplementation (Capitation and other programs encouraging economical use of benefits will rapidly become more common. Extension of covered benefits to nursing home and related long-term services is likely.)

— Opportunities for additional contribution by employees

— Accounting for unvested liabilities

— Funding of unvested pension liabilities

— Use of unvested funds in hospital finance

— Division of investments between equity and fixed-dollar obligations and selection of those investments

— Incentives to encourage or discourage retirement (Age 65 is an arbitrary and increasingly irrelevant standard. Federal law allows most older workers, including hospital workers, the right to continue work without a mandatory retirement age.)

Many of these issues can be and frequently are delegated to pension management firms or fund trustees. Others are important parts of a well-planned work force management program which must be handled by the human resources system. In addition to these financial, technical, and motivational concerns, most hospitals accept an obligation to provide retirement counselling, including education to help the employee manage pensions and health insurance benefits.

Retired workers represent large future liabilities which for many hospitals may not be fully recognized on current balance sheets. At the time of a female employee's retirement, the hospital typically commits itself to pension payments and support of Medicare supplementary health insurance for a period averaging nearly 15 years. ERISA requires a trust fund to support pension payments, but the health insurance supplement payment is generally not funded. Also, many hospitals have felt obligated to adjust pensions for very old workers, because inflation has eroded their buying power below subsistence levels. Such adjustments are, by definition, not funded.

Although hospitals are currently using retirement bonuses as a method of work force reduction, at other times it may pay hospitals to retain older workers. In general, they are more amenable to reduced hours, have reliable work habits, and are less likely to have unpredictable absences.

Economic, Legal, and Social Considerations in Compensation. Employment is an exchange transaction governed primarily by an economic marketplace. Compensation, including benefits, is a major part of the economic agreement. It follows then, that the market is the best and usual source of information on compensation. Hospitals depart from the market price for labor at their peril: a lower price may not attract enough qualified personnel, and a higher one may waste the owners' funds. Deliberate departure from market prices should be justified by some proven benefit; accidental departure should be minimized. Thus the importance of wage and salary surveys is emphasized. These are often available for purchase, particularly for national markets; however, continuing contact with appropriate markets is one of the important functions of the human resources system.

Legal restrictions are also important. Hospitals are subject to federal and state laws governing wages, hours, and working conditions. As noted, they are also obligated to follow equal opportunity and affirmative action regulations. The human resources department is usually accountable for compliance with most of these regulations and for instructing others when it is not accountable. It also is generally accountable for all records and documentation in support of compliance.

Social considerations are more complex. Many people who are concerned with hospitals are also concerned with related issues of a good society, such as the availability of meaningful work for all, the adequacy of low wages and pensions, the equity of payment for equivalent work, and the avoidance of exploitation of minorities or subgroups of the society. These questions are rarely addressed straightforwardly. In particular, efforts to improve compensation are often associated with reductions in the number of jobs available, possibly by reducing the competitiveness of the hospital. Well-run hospitals tend to do the following:

— Comply with market trends

— Comply with applicable laws and regulations

— Take limited advantage of low-risk ways to increase employment or compensation to disadvantaged groups

— Advocate as an organization more significant redress of these important social problems

— Adopt riskier programs for addressing social problems only as part of an explicit mission implemented through the five-year plan

This posture makes the hospital a passive rather than an active force in resolving social problems related to work. It also means that a more active position will require board debate and approval. Few hospitals currently make these issues part of their formal mission.

Collective Bargaining Agreements

Extent and Trends in Collective Bargaining. Hospitals are subject to both state and federal legislation governing the right of workers to organize a union for their collective representation on economic and other work-related matters. Federal legislation generally supports the existence of unions; state laws vary. As a result of the extension of federal law to hospitals and of the increased availability of funds, hospital organizing drives became more common and more successful around 1970. By 1980, 20 percent of all hospital employees were unionized. Unskilled workers and building trades were the most likely to be organized. Nurses were next most likely; other clinical professionals were rarely organized. Small numbers of house officers were union members. Periodic efforts to organize attending physicians had gained little headway, but a group called the Union of American Physicians and Dentists claimed about 8 percent of doctors as members, with rapid growth in 1985.[2] The likelihood of unionization differed significantly by state, with the northeastern states and California most likely, and was far more common in urban areas.

With the recession of 1981–1983, the prevailing attitude toward unionization in the United States appears to have changed. Both total number and percentage of employees in unions declined, organizing drives encountered greater resistance, management strategies to resist or even eliminate unions became more aggressive, and contract settlements became less generous. The causes of the change are not certain, but increased recognition of international competitive pressures seems to have been important. The change may have occurred in hospitals as well, although in 1986 unions were reported to be increasing their membership efforts.[3] The economic benefits of unionization for hospital employees have been diminished by the competitive environment.

Although views on the meaning and value of unions differ, one important view is that they are at best unnecessary and often dysfunctional for the long-term benefit of both corporation and employee. Recent trends suggest that this view has been prevailing. An alternative view notes that unions have been a strong positive force for improving working conditions, and that the concept of representation is consistent with employee participation as a means of improving motivation.

For most hospitals, a position that avoids or diminishes the influence of unions is likely to be consistent with the exchange environment. The hospital's relation to unions is actualized through its position on work-related concerns of employees, its response to organizing drives, and its negotiation and administration of union contracts. In both pro-union and antiunion communities, the true goal of the well-run hospital is to minimize employee dissatisfaction and conflict; the presence of the union affects the means more than the end. Despite the traditional labor organizer's rhetoric, neither the union nor the hospital may have much control over the exploitation of the worker.

Work-Related Employee Concerns. Union organization drives and collective bargaining tend to be strong where employees perceive a substantial advantage to collective representation. This perception is stimulated by evidence of careless, inconsiderate, or inequitable behavior on the part of management in any of the key concerns of the work place: output expectations, response to workers' questions, working conditions, and pay. It is possible to diminish both the perception of advantage and the real advantage of unionization by consistently good management. Many companies have existed for decades in highly unionized environments without ever having a significant union organization.

For a hospital which wishes to avoid conflict with existing unions, reduce the risk of organization, and diminish the influence of collectively bargained contracts, the first step is to make certain there is little room for complaint about the key concerns of the work place and no obvious opportunity for improvement. The union then has nothing to offer in return for its dues, and its strength is diminished. The first task of the human resources department in this regard is to achieve high-quality performance on its functions. The second is to assist other systems of the hospital to do the same, and the third is to present the hospital so that its performance is recognized by workers.

Organization Drives and Responses. Organization drives are regulated by law and have become highly formal activities. The union, the employees, and management all have rights which must be scrupulously observed. The regulatory environment presumes an adversarial proceeding. Under this presumption, management is obligated to present a reasonable argument on behalf of independence from the union and to take legal actions which limit the organizers to the framework of the law. If management fails in this duty, the rights of employees and owners who do not wish union representation are not properly protected. Well-run hospitals respond to organizing drives by hiring competent counsel specifically to fulfill their adversarial rights and obligations. They act on advice of counsel to the extent that it is consistent with their general strategy of fair and reasonable employee relations. They avoid responses which might be interpreted as unfair or vindictive by significant numbers of employees.

Negotiations and Contract Administration. Like many other aspects of unionization, bargaining procedures are also carried out in an adversarial environment. Well-run hospitals use experienced bargainers and have counsel available for the more complex formalities. Once again, management is obligated to represent owners and employees who are not present at the bargaining table. Hospitals with existing unions pursue a strategy of contract negotiation which attempts to minimize or eliminate dissent. They will accept a strike on issues which depart significantly from the current exchange environment for workers or patients, but as a strategy they avoid strikes whenever possible.

Under certain circumstances, management must pursue contracts which reduce income or employment for union members. Two rules govern such a case for the well-run hospital: it must apply equally to nonunion workers, and it must be well justified by external forces in the exchange environment.

Contract administration is approached in a similar vein, but the adversarial characteristic of organizing and bargaining should not carry over into the work place. The well-run hospital maintains a posture of collaboration in its primary work groups. The objective is to comply fully with the contract but to minimize literal interpretation. Considerable supervisory education is necessary to implement this policy. Supervisors should know the contract and abide by it, but whenever possible their actions should be governed by fundamental concerns of human relations and personnel management. Any distinction between unionized and nonunionized groups should be minimized.

Organization and Personnel

Human Resources Management as a Profession

Human resources management emerged as a profession after World War II, in response to the complexities created by union contracts, wage and hour laws, and benefits management. Hospitals were sheltered from these developments for several years, but as the need arose they moved to establish an identifiable human resources system and to hire specially trained leadership for it. Although there is no public certification for the profession, there is an identifiable curriculum of formal education and a recognizable pattern of professional experience. Hospital practitioners have an association, the American Society for Healthcare Human Resources, a unit of the American Hospital Association. Well-run hospitals now recruit their human resources director or vice-president from persons with experience in the profession generally and, when possible, with experience in hospitals. Larger hospitals often have several professionals in this field.

Professional training and experience contribute to mastery of the several areas in which laws, precedents, specialized skills, or unique knowledge define appropriate actions. These areas now include recruitment, collective bargaining, supervisory education, wage and salary administration, and benefits management. It is likely that work force planning and knowledge of the job markets of the hospital professions benefit most from human resources managers with hospital experience.

Organization of the Human Resources Department

Internal Organization. The human resources department is organized by function, in order to take advantage of the specialized skills applicable to its more time-consuming activities. The common sections in smaller hospitals are

— Compensation
  • Wage and salary administration
  • Benefits administration

• Work force maintenance

Collective bargaining is added as a section in hospitals with substantial unionization. Larger hospitals subdivide these sections along functional lines. Work force planning is generally handled by an ad hoc team led by the vice-president for human resources.

Division of Responsibility with Other Systems. The more controversial organizational problems relate to the division of human resources functions between the department and the line department or unit accountable for the member's costs and output. Whether the human resources department is involved or not, the functions of the human resources system must be performed for all hospital members. Even volunteers require selection and orientation. Although they receive no wages, they are often given some benefits. The question of what benefits they will receive is, of course, a compensation issue. Attending physicians are subject to extensive recruitment and selection and often receive monetary compensation and substantial benefits. By the same token, all hospital members require supervision by and assistance from their accountable line unit. Thus the question of the exact domain of the human resources department is inevitably a matter of judgment.

Well-run hospitals have identified the question as one of appropriate joint contribution to the needs of the member. They seek the solution not in the assignment of certain member groups to either the line or the human resources department, but rather in the identification of the amount and kind of contribution each unit can make in completing each function. This approach recognizes that the goal is to perform each function well for each member of the hospital work force and that the human resources system must be a collaboration between the department and the line unit involved. In judging the assignment of specific functions, one bears in mind the human resources department's contributions: uniformity, economy, and specialized human resources skills. The line unit's contributions are professional and technical knowledge of the specific tasks.

In the 1970s, a national movement toward equity and uniformity in work-related issues led well-run hospitals to expand the human resources department's role. Equal opportunity laws, growing collective bargaining, increased exposure to workers' compensation liability, increased regulation of occupational safety, and requirements for due process in privileging physicians all suggested increased centralization of work force management functions. On the national scene, recognition of the costs of these objectives has led to significant retrenchment. From this one might infer that the centralization of human resources functions has peaked; the role of the line may grow slowly in coming years.

At present, the major functions tend to be distributed as follows in well-run hospitals:

— *Work force planning.* Line units are generally responsible for short-term forecasts and the relationship between workers and output. Long-term forecasts of output are developed centrally by the governance system. The human resources department is responsible for extending the work force requirement to the horizon of the long-range plan. These extensions are reviewed by the line units, and discussions of specific adjustments are joint. Governance system members resolve disputes.

— *Work force maintenance activities.* These activities include the following:

  • *Recruitment and retention*—Recruitment activities are decentralized to the line units for all supervisory and professional positions, with active participation of the human resources department. Retention is even more decentralized, with participation of the human resources department limited to major work force reductions and review for compliance with due process and equal opportunity regulations.

  • *Employee services*—These services are centralized.

  • *Grievance administration*—Formal procedures are always centralized. Informal procedures are decentralized, with the human resources department available for advice.

  • *Supervisory training and counselling*—These services are centralized.

— *Compensation.* Compensation is a centralized service except for three specific contributions from the line units:

  • *Job content and description*

  • *Advice on professional markets and competing offers*

  • *Recommendations for individual merit increases*

— *Collective bargaining agreements.* These are centralized, but line units have a strong advisory role.

Measures and Information Systems

The growth of both centralized and decentralized roles in human resources activities demands quantitative assessment of the human resources system as well as the human resources department. Overall human resources performance must be assessed because of exchange pressures. A high-quality work force requires competitive planning, recruitment, wages, benefits, and employment services. The global measure of quality can be member satisfaction. When members are satisfied, and management is satisfied with members, one may infer that the human resources function has been properly performed. The more human resources functions are decentralized, the more complex the supporting information system must be. The human resources department itself must be assessed to establish expectations for demand, output, quality, and efficiency. When human resources department costs are accounted to line units through transfer pricing, the department must have as comprehensive an information system as an independent consulting company.

Measurement of Human Resources System Performance

It is possible to measure many closed system parameters of the human resources system using sophisticated accounting and satisfaction surveys. Precise definitions of the concepts being measured are easily obtained. Many are defined in accounting practice; several others are defined for the industry by common statistical usage.[4] Figure 14.1 lists many of the commonly used measures for assessing the system. It also lists the much rarer measures for transfer pricing of human resources department services.

Figure 14.1 emphasizes outcomes measures of quality. It suggests the use of satisfaction surveys for line managers and for hospital employees, supplemented by several less costly measures arising out of routine information systems. The cost of the special surveys can be minimized by reducing the frequency of them. The less costly process measures of quality serve as a guide to the necessity for surveys.

Information Systems

Structure. The information systems of human resources management are built around the list of approved positions, the file of employed or member personnel, and the payroll. Records of the current status of the human resource—personnel activity, costs, and needs—are taken from these sources. The human resources plan is a deliberate forecast of these measures, and the controls exercised by both line departments and the human resources department are supported by these data. Labor skills, costs, turnover, absenteeism, benefit usage, and vacancies are calculated from these basic files.

Automation of these records has progressed quite far in well-run hospitals. Although most applications are limited to paid employees, it is a simple matter to extend coverage to volunteers and physicians.

Flexible, detailed payroll systems not only support pay disbursements and cost reports for each primary monitor or supervisor, but also generate records of payroll deductions and benefit coverage. The list of approved positions is embedded in the payroll system. A second automated file extends the historical dimension and documents the work record of every current employee. The records in it are supplemented with non-pay-related transactions, particularly a record of continuing education and skill profiles. A third file accumulates utilization of services and benefits. It requires posting of claims and use data for each of the actuarially oriented benefits, including health insurance, workers' compensation, sick pay, and accident and disability. A fourth file, similar in concept to the third, records occupational hazards, incidents, exposures, and process measures of risk. Finally, a fifth set of information, rarely automated, describes competitive conditions, including wage and benefits surveys.

Data base management is increasingly useful for automated records. It permits retrieval by any dimension of the work force, in essentially limitless combinations. This capability encourages aggressive search for improvement. It is possible to array health insurance utilization by diagnosis, skill level, and department, for example, in a search for preventable expenditures. Identification of professionals claiming a certain skill, such as nurses trained in parenteral fluids administration, can be almost instantaneous.

Ethical Issues. Important ethical questions are raised in connection with the information in these files. The records involved are usually viewed as confidential. Unguarded automated systems can make large quantities of information public. At the simplest ethical level, human resources files must be guarded against unauthorized access and misuse.

More serious questions arise when basic concerns have been met. Prevention of turnover, accidents, absenteeism, and illness is a socially useful goal of human resources management. It is clearly proper, even desirable, to study variation in absenteeism and turnover as measures of supervisory effectiveness that can be improved by counselling and education. Yet actions based upon analysis of absenteeism by worker characteristics such as age, sex, or race can be both unethical and illegal. Individuals' records of illness and disability can be used to deny promotion or employment. Some companies have attempted to deny employment opportunities in situations where there was high risk of occupational injury. For example, such an approach would deny employment in operating rooms to female nurses in their childbearing years, because there are known pregnancy risks related to exposure to anesthesia.

Figure 14.1

Measures of Human Resources System Performance

Output Measures
  Employment counts
    Number of employees
      Full-time
      Part-time
      Full-time-equivalent (FTE)
    Candidates recruited
    Placements
    Outplacements
      Retirements
      Other
Resource Consumption Measures
  Operating budget of human resources department
  Work force costs
    Total payroll
    Costs of nonsalary benefits
    Retirement costs and liabilities
    Costs of contract labor
Resource Conservation Measures
  Transfer prices for services sold to other units
    Recruitment services per new hire
    Compensation services per employee
    Training services per enrollee
    Other general services (employee services, grievance administration, supervisory training and counselling, occupational health and safety) per employee
    Contract negotiation services per contract
  Implied profit from successful "sales"
Efficiency Measures
  Work force maintenance—human resources department cost per FTE
    Recruitment—cost per position filled
    Supervisory training—cost per supervisor
    Other work force maintenance—cost per FTE
  Compensation
    Retirement and pensions—human resources department costs per retiree
    Other compensation management—human resources department cost per FTE
    Collective bargaining—human resources department cost per FTE in bargaining group   *Continued*

One must note that in almost all cases harm results from the use of information rather than the acquisition of it. In fact, knowledge of age-, sex- and race-related hazards can only be deduced from studies of their specific impact. Thus denial of the value of all or part of the information potential is also unethical—it theoretically causes the hospital to do less than it should on behalf of all workers. A sound policy must

Figure 14.1 Continued

Quality Measures
  Outcomes measures
    Employee satisfaction surveys
    Management satisfaction surveys
    Retention and turnover
      Turnover ratios
      Average length of service
    Grievances
      Recorded (count)
      Resolved (count, percent)
      Arbitrated (percent in management's favor)
    Work force productivity
      Absenteeism
      Nonproductive time
    Recruitment effectiveness
      Number of qualified candidates
      Delay in recruitment
      Rank of candidate accepting employment
    Compensation
      Variation from survey compensation level
  Process measures
    Percent on time for each major function
    Percent completion for each major function
    Inspection and oversight

balance the advantages of investigation against its dangers. The well-run hospital attempts to use information from personnel files constructively and judiciously. These rules help:

— Information access is limited to a necessary minimum group. Those with access are taught the importance of confidentiality and the hospital's expectation that individuals' rights will be protected.

— Formal approval must be sought for studies of individual characteristics affecting personnel performance. Often a specific committee including members of the hospital's ethics committee reviews each study. Criteria for approval include protection of individual rights, scientific reliability, and evidence of potential benefit.

— Actions taken to improve performance are reward- rather than sanction-oriented. Considerable effort is made to find nonrestrictive solutions. (In the operating room example, avoidance of the more dangerous gases would be one such solution, improved air handling another, and concentrating use in one location a third. While none of these may be practical, all should be considered before a restrictive employment policy is established.)

— When used, sanctions or restrictions offer the individual the greatest possible freedom of choice. The right of the individual to take an informed risk should be respected, although it may not reduce the hospital's ultimate liability. (In the operating room example, a nurse may accept employment with a full explanation of the risks as they are currently known. The complex probabilities of pregnancy, stillbirth, and infant deformity clearly depend on her personal life-style and intentions. Weighing them would be her moral obligation. Legally, the hospital's liability for later injury might be reduced by evidence that full information was supplied about the hazards involved, although such an outcome is not certain.)

Use of the Information System for Analysis. The information system described above, plus the normal cost accounting system, can provide most of the measures suggested in figure 14.1 at negligible cost. Thus expectations can be set each year in the annual budgeting exercise, and reports of achievement can go routinely to sections of the human resources department. As usual, it is anticipated that expectations will be met. Improvement will occur by learning how to exceed the current expectation and will be recognized by reward.

The same measures should be reported to line supervisors. Most issues of the human resources system are the result of joint action. While it is sometimes difficult to analyze the independent effect of the line and the human resources department, review of departmental performance over a representative group of line managers can often suggest improvements the department can make. (Difficulties in proving association are reduced by taking the reward-oriented approach to the use of measures.)

Special attention will be required to obtain user evaluations. Formal surveys of employees' and line supervisors' perceptions of the department may be infrequent, but they should be conducted often enough to assure that the department recognizes its obligation to be responsive to these groups. The need for this measure increases with transfer pricing. The human resources department sells its services to other departments, which respond by minimizing unnecessary use of the department. The transfer price may be compared against market evidence, but the human resources department inescapably has a monopoly on most activity. Thus the surveys of user opinion are an important safety valve as well as a guide to outcomes quality.

Management Issues

The competitive environment for hospitals will demand extraordinary efforts to improve human relations. All hospitals must make major changes in labor efficiency and cost. The best will understand that the loyalty, skill, and motivation of the work force are also critical and that any effort to address the problems of costs must involve increasing the contribution and the compensation of many workers. Pursuing these concepts will improve hospital efficiency while simultaneously making workers increasingly valuable to themselves and to the hospital. Badly managed hospitals will take hasty, ill-considered actions devastating those persons who are terminated and demoralizing those who remain. The demoralization will generate problems of cost, efficiency, quality, and attractiveness to patients and doctors.

The well-run hospital will be competent in each of the functions of the human resources system, placing special emphasis on work force planning, benefits management, and supervisory training. It will have the necessary information systems, including data base management systems for retrieval and analysis of human resources data. It will have automated personnel scheduling for its clinical personnel and other workers whose long hours of service and variable work loads complicate scheduling. It will have measures of quality and efficiency for the human resources department itself, emphasizing service to other systems and outcomes quality. Beyond that, four areas appear to be emerging:

1. Worker-set expectations and improvements

2. Incentive compensation

3. Trends in the use of part-time and temporary workers

4. Transfer pricing

Worker-Set Expectations and Improvements

That there are many dimensions to a sound and fruitful relationship between an individual and an organization is no longer a matter for argument. It has been repeatedly documented that the relationship is enhanced by worker participation; supervisory responsiveness; recognition of contribution; promptness, candor, and equity in resolving difficulties; and consideration of the worker's basic economic needs. The problem is to sustain these desiderata in the face of ongoing external pressures.

Well-run hospitals continuously reinforce the concepts through supervisory training, measurement systems, and incentives. Some hospitals have gone beyond this, to experiment with greatly enhanced worker participation. The central concepts underlying this approach are equality and teamwork, the notions that both the power of the team and the rewards to individuals from participating on the team significantly exceed what can be obtained through conventional methods of supervision. The approach delegates decision making to the workers themselves.

The power of such an approach is tantalizing. Examples of success have existed for decades in other industries. Some may exist in hospitals, although there is no documentation. Certain difficulties are apparent:

— Worker participation requires a strong corporate culture to overcome conventional beliefs about the work place. The workers themselves must be convinced of the virtue and reality of contribution, and all supervisors must understand the importance of supporting that belief. The authoritarian attitude which has characterized the clinical professions, both within their individual cultures and among them, is a major barrier.

— Delegated decisions must be clearly defined. First-line worker groups must understand a discrete domain and perceive credible responses to questions about the external world. Lack of articulate, rational expectations about many hospital activities discourages workers and causes anxiety among supervisors. (The best way to understand this problem is to listen to the answers given by authoritative professionals to some typical questions, for example, "Why are patients awakened at six o'clock?" "Is nursing or social work responsible for discharge placement?" "What consultative services should be provided in pharmacology, pathology, and imaging?" In many hospitals the answers are superficial, ambiguous, or even evasive. Only when management is willing to examine such issues rationally will worker contributions be valuable.)

— The expectations for the small group must be relatively well measured. Until recently, quality assessment was so subjective that many efforts at economy and efficiency failed on arguments about perceived loss of quality. As the parameters of the closed system are more carefully defined and measured, it is possible to state more precise expectations and to test proposals empirically.

— There must be rewards for successful effort. The environment prior to competition offered little incentive for improving performance. In important respects it encouraged separatism and protectionism among professions and nonprofessional workers. Competition is so recent that few, if any, hospitals have changed that culture or devised a reward structure for effective improvement.

Well-run hospitals are beginning to address these difficulties. New information technology and the competitive marketplace combined should stimulate progress. Well-designed incentive compensation will also help. A supportive human relations environment will probably prove to be the critical factor.

Incentive Compensation

A management scheme built on rewards and the search for continued improvement rather than sanctions must develop a system of compensation which supplements personal achievement and professional recognition. Hospitals have far to go in this regard. Despite a few developmental efforts,[5] there is virtually no record of continued incentive compensation, even for the upper levels of management.

One approach is to recognize that starting wages and salaries should be based solely upon market conditions, but that subsequent adjustments in compensation are most appropriately based on two factors: the employee's unique contribution and shifts in the market that are major enough to require readjustment of the starting rate. In effect, each individual has the opportunity to earn a differential over market by her or his contribution to hospital goals. Certain constraints must be recognized in designing a system of this type:

— The resources available will depend more on the hospital's overall performance than on any individual's contribution.

— The resources available for rewards may be severely limited through factors outside the hospital's control.

— Equity and objectivity will be expected in the distribution of the rewards.

— The individual's contribution will be difficult to measure.

— Group rewards attenuate the incentives to individuals. The larger the group, the greater the attenuation.

These problems afflict any effort at incentive compensation, yet such compensation is commonplace in private organizations. Well-run hospitals are beginning to experiment with it. It is likely that successful designs will have the following characteristics:

— The use of incentive compensation will begin at top governance levels and be extended to lower ranks with experience.

— Annual longevity increases will disappear as incentive pay increases.

— Incentives will be limited by difficulties in measurement and administration, but will reach 25 to 50 percent of total compensation.

— Incentives will be related to overall hospital performance but will be awarded to individuals based upon their perceived contribution.

— Assessment of contribution will be retrospective but will be based upon achievement of improvements in expectations set in the preceding budget negotiation.

A bolder scenario assumes a prompt move to worker-set expectations. Approaches such as the Scanlon Plan[6] suggest that primary worker groups can effectively set expectations consistent with the needs of the larger organization and that the effort to do so will lead to measurable improvement in achievement. Those gains can then be used in part to reward the workers. Despite a 50-year history, Scanlon plans have worked best where achievements are well defined and work groups are small. It has yet to be proved that the approach can work in complex, multiprofessional organizations with relatively ambiguous goals; however, the time is ripe for experimentation.

Trends in the Use of Part-Time and Temporary Workers

Hospitals have traditionally structured their work forces around full-time employment. The 8-hour day and the 40-hour week became common after World War II and were reinforced by the extension of the federal wage and hour law to hospitals. Various other patterns have been of passing interest and found roles in specialized settings such as emergency rooms.[7] Part-time and temporary workers are also used in hospitals. The exact extent to which they are used is not clear, because there are no uniform definitions of temporary and because workers obtained from labor agencies are not employees and are therefore not measured as labor in the accounting system.

It is likely that the balance will shift away from full-time, permanent employees to part-time and temporary workers. With this change will come more experimentation with scheduling, off-site work assignments, and other flexible arrangements. Highly competitive service industries such as fast food restaurants rely heavily on part-time workers. If such workers can produce a product of acceptable quality, they offer significant cost advantages. They tend to average very near the starting rates, sharing neither in tenure nor incentive gains. They require few employment services. They share less than proportionately in benefits. Overtime can be reduced by increasing the number of workers at straight time.

There is already widespread attention to the social consequences of using temporary workers. The cost savings occur largely because these workers do not share in the social benefits which the nation deliberately built into the employment relationship. Health insurance and pensions are the two most important of these. A hospital which increases its ratio of part-time to full-time workers to some extent undermines its stated motives regarding Samaritanism, personal health service, and public health. Yet it offers employment that is competitive with other opportunities. There is some possibility that life-styles are changing from the emphasis on full-time, lifetime work, which was the norm for past generations. Other methods besides employment may emerge to support these social benefits.

A second serious drawback to the use of part-time and temporary personnel is the need for training. In the complex hospital environment, where different professions rely on mutually coordinated efforts, inexperience is costly and can be dangerous. Even if one has the appropriate formal training, it takes more experience to give good health care than to make good hamburgers. Automation is ameliorating, but not eliminating, this problem:

— Personnel scheduling systems permit more flexibility in hours and can handle larger numbers of individuals for each position to be filled.

— Individual experience records permit more complete and precise identification of skills and the development of profiles for multiple assignments.

— Computerized work stations permit easy retrieval of methods and procedures, and they prompt users on specific activities that might otherwise be overlooked.

— Some computerized clerical work can now be done at home.

A reasonable forecast suggests that well-run hospitals will minimize or eliminate reliance on agency personnel and develop internal pools of part-time workers. As this scheme matures, three further developments may emerge:

1. Part-time workers may agree to continuing contracts to work under specified conditions of notice and duration, allowing the hospital to formalize a pool of available workers for a variety of skills.

2. Workers seeking full-time employment may be willing to accept limited benefits for an initial period, with enhanced security and benefits under a "tenured" contract awarded for merit after several years.

3. Combining these two trends, beginning workers may be offered less than full-time employment, with the opportunity for increased or more predictable employment used as an explicit reward for learning, experience, and good performance.

Transfer Pricing

The human resources department has traditionally been an overhead, or non-revenue-generating, center in hospital accounting. There are two difficulties with this concept. One is that neither the executive nor the human resources department itself has anything but a crude guide to the value of its contribution. This lack of clarity impairs decisions at the margin, that is, how to evaluate the merit of an incremental change in the size of the department. The other is that the cost of human resources appears as a fixed item to the line units, which therefore have no incentive to investigate and reduce unnecessary expenditures. Yet in fact expenditures on human resources can be reduced by reducing turnover, changing recruitment patterns, revising benefit design and management, reducing grievances, and eliminating union disputes.

A possible solution to this problem is the use of transfer prices to allocate departmental costs to line units. Prices must be established in some rational way for as many as possible of the department's services. The approach is the same as that used by a lawyer, outside arbitrator, or consultant selling services to an independent buyer. Fees are established initially on relatively imprecise cost accounting and are refined later on "market" responses, as well as more accurate costing. Priced functions are treated as purchased services by the line department and as revenue sources by the human resources department. Services which are difficult to price for an individual unit, such as wage and salary surveys and occupational health and safety, can either be distributed as overhead in the same manner as before, or "sold" to the governance unit. Several possible cost measurement concepts supporting transfer pricing are shown in figure 14.1. The transfer price list for human resources department sales to middle managers in other systems might look like this:

— *Recruitment services,* fee based on actual costs incurred per position posted

— *Employment and orientation,* standard fee per hire or per participant, based on average costs

— *Promotion and termination,* standard processing fee based on average cost per occurrence

— *Employee services,* annual or monthly fee based on average cost per employee

— *Grievance administration,* fee per formal grievance processed, based on actual costs and including a markup for general costs of the grievance system

— *Benefits administration,* actual costs of benefits per employee, to a preset limit, plus an average cost for administration and an average cost for catastrophic events, such as a serious disease or accident, which would exceed the individual employee limit

— *Other services,* (wage and salary administration, supervisory training, employee counselling, and collective bargaining), the costs of which are borne by the executive office on behalf of the institution as a whole

The transfer price scheme clearly requires a robust accounting system to provide human resources department managers with the information they need to control their own costs. It demands an extensive information system for measuring departmental quality as well. In addition to these relatively technical requirements, the scheme will test the balance of assignment of human resources functions between line units and the department. Some line units will seek to minimize their transfer costs by undertaking many functions on their own. While this may be satisfactory, there are legitimate concerns about the cost of failure; it takes many years of effort to build high morale and a responsive, motivated work force, but only a few months to destroy one. Perhaps the biggest drawback is the size of the gain. The entire cost of the human resources department is a relatively small percentage of labor costs. When the human resources department has superior management and is located in a similarly managed general environment, the problems associated with transfer pricing might be easily managed. Particularly in the context of multihospital systems, centralized or regional human resources departments might meet the challenges.

Notes

1. American Hospital Association, *Hospital Statistics* (Chicago: AHA, 1984 and preceding years).
2. *Washington Report on Medicine & Health,* 24 February 1986, p. 2
3. *Washington Report on Medicine & Health,* 3 March 1986, p. 3.
4. *See Hospital Statistics.*

5. L. Shyavitz, D. Rosenbloom, and L. Conover, "Financial Incentives for Middle Managers: Pilot Program in an Inner-City Municipal Hospital," *Health Care Management Review* 10 (Summer 1985): 37–44.

6. C. F. Frost, *The Scanlon Plan for Organizational Development* (East Lansing, MI: Michigan State University Press, 1974). Also see B. E. Moore and T. L. Ross, *Scanlon Way to Improve Productivity* (New York: Wiley Interscience, 1978).

7. B. Arnold and M. E. Mills, "Core-12: Implementation of Flexible Scheduling," *Journal of Nursing Administration* 13 (July-August 1983): 9–14.

Suggested Readings

American Society for Hospital Personnel Administration. *Fairshakes: The Health Care Compensation Handbook.* Chicago: Pluribus Press, 1983.

Metzger, N. E., ed. *Handbook of Health Care Human Resources Management.* Rockville, MD: Aspen, 1981.

Shortell, S. M. "Theory Z: Implications and Relevance for Health Care Management." *"Health Care Management Review,"* (Fall 1982): 7–21.

15

Plant Services

The plant of the modern hospital is a closely controlled, largely self-contained physical environment. It monitors and controls temperature, humidity, contaminants, wastes, dangerous chemicals and sources of energy, and human traffic. Given a continuous supply of water, energy, food, and other resources, it provides complete environmental support not only for patients, but for staff and visitors as well. In these respects it is no different from any large hotel or office building. The uniqueness of the hospital environment lies in the specifics of environmental control for patient care. To protect and improve health, unusual hazards are created and controlled, and narrow tolerances are achieved.

The plant system is the second largest of the hospital systems in terms of personnel. Housekeeping and food service often rank just behind the two largest clinical departments, nursing and laboratory, in employees and costs. Most plant services and some plant personnel must be available around the clock, and most services affect everyone and everything in the hospital.

Consistent with the plan of the book, this chapter attempts to describe the plant system as it contributes to the other four systems of the hospital, governance, finance, clinical, and human resources. It emphasizes what the chief operating officer and the heads of the clinical departments must expect from plant services, rather than what plant services may traditionally have provided. The focus is upon:

— What must be done, with attention to the total requirement rather than the part traditionally assigned to plant departments

— The skills and organization required in plant systems
— The measures that show how well the job has been done and
   areas needing improvement
— Some issues in plant systems management which appear to be
   arising in well-run hospitals

With this focus on what is expected of the plant system, the chapter can also assist people who work within that system to understand what is expected of them and how their contribution is judged. They must know a great deal more about the components of the plant system. There is a substantial library on the components which this chapter does not replace; some of the more general works are cited at the end of the chapter.

Purpose

Smooth, continuous operation of the hospital plant is occasionally a matter of life and death. Certain hazards, if uncontrolled, can cause loss of life among employees, visitors, and patients. The well-run hospital uses carefully designed, conscientiously maintained programs to reduce these risks to near vanishing. The plant and the plant services determine in large part what impressions people form about the hospital. They are thus an important element in the promotional activity of the hospital, not only in regard to patients but also in the recruitment of hospital team members. Beyond the minimum required for safety, the well-managed hospital strives to operate a plant system which is reliable, convenient, attractive, and yet economical, because these are the expectations of the hospital members and customers.

> **The purpose of the plant system is to provide the complete physical environment required for the hospital's mission, including all buildings, equipment, and supplies; to protect hospital members and visitors against all hazards arising within the hospital environment; and to maintain reliable plant services at satisfactory levels of economy, attractiveness, and convenience.**

Functions

The numerous activities constituting the plant system can be grouped into four major categories:

1. Facilities services (operation of buildings, utilities, and equipment)

2. Maintenance services (housekeeping, groundskeeping, and environmental safety)

3. Guest services (support for workers, patients, and visitors)

4. Supplies services (materials management)

Facilities Services

The plant system obviously begins with operation of the plant itself. In the well-run hospital, plant operation begins with adequate planning for space and equipment and continues through construction, maintenance, and renovation. Hospital plants are built by their users, thus plant operation includes the development of architectural specifications and the management of construction contracts. Plant operation also includes acquiring and distributing utilities. In addition to the usual conditioned air, electricity, and water, hospitals provide high-pressure steam, oxygen, and suction to several different locations. The important components of facilities services are shown in figure 15.1.

Planning and Space Allocation. The criterion for allocating space is conceptually simple. Each space should be used in the way which optimizes achievement of the hospital's mission. In reality, this criterion is quite difficult to apply. Hospital activities tend to expand to fill the available space. As a result, there are always complaints of shortages of space and an agenda of possible reallocations or expansions. Space is highly valuable and unique; the third floor is not identical to the first. Space also confers prestige and symbolic rewards; space next to the doctors' lounge is more prestigious than space adjacent to the employment office. As a result, space allocation decisions tend to be strenuously contested.

Well-run hospitals address this problem by incorporating space use as part of their long-range plan, using the capital budget review and planning committees as the arbiters of decisions concerning space. Then each unit seeking substantial additional space or renovation must prepare a formal request, following the procedures for new proposals outlined in chapter 7. The request must gain approval twice; first from the space management office and then against competition with other capital opportunities. The following guidelines assist in space management:

— Space management is assigned to a single office which permits occupancy and controls access to space.

— A key function of the space management office is the preparation of the long-range space plan. Planning and marketing staff assist in the preparation. The draft plan is derived from the

Figure 15.1

Facilities Services (Operation of Buildings, Utilities, and Equipment)

Planning and Space Allocation
Construction, Maintenance, and Repair Services
    Construction and major renovation management
    Plant maintenance and refurbishing
    Preventive maintenance
    Repair of conventional equipment
    Maintenance of specialized technical equipment
        Medical equipment
        Electronic equipment
        Other specialized machinery
            Vehicles
            Laundry machinery
            Elevators
Provision of Utilities
    Electrical service
        Reliability of service
        Emergency generation
        Cogeneration
    Heating and air conditioning
        Routine heating and air conditioning needs
        High-pressure steam
        Special air control problems
    Communications support
        Telephone, television, and computer wiring
        Radio communication
        Pneumatic tube systems
    Patient-related utilities
        Oxygen
        Suction

---

hospital's long-range plan, and the final version becomes part of it. The space plan includes:

- Forecasts of patient activity translated to growth and shrinkage of major types of space use

- Strategic acquisitions, divestitures, and new programs, translated into requirements for space

- Routine replacement, renovation, and refurbishing requirements

- Plant revisions indicated by approved new services and technology, the physician recruitment plan, and the human resources plan

— The draft plan is incorporated into the long-range planning approval and annual review processes. These processes assure widespread knowledge and discussion of the space plan. The implications of the space plan for the long-range financial plan are extensive, and they are included in the review discussion. The space plan is approved as part of the package believed to implement the hospital's mission best.

— Specific space allocation decisions are made like other capital investment decisions, via formal proposals documenting costs and benefits heard by the series of committees which reviews these proposals. A cost-benefit ratio is used in making space decisions, evaluating benefits in terms of the hospital's mission. The space plan helps in maintain consistency in the allocations (see chapter 7).

— The decisions are implemented by the plant department, including the space management office and the construction and renovation management office.

Construction, Maintenance, and Repair Services. As figure 15.1 shows, a substantial amount of plant system activity is devoted to building, maintaining, and rebuilding the actual plant and its major equipment.

All parts of the hospital facility are subject to safety and convenience regulations, with patient care areas having the highest standards. Most of the regulations are contained in the **Life Safety Code** and other codes developed by the National Fire Protection Association.[1] Licensure, JCAH, and Medicare certification requirements enforce compliance.

These regulations require routine inspection and maintenance. They often dictate important specifications of new construction. They require revision of previously approved construction when a renovation is made to the general area containing conditions no longer in compliance with the current code. They occasionally require renovation specifically to meet changes in the code. The length of time before compliance with current codes becomes mandatory is variable, depending upon the severity of the hazard. The degree of departure from current code is an important factor in renovation and remodelling plans.

Major construction and renovation usually call for extensive outside contracting. Hospitals usually retain an architect, a construction management firm, and a general contractor, although some firms supply combinations of these services. Construction financed directly by public funds, such as that of public hospitals, usually must be contracted via formal competitive bids. Private hospitals frequently prefer more flexible arrangements, negotiating contracts with selected vendors. Formal bidding may reduce collusion and fraud, but there is no evidence that it necessarily saves construction costs or total costs, including later maintenance and operation.

Smaller projects are often handled by the hospital staff. As an interim step, the hospital can provide design and construction management, preparing the plans and contracting with specific subcontractors.

Maintenance and repair services should emphasize prevention. Most equipment requires periodic inspection and adjustment. When the cost of downtime is included, it is usually preferable to fix or replace equipment before it is broken. Well-managed plant systems schedule preventive maintenance for all the mechanical services. A significant fraction of mechanics' time is devoted to preventive maintenance, and adherence to the schedule is one of the measures of the quality of the department's work.

The technical requirements of hospital equipment dictate that contracts with outside vendors be used for many of the more specialized items. Contracts should weigh responsiveness and downtime appropriately and should be for relatively short periods, to permit prompt change of vendor if necessary. One issue is the question of who should initiate and supervise maintenance contracts. Well-run hospitals tend to place the responsibility on the line unit using the equipment, unless the equipment is for general use, such as elevators, or the same item is used in several units, for example, typewriters and personal computers. It is important that the line unit also bear some accountability for the cost and management of the maintenance contract. All the actual contracting is centralized through materials management.

Provision of Utilities. Most hospitals operate a sophisticated utility system that provides air, steam, and water at several temperatures and pressures in response to automatic or user-determined requirements. Utilities are more elaborate than those usually found in public buildings of similar size because of the need to overcome failure in an emergency and to meet more demanding operating conditions. For example, hospitals supply high-pressure steam for sterilizing laundry and equipment, and the use of higher pressures requires continuous surveillance by a licensed boiler operator.

Electrical systems are particularly complex. Two or three substations are desirable, with feeds approaching the hospital from opposite directions. In addition, the hospital must have on-site generating capability to sustain emergency surgery, respirators, safety lights, and communications. Several areas must switch to the emergency supply automatically, requiring them to be separable from other, less critical uses.

Many hospitals use their heating boilers to generate electrical power, a practice called *cogeneration*. The hospital's system is integrated with the public utility supplying electricity, and the utility buys any surplus the hospital generates. Alternatively, if the hospital is located close to a generating plant, it may buy steam from the utility, avoiding the cost of maintaining its own boiler.

Several other problems complicate the hospital's utility supply. Operating and delivery rooms, and certain other sites, require special air handling units that filter out most bacteria and that maintain higher pressures within the suites than in surrounding spaces. Most hospitals pipe oxygen and suction to all patient care areas. Many also pipe nitrous oxide to surgical areas. Hospitals generally have a radio paging system and several external two-way radios for use in disasters or when telephone service is interrupted. "Telephone" service itself is becoming more complicated as it becomes more related to computer communication. Optical fiber networks are now recommended to replace conventional internal telephone wiring. Many hospitals use pneumatic tubes to transport small items such as paper records, drugs, and specimens. A few use automated cart systems with signal wires embedded in the floor.

Maintenance Services

Housekeeping and Groundskeeping. The array of activities involved in housekeeping, groundskeeping, and environmental control is shown in figure 15.2. In well-run hospitals these activities are supported by specialized equipment, training, and supplies. They are conducted to explicit standards of quality and are monitored by inspectors using formal survey methods. Decorating and landscaping are done with an understanding both of public taste and of the cost of specific materials. These activities also interact with important programs for environmental safety.

Housekeeping, groundskeeping, landscaping, and interior decorating are subjects upon which everyone feels comfortably expert. That comfort is misplaced. It can cause a glib superficiality which proves costly and occasionally dangerous. It is one thing to know how to empty the trash and sweep floors. It is quite another to know how to maintain a campus of up to a million square feet efficiently at standards assuring bacterial and other hazard control. Thus the first rule of housekeeping and groundskeeping management is to find a competent, experienced professional to do it.

Cleaning service, like food service and some equipment maintenance, is frequently subcontracted (guidelines are given later in this chapter). The most common contracts are for management-level services; hospital employees are paid by the hour. Large hospitals, and those

624 HUMAN RESOURCES AND PLANT SYSTEMS

Figure 15.2

Maintenance Services (Housekeeping, Groundskeeping, and Environmental Safety)

Housekeeping
    Interior decorating
    Routine cleaning
        General patient areas
        High-risk patient areas
        Nonpatient areas
    Solid waste removal
    Special problem areas
        Odor control
        Sound control
Groundskeeping
    Landscaping
    Grounds maintenance
Environmental Safety
    Physical control of chemical, biological,
        and radiological hazards
    Contaminant storage
    Contaminant waste removal
    Special cleaning and emergency procedures
    Facility safety
        Inspection and hazard identification
        Hazard correction

with access to central services for training and development of methods, may be able to justify their own management. Smaller hospitals may argue that their problems are less demanding and that they do not yet need the more sophisticated service, although that argument may not hold up in the future.

Environmental Safety. There are several hazardous materials in hospitals and four basic approaches to control of them. These approaches are assigned to different units in most hospitals.

1. *Restricting exposure at the source*—The cheapest way to deal with a specific chemical contaminant is frequently to replace it. Most of the chemicals used in hospitals are selected as part of the clinical diagnosis and treatment, however, so review of the necessity for using dangerous chemicals is usually a medical question.

    Restricting exposure to bacteriological contaminants is more difficult, and building design and operation are frequently important in that effort. Human vectors in the spread of infection are also important. Special gowns and techniques are used to protect hospital members and to prevent the spread of infection to other patients. Development of control systems and monitoring of actual infection rates is a clinical function usually assigned to an infection control committee. It is wise to have at least one plant person on the infection committee. Larger hospitals may have one from plant operations, a second from housekeeping, and a third from central supply services.

2. *Cleaning and removal*—Throughout the hospital, construction materials and cleaning methods must reflect the need for bacterial and chemical decontamination. The housekeeping department is usually responsible for cleaning and removing hazardous substances. All horizontal surfaces are major sources of bacterial cross contamination; in some areas, such as the operating rooms, more extensive attention is needed. There are occasionally special problems of chemical contamination as well, such as from the use of radioactive isotopes. Hospital trash contains both chemical and unusual bacteriological contaminants. It must be removed safely and disposed of acceptably. One of the greatest risks is to the initial handlers, who must be taught how to remove the trash without exposing themselves. In addition, housekeeping personnel can be a source of contamination. They must be trained to follow the procedures for restricting exposure as completely as any other hospital members.

3. *Attention to exposed patients, visitors, and staff*—Trauma or infection results from exposure to contaminants. Diagnosis and treatment of it is a proper function of physicians. Hospitals must provide workers' compensation for any employee injury resulting from exposure. Although workers are entitled to their choice of physician, many hospitals use a clinical member of the infection committee to examine any person believed to be injured and to provide care to those who will accept it. Concentrating cases in a single doctor provides continuity and promotes thorough understanding of hospital hazards.

4. *Epidemiological analysis of failures*—Epidemiological studies are an important part of an infection control program. Studies of the incidence of specific illnesses can detect incipient epidemics and may be the only way to reveal certain problems of chemical contamination. The information necessary for epidemiological studies frequently requires the assistance of a physician. Much of the work can be done by any interested person who can understand the statistical concepts involved. It is often assigned to a member of the infection committee.

Figure 15.3

Guest Services (Work Force, Patient, and Visitor Support)

Security Services
  Guards
  Employee identification
  Facility inspection and monitoring
Food Service
  Cafeteria and vending service
  Patient food service
    Routine patient service
    Therapeutic diets
Communication and Transportation Services
  Telephone and television service
  Telephone operations
  Messenger service
  Tube transport system
  Reception and guidance
    Signage
    Parking
    Reception desks
    Telephone reception

Guest Services

Large numbers of patients, visitors, and staff become the guests of the hospital and require a variety of physical services. People expect to come to the hospital; park; find what they want; get certain amenities such as waiting areas, lounges, and food; and leave without even recognizing that they have received service. Those telephoning expect a similarly complete but unobtrusive response. The hospital's attractiveness is diminished if the services listed in figure 15.3 are either missing or intrusive. The personnel delivering the services are in constant contact with the hospital's important constituencies. Their effect upon exchange partners' satisfaction is almost as great as nursing's.

Guest services frequently involve multiple locations and small work groups, but they require coordinated management and a significant investment in centrally operated support systems. For example, receptionists and security personnel need current knowledge of the location of each inpatient and each special event or activity. Coordinated management can stress the importance of a satisfactory overall impression. It may also contribute to efficiency by allowing overlapping functions to be eliminated. Relations with housekeeping, security, and plant operations also require coordination.

Reception. In a large hospital, several dozen people have reception jobs that involve primarily meeting and guiding the hospital's guests. Each visitor or telephone contact must be guided efficiently to his or her destination. Delays and missteps cost the hospital as well as the visitor. Signs and display of telephone numbers (as in the Yellow Pages) aid efficient routing. Those persons who require more detailed assistance expect it to be given cordially, promptly, and accurately.

Messenger Services. Patients and large physical items must be moved around the hospital, and training in guest relations, emergency medical needs, and hospital geography are necessary to do the job well. Because requests are usually unforeseen and because it is difficult to supervise messengers, there are important efficiencies in pooling messenger needs. Very large hospitals may have more than one pool, but smaller ones usually combine all messenger and reception activities under one supervisor.

Security Services. Security services are necessary in most urban settings to protect employees, visitors, patients, and property. High-quality security services are preventive. Security involves controlling access to the hospital, monitoring live and by television, traffic flow, employee identification, and lighting to create an environment both reassuring to guests and discouraging to persons with destructive intentions. Employee education is helpful in promoting safe behavior and prompt reporting of questionable events. Uniformed guards are the final element of a high-quality program, not the initial one. They serve three functions:

1. To provide a visible symbol of authority
2. To respond to questions and concerns
3. To provide emergency assistance in those infrequent events which exceed the capability of reception personnel

Emergency assistance should normally follow a previously developed security plan. The recurring major hazards of public areas should be addressed in the plan. These include armed and unarmed criminals, political protesters, and the insane; bomb threats, fires, and serious accidents involving damage or release of toxic materials. The security plan for major community disasters is particularly taxing and is part of the hospital disaster plan (see chapter 6).

Security is frequently a contract service, although it obviously must be coordinated with local police and fire service. Municipal units sometimes provide the contract service, particularly in government hospitals. The voluntary hospital usually does not pay local taxes in support of local fire and police service; as a result, there is often a question about the extent to which taxpayer services should be provided to the hospital.

Food Service. The preparation of hospital food has become a service similar to the food services of hotels, airlines, and resorts, rather than a clinical service. It must be conducted to high standards of quality, beginning with control of bacterial hazards and safety in preparation and distribution. Several foods are ideal media for bacterial growth. Employee handwashing and medical examinations are important to avoid systematic bacterial contamination. Further, careful food handling is necessary to prevent acute food poisoning. Kitchens include an unusual number of burn, fall, and injury hazards. Food service must also provide inexpensive, nutritious, appealing, and tasty meals that encourage good eating habits. It must supply them to remote locations and, either directly or by arrangement with nursing, deliver them to many people who are partially incapacitated.

Hospitals typically serve several meals to each patient on census. Patients expect a choice of entrees, appetizers, and desserts. Their meals must also be provided to a variety of clinical specifications. Soft, low sodium, and sodium-free diets constitute up to half of all patient meals; however, bulk foods meeting these specifications can be prepared by personnel without clinical training. In addition to the meals patients eat, about an equal number of others are provided to members and guests, usually in cafeterias. Visitors and employees expect greater variety, a range of prices, and service at odd hours. Hospitals now generally encourage visitors to eat in the cafeteria once reserved for doctors and employees. In addition, it is common to operate a snack bar or coffee shop and a variety of vending machines offering snack food and soft drinks. (Well-run hospitals do not permit the sale of cigarettes, however.)

These concerns are relatively easy to meet through sound general procedures. Food service is frequently contracted. Contract food suppliers meet the quality and cost constraints through centralized menu planning, well-developed training programs for workers and managers, and careful attention to work methods. Nutritional education and consultation and the preparation of special diets to meet medical needs is available through the clinical dietetics service. These professional nutritionists have an important advisory role in menu planning, but they have limited contact with the mass feeding operation.

Supplies Services

A hospital spends several million dollars each year for supplies, roughly the same as a small retail store. Like other industries, hospitals use office supplies, foodstuffs, linens and uniforms, fuels, paints, hardware, and cleaning supplies. The raw materials of the health care process are unique—implants, whole blood, specialized dressings, single-purpose medical tools, and a large variety of drugs. Most supply costs are represented in the following inventories, which are either large volumes of inexpensive items, like foodstuffs, or relatively small volumes of very expensive items, like implants:

— Surgical supplies and implants

— Anesthesia gases

— Drugs, intravenous solutions, and pharmaceuticals

— Foodstuffs

— Linen

— Dressings, kits, and supplies for patient care

Nature of Supplies Use in Hospitals. Supplies must be purchased, stored, protected, processed, and distributed. Costs are involved in each of these steps. The objective of the materials management function is to acquire and deliver to the user all necessary supplies, on time, at the minimum possible cost. There is no benefit to be gained from delivering either more or earlier than needed, while there are significant costs to being late, wrong, or incomplete. The most basic measures of quality of materials management are the accuracy and promptness of delivery. Costs of failure on these two criteria are so high that system design in the well-run hospital strives for virtually flawless performance. Satisfaction of users is a less vital but still important element of quality.

Improving the Materials Management Function. The materials management function includes the activities shown in figure 15.4. Many of these items conflict with one another. For example, larger order quantities save delivery costs but increase warehouse costs, and cheaper distribution systems may increase user dissatisfaction or waste. Thus the problem of materials management is to achieve the balance among various costs which is lowest overall. This is generally done by considering the management problem in the four major categories above and by centralizing almost all purchases of recurring supplies.

In the well-run hospital, only nonrecurring items are purchased directly by line departments; all recurring items go through a central materials management function. The line departments assist in writing the

Figure 15.4

Materials Management Activities

Purchasing—the cost of goods purchased is minimized by
Standardization of items and reduction in the number of items
Competitive bidding
Annual or periodic contracts for larger volumes
Group purchasing with other hospitals

Receipt, Storage, and Protection—each order received must be verified, off-loaded, and put in a safe place. Verification includes not only the counts received, but also compliance with a duly authorized order and, in some instances, quality control sampling. Storage requirements vary with the products, which must sometimes be maintained under special temperature, humidity, light, and fireproof conditions. Storage must also protect products from theft and provide safety to handlers and bystanders. Costs are minimized by
Control of shipment size and frequency
Reduction of handling
Elimination of waste through damage or theft
Economical warehouse operation
Reduction of inventory size

Processing—foodstuffs, surgical supplies, and linen require significant processing on site in the form of reassembly, wrapping, or cleaning and sterilization. Hospitals once reprocessed or manufactured large amounts of their materials, but high labor costs and product liability considerations have made purchase more attractive. Even linen is frequently replaced by paper, and preprocessed foods have replaced many raw items. Both laundry and food service are frequently contracted *in toto.* Costs are minimized by
Replacement of processing by purchase of processed goods
Reduction of processing costs by improved methods
Reduction of reprocessing, or turnaround, time by improved methods

Distribution—items disbursed from inventory must be delivered to an appropriate user, charged to a cost account, and, in many cases, billed to a patient or other revenue account. Protection is required throughout. Costs are minimized by
Elimination or automation of ordering
Reduction of delivery costs by improved methods
Reduction of end user inventories
Reduction of waste and unauthorized use

Income can be temporarily increased by improved records for posting patient accounts. (Well-run hospitals set charges for supplies on the basis of a percentage markup over purchase costs. The markup is a function of three factors: competition, if any; hospitalwide financial needs; and purchasing and distribution costs, including waste. If waste and unbilled items are reduced, the markup should be adjusted in the next budget year. Thus the increase in income from elimination of billing errors disappears after one budget cycle.)

---

purchase specifications, including any special handling needs. They cooperate with materials management, which can help minimize costs through knowledge of the market, understanding of the implications of limiting specifications, and knowledge of the distribution system. Although line departments often desire direct purchasing and decentralized inventories, the trend has been steadily toward centralization. Drugs, surgical supplies, and foodstuffs were the last inventories to be centralized.

Objections to standardization and centralization tend to disappear in well-run hospitals, where incentives for efficiency and cooperation overcome line objections to perceived loss of authority and contact with salesmen. (In some cases, direct contact with salesmen has been known to involve bribes and kickbacks as well.) On the other hand, well-run hospitals recognize that centralization is a mixed blessing. They are not reluctant to relax standardization and group purchasing rules which are viewed as onerous by their line managers, and they avoid situations which will unnecessarily impair a supplier's viability. Permitting override of centralization for good cause and allowing line personnel to see salesmen when they request it makes central standards and systems more acceptable and, in the long run, more effective.

Well-run hospitals are also reducing materials management costs by group purchasing and large volume contracts. All belong to at least one cooperative or corporate buying group. Groups negotiate discounts from suppliers by aggregating the buying power of several hospitals. To make effective use of group purchasing, both specifications and delivery arrangements must be standardized among hospitals.

Distribution improvements in well-run hospitals have focused on exchange cart replacement of routine items, automated ordering of items billed to patients, and minimization of inventories. Exchange carts permit materials management to control the inventory at line sites. Daily or weekly needs are generously estimated and delivered on a cart. (Shortages are costly and destructive and must be avoided.) The old cart is removed and refilled for the next delivery, with the result that older material is used promptly, cost accounts are exact, and line hoarding is discouraged. Waste is reduced because the most exposed inventory, that which is decentralized to patient care units, is minimized. For more expensive items, patient order entry systems permit automatic posting of a supply order and a patient charge. This allows control of dispensing, accurate current inventory counts, and improved revenue control. Central inventories are minimized through analysis of optimal order quantity. The three systems in combination significantly reduce the waste, handling costs, and inventory requirements.

Inventories can be further reduced by arrangement with the supplier. Some will deliver daily, and most will guarantee delivery of critical items in a very short time. This practice is like an exchange cart for the hospital as a whole. Although suppliers have offered management contracts for the entire materials management function, these have not been popular, because they introduce problems of price and control.

Purchasing of Services. Although the term *materials* and most of the real activity of materials management deals with goods, some of the same principles can be applied to the purchase of services. Hospitals purchase many services, ranging from ad hoc consultants to part-time temporary labor. Where these can be standardized and negotiated in larger volumes, price and quality advantages usually accrue. The best examples are probably maintenance contracts, service contracts for plant services such as food and housekeeping, and recurring contracts for standardized labor, such as clerical personnel. Centralization has the added benefit of improving accountability.

Personnel Requirements and Organization

Personnel Requirements

Managers and Professional Personnel. There are few widely recognized educational programs in plant management. The professional societies have not offered registration as a guide to qualifications, but they do suggest that active membership should be a criterion.[2] As a result, job descriptions depend heavily on prior experience. Contract management firms have extensive on-the-job training and may be the best source of managers.

A bachelor's degree in engineering is generally considered necessary for building maintenance managers, particularly if construction responsibilities are included. Some large hospitals also employ architects, a profession with both formal education and licensure. Although there are licensure requirements for professional engineers and architects in consultative practice, the requirements do not apply to employment situations.

Materials managers should acquire general business knowledge. Course work in law and business is certainly an asset, but much of the knowledge needed can also be acquired by well-supervised experience.

Several professions are involved in environmental safety. Infection control is often the concern of a medical or nonmedical epidemiologist. Both have formal educational requirements. The physician is frequently privileged in communicable disease and in any case should be subject to routine credentials review. Medical advice on the selection of a nonmedical epidemiologist is highly desirable. Hospitals with high-voltage radiation therapy services usually employ a radiation physicist, who can also assist with radiation safety. Large hospitals employ toxicologists to assist with control of chemical contamination. There is a specialty known as safety engineering. Consultative services in all of these areas are often available through the local public health department.

Employees. The traditional building trades and stationary engineers provide apprenticeships and are usually licensed by local or state authorities. Security personnel are frequently former police and may have attended college programs in police work. Job descriptions in these fields normally require the appropriate license or certificate and consider relevant prior experience favorably.

All other employees are recruited as unskilled labor or, in the case of materials management, clerical labor. Even if they have had prior experience, they must be trained on the job in the policies of the hospital. Although the tasks are repetitive, there are clear advantages to the correct use of tools and supplies, and process control is usually important to both efficiency and quality.

Ability to train and motivate unskilled personnel in the proper procedures is a major asset of contract management. Hospitals which employ their own managers must acquire comparable sets of training materials and task descriptions. This usually requires consultation; it is rare that a local housekeeper, plant engineer, or materials manager will have the skill to develop them. Much of the scheduling, quality control, and communications activity can now be automated. Automation of materials management is extensive. Commercial programs for energy control, preventive maintenance, menu planning, and housekeeping work scheduling are becoming more widely available. Software from commercial vendors is almost always preferable, because even extensive modifications are cheaper than independent development.

Use of Contract Services

Hospitals have always used contract services extensively. From one perspective, the entire tradition of medical privileges is a contract service. Laboratory and radiology involve medical contracts, and major construction usually involves contracts with a planning consultant, an architectural firm, and a builder. It is not surprising, therefore, that, when specific technologies began to emerge for laundry, housekeeping, groundskeeping, specialized equipment maintenance, food service, and security, hospitals turned quickly to contracts, which provided inexpensive access to them.

Extent of Contracting. Service contracts vary from arrangements with individuals which substitute for employment to complex long-term commitments between corporations. Retainers or fees for legal counsel are examples of the first, especially if they are with one attorney rather than a firm. A large-scale construction contract or a contract to operate an entire hospital is an example of the other extreme. Awarding and administering service contracts depends upon their complexity and uniqueness. Contracts for plant management and its major functions can be delegated to middle management once initial criteria and procedures are approved by the governing board. Many service contracts can be effectively assigned to materials management for execution. The list of such contracts is quite long, and growing. Examples include:

— Sporadic or infrequent services, such as snow removal, grounds care, and maintenance on specialized equipment

— Contracts related to purchases, usually for maintenance of equipment or software

— Contracts for specified discrete tasks, such as job classification and salary surveys, preventive maintenance, or construction

— Contracts for continuing services, such as housekeeping, food service, laundry, data processing, and in-service education

All forms of contracting seem to have been increasing, but the last has risen from near zero to a substantial fraction of hospital expenditures. Although exact figures are difficult to obtain, the total for continuing services is probably 3 to 5 percent of hospital expenditures, substantially over $5 billion a year.

Continuing Service Contracts. By specializing in a function and building up experience and activity in that area, the contractor can:

— Develop a cadre of experienced people who are well equipped to solve whatever problems may arise

— Develop more efficient methods
  • Specify better tasks, tools, and supplies
  • Train personnel more effectively
  • Develop more precise measures of quality and efficiency

— Learn more effective ways of motivating personnel

— Take advantage of larger volumes
  • Gain lower prices on supplies and equipment
  • Support more cost-effective substitution of capital for labor

There is clearly no magic on this list. It is the same set of factors that supports any industrial specialization. Different services have different profiles of specific advantages. In each case, success is proved by growth in the marketplace.

There are also well-known disadvantages to specialization. The savings may not be passed back to the hospital. Successful contract suppliers grow and may not be as efficient as they once were. Growth can create personnel shortages, unexpected problems, overcommitment, inflexibility, and loss of motivation. Thus there is always a point of equilibrium at which contracting and not contracting are equally appealing. The equilibrium is subject to adjustment with changing conditions. At the moment, the equilibrium is shifting away from hospital employment in plant systems and toward contract services.

Assuming that the underlying economic advantage of a specific form of service contract is proven, other potential disadvantages are related to the consequences of the contract itself, rather than to the service in question.

— Incomplete or incorrect specification of the desired service may lead to excessive cost or dissatisfaction.

— Ineffective supervision of the contract may lead to suboptimal achievement of its terms.

— Monopoly or ineffective negotiation may leave most of the savings with the supplier.

— Poorly designed incentives may encourage the supplier to be inefficient or to produce unsatisfactory quality.

— Factors outside the hospital, such as unexpected growth, may affect the supplier's ability to deliver the anticipated efficiencies.

Criteria for Successful Contracting. Well-run hospitals negotiate contracts for continuing services in a way that will exploit the advantages and disadvantages to their overall benefit. This is not necessarily to the supplier's disadvantage; the best contracts are frequently those in which both parties win. The following conditions make a successful result more likely:

1. The hospital has a full, clear, and realistic understanding of the service desired:
   a. Descriptions of the scope of work are unambiguous.
   b. Systems are in place to measure supplier's performance with regard to demand, output, quality, and cost.
   c. Quantitative expectations on these parameters have been developed from the hospital's experience.
2. Resources which the hospital must supply are available:
   a. Facilities and equipment are scheduled for the contractor's use.
   b. Systems for supplying orders and other necessary communications are in place.

      c. Terms, methods, and personnel for contract supervision can be specified.

      d. Programs for the transfer of activity have been developed.

3. There is a competitive market. Several suppliers have records of effective performance in similar situations and demonstrate both interest and capability in the service to be performed.

4. An initial request for proposals is used to evaluate suppliers and to improve the quality of the specifications:

      a. Invitations include all potentially qualified bidders.

      b. Initial specifications avoid accidental or arbitrary restriction of bidders or of potential gains. The scope of work is pragmatically defined to cover items which are essential to the hospital and also achievable by a satisfactory number of bidders.

      c. Suppliers are encouraged to respond with modifications or extensions of the initial specifications; these can be evaluated on their merits.

      d. Further discussion with suppliers can help develop the best possible final specifications.

5. Qualified suppliers are selected from the initial round and asked to submit more detailed proposals, including competitive prices:

      a. Sufficient bidders are invited to the second round to encourage competitive pricing.

      b. Format for the final proposal is specified closely enough to permit direct comparison of bids.

      c. Opportunity to price alternatives and options separately remains.

      d. Contract length is kept to a relatively short period, or termination on short warning is permitted, to provide continuing incentive for achieving the hospital's expectations.

The obvious difficulty with these criteria is that they fail to cover realistic situations in which the hospital is justified in seeking a service contract. They say, in effect, that when there are several well-managed suppliers, a hospital with a service that is already well managed can negotiate a good contract. While this is true enough, it overlooks situations in which the hospital must correct serious weaknesses in plant systems services and situations in which one dominant service contractor has developed an exceptional record. Some issues to consider in those situations are as follows:

— In effect, the competition can be against the hospital's own per-formance. The contract must be judged on marginal rather than optimal standards.

— The expertise of the supplier can often be used to strengthen the hospital's capability in setting expectations and establishing measures of performance. This can be done either through short-term consulting contracts prior to a longer-term commit-ment or through contracts which specify the development or improvement of performance measures and expectations dur-ing an initial period.

— A poorly run hospital or a hospital with a poorly run service may have to sacrifice price for quality. For most plant services, the highest cost of poor performance is loss of customer satis-faction, whether the customer is the hospital's own members or its patients and visitors.

— A hospital which assists a new company or pioneers in new areas of contract services should anticipate extra benefits in the form of price reduction or profit sharing on future sales.

Organization of Plant Services

Comprehensive Accountability. Traditionally, hospitals have had chief engineers, purchasing agents, housekeepers, security officers, food serv-ice heads, and central supply supervisors with departmental status who report to deputy operating officers in large hospitals and the chief oper-ating officer in smaller ones. Communications services and other sup-port activities tended to be assigned expediently. Single accountability, that is, concentrating plant services under one manager reporting to the COO, seems to have been rare, but it is likely to become more com-mon.

Plant systems organization should be flexible for hospital size and extent of outside contracting. Figure 15.5 shows a general model for plant systems organization in a large, well-run hospital with extensive contracting. Figure 15.6 shows one for a smaller hospital. These models accomplish the general goal of grouping similar activities under a mid-dle manager who can encourage patience and present the group's prob-lems to others. Given the diversity of plant systems activities, some such grouping is probably desirable, although it should be noted that several of the activities shown in the figures are small organizations within themselves with at least one level of middle management over their responsibility center managers.

Specific hospitals should adjust their organization to reflect skills of specific individuals, and titles should follow local customs. The ad-

Figure 15.5

Organization of Plant Systems Organization in Large Hospitals

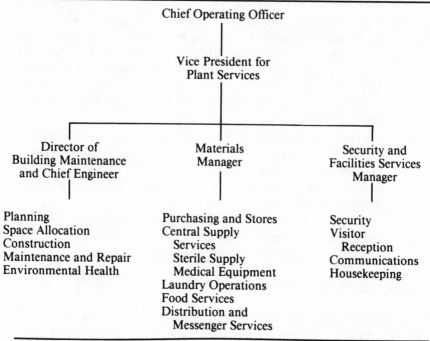

justments for contracting would depend on the service. Locally run services would be less likely to be assigned to the materials manager.

Plant System Organization. When a single plant management position is established, it is often accountable for less than the full set of plant functions. If the manager is successful, a more comprehensive structure should evolve, because there are frequent and important cross communications and management issues among the plant functions. Most of them have important implications for guest relations and promotion. Several of the services within the plant system depend heavily on utilities and plant maintenance. Housekeeping, laundry, food service, security, and several specialized maintenance functions are often supplied by outside contract. Where functions are contracted out, detailed technical knowledge may be less necessary than general contract management skill.

Debate on the content of the plant system is more strenuous regarding guest services and materials management than activities more obviously related to the physical facility. The practice of recognizing

Figure 15.6

Organization of Plant Systems in Smaller Hospitals

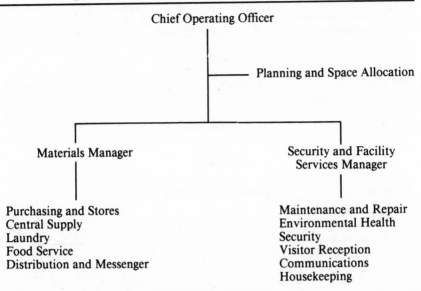

food service as a clinical subsystem is on the wane, but it is often elevated to higher status than other guest services. Despite tradition, the guest services group shares many common concerns, and it can improve both quality and efficiency by coordinating activities.

The most debatable question appears to be the organizational locus of materials management. Surprisingly, leading materials managers themselves feel that the "importance placed on materials management . . . was related more to who reports to the materials manager than to whom the material manager reports. . . ."[3] One option would be to treat the unit as part of finance, but this places product delivery in what is otherwise an information-processing activity, creating few promotional opportunities for the successful manager. The concept of separation of duties to discourage fraud and abuse also militates against the close association of materials control and accounting. A second option would be for the materials manager to report directly to the COO. A third is the hierarchy suggested here, reporting to the manager of plant services, who reports to the COO.

Within the materials management organization itself there seems to be virtue in centralization of authority. The managers surveyed by Holmgren and Wentz saw all plant services except housekeeping, security, and maintenance as their "ideal" domain.[4] They also believed they

Table 15.1   Examples of Demand Measures for Plant System
Functions

Service Requested	Resource Required	Duration
Surgical operations	Type of room required	Hours per room
Heating	Degree-days	n/a
Maintenance (cleaning per week)	Cleaning Service	Required hours per service
Safety inspection	Specific type required	Hours per inspection
Guest service	Meals per day, specific type required	n/a
Security	Guards per location	Shifts
Supplies	Supplies per day, specific type required	n/a

n/a: Not applicable.

should control all inventories, including drugs and foodstuffs, although they conceded the need for clinical functions in the dietary and pharmacy departments. Although materials management can easily include supervision of annual contracting for housekeeping and similar services, it seems unlikely that other guest services would be grouped with materials services.

Measures of Performance

Plant services must first be reliable and safe, then satisfactory to hospital members and visitors, and finally efficient. Measures for the closed system parameters are well developed and can usually be transferred easily from industrial sites or between hospitals.

Measures of Output and Demand

Output and demand for plant system services are usually measured identically; output is simply that portion of demand which is filled. Demand is measured differently for each of the four functions of the plant system, using various combinations of patient or service requests, specific facility required, and duration, as reflected in the examples shown in table 15.1.

In general, demand expectations are useful for all three measures: service requested, resource requested, and duration. Service requested is least subject to control within the plant system, and design modifications and changes in performance can reduce resource requirements and duration. Annual review of expectations can encourage attention to improved productivity in all three areas if the distinction is emphasized in the measurement system.

To establish resource expectations, it is necessary to express demand in resource units. This is usually possible by taking the product of service requests times duration for each identified physical resource. Questions of random and cyclic fluctuation are important. The expectations for plant systems consist of a large set of numbers arranged to reflect the specific physical resources, the numbers of services requested, and the duration of service. Forecasts for values, such as frequency distributions, ranges, or categories of demand, are frequently required to set sound expectations.

Forecasting for Physical Facilities. Most physical facilities must be large enough to meet peak, rather than average, load. Correctly forecasting space and facility requirements is an important part of the space planning function. Forecasts are prepared for service requests in relevant categories by studying trends and constructing models relating that category to larger aggregates. It is common to forecast population, admissions, admission categories, and specific service requirements by analyzing trends in the relationship. For example:

Number of Orthopedic Surgeries = (Population) ×
(Admissions/Population) × (Percent of Admissions in
Orthopedics)

Number of Hip Replacements = (Number of Ortho. Surgeries) ×
(Percent of Ortho. Surgeries in Hip Replacement).

Or:

Number of Hip Replacements = (Population over 65) ×
(Hip Replacements/Population over 65)
+ (Population under 65) × (Hip Replacements/Population
under 65).

Often several methods are used to improve confidence in the forecast.

Methods for the actual calculation will get quite complex. Nominal categories of resources will be used (see chapter 3). For example, surgeries will be categorized by type of room and square feet required. Duration of operation will be studied through simulation modelling. Trade-offs will be required among satisfaction with specific room designs, satisfaction with anticipated delay for service, and efficiency.

Trade-offs between current efficiency and future flexibility must also be evaluated. A suite designed for a certain distribution of demand among specialties might be highly inefficient for other patterns of demand.

Estimating Demand for Inventories and Supplies. Many activities of the plant system require short-term forecasts, with horizons ranging from hours to months. Efficiency in supply and service processes such as housekeeping, heating, and food service depends upon careful adjustment to variation in demand. Well-run hospitals are supplying current estimates of demand for services like these from order entry and nursing scheduling systems. (Several kinds of service are related to patient acuity.) It is likely that, in the future, patient scheduling systems will be used to forecast demand for these services.

Inventory management calls for slightly longer term forecasts. The key to efficiency and quality of service is accurate forecasts of demand at the most detailed level possible. These forecasts can be used to operate exchange cart deliveries, minimizing out-of-stock items and emergency trips, and to maintain optimum inventory levels and ordering cycles. In well-run hospitals, they are prepared from past experience, carefully analyzed for trends, cycles, and random variation. The preparation of these forecasts is normally the obligation of the materials management unit, with guidance from finance and planning. Experienced materials managers can often make useful subjective refinements to statistically prepared forecasts.

Measures of Resource Consumption

Functional Accounting Costs. Although many plant services process resources for other systems (for example, fuel is processed to heat by the heating system), the costs of all the resources involved should first be accounted to a plant system responsibility center. When the goods or services are transferred or sold to another responsibility center, a separate accounting transfers some of the cost incurred to the final user. Either cost accounting or, as discussed earlier, transfer pricing can be used to distribute the cost to the final users. This system permits double accountability for the costs. The using responsibility center is accountable chiefly for the quantities used; the plant responsibility center can be held accountable for the total cost of operating the unit, including purchase price, inventory level, and waste of inventoried items, as well as labor and materials consumed by the unit.

Cost accounting focuses on the efficiency of the plant system itself and encourages plant system managers to assist final users in reducing the quantities they use. However, standard cost accounting practices have some important deficiencies. Capital costs are accounted at straight-line depreciation of original purchase price, without interest, often resulting in substantial understatement. Inventory costs are rarely adjusted for the value of money invested in inventory. Only the most elaborate cost accounting systems incorporate all the other costs of maintaining the plant service. A rental concept of capital (that is, the current market cost to rent the facility or equipment involved) may be more useful, particularly in deciding whether to continue operating plant system units or to contract services. Similarly, inventory handling costs can include the interest earned on capital rather than the amount invested.

Fixed and Variable Costs. Traditional functional accounting also has inaccuracies because it fails to identify fixed and variable costs. Flexible budgeting and cost accounting techniques are particularly appropriate for plant units with high variability in demand, such as food service, laundry service, and heating. Fixed cost elements, that is, those not sensitive to changes in demand, are budgeted annually and minimized principally through changes in work processes. In the case of variable cost items, including some labor costs and most supplies consumed, the plant responsibility center manager can be held accountable for units used and price, while the line manager is responsible for volume. By identifying the elements of cost variation, one can deal with each as a separate management problem.

Sunk Cost Management. For many plant and equipment items, the opportunity for eliminating fixed costs occurs only once in a long while. Once a laundry or a steam boiler has been installed, for example, recovery of the construction and equipment costs is difficult or impossible. The opportunity to make major changes in the system, such as purchasing services from outside sources, occurs only when the equipment has worn out. Such costs are said to be *sunk.* Although many costs are sunk for long periods of time, some sunk costs emerge every year, as equipment needs to be replaced. The plant system manager has realistic opportunities for minimizing sunk costs, and the incentives offered him or her should encourage aggressive search for them. Many of these opportunities require close coordination of planning and plant system management.

Joint and interrelated projects are identified and developed utilizing advance forecasts of obsolescence or replacement. Sunk costs are minimized by:

— Accurate forecasts of future demand

— Exploration of substitute, shared, or contract opportunities

— Design efforts to minimize long-term investment

Measures of Efficiency

Intermediate Product Efficiency Measures. Efficiency measures should reflect both the intermediate, or internal, efficiency and the efficiency of production of the final product. The intermediate product efficiency is expressed as cost (or physical unit of resource) divided by number of such units produced, for example:

— Energy consumption per square foot of floor space
— Labor cost per pound of linen
— Raw food cost per meal served
— Materials handling costs per pound of supplies purchased

It is a relatively simple matter to generate these measures for many plant service responsibility centers. Comparative and scientific standards for these values are widely available. Labor standards for laundries, kitchens, and the like and cost standards for energy use, construction, renovation, and security are supplied by numerous consultants.

Final Product Efficiency Measures. The weakness of intermediate product efficiency has been noted in connection with clinical support services. It is all too easy to achieve high internal efficiency without a corresponding return to the consumer of the final product. If plant services are provided in excessive quantities, even if very efficiently by internal standards, they will add excess costs to the final product. Final product efficiency must be calculated on the basis of a completed product or total inpatient service, such as energy consumption per discharge or laundry cost per clinic visit. The numerator of the efficiency ratio is the resources consumed; the denominator is a total measure of a discrete episode of patient care. It should be possible to differentiate the numerator whenever important denominators are counted, for example, "energy consumption in the outpatient building per visit" and "energy consumption in the inpatient building per discharge." A less desirable substitute adjusts the denominator to reflect an index of multiple products, for example, "adjusted discharges," as defined by the AHA, include a weighting for outpatient activity.

Some problems become easier with a final product approach. While the internal efficiency remains problematic, many final product cost efficiencies, such as security costs per discharge or space management cost per discharge, are easily measured. Most important, it is final product efficiency which meets exchange demands and therefore must

Figure 15.7

Measures of Quality for Plant Systems

Outcomes Measures
  Complaints
  User satisfaction surveys
  Incident rates
  Crime and property loss rates
  Inventory loss rates
  Licensure, accreditation, and inspection reports and citations
    Occupational Safety and Health Administration
    Environmental Protection Agency
    Joint Commission on Accreditation of Hospitals
    State and local health departments
Process Measures
  Inspections
  Work reports on conditions and problems encountered
  Delays and incomplete work
  Automated monitoring

---

be used to guide the expectations for each plant service unit. That is, the true performance requirements for a plant system are set by exchange demands, the price the public is willing to pay for the service. Efforts to understand efficiency requirements in terms of history or technology rather than willingness to pay can be seriously misleading.

Measures of Quality

Plant systems generally are not lacking for quality measures. The major sources are users, outside inspectors, inside inspectors, and work records; the number and variety of examples has grown steadily in recent years. Line managers, particularly in nursing, should be encouraged to report any maintenance failure that is likely to reduce patient satisfaction or safety promptly. Repeated reports on the same problem indicate a major deficiency in quality. Figure 15.7 shows important measures of quality that are available to almost any hospital.

Process measures are useful in monitoring day-to-day activity. Inspections are critical to laundry, food service, supplies, maintenance, and housekeeping. Subjective judgment is usually required, but it is improved by clear statements of process standards for cleanliness, temperature, taste, appearance, and so on. The frequency of inspection is adjusted to the level of performance, and performance is improved by training and methods rather than negative feedback. Work reports, like incident reports, reveal correctable problem areas in plant maintenance and materials management.

Back orders, incomplete work, and delays in filling orders can be reported as incidents or as ratios of days' work outstanding. These are essentially failure statistics, and they need to be classified by severity or importance. Being out of stock, particularly of critical items, can be treated similarly. Many utilities services are now automated, so permanent records exist of environmental conditions. Under automated order systems and electronic accounting of supplies use from exchange carts, out-of-stock items and back orders can be reported automatically as well.

Given this wealth of information, outcomes measures can be used for annual budget and expectation setting. The following might be reasonable budget goals:

— Outcomes measures:
- Maintain or improve the standard of service reflected in user surveys and complaints.
- Make selected improvements over past failure rates.
- Have no major deficiency on any outside inspection.

— Process measures:
- Make selected improvements over past averages.
- Improve overall consistency and eliminate selective failures.

Measures of Revenue and Resource Conservation

Traditionally plant services have been viewed as overhead costs. Consistent with that thinking, the services were not charged directly to patients, but were recovered as a surcharge. The physical plant of a hospital was understood to be a common rather than a specific resource which therefore should be financed on a collective rather than an individual charge. Charges for parking were one of the first departures from this view, although it still applies in many areas. The now common parking charge is slightly annoying, but renting a chair in the lobby or the use of the elevator seems absurd!

Patient Charges and Transfer Pricing. There is merit to pricing and charging for plant services as used. Uniform surcharges may be inequitable, as, for example, "free" parking is inequitable to the visitor who comes by bus or taxi. Goods and services perceived as free tend to be unappreciated and wasted. Sales and purchase opportunities for plant services may exist outside the hospital. Finally, profit is a measure of contribution which can serve as a reward for those providing the service. As a result of these considerations, more highly automated accounting capability has been used for more precise costing and charging records, and competitive contracting with hospitals has emphasized precision and detail in patient charges.

The trend toward more precise charging for plant services can be extended to the development of transfer prices for line responsibility centers. A line manager can thus be held accountable for the cost of materials management, just as he or she is for supplies, and for housekeeping and repairs, just as for direct labor costs. The management of plant services becomes part of the responsibilities of the supervisor, exactly as a resource purchased from outside would. At the same time, the plant service manager must compare his or her price against outside competition. Thus both service users and service providers are led to opportunities for improved efficiency that they might otherwise have overlooked.

Sale of Goods and Services to Other Departments. Corporations selling plant services—building management, food service, parking services, security, and so on—became more popular in hospitals in the 1960s. The merits of contract services per se are discussed above, but two implications arise simply from the existence of them. One is that the charges they submit can be passed directly to the user department if desired. The purchase of housekeeping is no different from the purchase of supplies or an educational program. The second is that if an outside vendor can sell the service, at least conceptually the hospital can sell it as well. Cooperative laundries and computer services were established in many cities during the 1960s and 1970s, on the theory that not-for-profit corporations could attain the same efficiency as commercial vendors. Larger hospitals also began to sell services directly to smaller ones. As a result, by the 1980s about a third of all hospitals were involved in shared services.

Revenue Measurement in Plant Systems. The implication of these changes combined is that all well-run hospitals will sell or transfer price most plant services in the future, generating direct costs to line units and revenues for plant systems. Growing experience with shared services and expanded accounting capability make such a policy feasible. The incentive requirements of the new competitive environment make it desirable.

Revenue measurement for plant systems will require extensive changes in accounting, budgeting, and management practices. There are three steps to an improved system; these will take even an excellent hospital several years to complete:

1. Accounting records must show where plant services were actually distributed. Use of utilities must be metered, and housekeeping, security, repair, and maintenance activity and supplies must be accounted to final users. Some activities are truly common. Costs for these could either be distributed to user groups according to conventional cost accounting or transferred to the governance system and reflected in the line units only as part of the expectations for unit operating profits. (In this approach, common in for-profit holding companies and subsidiaries, the governance system would have revenues from its subordinate units, a variety of direct costs, and an accountability for net hospital profit.)

2. Cost accounting records within the plant services must be revised so that accurate and complete costs can be assigned to each type of transaction, such as security service, receptionists, and so on. This is a routine accounting function in retail stores, for example, and in construction contracting.

3. Prices for plant goods and services must be initially estimated by the accounting system. In competitive markets, prices are set by the market, but accounting information is used to set initial offerings. Well-run hospitals will recognize this important fact and will examine competing sources of plant services closely. Thus the transfer price for housekeeping service may initially be estimated from cost budget data, but the final price should be the lowest of the available offers. Revenues must be posted to plant systems with equal amounts posted as costs to line or final user systems instead of the less specific overhead allocations previously used. This step changes the line departments' costs to a volume basis and simultaneously allows the plant responsibility centers to earn revenues and have measures of profit.

The third step introduces a major managerial change. If the plant unit cannot produce at competitive prices, transfers and sales should be posted at market, and the unit will show a loss. Obviously, repeated losses require investigation and correction. Four theoretical solutions exist for such a case:

1. Discontinue the service and purchase from the lowest acceptable bidder.

2. Improve internal efficiency so that the service becomes competitive.

3. Enlarge the revenue base, distributing fixed costs more broadly and permitting a lower unit price.

4. Subsidize the service for some corporate purpose outside the immediate needs of either the plant services or the user departments. The cost of the subsidy, of course, should be accounted to the purpose, not distributed directly to the users.

The last should clearly be a rare, unusual, and transient event. To deliberately and indefinitely operate a plant system at higher than alternative costs is obviously not consistent with reasonable missions.

Management Issues

The subsystems supporting plant service functions have undergone substantial revision in recent years. Well-run hospitals have developed comprehensive materials management programs with effective purchasing and handling activities. They use generic specification of items, group purchasing, exchange cart distribution, and full costing of supplies to improve internal efficiency and, to a lesser degree, final product efficiency. Energy conservation programs have significantly reduced energy requirements (but not energy costs). Security services are prepared to cope with a variety of threats and problems unforeseen two decades ago. Environmental hazard controls are much more prominent in hospitals than in many industries. While the controls are imperfect, the hazards from the physical environment are probably smaller than those most people encounter in their own homes.

Many of the recent advances rely on contract or shared services, apparently reflecting accurately the contributions of larger scale in plant systems. The next round of gains may be from centralized multihospital systems for plant management.

One important frontier is the interaction between plant services and rest of the hospital. The formal and informal communications that bind the plant system to the total operation are not as strong as they should be. Plant services, even when they fail, are too often ignored; when they are effective, they are too faintly praised.

A second frontier is the organizational structure of plant services. Hospitals now frequently purchase services from outside vendors and from each another. Whether competitive markets exist for these services is not clear. Newer approaches emphasize more use of joint and subsidiary corporations and stress the advantages of operating in a competitive market that are believed to result.

Motivating Efficiency, Economy, and Quality

Satisfaction of customer requirements, including both price and quality, should be the consuming goal of all plant services. The customers of plant services include members of the hospital, patients, and visitors. It is easy to reduce quality of plant service under severe cost constraints. Attractive, convenient, comfortable plant services are a competitive asset. Without them, hospital market share may fall. As it does, volume declines, forcing fixed costs per discharge up. Thus final product efficiency may depend more on the quality of plant service than on its intermediate product efficiency. Some hospitals may even wish to increase plant system costs to gain an advantage in the market.

Well-run hospitals are now on a path toward holding plant services responsible for meeting market demands for cost and quality. Measurement of achievement, annual expectation setting, training, methods and equipment, and reward are the tools for improving both. At present, the move to independent pricing of plant services is not yet widespread. Similarly, most hospitals do not measure whether the service offered is satisfactory to the patient or visitor, or to the line department acting in their behalf. Well-run hospitals are steadily improving these tools, however.

Improving Measurement Systems. The well-run hospital has moved, or is moving rapidly, toward:

— Transfer pricing for plant services

— Final product measures of efficiency

— Periodic user satisfaction surveys supplementing external agency surveys

— Formal complaint or incident reporting mechanisms, with rapid follow-up

— Inspection activities to assure process quality

Such a balanced and comprehensive information system provides:

— Data for setting quantitative expectations for demand, cost, quality, and efficiency

— Routine assessment of performance

— Early warning of change in either customer expectation or unit activity

— Support for appropriate distribution of rewards

— Data for evaluating offers from alternate suppliers

Setting Annual Expectations. The annual budget exercise, tied to the long-range plan, should address the comprehensive performance of each responsibility center. Most plant units should be able to improve some dimension of performance each year. Failure to improve, or to remain competitive with alternate suppliers, suggests the need to restructure the service or to change suppliers.

Evaluating Long-Term Opportunities. Long-range issues involve questions of capital replacement. Opportunities for making major improvements in overall efficiency and quality often require extensive recapitalization and therefore must be integrated with the hospital's overall replacement schedule. Plant services frequently figures in expansion and renovation of space for other activities. Contract services for warehousing, utilities, and laundry may be significantly more competitive when opportunity costs of existing space and replacement capital costs are included. Recovering space from plant use may take several years to achieve, particularly if the hospital's obligations to loyal workers are honored. The annual planning process should include review of the facilities and equipment plan and explicit evaluation of opportunities to purchase plant services from outside vendors.

Revising Methods, Equipment, and Training. Most improvements in efficiency are related to changes in work methods rather than to just better motivation of workers. Methods for most plant activities are dictated by the equipment. Automation has made substantial gains, but it probably will make still more, particularly in scheduling and optimizing work routines.

The way in which new methods and equipment are introduced is often critical to their success. Worker participation in selecting and evaluating a new method is useful. Training, incentives, and handling of redundant employees should be considered in evaluating and installing an improved method.

Training must emphasize correct methodology. Orientation to the goals of the unit and to using the reported measures is also important. Customer relations are included in almost all plant system jobs. Training programs in responding to the desires of patients, visitors, and fellow workers, often called guest relations programs, are obviously appropriate. Security personnel need training beyond that in order to deal with disturbed, impaired, or potentially criminal persons while simultaneously providing assistance and reassurance to the anxious and innocent.

Increasing Incentives and Rewards. If attention is paid to measures, goals, and methods, the gains from reward systems are greatly increased, both for the worker and for the hospital. Three desirable guidelines are that most expectations should be met, rewards for good performance should be frequent and generous, and sanctions should be rare. (Not surprisingly, this is as true for the plant system as for the medical staff.)

The most important incentives are nonmonetary. Pride of achievement is probably the most important. It is supported by prompt reporting of formal measures, well-designed methods, appropriate training, and responsive supervision. Recognition of achievement includes both verbal and nonverbal responses of the supervisor. The amount of recognition should be tailored to the level of achievement: any positive response should be recognized by the supervisor, above average results by co-workers, and extraordinary achievement by the hospital at large.

The role of the supervisor is critical in pride of achievement and recognition. One essential job of the first-line supervisor is to provide the proper tools, supplies, and training. A second, related one is to answer all questions promptly and appropriately. A third is to recognize achievement. Well-run hospitals build supervisor understanding and capability with training programs.

Explicit monetary incentives, beyond the basic contract for compensation and employment, appear to play a relatively minor role in motivating workers. For example, they cannot overcome disincentives from poor supplies or equipment. Nor do they effectively replace pride of achievement. They are most powerful as supplements to nonmonetary incentives, where even a small payment serves to show the seriousness of management intent.

Monetary incentives can be dysfunctional and can be defeated by worker resistance. Many piece-rate and intermediate efficiency-oriented standards ignore quality and customer satisfaction. They can be defeated by collusion, by exaggeration of supply and equipment problems, and by grievances. They can be dysfunctional when they encourage unneeded output or disregard of customer wants.

Corporate Structures for Improving Plant Services

Plant services are conventionally structured as components of the larger hospital organization. In recent decades, many of these components have been purchased. The issues of transfer pricing, competitive bidding, and obligations for both economy and quality suggest still greater autonomy of plant activity. It is likely that the best corporate structure has not yet been devised. Several possibilities seem to merit further development:

— Any one of the four functions (facility services, maintenance services, guest services, and supplies services) might be assumed by a freestanding or subsidiary corporation. That corporation might be provided with target prices and monetary incentives and might provide itself with information systems and systems for improving economy and quality. Scale would come from the sale of services to several hospitals, either in a region or in a multihospital system.

— The four functions might all be assumed by a single corporation, or other groupings might be formed. Supplies services is probably the least associated with the others and the most likely to be organized separately. In a competitive environment, materials management services, including exchange cart delivery, could be purchased by the hospital. The hospital would transfer all inventories and processing and distribution equipment to the books of the service corporation. The hospital might retain its ability to select vendors and approve purchase contracts. Similar corporations might provide maintenance and guest services.

— Sale and lease-back of equipment groups or entire facilities might prove more attractive to the not-for-profit organization than ownership either of buildings or of plant service corporations.

All of these models assume that an organization specialized in plant services can meet both quality and economy constraints. The larger and more at arm's length the plant services contracts, the greater the need for formal measures of quality to protect the hospital's interests and the more valuable the internal systems and efficiency to the supplier corporation. The models also assume the existence of a competitive market to permit comparison of performance. Finally, their attractiveness results from a combination of legal, financial, and management factors. In particular, they depend on the treatment of capital by major buyers. The current system, a mix of the cost pass-through still used for Medicare capital payments and various price structures, gives hospitals no clear incentive for exploring the larger opportunities. That situation is temporary, however.

Notes

1. National Fire Protection Association, *Code for Safety to Life from Fire in Buildings and Structures* (Boston: NFPA, 1981). See also other NFPA publications, such as *Life Safety Code Handbook,* 1982, and *Standard for Health Care Facilities,* 1984.
2. American Hospital Association, *Hospital Engineering Handbook* (Chicago: AHA, 1974), pp.20–21; John H. Holmgren and Walter J. Wentz, *Material Management and Purchasing for the Health Care Facility* (Ann Arbor, MI: AUPHA Press, 1982), pp. 243–49.
3. Holmgren and Wentz, p. 6.
4. Holmgren and Wentz.

Suggested Readings

American Hospital Association. *Hospital Engineering Handbook.* Chicago: AHA, 1974.

American Hospital Association and National Safety Council. *Safety Guide for Health Care Institutions,* 3rd ed. Chicago: AHA, 1983.

Colling, Russell L. *Hospital Security,* 2d ed. Boston: Butterworths, 1982.

Holmgren, J. H., and Wentz, W. J. *Material Management and Purchasing for the Health Care Facility.* Ann Arbor, MI: AUPHA Press, 1982.

Rohde, D. J., Prybil, L. D., and Hochkammer, W. O. *Planning and Managing Major Construction Projects, A Guide for Hospitals.* (Ann Arbor, MI: Health Administration Press Perspectives, 1985.

Wenzel, R. P. *CRC Handbook of Hospital-Acquired Infections.* Boca Raton, FL: CRC Press, 1981.

Glossary

accountability—the notion that the organization can rely upon the individual to fulfill a specific, prearranged expectation.

accountability hierarchy—the structure of reporting, formal information flow, and accountability for expectations which defines a bureaucratic organization.

activity or procedure expectation—expectation for component tasks of clinical care, such as injections or physical examinations.

acuity—a measure of how sick patients are, used to establish nurse staffing needs.

American Osteopathic Hospital Association (AOHA)—A voluntary national organization of hospitals emphasizing privileges for osteopathic physicians. AOHA offers inspection and accreditation services similar to those of the Joint Commission.

apex—the uppermost levels of a bureaucratic organization concerned principally with functions of governance, planning, and finance.

attending physicians—those doctors having the privilege (q.v.) of using the hospital for patient care.

blended model—a theory of organization of hospital governance which blends the committee and corporate model approaches.

budget guidelines—desirable levels of key financial indicators established at the start of the budget process by the governing board.

bureaucratic organization—a form of human endeavor where groups of individuals bring different skills to bear on a single objective in accordance with a formal structure of authority and responsibility.

case manager—an individual who coordinates and oversees other health care professionals in finding the least costly method of caring for specific patients.

census—number of patients in a hospital or unit.

certificates of need—franchises for new services and construction or renovation, issued by many states.

chief executive officer (CEO)—the agent of the governing board holding the formal accountability for the entire organization.

clinical expectation—a consensus reached on the correct professional response to a specific, recurring situation in patient care.

clinical nurse practitioner—nurse with extra training who accepts additional clinical responsibility for medical diagnosis or treatment.

clinical support service—(1) a unit organized around one or more medical specialties or clinical professions providing individual patient care on order of an attending physician such as laboratory or physical therapy, or (2) a general community service, such as health education, immunization, and screening, under the general guidance of the medical staff.

clinical system—the part of a health care organization which provides hands-on patient care and monitors it to ensure both quality and effectiveness.

closed system activities—those looking inward on what the organization is doing and comparing that to expectations.

closed system model—a representation of the way a unit of a formal organization makes a predictable response to external stimuli. Predictable responses are necessary to allow units to interact.

collateral organization—the broad group of organizational activities such as committees, conferences, task forces, and retreats, which are established for the purpose of attacking problems crossing several organizational units.

community—a group of geographically related individuals and organizations sharing some resources. Hospitals are usually among the shared resources of a community.

conditional expectations—expectations using a branching logic which incorporates alternative conditions for certain actions.

conjoint medical staff—a flexible and pluralistic relationship between doctors and the hospital that assumes increasingly close affiliation.

controlled substances—drugs regulated by the federal government, such as narcotics.

corporate model—a theory of organization emphasizing a powerful chief executive, resembling the prevailing styles of large industrial and commercial corporations.

credentialing—the process of privilege (q.v.) review.

cybernetic—a characteristic of organizations reflecting purposive search: the establishment of goals, measurement of progress, and correction of activity to improve progress (from *cybernos,* helmsman).

data base management—method of storing and retrieving electronic data files.

department—a unit of the accountability hierarchy, such as "housekeeping department." Also an organization of doctors in a major specialty, as in "obstetrics department."

discharge planning—a part of the patient group protocol and the nursing care plan which identifies the expected discharge date and coordinates the various services necessary to achieve the target.

elective—demand which can be met at an indefinite time.

emergency—demand which must be met in a short time period.

environmental assessment—the process of surveillance (q.v.).

exchange—an exchange is mutual or reciprocal transfer that occurs when both parties believe themselves to benefit from it. It results in a relationship between an organization and its environment, such as employment, sales, donations, purchases, etc.

exchange partners—individuals or groups participating in exchanges with the hospital.

expectations—specific statements about the desired parameters of the closed system model; work goals for organization units and their members.

final products—sets of clinical services reaching generally recognized end points in the process of care such as hospital discharge.

finance system—the part of a health care organization which collects and manages the funds the organization needs, but which also monitors the proper use of resources and maintains much of the internal information system.

for-profit hospitals—those owned by private corporations which declare dividends or otherwise distribute profits to individuals. Also called *investor owned*. They are usually community hospitals.

formulary—a list of drugs the hospital will inventory, and rules governing prescription and administration of these drugs.

general ledger transactions—financial transactions which are internal rather than external exchanges. They often deal with resources that last considerably longer than one budget or financial cycle.

governance system—the part of a health care organization which monitors the outside environment, selects appropriate alternatives, and negotiates the implementation of these alternatives with others inside and outside the hospital.

government hospitals—those owned by federal, state, or local governments. Local government includes not only cities and counties, but also, in several states, hospital authorities that have been created from smaller political units. Local government hospitals are counted as community hospitals. State mental hospitals and federal hospitals are not counted as community hospitals.

grand rounds—didactic presentations on clinical subjects of general interest.

gross revenue—the sum of all posted charges in a specified time period.

health maintenance organizations (HMOs)—health insurance plans emphasizing comprehensive care under a single insurance premium.

Health Systems Agencies (HSAs)—local or regional public organizations advising state agencies on issues of hospital and health care planning. HSAs were widespread in the 1970s but have become less common after the end of federal support in 1986.

hierarchical data system—structured retrieval system for automated data using a pre-arranged set of retrieval categories or definitions.

homeostasis—in biology a "state of physiological equilibrium produced by a balance of functions and of chemical composition within an organism" and more generally a "tendency towards relatively stable equilibrium between interdependent elements."

horizontal integration—integration of organizations providing the same kind of service, such as two hospitals or two clinics.

hospital-based specialists—those physicians providing consultative care to attending physicians such as pathologists, radiologists, and anesthesiologists.

house officers—licensed doctors pursuing postgraduate education.

human resources system—the part of a health care organization which recruits and supports the hospital's employees and other workers, such as doctors and volunteers.

incident report—written report of an untoward event that raises the possibility of liability of the organization.

independent practice associations (IPAs)—health insurance plans providing care for an annual premium (see HMO), but paying their affiliated doctors on a fee-for-service basis.

influence—the ability to affect an organization's or an activity's success. Influence is usually gained by controlling a resource.

influentials—exchange partners having above-average influence on the affairs of the hospital.

information system—an automated process of capture, transmission, and recording of information important to management in a permanently accessible manner.

intermediate product protocol—consensus expectation which establishes the normal set of activities for a complex procedure such as a surgical operation.

intermediate products—outputs of component processes of care, such as admissions, patient days, inpatient meals, and laboratory tests. Commonly treated as inputs to final products.

inurement—an illegal diversion of funds of a not-for-profit corporation to an individual, particularly to persons in governance or management.

Joint Commission on Accreditation of Hospitals (JCAH)—a national organization of representatives of health care providers: American College of Physicians, American College of Surgeons, American Hospital Association, American Medical Association, and consumer representatives. The JCAH offers inspection and accreditation on quality of operations to hospitals and other health care organizations.

joint venture—an activity between two or more corporations or individuals and corporations involving mutual contribution of capital to some activity or program with the promise of future return.

Life Safety Code—safety and convenience regulations developed by the National Fire Protection Association.

line-units—units of the accountability hierarchy directly concerned with the principal product or outcome of the organization. In hospitals, these are the clinical units: the medicine, nursing, and the clinical support services.

management by objective (MBO)—agreement in advance between the responsibility center manager and the supercontroller as to the accomplishments, documents, or projects to be completed within the period.

management letter—comments of external auditors to the governing board which accompany their audited financial report.

market oriented—a style of management identifying the interests of the community and searching for ways the hospital can meet them.

marketing—see planning-marketing.

Medicaid—governmental assistance for care of the poor and occasionally the near-poor established through the state/federal program included in Public Law 89-97, Title 19.

Medicaid agency—the state agency handling claims and payments for Medicaid.

medical staff organization—the structure which both represents and governs physicians and affiliate staff members.

medical staff recruitment plan—an element of the long-range plan establishing both the size of the medical staff and the services the hospital will provide.

Medicare—Social Security health insurance for the aged established in Public Law 89-97, Title 18.

Medicare intermediary—the private agency handling claims and payments for the federal Medicare program. Often the local Blue Cross and Blue Shield Plan.

members—those people who participate in the hospital's closed system activities. Members are employees, doctors, trustees, other volunteers, and other nonemployed providers of care, chiefly dentists, psychologists, and podiatrists.

mission—a statement of the good or benefit the hospital intends to contribute, couched in terms of an identified community, a set of services, and a specific level of cost or finance.

net revenue—income actually received as opposed to what is initially posted; equal to gross revenue minus adjustments for bad debts, charity, and discounts to third parties.

not-for-profit hospitals—those owned by corporations established by private (non-governmental) groups for the common good rather than for individual gain. Most are community hospitals.

nurse anesthetist—nurse with special training who admininisters anesthesia.

nurse clinician—specialist in the nursing problems of patients with certain diseases such as pediatrics or medicine.

nurse midwife—nurse with special training who practices uncomplicated obstetrics.

nursing—the provision of physical, emotional, and educational services to support or improve the patient's equilibrium with his or her environment and to help the patient regain independence as rapidly as possible.

open systems activities—outwardlooking activities, those through which the organization selects its exchanges.

opportunity cost—the cost of committing a resource and thereby eliminating it from other potential uses or opportunities.

optimization—allocation of scarce resources to maximize achievement of some good or benefit.

patient group protocol—a formal or informal consensus on the appropriate pattern of diagnosis, treatment, and follow-up for a specific set of diseases. Usually formalized by the medical specialty most familiar with the disease, assisted by others who frequently treat the disease.

patient ledger—account of the charges rendered to individual patients.

peer review—evaluation of the credentials of applicants and annual review of the performance of physicians with privileges. Also, any review of professional performance by members of the same profession.

Peer Review Organizations (PROs)—organizations led by doctors, which do not insure or provide care, but which audit the quality of care and the use of insurance benefits for Medicare and other insurers.

planning—see planning-marketing

planning-marketing—the process which identifies changing opportunities for the hospital to serve its community, develops alternative ways to meet those opportunities, selects among these, and coordinates and implements the desired changes. Also, a unit of the governance system which is accountable for managing the planning-marketing process.

plant system—the part of a health care organization which operates and maintains the physical facilities and equipment.

position control—a central review of the number of positions created and persons hired to fill them.

preferred provider organizations (PPOs)—insurance plans that encourage subscribers to seek care from selected hospitals, doctors, and other providers with whom they have established a contract. The contract generally includes both price and utilization restrictions, and the subscriber is rewarded with a higher level of insurance coverage.

primary monitor—see responsibility center manager.

privileges—rights granted annually to physicians and affiliate staff members to perform specified kinds of care in the hospital. The extent of privileges is determined by professional peers, based upon education and past performance.

proactive—emphasizing foresight and placing the thinking of management ahead or in the future compared to the present.

Professional Standards Review Organizations (PSROs)—a physician-controlled group responsible for monitoring both the quality and the appropriateness of hospital care. PSROs were replaced by Peer Review Organizations in 1983.

programmatic proposals—proposals for resource allocation usually arising from the units or departments tending to affect only the nominating department, which can be evaluated in light of the existing mission and long-range plan.

Prospective Payment System (PPS)—nationally promulgated price structure for Medicare patients.

relational data system—a flexible retrieval system for automated data which allows the retrospective establishment of a category or definition.

responsibility center (RC)—the smallest formal unit of organizational activity, usually the first level at which a supervisor appears.

responsibility center manager (RCM)—the supervisor of a responsiblity center. Also called a primary monitor or first-line supervisor.

section—an organization of members of a given medical subspecialty.

staff units—units of the accountability hierarchy which serve technical or support activities for the line.

stakeholders—those exchange partners whose views are sufficiently important to directly affect the hospital's success.

strategic opportunities—opportunities which involve quantum shifts in service capabilities or market share, usually by interaction with competitors or by very large scale capital investments. Mergers, acquisitions, and joint ventures are generally strategic opportunities.

strategic plan—a document incorporating the mission, environmental surveillance, and previous planning decisions used to guide annual and non-recurring resource allocation decisions.

strategic responses—decisions about the future of the hospital at the level of mission or long-range plan which may result in substantial changes in the relation of the hospital to its environment.

structural measures—measures of compliance with static expectations such as those relating to physical facilities or the formal training of individuals.

supercontrollers—managers who supervise responsibility center managers.

surveillance—a sensory function identifying changes in the environment, and perspectives of others in the community on these changes, with particular attention to those changes affecting customers, competitors, and members of the hospital.

third-party administrators (TPAs)—organizations which process claims and sometimes also control use of benefits for employers who are carrying their own insurance.

transfer price—imputed revenue for a good or service transferred between two units of the same organization, such as housekeeping services provided to nursing units. Where the service is not sold directly to the public, the price is established by complex cost-accounting and comparison against available market information.

unbundling—the selection of physician contract options or the organization of clinical support services to maximize revenue.

urgent—demand which may be met within a few days but which cannot be deferred indefinitely.

valuation premises—a set of assumptions about resource allocation decisions which are independent of the specific opportunity or alternative. They include attitudes on risk and liquidity and perspectives on time horizons and the intrinsic merit of certain kinds of action, e.g., prevention versus use.

vertical integration—the affiliation of organizations providing different kinds of service such as hospital care, ambulatory care, long-term care, and social services.

ward rounds—educational review of actual cases in the hospital.

working capital—a firm's investment in short-term assets—cash, short-term securities, accounts receivables, and inventories.

Index

About the Author

John R. Griffith, M.B.A., is Andrew Pattullo Collegiate Professor, Department of Health Services Management and Policy, School of Public Health, The University of Michigan. He is a graduate of The Johns Hopkins University and the University of Chicago. Before joining the Department in 1960, he was associated with The Johns Hopkins Hospital and Strong Memorial Hospital at the University of Rochester. He was director of the Program and Bureau of Hospital Administration (now titled the Department of Health Services Management and Policy) from 1970 to 1982. He has served as president of the Association of University Programs in Health Administration, chairman of the board of Medicus Systems Corporation, and chairman of the board of Health Administration Press. He has been active on the editorial boards for many of the scholarly journals in health care administration. He has been a consultant to federal, state, and local governmental agencies and private hospitals and corporations. He has directed the annual Blue Cross Blue Shield National Health Care Institute since 1970. He is the author of five books and monographs, and has written numerous articles for both scholarly and professional publications, principally in areas related to improving hospital utilization and productivity. Professor Griffith is a Fellow of the American College of Healthcare Executives and the American Public Health Association.